Series Editors:
David R. Beukelman, Ph.D.
Joe Reichle, Ph.D.

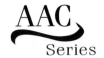

Exemplary Practices
for Beginning Communicators

Also in the Augmentative and
Alternative Communication Series:

*Augmentative and Alternative Communication
for Adults with Acquired Neurologic Disorders*
edited by David R. Beukelman, Ph.D.,
Kathryn M. Yorkston, Ph.D.,
and Joe Reichle, Ph.D.

Series

Exemplary Practices
for Beginning Communicators
Implications for AAC

edited by

Joe Reichle, Ph.D.
University of Minnesota–Twin Cities

David R. Beukelman, Ph.D.
University of Nebraska–Lincoln

and

Janice C. Light, Ph.D.
The Pennsylvania State University–University Park

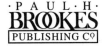

·P A U L·H·
BROOKES
PUBLISHING C⁰

Baltimore • London • Toronto • Sydney

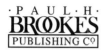

·P A U L·H·
BROOKES
PUBLISHING C⁰

Paul H. Brookes Publishing Co.
Post Office Box 10624
Baltimore, Maryland 21285-0624

RJ
496
.C67
E945
2002

www.brookespublishing.com

Typeset by Integrated Publishing Solutions, Grand Rapids, Michigan.
Manufactured in the United States of America by
The Maple Press Company, York, Pennsylvania.

The vignettes in this book are based on the authors' experiences. Some of the
vignettes represent actual people and actual circumstances. The names and other
identifying information of individuals have been changed to protect their identities.
Some of the vignettes are composite accounts that do not represent the lives or
experiences of specific individuals, and no implications should be inferred.

Library of Congress Cataloging-in-Publication Data

Exemplary practices for beginning communicators : implications for AAC /
edited by Joe Reichle, David R. Beukelman, Janice C. Light.
    p.   cm. − (AAC series)
    Includes bibliographical references and index.
    ISBN 1-55766-529-X
    1. Communicative disorders in children.   2. Handicapped−Means of
communication.   3. Handicapped children.   4. Communication devices
for the disabled.   I. Reichle, Joe, 1951−   II. Beukelman, David R., 1943−
III. Light, Janice C. (Janice Catherine)   IV. Series.
RJ496.C67 E945 2001
618.92′855−dc21
                                                                    2001037983

British Library Cataloguing in Publication data are available from the British Library.

Contents

Series Preface

The purpose of the *Augmentative and Alternative Communication Series* is to address advances in the field as they relate to issues experienced across the life span. Each volume is research-based and practical, providing up-to-date and groundbreaking information on recent social, medical, and technical developments. Each chapter is designed to be a detailed account of a specific issue. To help ensure a diverse examination of augmentative and alternative communication (AAC) issues, an editorial advisory board assists in selecting topics, volume editors, and authors. Prominent scholars, representing a range of perspectives, serve on the editorial board so that the most poignant advances in the study of AAC are sure to be explored.

In the broadest sense, the concept of AAC is quite old. Gestural communication and other types of body language have been widely addressed in literature about communication for hundreds of years. Only recently, though, has the field of AAC emerged as an academic discipline that incorporates graphic, auditory, and gestural modes of communicating. This series concentrates on achieving specific goals. Each volume details the empirical methods used to design AAC systems for both descriptive groups and for individuals. By tracking the advances in methods, current research, practice, and theory, we will also develop a broad and evolutionary definition of this new discipline.

Many reasons for establishing this series exist, but foremost has been the number and diversity of the people who are affected by AAC issues. AAC consumers and their families, speech-language pathologists, occupational therapists, physical therapists, early childhood educators, general and special educators, school psychologists, neurologists, and professionals in rehabilitative medicine and engineering all benefit from research and advancements in the field. Likewise AAC needs are not delineated by specific age parameters; people of all ages who have developmental and acquired disabilities rely on AAC. Appropriate interventions for individuals across a wide range of disabilities and levels of severity must be considered.

Fundamentally, the field of AAC is problem driven. We, the members of the editorial advisory board, and all professionals in the field are dedicated to solving those problems in order to improve the lives of people with disabilities. The inability to communicate effectively is devastating. As we chronicle the advances in the field of AAC, we hope to systematically dismantle the barriers that prevent effective communication for all individuals.

Editorial Advisory Board

About the Editors

Joe Reichle, Ph.D., Professor, Department of Communication Disorders, University of Minnesota, 164 Pillsbury Drive SE, 115 Shevlin Hall, Minneapolis, Minnesota 55455. In addition to his work as Professor, Dr. Reichle is Associate Chair of the Department of Communication Disorders at the University of Minnesota. He is currently responsible for the master's, doctoral, and postdoctoral personnel preparation programs in the area of AAC. Dr. Reichle has worked for 20 years in general and special education programs serving school-age children with moderate to severe developmental disabilities and providing services to families, teachers, therapists, and paraprofessionals. In addition to his interest in communication intervention, Dr. Reichle is a recognized expert in communicative approaches to managing challenging behavior. He has served as a co-principal investigator of model in-service projects and outreach projects, which have been designed to develop technical assistance teams in local school districts to serve children with severe challenging behavior in inclusive classroom environments. Dr. Reichle has published numerous articles about AAC and challenging behavior and, along with Dr. Steven F. Warren, served as series editor of the *Communication and Language Intervention Series* (Paul H. Brookes Publishing Co.).

David R. Beukelman, Ph.D., Professor, Department of Special Education and Communication Disorders, University of Nebraska, 202F Barkley Memorial Center, Post Office Box 830732, Lincoln, Nebraska 68583. Dr. Beukelman is Barkley Professor of Communication Disorders at the University of Nebraska. He is also Director of Research and Education of the Communication Disorders Division, Munroe-Meyer Institute for Genetics and Rehabilitation at the University of Nebraska Medical Center in Omaha, Nebraska, a research partner in the Augmentative and Alternative Communication Rehabilitation Engineering Research Center (AAC-RERC). In addition, Dr. Beukelman is Senior Researcher in the Institute for Rehabilitation Science and Engineering at the Madonna Rehabilitation Hospital in Lincon, Nebraska. He is co-author of the textbook *Augmentative and Alternative Communication: Management of Severe Communication Disorders in Children and Adults* (2nd ed., 1998, Paul H. Brookes Publishing Co.). Dr. Beukelman also served as editor of the *Augmentative and Alternative Communication Journal* for 4 years.

Janice C. Light, Ph.D., Professor, Department of Communication Disorders, The Pennsylvania State University, 110 Moore Building, University Park,

Pennsylvania 16802. Dr. Light is actively involved in research, personnel preparation, and service delivery in the area of AAC. Her primary interest has been furthering understanding of the development of communicative competence and self-determination in individuals who use AAC, and she is co-author of the book *Building Communicative Competence with Individuals Who Use Augmentative and Alternative Communication* (1998, Paul H. Brookes Publishing Co.). Dr. Light is the principal investigator on several federally funded research grants to improve outcomes for individuals who have significant communication disabilities through the use of AAC. She is also one of the project directors in the Augmentative and Alternative Communication Rehabilitation Engineering Research Center (AAC-RERC), a virtual research consortium funded by the National Institute on Disability and Rehabilitation Research. In 1996, Dr. Light was recognized as the Don Johnston Distinguished Lecturer by the International Society of Augmentative and Alternative Communication for her leadership in the AAC field. In 1999, she received the Dorothy Jones Barnes Outstanding Teaching Award at The Pennsylvania State University.

About the Contributors

Wendy K. Berg, M.A., Research Psychologist, The University of Iowa, 100 Hawkins Drive, Room 251, Iowa City, Iowa 52242. Ms. Berg is an investigator on two research grants to evaluate the use of concurrent operant procedures as methods for augmenting functional analysis results for prescribing treatment. Her research interests include developing alternative assessment procedures for identifying factors that influence both appropriate behavior and problem behavior.

Nancy C. Brady, Ph.D., Assistant Research Professor, Kansas Center for Research on Mental Retardation and Developmental Disability, The University of Kansas, 1052 Dole, Lawrence, Kansas 66045. Dr. Brady conducts research on the acquisition and use of communication systems by individuals with severe disabilities.

Melissa Cheslock, M.S., CCC-SLP, Speech-Language Pathologist, Project Coordinator, Language Intervention for Toddlers, Department of Communication, Georgia State University, One Park Place South, Atlanta, GA 30303. Ms. Cheslock has extensive clinical experience working with young children with developmental disabilities and their families. Her work has primarily focused on providing augmentative and alternative assessment and intervention services to enhance and encourage communication development in children.

Albert M. Cook, Ph.D., PE, Dean, Faculty of Rehabilitation Medicine, University of Alberta, 3–48 Corbett Hall, Edmonton, Alberta T6G 2G4, Canada. In addition to his work as Dean of the Faculty of Rehabilitation Medicine at the University of Alberta, Dr. Cook is associated with the Assistive Device Service at Glenrose Rehabilitation Hospital in Edmonton. He has worked with interdisciplinary clinical and research teams on developing assistive devices and assessing the effectiveness of technology used by people with disabilities.

Cynthia J. Cress, Ph.D., CCC-SLP, Assistant Professor, Department of Special Education and Communication Disorders, University of Nebraska–Lincoln, 202G Barkley Memorial Center Lincoln, Nebraska 68583. As Assistant Professor at the University of Nebraska–Lincoln, Dr. Cress specializes in language, AAC, and early intervention. She researches patterns of communication in infants and toddlers with physical impairments who will need to use

AAC. For 15 years, Dr. Cress has provided clinical services for children and adults who use AAC.

Patricia Dowden, Ph.D., CCC-Sp, Clinical Assistant Professor, Speech and Hearing Sciences, University of Washington, 1417 NE 42nd Street, Seattle, Washington 98105. During Dr. Dowden's 20 years of practice, she has directed several assistive technology clinics and worked directly with AAC users of all ages. She teaches courses in augmentative communication both online and on campus.

Kathryn Drager, Ph.D., Assistant Professor, The Pennsylvania State University, Department of Communication Disorders, 110 Moore Building, University Park, Pennsylvania 16802. Dr. Drager's primary areas of interest include AAC applications for children and adults and the communicative function of challenging behaviors.

Erik Drasgow, Ph.D., Assistant Professor, Department of Educational Psychology, University of South Carolina, 235-I Wardlaw, Columbia, South Carolina 29208. Dr. Drasgow's areas of interest include language intervention for individuals, special education law, and functional assessment and behavior support plans for students with emotional or behavioral disorders.

Michelle Gutmann, M.S., CCC-SLP, Speech-Language Pathologist, Department of Special Education and Communication Disorders, Barkley Memorial Center, University of Nebraska–Lincoln, Lincoln, Nebraska 68583. Ms. Gutmann has 9 years of experience in AAC. She has worked with both adults and children in a variety of settings, including a mobile adult AAC service, a pediatric rehabilitation center, and a clinic for people with amyotrophic lateral sclerosis. Ms. Gutmann is currently pursuing her doctorate.

James W. Halle, Ph.D., Professor, Department of Special Education, University of Illinois at Urbana-Champaign, 1310 South Sixth Street, Champaign, Illinois 61820. Dr. Halle's research program focuses on the communication efforts of children who lack language and the ways in which partners respond to these efforts. Central to his research is the analysis of variables that comprise the social context of communication and mediate its generalized use. His recent work encompasses conceptualizing challenging behavior as communicative repair.

Jay W. Harding, Ed.S., Program Associate, The University of Iowa, 100 Hawkins Drive, Room 251, Iowa City, Iowa 52242. Mr. Harding is currently the project coordinator of a federally funded research project evaluating the influence of choice making with young children who exhibit severe challenging behavior.

Kerri Harwood, Ph.D., Adjunct Assistant Professor, Peabody College, Vanderbilt University, Box 328, Nashville, Tennessee 37203. As a special educator, Dr. Harwood has worked extensively with students with multiple disabilities. Her interests include nonsymbolic communication intervention, AAC, and literacy instruction for AAC users.

Katherine C. Hustad, Ph.D., CCC-SLP, Assistant Professor, Department of Communication Disorders, The Pennsylvania State University, 110 Moore Building, University Park, Pennsylvania 16803. Dr. Hustad's primary areas of interest include the integration of AAC and natural speech, interventions for improving speech intelligibility in individuals with chronic dysarthria, and linguistic variables that influence intelligibility/comprehensibility. As a clinician, Dr. Hustad has worked for 9 years in a variety of settings—in pediatric rehabilitation, at a regional AAC center, and at a university-based clinic—and she has served as a vocational rehabilitation consultant. Her clinical work has focused on AAC applications for children and adults with neuromotor disorders.

Amy M. Hyatt, Graduate Student, Department of Educational Psychology and Special Education, Georgia State University, One Park Place South, Atlanta, GA 30303. As a graduate student in the Communication Disorders Program at Georgia State University, Ms. Hyatt's interests include language assessment and intervention for preschool children.

William J. McIlvane, Ph.D., Director, Mental Retardation Developmental Disabilities Research Center, Shriver Center, University of Massachusetts Medical School, 200 Trapelo Road, Waltham, Massachusetts 02452. As Director of the Shriver Center's Mental Retardation Developmental Disabilities Research Center, Dr. McIlvane directs an interdisciplinary program of research. This program addresses basic learning processes in individuals with severe mental retardation, brain activity correlates of behavior, animal models of fundamental cognitive processes, and related research-to-practice and technology transfer activities.

Pat Mirenda, Ph.D., Associate Professor, Department of Educational and Counselling Psychology and Special Education, The University of British Columbia, 2125 Main Mall, Vancouver, British Columbia, V6T 1Z4 Canada. Through the years, Dr. Mirenda has concentrated on AAC for people with developmental disabilities. In addition, she has focused on the integration and inclusion of augmented communicators in general education classrooms.

Dr. Mirenda is the editor of the journal *Augmentative and Alternative Communication*. She is also co-author of the book *Augmentative and Alternative Communication: Management of Severe Communication Disorders in Children and Adults* (2nd ed., 1998, Paul H. Brookes Publishing Co.).

Toni B. Morehouse, M.A., CCC-SLP, Speech-Language Pathologist, University of Nebraska–Lincoln, 253 Barkley Memorial Center, Lincoln, Nebraska 68583. Ms. Morehouse is a lecturer in the Department of Special Education and Communication Disorders at the University of Nebraska–Lincoln. Her primary areas of interest are preschool language, phonological disorders, and phonological awareness. She has worked with children for more than 25 years as a public school speech-language pathologist and as a supervisor in the University of Nebraska–Lincoln speech-language clinic.

Mark F. O'Reilly, Ph.D., Lecturer, Senior Psychologist, National University of Ireland–Dublin, St. Michael's House, Belfield, Dublin 4, Ireland. Dr. O'Reilly is Lecturer in psychology at National University of Ireland, Dublin, and Senior Psychologist with St. Michael's House, Dublin, which provides services for people with cognitive disabilities. His interests include assessment and treatment of behavior difficulties with people with severe disabilities, assistive technology for people with multiple disabilities, and social skills interventions to promote inclusion in typical life settings for people with disabilities.

Arielle R. Parsons, M.S., Speech-Language Pathologist, private practice, Piermont, New York. Ms. Parsons received a master's degree in communications disorders from The Pennsylvania State University. She is an independent speech-language pathologist in the greater New York area.

Mary Ann Romski, Ph.D., Professor, Department of Communication, Georgia State University, One Park Place South, Atlanta, GA 30303. Dr. Romski's research has focused on studying the language acquisition process of children with developmental disabilities who use augmentative communication devices.

Rose A. Sevcik, Ph.D., Associate Professor, Department of Psychology, Georgia State University, One Park Place South, Atlanta, GA 30303. Dr. Sevcik's research interests include language and communication acquisition and impairments, mental retardation, and reading development and disorders.

Ellin B. Siegel, Ph.D., Associate Professor, Department of Special Education and Communication Disorders, University of Nebraska–Lincoln, 202 Barkley

Memorial Center, Lincoln, Nebraska 68583. Dr. Siegel directs the graduate programs in severe disabilities and vision impairments. Dr. Siegel also co-directs the Augmentative and Alternative Communication Center at Barkley Memorial Center. Dr. Siegel's research, presentations, and publications have focused on early communication strategies and augmentation for learners with severe disabilities, autism, and dual sensory impairments.

Jeff Sigafoos, Ph.D., Professor, Department of Special Education, The University of Texas at Austin, George I. Sanchez Building, Austin, Texas 78712. As Professor in Special Education at The University of Texas at Austin, Dr. Sigafoos's research is focused on teaching beginning communicators to use AAC and on the treatment of severe behavior problems in children with developmental disabilities.

Bonnie L. Utley, Ph.D., Associate Professor, School of Education, University of Colorado at Denver, 1200 Larimer Street, North Classroom Building, Denver, Colorado 80204. Dr. Utley has served the education field for almost 30 years. She has worked extensively in the area of low-incidence disabilities as a practitioner, researcher, and technical assistance provider. She currently prepares both general and special educators for service within inclusive schools.

David P. Wacker, Ph.D., Professor of Pediatrics and Special Education, The University of Iowa, 100 Hawkins Drive, Room 251, Iowa City, Iowa 52242. Dr. Wacker has conducted numerous studies on interventions for children who display problem behavior, and he provides psychological services for children with behavior disorders in two outpatient clinics at The University of Iowa's Department of Pediatrics. He recently completed a 3-year service as editor of the *Journal of Applied Behavior Analysis*.

Steven F. Warren, Ph.D., Director and Professor, Schiefelbusch Institute for Life Span Studies, The University of Kansas, 1000 Sunnyside Drive, 1052 Dole, Lawrence, Kansas 66045. In addition to his work as Director of the Schiefelbusch Institute for Life Span Studies, Dr. Warren is Professor of Human Development and Family Life at The University of Kansas. He has conducted extensive research on early communication and language intervention approaches. Dr. Warren is a series editor for the *Communication and Language Intervention Series* (Paul H. Brookes Publishing Co.).

Krista M. Wilkinson, Ph.D., Assistant Professor, Communication Sciences and Disorders Department, Emerson College, 120 Boylston Street, Boston, Massachusetts 02116. In addition to her faculty appointment at Emerson College, Dr. Wilkinson holds a research appointment at the Shriver Center of the University of Massachusetts Medical School. She studies vocabulary learning in young children with and without developmental disabilities.

Paul Yoder, Ph.D., Research Professor, Peabody College, Vanderbilt University, Box 328, Nashville, Tennessee 37203. For more than 16 years, Dr. Yoder has been studying adult–child interaction as it relates to children's communicative and language development.

Acknowledgments

We are grateful to the beginning communicators who use AAC, their families, and the professionals who have shared their experiences with us. They have provided us with many valuable insights that have guided our research and practice. We also thank the many students at our universities who have asked important questions and have assisted with our research to advance the field. We acknowledge the support that we have received over the years to develop the AAC programs in our universities. The AAC program at the University of Minnesota has been supported through funding from the U.S. Department of Education (USDE) and the National Institute on Disability and Rehabilitation Research (NIDRR). The AAC program at The Pennsylvania State University has been supported through funding from USDE, NIDRR, the AAC Rehabilitation Engineering Research Center (AAC-RERC), and the Pennsylvania Office of Vocational Rehabilitation. The AAC program at the University of Nebraska has been supported through funding from USDE, NIDRR, AAC-RERC, and the Barkley Trust. We thank Paul H. Brookes Publishing Co. for supporting the *AAC Series* and this specific volume in the series.

Introduction

Augmentative and alternative communication (AAC) is an area of study that examines methods to supplement or replace spoken communication. Both gestures (e.g., natural gestures, sign systems, sign language) and graphics (e.g., traditional orthography, photographs, line drawings) may either supplement speech or act as a primary communicative mode. In addition, gesture or graphic mode communication can play an important role in producing and/or comprehending speech. AAC applications can be as simple as a pointing gesture or as technologically sophisticated as an electronic communication device that produces synthesized digitized speech and offers predictions about the remaining elements of a message that is being formulated.

Guidelines generated by the National Joint Committee for the Needs of Persons with Severe Disabilities (1992) reminded us that all individuals have the basic right to communicate. Unfortunately, more than 2 million Americans with significant communication disabilities, struggle daily to utilize that right. A number of conditions underlie the possible need for strategies to augment or replace spoken language. People with congenital as well as acquired disabilities can benefit from the careful and thoughtful application of AAC strategies. In *Exemplary Practices for Beginning Communicators: Implications for AAC*, the emphasis is on individuals with congenital disabilities, although the authors fully recognize that many people with acquired disabilities must grapple with the role that AAC might play in their rehabilitation.

The AAC field remains in its infancy in spite of dramatic growth since the mid-1970s. Although the knowledge base addressing assessment and intervention strategies has increased significantly in a wide variety of disciplines that are relevant to AAC, some of the most impressive advances have been in the capability to serve the earliest communicators. The Individuals with Disabilities Education Act (IDEA) of 1990 (PL 101–476) and subsequent amendments provided an important impetus for practitioners and researchers representing a number of disciplines to begin considering more functionally what and how to establish a beginning communicative repertoire. This book is dedicated to advancing the understanding of how to approach the task of initiating functional strategies that establish beginning communication skills in a timely manner among individuals who are at risk for developing speech comprehension and production skills.

Exemplary Practices for Beginning Communicators: Implications for AAC emphasizes the importance of developmentally and chronologically appropriate clinical and educational practices. Yet, the book's authors also recognize that many individuals with multiple disabilities present challenges to interventionists that may require looking beyond typical patterns of development to derive functional assessment and intervention. Although many of the chapters in this book address young children who are acquiring their first communication system, several of the chapters directly address aspects of initial communication in individuals who already have started to acquire a language system that does not efficiently meet daily communicative needs. In addressing the chronological range of individuals who may be candidates for an AAC system, we believe that the term *nonlinguistic,* as opposed to *prelinguistic,* is more accurate for older individuals with developmental disabilities. In this book, both of these groups are considered as candidates for beginning AAC systems.

The framework for this book's discussion of beginning AAC applications is based on a transactional model of communication development. The acquisition of communication skills is a dynamic process of bidirectional influence between the speaker and the listener(s). Furthermore, many of the contingent exchanges between a beginning communicator and his or her partner may involve a partner's reaction to idiosyncratic or socially unacceptable behavior. If a history of contingent reinforcing responses to these behaviors occurs, then it is probable that a socially unacceptable repertoire will develop. Many learners have some portion of their communicative repertoire that is idiosyncratic or socially unacceptable. In either case, the interventionist will need to consider establishing clearer and/or more socially acceptable alternatives. Some individuals may also have a history of producing communicative overtures that are inaccurately deciphered by their partners. Consequently, a history develops in which their communicative overtures do not culminate in the desired outcome. Over time, these individuals may increasingly exhibit characteristics that are associated with learned helplessness and social passivity. Therefore, people who are likely to interact with individuals who use AAC systems are also candidates for intervention.

Formulating and implementing an intervention strategy is an immense responsibility for professionals and family members. Experience suggests that "camps" of professional points of view often tend to create a challenge in matching the most efficient intervention protocol to a particular learner. Common areas of professional conflict are the selection of communicative functions and related vocabulary, the density of instructional opportunities to provide, and the degree to which overt discriminative stimuli are delivered to convey to the learner that he or she has an opportunity to communicate. Being acquainted with only one intervention approach represents a danger to interventionists. In addition, consumers and family members play a critical role in steering professionals toward intervention approaches that are not only effective but also meet rigorous standards of practicality. In the AAC discipline, social validity is the glue that binds effective components of intervention packages. Consequently, we believe that the following questions should be addressed:

1. What communicative functions and related vocabulary would be most important to the learner and significant communication partners?
2. How overt do the cues and prompts need to be to demonstrate AAC's efficiency to the learner?
3. How can the learner be supported to enable effective communication in his or her current situation while having opportunities to learn more effective methods to enhance learning?
4. What cues and prompts will be available in the natural environment to maintain the skill that is taught?
5. What situations should be emphasized during intervention to fully sample the range of situations in which the new communicative behavior could be used?
6. How will situations be handled in which the learner's communicative overtures cannot be reinforced?

By carefully addressing these issues, it is likely that an interventionist may blend a number of instructional techniques into a plan that is customized to meet each learner's specific needs.

Wetherby, Warren, and Reichle (1998) described the development of communication as a continuous, three-stage, ontogenetic process that involves a transition from perlocutionary (preintentional) to illocutionary (intentional) preverbal communication to locutionary or symbolic communication. In *Exemplary Practices for Beginning Communicators: Implications for AAC*, we consider these areas. Yet, equally important for a prospective AAC user is the method that he or she will use to express and receive communicative acts. It would be tidier if a linear sequence of steps could be arranged to guide the interventionist in selecting the content of a beginning strategy to establish a communicative repertoire. In reality, however, the interventionist must consider a number of areas somewhat concurrently if a plan of action is to be developed and executed in a timely manner.

Timeliness in implementing an AAC system is paramount. The earlier that graphic and/or gestural mode supports are put into place, the greater the preventive value. By prevention, we mean that having a compromised ability to comprehend and produce speech does not mean that a learner cannot proceed in gestural and/or graphic modes to acquire intelligible communicative acts and corresponding vocabulary. The greater the range of socially acceptable and readily decipherable communicative behavior that can established, the less ominous is the task of mapping that system to speech. Often, parents and interventionists are reluctant to consider implementing AAC because they fear that it will impede the learner's development of speech. Although this concern is understandable, the literature does not support it. Research suggests that a substantial proportion of children who receive graphic mode intervention subsequently begin to acquire and expand their speech repertoire. It is possible that voice output communication aids may provide an important opportunity for beginning communicators to acquire an understanding of spoken words, which, in turn, may facilitate the acquisition of communicative production. Since the mid-1980s, we have turned to the literature on matching law to explain the learner's allocating communicative acts to speech and moving away from graphic and gestural modes over time. Matching theory suggests that individuals allocate their responses to the most efficient alternative (Mace & Roberts, 1993). For example, when speech is compared with graphic symbols, it is clear that speech is a faster communication mode. Speed allows the individual to communicate in real time. Although researchers are still investigating these phenomena, we feel comfortable concluding that postponing the implementation of AAC creates greater risk than aggressive implementation.

This book contains a well-integrated mixture of cutting-edge information that addresses the range of communicative content means and contexts that must be considered to establish an initial functional communicative repertoire. Our goal is to present a scholarly discussion of strategies and issues that should be thoughtfully discussed if the field is to advance scientifically in its knowledge of the best options for establishing beginning AAC systems.

OVERVIEW OF THE CHAPTERS

Chapter 1 provides an overview of intervention strategies that are often implemented to establish an early communicative repertoire. This overview delineates some important areas that should be considered for improving the efficacy of AAC applications.

Chapter 2 offers an overview of graphic and gestural means for focusing on more subtle environmental variables that can influence the learner's propensity to act on communicative opportunities. This chapter emphasizes strategies that maximize opportunities to move from perlocutionary to illocutionary communicative acts. Intrinsic considerations, such as the learner's state, are considered as well as external considerations, including the physical and social features of communicative environments.

Chapter 3 offers a review and discussion of what is known about the effect of partner responsiveness on the emergence of a beginning intentional communicative repertoire. The chapter authors offer insight into the role that several distinctly different intervention strategies—including prelinguistic milieu teaching, picture exchange communication intervention, and responsive teaching—may have during the development of a beginning productive repertoire.

Chapter 4 addresses learners who already have intentional communication skills that may be clearly decipherable by a listener but are socially unacceptable. The chapter authors provide a discussion of how to determine the social functions of challenging behavior. In addition, they address how to arrange the environment so that the beginning communicator sees socially acceptable communicative behavior as an efficient alternative to socially unacceptable communicative forms.

Chapters 5, 6, and 7 consider strategies to establish basic communicative functions that emerge fairly early in the repertoires of typically developing individuals. Chapter 5 discusses strategies to teach requesting as a means to gain access to desired items and activities. This chapter addresses rudimentary topics, such as ensuring that the interventionist has identified a range of reinforcing items and activities. Chapter 5 emphasizes the importance of teaching the learner when he or she can act independently versus when he or she needs to engage in a communicative request as a mediating response. In this context, the chapter authors discuss the importance of complementing independent actions with the conditional use of communicative behavior. Equally important is the selection of symbols that will be used to represent communicative functions. The authors address how the specificity of symbols can influence acquisition opportunities, maintenance, and generalization.

Chapter 6 addresses the necessity of empowering beginning communicators to escape and avoid objects, activities, and people without resorting to problem behavior. The chapter authors describe a number of subtly different communicative functions, which include protesting, requesting a break, requesting assistance, and requesting a work check. All can serve an escape function but may differ in their efficiency depending on a particular communicative situation. Chapter 6 also builds directly on information presented in Chapter 4, discussing the importance of identifying the social function of inefficient or inappropriate communicative behavior and then matching a socially acceptable alternative to the derived function. Chapter 6 addresses the need to balance the communicative power to opt out of activities and to learn self-regulation of one's behavior. The authors express the point of view that self-regulation must be carefully coordinated into the introduction of any communicative function. Although the empirical literature is only beginning to address the coordination of empowerment and self-regulation, discussing potentially viable intervention strategies to achieve a balance between the two is critically important.

Chapter 7 takes the position that initial intervention strategies may place an inordinate emphasis on the communicative functions of requesting and protesting. The chapter authors point out that important communicative opportunities may be lost because learners do not have adequate opportunities to use their communicative skills to achieve social closeness. They make a compelling argument for the early acquisition of communicative functions that focus on interpersonal contact with other individuals. The observations made in Chapter 7 have significant implications for selecting which communicative functions to introduce. Care must be taken early in the assessment process to carefully gauge the learner's interest in social contact with others. If this contact is currently met by using idiosyncratic or socially marginal strategies, then communicative forms to express social closeness become an intervention priority. Yet, if the learner appears to show little interest in achieving or maintaining social closeness, intervention in this area is still in order. The available literature makes it very clear that children with significant developmental disabilities tend to have fewer opportunities to engage in social interactions with others. In part, this may be due to their partners' inability to identify emitted social overtures. Over time, with this lack of listener responsivity, the learner's social overtures may decrease. Chapter 7 suggests strategies that may improve partners' responsivity to overtures for social closeness.

Chapter 8 provides a broad working definition of AAC that includes modifying the environment as well as the behavior of prospective communicative partners. These strategies become components of AAC strategies if they would not necessarily occur during typical communication patterns between speaking individuals. In describing a range of strategies, Chapter 8 discusses efficacy research in AAC and provides vignettes that support combining behavioral and symbolic forms of AAC.

Chapter 9 discusses strategies for selecting which type of graphic symbol is most efficient for the learner, the conditions under which speech output might be helpful, and the role of dynamic and fixed displays in acquiring new symbols. The chapter's discussion of specific suggestions about teaching, implementing, and troubleshooting procedures is particularly valuable. These suggestions focus on establishing an initial repertoire of discriminations that are required to utilize a beginning graphic mode communication system for people who have significant developmental disabilities.

Chapter 10 explores the area of communicative repair as it pertains to beginning communicators who may benefit from AAC. The chapter authors review the literature that describes the repair strategies used by typically developing beginning communicators and apply this to beginning AAC users. Chapter 10 addresses a particularly important aspect, the range of repair strategies used and the extent to which specific repair strategies are associated with particular clusters of environmental stimuli.

Two chapters in this book address the issue of access for individuals who may have more significant sensory and/or physical disabilities. Chapter 11 addresses the role that vision impairment may play in the process of selecting and implementing the most efficient graphic mode AAC system. This chapter reviews the multiple dimensions of sensory functioning that apply to all beginning communicators who may be candidates for an AAC system. In doing so, the chapter author shares a sequence of critical questions that should be answered and corresponding assessment methods to be used in customizing a graphic mode communication system for an individual with moderate or severe disabilities. After reviewing basic sensory and motor characteristics of beginning communicators, the author offers assessment strategies to examine acuity, convergence, binocularity, presentation plane, and visually directed reaching.

Chapter 12 considers the range of selection techniques that may make it possible to overcome challenges when a learner cannot efficiently, directly select symbols from a graphic mode communication display. This chapter builds on information that would be obtained as a result of implementing the assessment strategies described in Chapter 10. Chapter 12 includes an overview of the potentially confusing terminology and definitions that pertain to selection techniques and activation strategies. A review of the research that has focused on selection techniques follows. The chapter concludes with a discussion of decision-making strategies that are designed to assist teams of professionals who are charged with the responsibility of customizing AAC technology for beginning communicators.

Chapter 13 tackles the topic of supplementing speech with AAC strategies. A number of individuals have communicative repertoires. Unfortunately, the intelligibility of their speech may be such that prospective communicative partners struggle to decipher messages. This chapter directly addresses the role of supplementing existing speech with graphic and gestural mode options. Particular attention is given to topic, alphabetic, and combined topic and alphabetic supplementing of spoken language. Chapter 13 also considers how the mode that is used in supplementing may affect communicative efficiency.

The final chapter in this book addresses a topic that is proving to be of increasing importance in the field's efforts to establish the most efficient path in creating a beginning communicative repertoire. Chapter 14 explores the relationship between comprehension and production in beginning candidates for an AAC system. The chapter authors directly examine the possible importance of comprehension skills in facilitating the acquisition of a productive communicative repertoire. They summarize their extensive research and educational/clinical experience in this area.

Exemplary Practices for Beginning Communicators: Implications for AAC is intended to stimulate future practice and applied research that is aimed at improving the field's ability to efficiently assist individuals in their effort to acquire an initial repertoire of functional communication skills. We discuss a number of areas that require further experimental scrutiny. Historically, this has been frustrating to a discipline that is focused on technical assistance and, to a great (and appropriate) degree, is consumer driven. We believe that continued improvement in our ability to establish beginning AAC skills rests in pursuing and expanding the respectful collaboration among consumers, practitioners, and researchers toward a common goal of enabling increasing numbers of individuals with disabilities to exercise their right to communicate.

REFERENCES

Individuals with Disabilities Education Act (IDEA) of 1990, PL 101–476, 20 U.S.C. §§ 1400 *et seq.*

Mace, F.C., & Roberts, M.L. (1993). Factors affecting selection of behavioral interventions. In S.F. Warren & J. Reichle (Series Eds.) & J. Reichle & D.P. Wacker (Vol. Eds.), *Communication and Language Intervention Series: Vol. 3. Communicative alternatives to managing challenging behavior: Integrating functional assessment and intervention strategies* (pp. 113–133). Baltimore: Paul H. Brookes Publishing Co.

National Joint Committee for the Needs of Persons with Severe Disabilities. (1992). Guidelines for meeting the communication needs of persons with severe disabilities. *Asha, 34*(Suppl. 7), 1–8.

Wetherby, A.M., Warren, S.F., & Reichle, J. (Vol. Eds.). (1998). *Communication and Language Intervention Series: Vol. 7. Transitions in prelinguistic communication.* Baltimore: Paul H. Brookes Publishing Co.

Exemplary Practices
for Beginning Communicators

1

A Continuum of AAC Language Intervention Strategies for Beginning Communicators

Mary Ann Romski, Rose A. Sevcik, Amy M. Hyatt, and Melissa Cheslock

One of the roles that augmentative and alternative communication (AAC) can play is to cultivate beginning communication skills. When AAC takes on this role for a beginning communicator, it must do so in concert with a language intervention strategy because communication competence usually does not emerge on its own. Language skills may not be waiting for the appropriate communication mode or device to be found.

Historically, the AAC field has focused much of its energy on assessment so that appropriate matches could be made between a communication mode and the communicator. This focus often resulted in beginning communicators being excluded from AAC interventions because it was thought that they did not have the prerequisite skills necessary to immediately begin using AAC (e.g., Chapman & Miller, 1980). Research has shown that all individuals can communicate when communication is defined along a continuum (National Joint Committee, 1992). The task, then, is not determining eligibility for AAC but rather ascertaining where along the communication continuum an individual will begin the AAC intervention process and what the desired language and communication intervention outcomes are.

In this chapter, we examine the continuum of language instructional approaches that are available for beginning communicators. The first section of this chapter provides a brief overview of the communication continuum and characterizes who is defined as a beginning communicator. The second section reviews the literature with respect to what is known about existing spoken language intervention approaches for children and adults at the very initial stages of communication and language development. Next, we discuss the role of

The preparation of this chapter was funded in part by National Institutes of Health (NIH) Grant No. DC-03799 and a Research Program Enhancement Grant from Georgia State University.

I

these spoken language intervention approaches, and other approaches, in AAC interventions for beginning communicators. We then consider some of the unique considerations that are related to AAC, including the mode of communication (unaided, aided), symbols, and selection technique. Finally, we provide some directions for future AAC research and practice.

AAC AND A CONTINUUM OF COMMUNICATION

An AAC system is an integrated group of four components that is used by an individual to enhance communication (American Speech-Language-Hearing Association [ASHA], 1991, p. 10). These four components are symbols, aids, techniques, and/or strategies. A *symbol* refers to the methods used for "visual, auditory, and/or tactile representation of conventional concepts" (ASHA, 1991, p. 10). Symbols are termed *aided* or *unaided*. Gestures, manual sign sets, and spoken words are unaided because their use does not rely on an external medium. Aided forms include visual graphic representations such as objects, pictures, photographs, line drawings, written words, and braille. Aided and unaided forms provide a mode by which individuals can communicate. They range along a representational continuum from nonsymbolic (e.g., signals—crying, physical movement) to iconic (e.g., real objects, photographs, line drawings, pictographic or visual-graphic symbols) to symbolic (e.g., spoken words, manual signs, arbitrary visual-graphic symbols, printed words) (see Sevcik, Romski, & Wilkinson, 1991, and Chapter 9 for a discussion of visual-graphic representational systems).

An *aid* is referred to as "a physical object or device used to transmit or receive messages. AAC aids are, for example, communication books, communication boards, charts, mechanical or electronic devices including those that speak and computers" (ASHA, 1991, p. 10). One striking characteristic of the AAC field at the beginning of the 21st century is the rapid development of new technologies. Technological advances have included significant improvements in speech output capabilities, portability, durability, financial cost, programming capabilities, and the variety of available input modes. These additions can provide a range of capabilities within one device that may enable an individual to use one piece of equipment for a longer period of time. The device market has also seen the emergence of many simple technologies that permit beginning communicators to gain access to communication from the earliest points in development. For example, activating a single pressure switch can produce speech and indicate the intent to communicate to a communicative partner.

A *selection technique* is the method by which an individual transmits messages. Selection techniques can be divided into two broad categories: direct selection and scanning. Direct selection allows the learner to communicate specific messages from a large set of options. Direct selection techniques include pointing, signing, natural gesturing, or touching. Some individuals use head pointers, head sticks, or eye gaze (or eye pointing) to select items. Scanning is a technique in which the message elements are presented to the individual in a sequence. The individual specifies his or her choice by responding "yes" or "no" to the person or the device that is presenting the elements. Scanning techniques include linear scanning, group-item scanning, directed scanning, and encoding (ASHA, 1991, p. 10). Encoding occurs when an individual uses a code to convey messages (e.g., Morse code). In general, a technique that requires fewer physical abilities requires more sophisticated cognitive abilities (e.g., encoding). Thus, a beginning communicator with both severe physical and cognitive disabilities may encounter more difficulty in finding a selection technique that permits him or her access to communication.

Strategies are specific ways in which the AAC aids, symbols, and techniques are used to develop and/or enhance communication. A strategy includes the intervention plan for facilitating an individual's performance (ASHA, 1991, p. 10). AAC intervention strategies must be considered with respect to the symbols that are employed and the aids and techniques that are used.

Communication can be defined in the broadest sense as "any act by which one person gives to or receives from another person information about that person's needs, desires, perceptions, knowledge, or affective states" (National Joint Committee, 1992, p. 2). Any intervention that uses AAC should incorporate the individual's full communication abilities. These abilities may include any existing speech or vocalizations, gestures, manual signs, and aided communication (ASHA, 1991). In this sense, then AAC is truly multimodal, thereby permitting a beginning communicator to use every mode possible to communicate basic wants, needs, and desires.

The ability to act intentionally on partners in one's environment and to affect the behaviors of those partners plays an important role in the language and communication development of typically developing children. As shown in Table 1.1, communicative intentions vary along a continuum from perlocutionary to illocutionary to locutionary (McLean & Snyder-McLean, 1988). During the perlocutionary stage, the individual's behavior has a single focus on an object or person with no apparent communicative intent, although the adult assigns "intent" to the behaviors observed. For example, the child is crying and the adult interprets the cry as hunger. The perlocutionary stage is followed by the illocutionary stage. During this stage, there is an alternating or dual focus on the referent object and adult. The behavior is directed at the partner and is persistent. The partner, or adult, "reads" the behavior as being intentional and responds in kind. Finally, during the locutionary stage, the individual uses specialized communicative forms (e.g., linguistic forms) from which the partner decodes the message and responds appropriately. The AAC modes that the individual uses to make his or her wants and needs known to his or her partner and the role the partner plays in the interaction will vary with

Table 1.1.   Continuum of communicative/linguistic skills

Communicative intentionality	Communicative role		Communicative form
	Child	Partner	
Perlocutionary			
Reactive	Passive	Active	Cry, eye gaze, laugh, movement, "fussing"
Proactive	Active	Active	Reach
Illocutionary			
Primitive	Active	Active	Physical manipulation
Conventional	Active	Active	Point, vocalization with inflection
Locutionary			
Emerging	Active	Active	Words, signs, graphic symbols combined with gesture and vocalization
Conventional	Active	Active	Words, signs, graphic symbols

From Romski, M.A., & Sevcik, R.A. [1995]. Communicative development of children with severe disabilites. In M. Smith & J. Damico [Eds], *Childhood language disorders* [p. 223]. New York: Thieme Medical Publishers; reprinted by permission.

the individual's status along the communication continuum. For example, some beginning communicators who have no conventional way to communicate may sometimes express their communicative wants and needs in socially unacceptable ways, such as aggressive or destructive behavior (e.g., Donnellan, Mirenda, Mesaros, & Fassbender, 1984; Doss & Reichle, 1991; Mirenda, 1997; see also Chapter 4).

Characteristics of Beginning Communicators

For purposes of this chapter, we define *beginning communicators* as individuals who come to the task of learning language with less than a 50 word/symbol vocabulary. We use this descriptor because it marks an important shift that occurs in typical language development known as the *vocabulary growth spurt*. During the period from birth to approximately 18–21 months of age, a young typically developing child advances through the perlocutionary and illocutionary stages of communication development. At about 9 months of age, the child begins to comprehend the speech of others in context; by 12 months of age, the child understands approximately 50 words. Somewhere between 12 and 15 months, the young child begins to produce first word approximations and slowly starts to develop a vocabulary. At about the same time that the young typically developing child attains a 50 word vocabulary (18–21 months), he or she also begins to combine words. Consequently, prior to the time that a child has 50 words, the focus of communication development is on the pragmatic (intentional communication, communication functions) and the semantic (vocabulary, semantic relations) aspects of language rather than on the grammatical aspects of language.

Even when this operational definition is applied, beginning communicators encompass a broad range of communicative profiles that vary depending on the blend of their biological status and their experiences in their environments. Individual profiles, in turn, will interact differentially with AAC instructional strategies to influence intervention outcomes. The individual factors that contribute to an individual's beginning communicative profile are cognitive development and related disabilities, communicative experience (which includes chronological age [CA]), vocal and gestural production skills, and speech comprehension skills. It is likely that beginning communicators have disabilities that have been present since birth because these individuals may have encountered difficulty with spoken communication from the onset of development. It is possible, however, that some children and adults with acquired disabilities, such as traumatic brain injury, could have profiles that also are consistent with the beginning stages of communication development.

The cognitive skills that a beginning communicator brings to the intervention task can vary from no evidence of cognitive disabilities to that of severe cognitive disabilities. It is likely that the beginning communicators that we are discussing in this chapter will have some degree of cognitive disability. Other disabilities related to severe levels of cognitive disability may include autism, cerebral palsy, genetic disorders, seizure disorders, sensory impairments, or challenging behaviors. These related disabilities may have additional influences on the individual's communicative profile (Guess & Horner, 1978; Snell, 1987).

When characterizing the factors that may affect communication acquisition, experience and chronological age are often overlooked. The chronological age range for beginning communicators begins with infants and toddlers with little communication experience to adults who have had a number of years of sometimes unsuccessful communication experiences and/or interventions. Each factor is intrinsic to the individual as a function of his or her biological makeup and experiences. Cognition and experience can combine in different ways with the selected AAC instructional approach to influence how the individual profits from a particular AAC experience. Because beginning communicators often demonstrate extremely limited productive language skills, it is frequently presumed that they are functioning at less than a 12- to 18-month-old developmental level. This assumption often provides an inaccrate, or at least incomplete, description of their competencies. In many respects, such individuals function well beyond the sensorimotor stage of development, as they have frequently developed and/or utilized a range of alternative ways, including some idiosyncratic means, with which to communicate within familiar environments (Romski, Sevcik, Reumann, & Pate, 1989). These natural communicative repertoires may have been employed for prolonged periods of time. Communication repertoires may include multiple conversational experiences, communicative partners, and environments and often do not resemble those of 12- to 18-month-old typically developing children. Often, repertoires are used in more variable contexts and perhaps less flexibly than those of young typically developing children. The effect of life experience beyond that of the early developmental period must be overlaid and considered as well in addressing an individual's communication competencies and needs.

Beginning communicators may have a wide range of vocal and gestural production skills. One of the most striking observations of the Romski and colleagues (1989) study was the extent to which school-age children vocalized naturally, though unintelligibly, prior to the introduction of an AAC device. The use of AAC interventions should not be contingent on failure to develop speech skills or considered a last resort. It appears that a more critical issue than which vocal skills a beginning communicator has in his or her repertoire at the onset of AAC intervention is whether AAC promotes or hinders the development of speech. A modest number of empirical studies report improvement in speech skills after AAC intervention experience (see Beukelman & Mirenda, 1998, and Romski & Sevcik, 1996, for reviews). There are no studies that support the belief that AAC intervention hinders the development of speech. Although vocal skills are not necessary for learning to communicate via an AAC system, studies suggest that the ability to vocally imitate at the onset of AAC intervention may play a role in the child's subsequent gains with speech in the context of the AAC system (e.g., Romski, Sevcik, Robinson, & Wilkinson, 1990; Yoder & Layton, 1988). Typically developing children use gestures for communication during the first year of life prior to the development of speech production skills (Goldin-Meadow, 2000; Hunt-Berg & Loncke, 2000). Gestural production skills are also an important consideration when examining the extant communication skills of a beginning communicator. To date, there is very limited information about the role that gestural production skills play for beginning communicators.

As part of their language profile, beginning communicators may evidence speech comprehension skills that range from no or minimal comprehension to comprehension skills that are equivalent to their chronological age (Nelson, 1992). Individuals who do comprehend some speech may have knowledge about the relationship between words and their referents in the environment (Romski & Sevcik, 1993) and use multimodal means to understand communication. Consequently, their auditory processing skills may be quite distinct from those of individuals who do not have such a foundation on which to build AAC skills. Individuals who do not understand spoken words confront a very different task. They must establish conditional relationships between the visual symbols to be learned and their real world referents while relying, almost exclusively, on the visual modality (Romski & Sevcik, 1996). AAC systems, then, can serve as both the input and output modes (see Chapter 14).

Thus, each beginning communicator presents a unique intrinsic profile with respect to cognitive development and related disabilities, communicative experience, vocal and gestural production skills, and speech comprehension skills. These distinctive profiles will interact with the chosen language intervention approach to produce a broad range of communication outcomes.

SPOKEN LANGUAGE INTERVENTION APPROACHES

The development of language intervention approaches for the treatment of language development difficulties in individuals who speak has been an area of remarkable and important developments (Bricker, 1993; Kaiser, 1993; Warren, 1993). This area of research was pioneered and developed beginning in the late 1960s (Schiefelbusch & Lloyd, 1974). Findings from developmental psycholinguistic research, combined with emerging behavioral instructional procedures, provided the foundation for developing language intervention protocols that taught individuals with developmental disabilities specific speech and language skills, initially through direct instruction (Guess & Horner, 1978; Miller & Yoder, 1972). Even then, an AAC approach, the Non-Speech Language Initiation Program (Non-SLIP; Carrier, 1974), was developed to teach grammatical skills to individuals who did not speak. This program employed plastic manipulable symbols to teach word order. Carrier (1974) reported that children with severe and profound mental retardation learned word order fairly efficiently by using this instructional program.

This emphasis on the formal aspects of language structure was followed by an increased interest in teaching semantic and pragmatic skills, on measuring generalization across environments, and on creating intervention approaches in the natural environment to promote a child's social competence (Kaiser, 1993; McLean & Snyder-McLean, 1988; Warren & Rogers-Warren, 1985; Warren & Yoder, 1997). These language intervention approaches included matrix training by using miniature linguistic systems (Wetherby & Striefel, 1978), milieu teaching (Kaiser, Yoder, & Keetz, 1992), parent-implemented interventions (Kaiser, 1993), and peer-mediated approaches (Goldstein & Kaczmarek, 1992).

Matrix training is a structured instructional approach using miniature linguistic systems that employ linguistic elements (e.g., nouns, verbs) arranged in systematic combination matrices. Typically, this approach was used to teach word combinations. Using 3 × 3 or 3 × 4 matrices, for example, a subset of the items was taught and then generalization to the remaining items was assessed. Studies typically reported that generalization was enhanced using matrix instruction (Wetherby & Striefel, 1978).

Milieu teaching is a naturalistic strategy for teaching functional language skills. Included in this class of language interventions are specific teaching techniques such as incidental teaching (e.g., Hart & Risley, 1975), mand-model (i.e., a request for the child to produce a communicative behavior) (e.g., Warren, McQuarter, & Rogers-Warren, 1984), and time delay (e.g., Halle, Marshall, & Spradlin, 1979). Typically, the language focus of these interventions was on the development of vocabulary or early two- and three-word semantic relations. Table 1.2 provides descriptions and comparison of each milieu technique and examples of outcomes from studies with individuals who speak.

Both parent-implemented and peer-mediated intervention approaches utilize milieu procedures as their foundation. Parent-implemented interventions can be utilized when parents or caregivers are taught a variety of the previously described milieu language teaching techniques (Kaiser, 1993). Peer-mediated intervention approaches involve teaching children without disabili-

Table 1.2. Milieu oral language teaching strategies and examples of outcomes

Milieu teaching	Definition	Communicators	Outcome
Incidental teaching	Interaction is between the unstructured situation, which is used by the adult to practice developing a skill or to communicate information.	Preschool children who were at risk (Hart & Risley, 1975)	Increased spontaneous language and the variety of words used
		Students with severe mental retardation (Haring, Neetz, Lovinger, Peck, & Semmel, 1987)	Increased frequency of initiations (Hart & Risley, 1975)
Mand-model	Interaction is initiated by the adult to increase opportunity for languages. The adult uses mands or verbal requests and provides models to teach a skill (Warren, McQuarter, & Rogers-Warren, 1984).	Children with moderate to severe language delays (Baer, Wolf, & Risley, 1968; Warren et al., 1984)	Accelerated generalization of trained language items in classroom and nonclassroom settings (Baer et al., 1968)
			Verbalization rates and language complexity increased (Warren et al., 1984).
Time delay	Interaction is a predetermined situation that is initiated when the adult approaches the child and delays desired material or assistance until the child makes the appropriate response (Halle, Baer, & Spradlin, 1981).	Children with severe mental retardation (Halle, Marshall, & Spradlin, 1979)	Increased language use and generalization across trainers
		Students with moderate disabilities (Halle et al., 1981)	Increased vocalizations in multiple settings

ties strategies that can be implemented to facilitate the occurrence of positive social-communicative interactions with children with disabilities (Ostrosky, Kaiser, & Odom, 1993). These approaches are each identifiable distinct language interventions with supporting empirical evidence that shows they work for individuals with specific developmental profiles, including some beginning communicators.

The downward extension of these milieu intervention approaches to infants and toddlers with developmental disabilities has been another important development in the field (Bricker, 1993). These language intervention approaches now include examinations of interventions that are targeted toward the development of intentional communication prior to the onset of speech (see Chapter 3). This prelinguistic milieu teaching method that incorporates some of the intervention procedures, such as responsive interaction with contingent imitation as a means of building routines and encouraging vocal imitation.

Overall, the field of child language disorders has developed by refining and expanding the content of intervention programs and the procedures that are used to present the content. Clearly, the field is on the verge of a new level of sophistication in spoken language intervention that will permit the experimental examination of the relationship between the intrinsic characteristics the child brings to the task and the extrinsic attributes of the interventions themselves.

EXTENSION AND EXPANSION OF LANGUAGE INTERVENTION STRATEGIES TO AAC

The majority of AAC research has centered on developing instructional approaches that are designed to replace or augment the existing receptive and expressive communication skills of beginning communicators (see Mirenda, Iacono, & Williams, 1990, and Romski & Sevcik, 1997, for reviews). For many individuals, spoken language has not been a successful avenue for communicative development, so specialized instruction via manual signs or visual-graphic symbols is required to acquire language. What role do the previously described spoken language intervention approaches play when translated into AAC language intervention approaches?

Contemporary theory and practice recommends that AAC should be implemented in natural environments (e.g., Calculator, 1988). AAC in the natural environment emphasizes the functional nature of language, the need for generalization of communicative repertoires to diverse contexts, and the need to increase the spontaneity of the communicative exchange. The matrix instruction approach provides a method by which to facilitate generalization of relational meanings, setting the stage for later grammatical development. The

Table 1.3. Selected AAC intervention studies

Study	Participants	Intervention approach	AAC Mode	Outcome
Karlan, Brenn-White, Lentz, Egger, & Frankoff (1982)	Three children ages 6–7 years with moderate to severe mental retardation	Matrix teaching	Manual signs	Significantly increased generalized and novel signed verb-noun phrase usage
Romski & Ruder (1984)	Ten children with Down syndrome in Early Stage 1, mean CA = 5 years, 7 months	Matrix teaching: comprehension	Manual signs	Significantly increased action + object combinations and generalization to untaught exemplars
Oliver & Halle (1982)	One 7-year-old child with mental retardation	Milieu teaching: time delay and incidental teaching	Manual signs	Increased sign initiations to means of 75% and 16% in two natural environments; decreased need for prompts
Hamilton & Snell (1993)	One 15-year-old adolescent with mental retardation and autism	Milieu teaching: teacher- and parent-implemented	Book with colored line drawings	Increased communication book use from 7% to 75% of all opportunities following 12 weeks of training in various environments
Glennen & Calculator (1985)	Two children—ages 12 years, 7 months, and 5 years, 9 months—with physical disabilities	Milieu teaching: expectant delay and structured communicative events	Board (using eye gaze)	Generalized initiations of object request to untrained vocabulary symbols following instruction
Angelo & Goldstein (1990)	Four children, ages 5–6 years, with mild to moderate mental retardation	Milieu teaching	Board with Rebus symbols and photos	Taught the participants three information request types: who, what, and where

Study	Participants	Intervention approach	AAC mode	Outcome
Kaiser, Ostrosky, & Alpert (1993)	Three teachers, six children with moderate to severe disabilities	Milieu teaching, environmental arrangement	Board, gestures	Facilitated learning for three children

CA = chronological age

milieu teaching strategy dovetails nicely with efforts to develop AAC skills in natural environments. In this section, we review literature that adapts spoken language intervention approaches to AAC and evaluates how successful they have been for beginning communicators. Table 1.3 provides selective examples of matrix instruction and milieu instruction spoken language strategies that have been adapted for use with AAC modes.

The matrix instruction approach has been adapted to incorporate manual signs in production and comprehension (Karlan, Brenn-White, Lentz, Egger, & Frankoff, 1982; Romski & Ruder, 1984). Karlan and colleagues used Signed English and a 64-item (8 × 8) matrix training approach to develop verb-noun phrase usage by three 6- to 7-year-old children with moderate to severe mental retardation. Two of the three children showed substantial gains in overall performance from 0% to 75% and 2% to 92%. The other child showed a slight increase in overall sign performance from 0% to 25%. Romski and Ruder also employed a 4 × 4 matrix training approach to teach the comprehension of semantic relations to ten children who had Down syndrome (mean CA = 5 years, 7 months) and were in Brown's Early Stage I (Brown, 1973). They employed three conditions: 1) no treatment, 2) speech alone, 3) speech + manual signs. Both treatment conditions were superior to the no treatment condition. Although they found no group differences between speech and speech + manual signs, there was substantial variability in the children's individual patterns of acquisition, with the majority of children taking fewer trials to reach criterion in the speech + manual sign condition.

The milieu approach has been adapted in at least five studies that focus on pragmatic or semantic intervention outcomes. Oliver and Halle (1982) adapted a milieu spoken language intervention composed of time delay and incidental teaching with manual signs for a 7-year-old boy with mental retardation. They showed that, using this intervention in two environments (exercise/play and lunch), the participant increased his manual sign initiations from a mean of 15% and 16% to a mean of 75% and 65%, respectively. The teacher's use of prompts also consistently decreased from a high of 89% to a low of 0%.

Angelo and Goldstein (1990) adapted the milieu teaching approach by replacing the spoken language component with a communication board containing Rebus symbols and photographs. They found that using the adapted milieu approach was effective in teaching four children (5–6 years old) with mild to moderate levels of mental retardation to request information using who, what, and where questions. The participants learned each request type within three to nine sessions. Each session consisted of 20 teaching opportunities. Participants generalized the use of a communication board to make requests in other environments.

Likewise, Glennen and Calculator (1985) implemented a communication board intervention using the milieu approach with two children–ages 12 years, 7 months, and 5 years, 9 months–who had physical disabilities. Both children used direct selection techniques and an eye-gaze response. To facilitate the participants' request for objects, Glennen and Calculator used expectant delays and structured communicative events. Not only did the participants' mean rate of initiating object requests increase, but also their frequency of communication board–conveyed messages increased.

Using a communication book with colored line drawings (predominantly Mayer-Johnson Picture Communication Symbols), Hamilton and Snell (1993) showed that using milieu techniques–such as expectant looking, questions, and a mand-model technique–improved the communication skills of a beginning communicator. Their adolescent participant with mental retardation and autism increased his communication book use from 7% of all opportunities to 75% of all opportunities after 12 weeks of milieu instruction in four different natural environments.

Kaiser, Ostrosky, and Alpert (1993) taught three preschool teachers to use environmental arrangement and milieu teaching strategies with three preschool children who did not speak and used a variety of AAC modes to communicate. The participating teachers learned and generalized the use of the milieu and environmental arrangement procedures to two environments in addition to the primary environment of intervention. The teachers maintained their use of the techniques across a 3-month maintenance period. The participating children demonstrated increases in total communication and the use of taught vocabulary following implementation of the milieu teaching strategies.

Overall, these studies have successfully demonstrated that beginning communicators can learn to use vocabulary to communicate when it is involved in spoken language interventions that have been adapted to utilize an AAC mode. Although the studies differ in the AAC mode (e.g., manual signs, communication board) and selection technique used, as well as in the characteristics of the children studied, they consistently reported positive and significant effects for most participants. Such positive findings appear to be the case whether intervention outcomes focused on pragmatic skills (e.g., requesting objects and information) or semantic skills (e.g., vocabulary development, semantic relations).

AREAS THAT NEED FURTHER INVESTIGATION
IN THE CONTINUUM OF AAC INTERVENTION

When the continuum of AAC language intervention approaches is considered, the previously described spoken language intervention studies fall short in shedding light on three particular intervention areas for beginning communicators: 1) prelinguistic augmented communication skill development, 2) communication with peers, and 3) communication with families. In addition to the approaches described thus far, there are other AAC intervention approaches for beginning communicators that contribute to the knowledge base and shed some light on these three areas. They focus on the development of communicative functions, vocabulary, and semantic relations; vary in the amount of direct instruction and structure they require; and often incorporate behavioral procedures as well information about the language and communication development of typical children (see Beukelman & Mirenda, 1998, and Reichle, York, & Sigafoos, 1991, for details about these approaches). Some of these approaches are discussed elsewhere in this book (see Chapters 6, 7, 9, and 14).

First, the communication intervention needs of beginning augmented communicators who are in the prelinguistic stage of communication development are not well represented in existing experimental studies. One challenging and frustrating lingering issue that may contribute to the lack of data is professional attitudes, philosophy, and beliefs about the use of AAC during the prelinguistic period. Although some of the existing research literature and recommended practices data support the notions that even very young children and other beginning communicators can use and benefit from AAC (e.g., Pierce, 1999; Romski & Sevcik, 1996), some professionals still believe that AAC is a last resort to be tried only after all other interventions have failed and the individual is still not talking (Romski, Sevcik, & Forrest, 2001). This belief may contribute to why AAC is often not incorporated into prelinguistic intervention strategies. Typically developing children primarily rely on gestures to communicate until about 12–13 months of age, when they increasingly use speech for communication (Goldin-Meadow, 2000). Using a developmental perspective, AAC interventions (e.g., gestures, devices, switches) can be viewed as tools to develop prelinguistic skills and set the stage for later vocabulary development regardless of whether the individual eventually talks.

Second, few investigations have addressed how well peers can implement AAC milieu approaches. A few studies indicate that AAC users can communicate with peers. Romski, Sevcik, and Wilkinson (1994), for example, found that the beginning communicators in their study directed a very small proportion (4%) of their communications to peers. The researchers suggested that special intervention attention may be required to facilitate communication with peers.

Third, few investigators have addressed strategies to coach parents and families in communicating with beginning communicators during daily activities. Kaiser (1993) reported that parents can be taught to implement milieu procedures, but it is unclear how easily these approaches can be translated to the needs of beginning AAC communicators. One intervention outcome concern requires addressing how easily families can incorporate language interventions into their daily activities. Another related concern is the location in which intervention occurs and the format in which it is implemented. Prevailing research and practice recommends that instruction take place in daily environments such as home, school, and the community (Calculator, 1988). In turn, evidence also supports the use of naturalistic communicative exchanges as formats for instruction within these environments (e.g., Beukelman & Mirenda, 1998; Guralnick, 2001).

The majority of existing studies have been short-term investigations. Yet, Romski and Sevcik (1996) conducted a 2-year study on the communication abilities of 13 school-age beginning communicators who had moderate or severe mental retardation and used the System for Augmenting Language (SAL). The SAL included five components: 1) speech-output communication device; 2) an appropriate arbitrary symbol vocabulary; 3) naturalistic communicative experiences during which the youth were encouraged, but not required, to communicate; 4) partners (teachers, parents, and siblings) who were taught how to use the device and how to provide both a symbol model and input via speech + symbols to the youth; and 5) a resource and feedback mechanism from investigators to monitor progress across the study. During naturalistic communicative experiences at home and school, the youth had opportunities to employ a range of communicative functions from greeting, requesting, and attention directing to answering and questioning. Romski and Sevcik found that the 13 youth integrated their use of the SAL with their extant vocalizations and gestures, resulting in a rich multimodal form of communication that they used to successfully and effectively communicate with adults (Romski, Sevcik, Robinson, & Bakeman, 1994) and peers (Romski, Sevcik, & Wilkinson, 1994). When considered as a whole, a broad range of language and communication intervention strategies are available to begin the language intervention process. There are, however, more options available for the beginning communicator who is on the verge of (or already) evidencing symbolic communication than for the beginning communicator who is at the prelinguistic stage.

Considerations that Are Unique to AAC Interventions

A number of considerations may be specific to the use of AAC for beginning communicators. Three important considerations in developing viable intervention strategies include decisions surrounding the use of technology, types of representations, and language and communication development issues.

Use of Technology   The use of any kind of technology is strikingly absent from the AAC modes that were used in the studies described in Table 1.3. This finding is in keeping with the general AAC literature. With the exception of a few studies (Locke & Mirenda, 1988; Romski & Sevcik, 1996; Romski, Sevcik, & Pate, 1988; Romski, White, Millen, & Rumbaugh, 1984), manual signs and low-technology communication boards have been the AAC modes of choice for individuals who have typically been considered beginning communicators. The prevailing belief has been that beginning communicators could not benefit from using more sophisticated technologies such as speech-output communication devices. There are at least two arguments against this still prevailing belief.

Romski and Sevcik (1996) argued that the use of a speech-output communication device was a critical component of their participants' successful use of the SAL. They contended that the speech output provided a link to the natural auditory world for the participants. Yet, no direct comparison of SAL acquisition (speech + symbols) with learning symbols alone was provided. Schlosser, Belfiore, Nigam, and Blischak (1995) conducted a study on three adults with severe mental retardation who would have been considered beginning communicators. The researchers compared the participants' acquisition of visual graphic symbols and speech output with the acquisition of visual graphic symbols alone. They found that the speech output + visual graphic symbols resulted in more efficient learning with fewer errors than the visual graphic symbols alone. These results support Romski and Sevcik's argument that speech output can play a critical role in AAC language learning.

Second, advances in technology afford new opportunities for both facilitating language learning and exploring additional dimensions of instruction for beginning communicators who are at the prelinguistic stage of development. One focus of intervention at the prelinguistic stage is developing an understanding that one can affect another's behavior through communication. New simple technologies may permit beginning communicators to effect changes in their environments that may lead to new understandings of intentional communication. For example, programming a simple "speaking" pressure switch to speak the word "cookie" and pairing it with the actual cookie may set the stage (with experience and practice) for an understanding that activating the switch gets the individual what he or she wants—the cookie. At the beginning of the prelinguistic stage, the individual may not necessarily understand that the word "cookie" elicits the communication partner's response. The individual does not have to have the skills in place for the use of simple technology to be initiated. Simple technology can be a tool, coupled with experience and practice, to facilitate the development of intentional communication, and it can set the stage for the later development of word meanings.

Types of Representations   Another consideration is the type of representation that is employed. This is another area in which there is substantial belief but not an equal amount of empirical data (Romski & Sevcik, 1997). The type of representation that is employed may interact with the intervention technique to affect the intervention outcome. In all of the adapted milieu studies, the types of representations that were employed were both unaided and aided, but all were either iconic or symbolic. Real objects (three-dimensional) and photographs (two-dimensional) were not included in these studies. The majority of research on the role of the representation itself has focused on how individuals with intact cognitive skills perceive symbols and/or learn the association between symbols and spoken words (Sevcik et al., 1991; see also Chapter 9). In fact, there is little empirical evidence about the role of the representational medium in language learning for the beginning communicator. Empirical evidence provides some support for a hierarchy of representations from real objects to arbitrary symbols such as printed words (e.g., Dixon, 1981; Mirenda & Locke, 1989; Sevcik & Romski, 1986). Yet, the data suggest that this hierarchy is also influenced by other factors (e.g., the spoken language comprehension skills that an individual brings to the task, the intervention strategy, the reinforcement value of the symbol). The beginning communicator actually highlights the issue of "When is a symbol a symbol?" because it is during this period of learning and development that symbolic communication skills are emerging. A symbol truly functions as a symbol when the relationship between the symbol and the referent is arbitrary. This type of relationship between symbol and referent emerges over time. Supporting the development of symbols is critical to later language development.

Several additional issues, which have not received research attention, interact with the type of representation and intervention to be used for beginning communicators. Using multiple modes of communication—combining unaided and aided types of representations (i.e., gestures with visual-graphic symbols)—has been advocated and seems to make sense developmentally. It is not known, however, whether combining types of representation is difficult for the beginning communicator. This next issue is one that combines technology with representation. With the development of computerized communication devices that have dynamic symbol displays, an understanding of the differences between using static and dynamic displays will be important to consider for the beginning communicator. A third issue is the quantity of symbols that are available to a beginning communicator. Do you begin with one symbol? Two symbols? Ten symbols? These are all empirical issues that require future research attention.

Language and Communication Development Issues   Two language and communication development issues that deserve highlighting are 1) vocabulary choice and 2) the relationship between comprehension and production. First, the choice of vocabulary and the meaning associated with the vocabulary item is an issue that is specific to AAC. Choosing vocabulary is a major AAC issue, especially because the chosen visual-graphic symbol vocabulary items are usually the only "words" that are available to the individual. Combining modes (gestures and visual-graphic symbols) may expand the available vocabulary. With a limited number of vocabulary items, should initial vocabulary be general ("snack") or more specific ("cookie," "juice," "chips")? How do you build a vocabulary? One symbol at a time?

In addition, does one symbol equal one word, as it does for typically developing children who are learning to talk? Or does one symbol equal one phrase? What effect does this choice have on the language and communication development of beginning communicators? If knowledge of typical language and communication development is employed to inform this discussion, then one symbol should equal one word unless the phrases are considered holistic, as sometimes is the case in early vocabulary development (e.g., "What is it?"). Often, however, AAC symbols are assigned multiword or phrase meanings (e.g., "I'd like a cookie," "Give me a hug"). One explanation for these clinical decisions is that rate of communication is a consideration. Having to use four touches or key presses to activate four symbols will negatively influence the speed of communication and the communication interaction. Using one symbol would also impede the naturalness of the communication interaction if an adult model is the standard. These issues must be balanced with the issue of whether an individual beginning communicator will advance beyond single-symbol use. If the individual is to learn semantic relations, then perhaps multiword or phrase symbols will be confusing. Although there are no empirical studies that address this aspect of AAC and language development, there are a number of complex issues and tradeoffs to consider as decisions about vocabulary are made. For example, the selection technique (e.g., direct selection, scanning) that is employed may influence a beginning communicator's access to communication. Beginning communicators with both severe physical and cognitive disabilities may encounter more difficulty in finding an access technique for communication because, as noted previously, a technique that requires fewer physical abilities requires more sophisticated cognitive abilities.

A second issue to be considered with respect to language development is the relationship of comprehension and production for the beginning communicator (see Chapter 14). A focus on comprehension may permit the individual to observe and to actively engage in the communicative process prior to actually taking on the role of speaker. Beginning communicators, similar to very young typically developing children, should be exposed to augmented language as input before they are asked to produce it. If the typical development literature is followed for beginning communicators, then an instructional focus on comprehension should proceed a focus on production. In general, AAC practice has followed an approach in which production (physical access to a device and the production of messages) precedes comprehension (Beukelman & Mirenda, 1998). For individuals who are first learning to use AAC, the field has not yet addressed how to incorporate both comprehension and production in AAC intervention efforts, including the sequence of introduction and the relationship between comprehension and production.

Future Research and Practice Directions   Language intervention approaches are at the center of potential AAC success for beginning communicators. The literature suggests that well-established spoken language approaches have had some utility for adaptation to AAC use. Studies have focused on beginning communicators who function at or close to the symbolic level. Much less evidence is available about the communication development of beginning communicators who are not functioning symbolically.

One particularly important yet challenging area of research need is that of language and communication measurement tools (Sevcik, Romski, & Adamson, 1999). Attention must be focused on the development of assessment tools that provide a fine-grained analysis of the child's language and communication skills across modes and that measure a range of intervention outcomes over time. Some outcomes of using AAC go beyond the development of specific comprehension and production vocabulary, and even grammatical skills, and have been somewhat elusive to quantitative measurement. Access to communication through AAC use can change the quality of an individual's life in inclusive environments regarding school and work, family interactions, and the perceptions and attitudes of others toward individuals who do not speak (Romski & Sevcik, 1996). Such communication access can also prevent the emergence of secondary disabilities (e.g., challenging behaviors). Creating tools that permit measurement of these elusive outcomes is important.

Another area of future investigation should be the identification of subgroups of beginning communicators. A great deal is known about the language and communication characteristics of beginning communicators, including the fact that they span the prelinguistic stage of development (from preintentional to intentional), as well as individuals who are beginning the symbolic stage. It may be possible to differentiate subgroups of individuals so that AAC interventions can be targeted and fine-tuned to fit particular subgroups (e.g., beginning communicators at the perlocutionary stage). It is also important to note that very little is known about the effects of gender and ethnicity in relation to AAC intervention outcomes. Wilkinson (1999) compared the communications of male and female adults with mental retardation and reported gender differences. The role of gender and ethnicity must continue to be woven into examinations of intervention outcomes.

With respect to practice implications, there are at least two broad considerations for clinicians. First, the communication device is a means to an end (gaining functional language and communication skills)—not the end in itself. Incorporating AAC for beginning communicators requires focusing on language and communication development within the context of the AAC mode. AAC is sometimes thought of as a separate area of practice and, thus, clinicians do not always incorporate the information that they know about language and communication development as they consider AAC assessment and intervention. It is imperative that these areas of knowledge be linked. Second, there is a strong history of empirical data to draw on as clinicians make practice decisions about intervention strategies for beginning communicators. Clinical decisions must be guided by empirical data in the context of clinical judgment, not merely by "beliefs."

CONCLUSION

Language intervention research has a more than 30-year history on which to build a continuum of AAC language instructional approaches for beginning communicators. Milieu teaching approaches offer a range of naturalistic interventions for beginning communicators. The translation of spoken language instructional approaches has merit for AAC, but there are considerations specific to AAC that make the translation a complex task. Further investigation is needed to explore the range applying these approaches in AAC intervention as well as their limitations. The most important practice implication is the link between the literature on spoken language interventions and AAC language interventions. In sum, beginning communicators highlight the continuum of communication and the resources available from the literature on language development and spoken language instructional approaches.

REFERENCES

American Speech-Language-Hearing Association (ASHA). (1991). Report: Augmentative and alternative communication. *Asha, 33*(Suppl. 5), 9–12.

Angelo, D.H., & Goldstein, H. (1990). Effects of a pragmatic teaching strategy for requesting information by communication board users. *Journal of Speech and Hearing Disorders, 55,* 231–243.

Baer, D., Wolf, M., & Risley, T. (1968). Some current dimensions of applied behavior analysis. *Journal of Applied Behavior Analysis, 1,* 37–49.

Beukelman, D.R., & Mirenda, P. (1998). *Augmentative and alternative communication: Management of severe communication disorders in children and adults* (2nd ed.). Baltimore: Paul H. Brookes Publishing Co.

Bricker, D. (1993). Then, now, and the path between: A brief history of language intervention. In S.F. Warren & J. Reichle (Series Eds.) & A.P. Kaiser & D.B. Gray (Vol. Eds.), *Communication and language intervention series: Vol. 2. Enhancing children's communication: Research foundations for intervention* (pp. 11–31). Baltimore: Paul H. Brookes Publishing Co.

Brown, R. (1973). *A first language.* Cambridge, MA: Harvard University Press.

Calculator, S. (1988). Promoting the acquisition and generalization of conversation skill by individuals with severe disabilities. *Augmentative and Alternative Communication, 4,* 94–103.

Carrier, J. (1974). Nonspeech noun usage training with severely and profoundly re-tarded children. *Journal of Speech and Hearing Research, 17,* 510–517.

Chapman, R., & Miller, H. (1980). Analyzing language and communication in the child. In R.L. Schiefelbusch (Ed.), *Nonspeech language and communication: Analysis and intervention* (pp. 159–196). Baltimore: University Park Press.

Dixon, L. (1981). A functional analysis of photo-object matching skills of severely re-tarded adolescents. *Journal of Applied Behavior Analysis, 14,* 465–478.

Donnellan, A., Mirenda, P., Mesaros, R., & Fassbender, L. (1984). Analyzing the com-municative functions of aberrant behavior. *Journal of The Association for Persons with Severe Handicaps, 9,* 141–150.

Doss, L.S., & Reichle, J (1991). Replacing excess behavior with an initial communica-tive repertoire. In J. Reichle, J. York, & J. Sigafoos (Eds.), *Implementing augmentative and alternative communication: Strategies for learners with severe disabilities* (pp. 215–237). Balti-more: Paul H. Brookes Publishing Co.

Glennen, S.L., & Calculator, S.N. (1985). Training functional communication board use: A pragmatic approach. *Augmentative and Alternative Communication, 1,* 134–141.

Goldin-Meadow, S. (2000). Beyond words: The importance of gesture to researchers and learners. *Child Development, 71,* 231–239.

Goldstein, H., & Kaczmarek, L. (1992). Promoting communicative interaction among children in integrated intervention settings. In S.F. Warren & J. Reichle (Series Eds. & Vol. Eds.), *Communication and language intervention series: Vol. 1. Causes and effects in com-munication and language intervention* (pp. 81–111). Baltimore: Paul H. Brookes Pub-lishing Co.

Guess, D., & Horner, R. (1978). The severely and profoundly handicapped. In E.L. Meyen (Ed.), *Exceptional children and youth: An introduction* (pp. 218–268). Denver, CO: Love Publishing.

Guralnick, M.J. (Ed.). (2001). *Early childhood inclusion: Focus on change.* Baltimore: Paul H. Brookes Publishing Co.

Halle, J., Baer, D.M., & Spradlin, J.E. (1981). Teacher's generalized use of delay as a stimulus control procedure to increase language use in handicapped children. *Jour-nal of Applied Behavior Analysis, 14,* 389 409.

Halle, J., Marshall, A., & Spradlin, J. (1979). Time delay: A technique to increase lan-guage use and facilitate generalization in retarded children. *Journal of Applied Beha-vior Analysis, 3,* 431–439.

Hamilton, B.L., & Snell, M.E. (1993). Using the milieu approach to increase sponta-neous communication book use across environments by an adolescent with autism. *Augmentative and Alternative Communication, 9,* 259–272.

Haring, T.G., Neetz, J.A., Lovinger, L., Peck, C., & Semmel, M. (1987). Effects of four modified incidental teaching procedures to create opportunities for communication. *Journal of The Association for Persons with Severe Handicaps, 12,* 431–439.

Hart, B., & Risley, T. (1975). Incidental teaching of language in the preschool. *Journal of Applied Behavior Analysis, 4,* 411–420.

Hunt-Berg, M., & Loncke, F. (2000). Gestures in AAC. *Augmentative Communication News, 13,* 1–4.

Kaiser, A. (1993). Parent-implemented language intervention: An environmental sys-tem perspective. In S.F. Warren & J. Reichle (Series Eds.) & A.P. Kaiser & D.B. Gray (Vol. Eds.), *Communication and language intervention series: Vol. 2. Enhancing children's com-munication: Research foundations for intervention* (pp. 63–84). Baltimore: Paul H. Brookes Publishing Co.

Kaiser, A., Ostrosky, M., & Alpert, C. (1993). Training teachers to use environmental arrangement and milieu teaching for nonvocal preschool children. *Journal of The As-sociation for Persons with Severe Handicaps, 18,* 188–191.

Kaiser, A.P., Yoder, P.J., & Keetz, A. (1992). Evaluating milieu teaching. In S.F. Warren & J. Reichle (Series Eds. & Vol. Eds.), *Communication and language intervention series: Vol. 1. Causes and effects in communication and language intervention* (pp. 9–47). Baltimore: Paul H. Brookes Publishing Co.

Karlan, G., Brenn-White, B., Lentz, A., Egger, D., & Frankoff, D. (1982). Establishing generalized, productive verb-noun phrase usage in a manual language system with moderately handicapped children. *Journal of Speech and Hearing Disorders, 47,* 31–42.

Locke, P., & Mirenda, P. (1988). A computer supported communication approach for a nonspeaking child with severe visual and cognitive impairments. *Augmentative and Alternative Communication, 4,* 15–22.

McLean, J., & Snyder-McLean, L. (1988). Applications of pragmatics to severely mentally retarded children and youth. In R.L. Schiefelbusch & L.L. Lloyd (Eds.), *Language perspectives: Acquisitions, retardation and intervention* (pp. 255–288). Austin, TX: PRO-ED.

Miller, J., & Yoder, D. (1972). A syntax teaching program. In J. McLean, D. Yoder, & R.L. Schiefelbusch (Eds.), *Language intervention with the retarded: Developing strategies* (pp. 191–211). Baltimore: University Park Press.

Mirenda, P. (1997). Supporting individuals with challenging behavior through functional communication training and AAC: Research review. *Augmentative and Alternative Communication, 13,* 207–225.

Mirenda, P., Iacono, T., & Williams, R. (1990). Communication options for persons with severe and profound disabilities: State of the art and future directions. *Journal of The Association for Persons with Severe Handicaps, 15,* 3–21.

Mirenda. P., & Locke, M. (1989). A comparison of symbol transparency in nonspeaking persons with intellectual disabilities. *Journal of Speech and Hearing Disorders, 54,* 131–140.

National Joint Committee for the Communication Needs of Persons with Severe Disabilities. (1992). Guidelines for meeting the communication needs of persons with severe disabilities. *Asha, 34*(Suppl. 7), 1–8.

Nelson, N. (1992). Performance is the prize: Language competence and performance among AAC users. *Augmentative and Alternative Communication, 8,* 3–18.

Oliver, C., & Halle, J. (1982). Language training in the everyday environment: Teaching functional sign use to a retarded child. *Journal of The Association for Persons with Severe Handicaps, 8,* 50–62.

Ostrosky, M.M., Kaiser, A.P., & Odom, S.L. (1993). Facilitating children's social-communication interactions through the use of peer-mediated interventions. In S.F. Warren & J. Reichle (Series Eds.) & A.P. Kaiser & D.B. Gray (Vol. Eds.), *Communication and language intervention series: Vol. 2. Enhancing children's communication: Research foundations for intervention* (pp. 159–185). Baltimore: Paul H. Brookes Publishing Co.

Pierce, P. (1999). *Baby power: A guide for families using assistive technology with their infants and toddlers.* Chapel Hill: The University of North Carolina Press.

Reichle, J., York, J., & Sigafoos, J. (Eds.). (1991). *Implementing augmentative and alternative communication: Strategies for learners with severe disabilities.* Baltimore: Paul H. Brookes Publishing Co.

Romski, M.A., & Ruder, K. (1984). Effects of speech and speech and sign instruction on oral language learning and generalization of action + object combinations by Down's Syndrome children. *Journal of Speech and Hearing Disorders, 49,* 293–302.

Romski, M.A., & Sevcik, R.A. (1993). Language comprehension: Considerations for augmentative and alternative communication. *Augmentative and Alternative Communication, 9,* 281–285.

Romski, M.A., & Sevcik, R.A. (1995). Communicative development of chidren with severe disabilites. In M. Smith & J. Damico (Eds.), *Childhood language disorders* (pp. 218–234). New York: Thieme Medical Publishers.

Romski, M.A., & Sevcik, R.A. (1996). *Breaking the speech barrier: Language development through augmented means.* Baltimore: Paul H. Brookes Publishing Co.

Romski, M.A., & Sevcik, R.A. (1997). Augmentative and alternative communication for children with developmental disabilities. *Mental Retardation and Developmental Disabilities Research Reviews, 3,* 363–368.

Romski, M.A., Sevcik, R.A., & Forrest, S. (2001). Assistive technology and augmentative communication in inclusive early childhood programs. In M.J. Guralnick (Ed.), *Early childhood inclusion: Focus on change* (pp. 465–479). Baltimore: Paul H. Brookes Publishing Co.

Romski, M.A., Sevcik, R.A., & Pate, J.L. (1988). The establishment of symbolic communication in persons with mental retardation. *Journal of Speech and Hearing Disorders, 53,* 94–107.

Romski, M.A., Sevcik, R.A., Reumann, R., & Pate, J.L. (1989). Youngsters with moderate or severe retardation and severe spoken language impairments I: Extant communicative patterns. *Journal of Speech and Hearing Disorders, 54,* 366–373.

Romski, M.A., Sevcik, R.A., Robinson, B.F., & Bakeman, R. (1994). Adult-directed communications of youth with mental retardation using the System for Augmenting Language. *Journal of Speech and Hearing Research, 37,* 617–628.

Romski, M.A., Sevcik, R.A., Robinson, B.F., & Wilkinson, K.M. (1990, November). *Intelligibility and form changes in the vocalizations of augmented language learners.* Paper presented at the ASHA Annual Convention, Seattle.

Romski, M.A., Sevcik, R.A., & Wilkinson, K.M. (1994). Peer-directed communicative interactions of augmented language learners with mental retardation. *American Journal on Mental Retardation, 98,* 527–538.

Romski, M.A., White, R., Millen, C.E., & Rumbaugh, D.M. (1984). Effects of computer-keyboard teaching on the symbolic communication of severely retarded persons: Five case studies. *The Psychological Record, 34,* 39–54.

Schiefelbusch, R.L., & Lloyd, L.L. (Eds.). (1974). *Language perspectives: Acquisition, retardation, and intervention.* Baltimore: University Park Press.

Schlosser, R., Belfiore, P., Nigam, R., & Blischak, D. (1995). The effects of speech output technology in the learning of graphic symbols. *Journal of Applied Behavior Analysis, 28,* 537–549.

Sevcik, R.A., & Romski, M.A. (1986). Representational matching skills of persons with severe retardation. *Augmentative and Alternative Communication, 2,* 160–164.

Sevcik, R.A., Romski, M.A., & Adamson, L.B. (1999). Measuring AAC interventions for individuals with severe developmental disabilities. *Augmentative and Alternative Communication, 15,* 38–44.

Sevcik, R.A., Romski, M.A., & Wilkinson, K. (1991). Roles of graphic symbols in the language acquisition process for persons with severe cognitive disabilities. *Augmentative and Alternative Communication, 7,* 161–170.

Snell, M. (1987). *Systematic instruction of persons with severe handicaps.* Columbus, OH: Charles E. Merrill.

Warren, S.F. (1993). Early communication and language intervention: Challenges for the 1990s and beyond. In S.F. Warren & J. Reichle (Series Eds.) & A.P. Kaiser & D.B. Gray (Vol. Eds.), *Communication and language intervention series: Vol. 2. Enhancing children's communication: Research foundations for intervention* (pp. 375–395). Baltimore: Paul H. Brookes Publishing Co.

Warren, S.F., McQuarter, R.J., & Rogers-Warren, A. (1984). The effects of mands and models on the speech of unresponsive language-delayed preschool children. *Journal of Speech and Hearing Disorders, 49,* 43–52.

Warren, S.F., & Rogers-Warren, A. (1985). *Teaching functional language.* Austin, TX: PRO-ED.

Warren, S.F., & Yoder, P. (1997). Communication, language, and mental retardation. In W. McLean (Ed.), *Ellis' handbook of mental deficiency, psychological theory and research* (pp. 379–403). Mahwah, NJ: Lawrence Erlbaum Associates.

Wetherby, B., & Striefel, S. (1978). Application of miniature linguistic system to matrix-training procedures. In R.L. Schiefelbusch (Ed.), *Language intervention strategies* (pp. 318–356). Baltimore: University Park Press.

Wilkinson, K.M. (1999). Gender differences in the use of linguistic devices by youths with mental retardation: A preliminary analysis. *American Journal on Mental Retardation, 104,* 227–235.

Yoder, P., & Layton, T. (1988). Speech following sign language training in autistic children with minimal verbal language. *Journal of Autism and Developmental Disorders, 18,* 217–229.

2

Overview of the Emergence of Early AAC Behaviors

Progression from Communicative to Symbolic Skills

Ellin B. Siegel and Cynthia J. Cress

This chapter focuses on children and youth who do not use or understand symbols and the rules of language. These communicators express themselves without symbols in the vocal mode (e.g., sounds) or the unaided mode (e.g., facial expressions, alertness, gestures). Intervention focuses on enhancing the quality of their nonsymbolic expressions and on expanding their repertoire to include symbolic communication across vocal, unaided, and aided modes. We use a developmental perspective to guide the interventionist to view the early communicator as an individual with diverse skills. This is accomplished through a tri-focal framework (Siegel-Causey & Bashinski, 1997) of assessment and intervention that is centered on the early communicator, his or her partner, and his or her environment. This framework concentrates on communication as a shared process. The National Joint Committee for the Communication Needs of Persons with Severe Disabilities defined *communication* as

> Any act by which one person gives to or receives from another person information about that person's needs, desires, perceptions, knowledge, or affective states. Communication my be intentional or unintentional, may involve conventional or unconventional signals, may take linguistic or nonlinguistic forms, and may occur through spoken or other modes. (1992, p. 2)

FOCUSING ON AAC FOR EARLY COMMUNICATORS

It is clear that *communication* is a broad concept that encompasses the use of multiple forms: symbolic expressions, nonsymbolic expressions, and other alternative or augmentative modalities. Augmentative and alternative communication (AAC) approaches have used multimodal interventions and build on individuals' full communication capabilities, including speech, vocalizations, gestures, and aided communication (American Speech-Language-Hearing Association [ASHA], 1991). It is important that AAC interventions for early communicators, or individuals who do not speak or use symbolic forms, emphasize 1) aiding these individuals to communicate as clearly as possible using nonsymbolic forms and 2) striving to make these forms as conventional as possible. Early AAC intervention is thus focused on helping individuals communicate in the present with nonsymbolic skills and on providing interventions that may aid them to acquire symbolic skills in the future.

Individuals who do not yet use symbols may rely on their own bodies, objects, partners, and current contexts to communicate. Their communication modes may include facial expressions, body movements, eye gazing, gesturing, and touching. This type of communication has been given many different names, such as *prelinguistic, nonsymbolic,* and *nonverbal;* we use the term *early communication.* Early communication that involves nonsymbolic behavior is viewed as a legitimate form of communication. Because many individuals with disabilities rely primarily on intentional nonsymbolic skills, it is crucial that early AAC interventions incorporate the individual's current communication repertoire and strive to expand it.

Early intervention for children with severe communication impairments is beneficial. It is recognized that during the first 5 years of life, tremendous growth occurs in communication and language skills. Disorders or delays in the early communication repertoire may interfere with further language development. A wide body of research (see Guralnick, 1997, for extensive research reviews) has demonstrated the effectiveness of early intervention and that such intervention is particularly important for children who may have communication difficulties, such as children with autism (e.g., Dawson & Osterling, 1997), motor impairments (e.g., Harris, 1997), Down syndrome (e.g., Spiker & Hopmann, 1997), and communication disorders (e.g., McLean & Cripe, 1997). Specialized AAC techniques are necessary to enhance early communication, and AAC strategies can be viewed as part of a continuum that can benefit diverse communicators.

Three primary criteria identify early communicators who are at high risk for being nonspeaking: 1) medical or health complications during pregnancy or birth, including anoxia and feeding difficulties; 2) delayed vocal output in each developmental stage from birth to 2 years of age; and 3) evidence of neuromotor deficits or conditions that are associated with unintelligible speech development (e.g., cerebral palsy, abnormal reflexes, severe oral apraxia) (McDonald, 1980). Although many individuals who fit this profile have multiple rehabilitative and medical intervention needs, it is also critical to include access to augmentative communication modes as early as possible. Yet, risk factors are not clearly identified for predicting communication in young children who are nonspeaking, and these factors are only beginning to be addressed by longitudinal research (Cress et al., 2000; Romski & Sevcik, 1996). Initial AAC evaluations and interventions may be postponed to coincide with a child's entry into preschool rather than being conducted earlier, when risk for being nonspeaking can be identified. Reasons for this delay include limited staff training in AAC, educational policies, a focus on physical and medical interventions, and a tendency to wait until vocal communication skills are at least 1–1.5 years behind those of chronological age peers (Blackstone, 1991).

Identifying the need for AAC with early communicators is often postponed until consistent delays in expected developmental milestones have been identified (Beukelman & Mirenda, 1998). Often, concerns that AAC may interfere with an individual's verbal expressive development contribute to the delay in identification. This view has been challenged, however, with assertions that AAC intervention also facilitates speech development when both communication systems are available to children (e.g., Silverman, 1995). In addition, individuals who are early communicators may not receive AAC intervention because of the perception that they are not "ready" for it. Previously, it was assumed that individuals need to demonstrate the prerequisites of sensorimotor stage V for sufficient symbolic understanding to begin to learn how to use AAC (e.g., Chapman & Miller, 1980; Owens & House, 1984). It was later recognized that individuals can acquire some of the presumed prerequisite skills much earlier through the functional use of AAC in naturalistic environments (Kangas & Lloyd, 1988; Reichle & Karlan, 1985). Over time, many researchers explored the scope of communication and language intervention on symbolic expression (learning to talk) to include a broader emphasis on the multiple processes of communication (comprehension) and partner roles (input). These historical shifts in emphasis have been well documented (Goetz & Sailor, 1988; McLean & McLean, 1993; Mirenda, Iacono, & Williams, 1990), and a literature base has emerged in support of the appropriateness of nonsymbolic intervention (e.g., Beukelman & Mirenda, 1998; Miles, 2000; Siegel & Wetherby, 2000; Siegel-Causey & Bashinski, 1997; Sigafoos et al. 2000).

No single disability or combination of impairments distinguishes which individuals communicate primarily in a nonsymbolic manner and, thus, need early AAC intervention. The individuals who use nonsymbolic communication form a heterogeneous group. They may have a physical disability (e.g., cerebral palsy), a cognitive impairment (e.g., mental retardation), sensory impairments (e.g., visual impairment, hearing impairment), and/or behavioral and social impairments (e.g., autism). One must focus on how each individual is able to communicate rather than on specific disabilities, although particular disabilities may influence communication. The following examples show ways in which early communicators with various disabilities might convey messages to others:

- Physical disability: Shawn uses eye gaze to choose which color paper to place on her collage. Her friend Ann interprets this signal and puts the selected paper on Shawn's wheelchair tray.
- Cognitive impairment: Eric nods and vocalizes when the teacher asks him if he has finished adding to his social studies journal and is ready to go to physical education class.
- Cognitive and motor impairments: Dan's muscle tone increases and he vocalizes when his mother picks him up and tells him that it is time to go swimming.
- Dual sensory impairment: Aileen reaches toward the two beverage containers that her peer Cody is holding. She explores both containers and selects the orange juice box by pulling it toward herself.
- Autism: Harris walks to his schedule shelf that holds objects representing each schedule change in his school day. He finds the wristband that he wears during physical education class in the next open box, which reminds him that this class will occur next. He puts the wristband on and walks towards the door where his classmates are lining up to go to the gym.

EXPANDING AAC INTERVENTIONS AND
RECOGNIZING THE INFLUENCES OF PARTNERS

The AAC discipline has traditionally focused on enhancing communication for individuals who are intentional and understand symbols. Symbolic methods (e.g., graphic symbol sets, voice output communication aids [VOCAs], sign language systems) are very effective for individuals who function beyond early communication levels. These symbolic strategies are not likely to match the expressive skills of individuals who are early communicators and may be neither symbolic nor intentional. Therefore, the strategies are most often used for exposure and/or as augmented input during these stages.

In the 1990s, however, there was a new emphasis on interventions for individuals who use nonsymbolic communication and their partners (Siegel & Wetherby, 2000; Siegel-Causey & Bashinski, 1997; Wilcox, Bacon, & Shannon, 1995; Yoder & Warren, 1993, 1998). Partners influence communication and play a critical role in interpreting early communication. If communicators convey information through eye gaze, body movement, or other behaviors, partners need to be able to recognize and value these expressions. At early communication stages, some of an individual's behaviors are signals that become communicative because the partners respond. Partner interpretations and responsiveness to early signals play an important role in the development of intentional communication (Dore, 1986; Yoder & Warren, 1999; Yoder, Warren, McCathren, & Leew, 1998). For instance, Yoder and Warren found that prelinguistic intentional communicators with developmental disabilities showed during a 12-month period a positive relationship between parent responsibility and later language development. Yoder and Warren concluded that partner and contextual influences on children's early language development predicted treatment prognosis. This suggests that interventionists need to rely on changing more than children's isolated behaviors to improve communication.

DEVELOPMENTAL PROCESSES IN EARLY AAC COMMUNICATORS

Early communicative behaviors, including spontaneous and nonintentional behaviors, support the development of later skills, including intentional and symbolic communication. Although symbolic communicative forms are an integral part of an individual's receptive communicative experience, it is important to provide an accessible communication mode that the individual can use and control. The following sections outline the progression of AAC behaviors that support later symbolic development.

Continuum of AAC: From Early Behaviors to Symbolic Communication

As observed in typically developing children, communication for individuals who rely on AAC progresses from spontaneous to intentional behaviors and then to intentional and symbolic communication (Bates, 1979; McLean & Snyder-McLean, 1987; Wilcox et al., 1995). *Spontaneous behaviors* include emotional reactions or posture shifts that arise in response to events or internal states without apparent goal-directed activity by the communicator. *Intentional behaviors* are goal-directed actions, such as reaching for a desired object, that are not directed communicatively toward a partner (Wetherby & Prizant, 1993). Examples of early communicative skills or qualities that reflect these levels of communication are provided in Table 2.1.

Both spontaneous and intentional behaviors have been referred to as *partner-perceived communication* (Wilcox et. al., 1995), as partners have the primary responsibility for assigning communicative meaning to these types of behaviors. Although few individuals produce all of their communicative behaviors at a single level, individuals may not achieve more complex communicative behaviors if they are not demonstrating key discriminative skills. For instance, individuals who do not direct their communicative signals toward a listener are producing intentional behaviors (partner-perceived communication) but are not intentionally communicating. The terms *partner-perceived communication, intentional communication,* and *symbolic communication* are used throughout this chapter to refer to concepts that Bates (1979) labeled respectively as *perlocutionary, illocutionary,* and *locutionary communication.*

It is important for communicative partners to recognize both the progression of communication behaviors and the continuum of forms that com-

Table 2.1.   Examples of communicative skills across levels of development

Partner-perceived communication	Intentional communication	Symbolic communication
Spontaneous behaviors		
Reflexive or environmentally triggered actions	Child directs behaviors toward adult with voice, gesture, or eye gaze	Child uses words, symbols, representational play, or gestures directed to partner
Partner interprets child's behavior as communicative	Child initiates communication and often persists to get desired results	Child responds to partner and expresses specific concepts
Adult responds communicatively to presumed unintentional child behavior	Child directs his or her behavior to adult with an identifiable message, even if the child is not yet linguistic	Child talks about concepts that are distant in time or space
Intentional behaviors		
Child directs behaviors toward toy or activity with implicit purpose		
Partner scaffolds most of child's communication		
Child acts toward toy (or parent as a "toy") and parent infers the communication act		

munication may encompass (see Table 2.2). First, communication is a multi-modal system that involves vocal, unaided, and aided systems. Vocal communication encompasses any voiced output (e.g., cry, vocalize) or babbling as well as speech. Unaided communication involves expression via one's body (e.g., gestures, sign language). Aided communication involves modes that are not part of the individual's own body and include commonly used AAC systems (e.g., objects, graphics, photos that are part of communication systems, VOCAs). Communicative partners and professional team members benefit from viewing these three modes as a continuum of behaviors from early communication to symbolic communication. One goal of AAC intervention is to help the individual move from his or her present communication level to a more conventional, symbolic system (e.g., sign language, picture symbols, VOCAs, written language).

The items listed within the three modes on Table 2.2 should be viewed as a possible order of acquisition and are displayed with nonsymbolic behavior on the left side, moving toward more symbolic behaviors on the right side. Individual learners may express themselves with a combination of nonsymbolic and symbolic modes and will not necessarily need intervention directed

Table 2.2. Progression of communication behaviors and a proposed continuum of forms that they encompass

Mode   Repertoire

Nonsymbolic ⟶ Symbolic

Vocal	Sounds	Babbling	Speech	Visual	Voice output communication aid (VOCA)	Sign language
Unaided	**Alertness**	**Facial expression/ affect**	**Body movement**	**Visual**	**Gestural**	**Sign language**
	Behavior state	Comfort/ discomfort	Body orientation and proximity	Eye gaze	Gestures	Manual signs
		Emotion	Body movement	Eye blink codes	Pantomime	Fingerspelling
					Yes/no headshakes	

	Objects	Photos/ pictures	Graphic symbol sets	Alphabet	Codes
Aided	**Objects**	**Photos/ pictures**	**Graphic symbol sets**	**Alphabet**	**Codes**
	Real objects	Color	Line drawings	Words	Color codes
	Partial objects	Black and white	Organizational symbol sets (PCS, Rebus)	Letters	Alpha codes
	Artificial association symbols				Alpha-numeric codes
	Textured symbols		Blissymbols	Morse code	Numeric codes
	Miniature objects		Arbitrary symbols	Braille	Iconic codes

Key: PCS = Picture Communication Symbols.
Note: Copyright © 2001 Ellin B. Siegel.

within a category. For example, an individual may 1) learn to express via real objects and then move on to partial objects (within a category), 2) move from using real objects to using both real objects or some expressions and artificially associated systems (within a category), or 3) move from real objects to photographs (one category to another). The view of vocal, unaided, and aided modes is presented to help interventionists assess the child's current expressions and then to develop interventions that encourage all three modalities, moving to a more symbolic repertoire.

Influences of Specific Disabilities on Early Communication Development

Strategies to encourage communication in an early communicator should account for challenges that result from that person's disability. Table 2.3 presents four types of impairments (physical, cognitive and/or language, sensory, and social/behavioral) that can influence communication, examples of possible communicative impacts for these impairments, and potential strategies to encourage communication for each type. For instance, physical and sensory impairments may interfere with both access and control of communicative events for different reasons. Also, individuals who have primary cognitive and/or language impairments in addition to physical impairments may approach language learning tasks in distinctly different ways from people with physical or sensory impairments only. Communicative strategies for individuals with impairments are described in the following vignettes:

- Physical disability: Shawn is in music class and is vocalizing to sing along with her classmates. When it is her turn to choose a song, Shawn's teacher plays a song excerpt on one cassette player and another excerpt on a second cassette player. Shawn indicates her choice by looking at the one playing the tape of the song that she prefers.
- Cognitive impairment: Eric is participating in a group project for science class. As the interaction with his peers progresses, he needs to know when to comment or express himself. When it is time for Eric to contribute his work to the group's diorama, his friend Mark tries to get Eric's attention. Mark has been instructed to use pauses to accommodate Eric's slower processing time. Mark waits 10 seconds because he knows that Eric will respond if he has a longer opportunity to figure out what he is to do next. Eric starts to put his work into the diorama and then looks up at Mark as a form of communication to be sure the work is going into the correct place.
- Cognitive and motor impairment: Dan is seated in his supported position in the kitchen as his sister finishes preparing dinner. His sister notices that Dan's vocalizations increase as he watches her, and she interprets this as Dan's interest in the dinner preparations. She brings the spaghetti bowl to

Table 2.3. Descriptions of disability influences and selected communication strategies

	Physical impairment	Cognitive and/or language impairment	Sensory impairment	Social/behavioral impairment
Areas influenced by disability	Access to materials and toys Control of the environment Expressive communication methods and experience Independence and exploration within activities Ability to produce sounds and learn phonetic skills	Slower processing time Short-term memory Generalizing across situations Processing and responding appropriately to complex stimuli Expected responses to environment	Gaining access to information in visual and/or auditory modalities (e.g., nonverbal, written) Recognizing and using social cues in various modalities Responding meaningfully to various forms of communication	Attending and responding appropriately to social and environmental cues Processing and discriminating among roles in social activities Sharing responsibility and control of communicative interactions
Strategies that encourage communication	Child-initiated routines and opportunities to take turns Encouragement of vocalizing Cause-and-effect learning and consequences Encourage phonetic information processing and sound play	Cognitive foundations of language, including cause and effect and means end Forming symbolic reference Adapting communication strategies to specific situations	Early vocalizing and sound/letter play Turn taking and interactive routines Responses to parent communication and environment	Turn taking Joint attention and reference Interactive routines

Dan, and they take turns adding the sauce and stirring. She imitates Dan's vocalizations and adds to them as turn taking progresses.

- Dual sensory impairment: Aileen's classroom job is handing out napkins for snack time. Aileen's friend Sam walks with her and pauses next to each person's chair. Aileen then reaches into the napkin basket and takes one out. Sam guides her to the place on the table in front of the next peer. This interaction encourages turn taking during an interactive routine.

- Autism: Harris enters his classroom after recess. He walks to his schedule shelf and puts his baseball cap in the small bag to the right of the shelf (represents tasks that are completed), then locates the next box that is open and finds a cassette tape. This tape indicates that he and his classmates have free-choice time. He walks over to the music area, stops, and begins tapping the cassette. His friend Joe taps Harris's shoulder and asks him to move out of the way. Harris moves toward the area with the tapes and cassette players.

Interactive Influences of the Early Communicator, the Partner, and the Environment

A complete description of any person's AAC system needs to include information about the individual's skills and priorities, partner skills and priorities, and environmental opportunities and limitations. This is particularly important for early AAC users, whose multimodal communication strategies may emphasize partner-perceived communication strategies. It is equally important to profile the ways in which a child can communicate and the ways in which the child does not yet successfully communicate.

The tri-focus framework (Siegel-Causey & Bashinski, 1997) incorporates concepts from various disciplines that are referenced to the learner, the partner, and the environmental context in which communication occurs. Figure 2.1 displays the interactive nature of the components. This framework emphasizes that communication interactions are experienced mutually by partners and the early communicator and that both parties are affected reciprocally. Thus, the focus of intervention is broadened to enhance the communication skills of the early communicators and their partners. In addition, this intervention approach addresses the influence of the physical and social aspects of the environment on communication interactions. *Physical aspects* include the specific environments (e.g., home, school), contexts (e.g., art, math, recess), and context attributes (e.g., lighting, noise level, available materials) of the interaction. *Social aspects* of the environment include peers and adults being in close proximity to the individual, nearby activity level, and the type of interaction that the learner is given (Ault, Guy, Guess, Bashinski, & Roberts, 1995). Figure 2.2 displays considerations to help partners plan assessment areas and related interventions. The circle displays the three components of intervention:

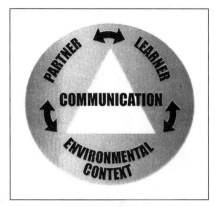

Figure 2.1. The tri-focus framework. (*Note:* Copyright © 1996 Ellin B. Siegel & Susan M. Bashinksi.)

1. *Partner*–broaden interaction style (use strategies that build early communication)
2. *Learner*–enhance partners' understanding of learner's communication (assessment)
3. *Environment*–improve contexts to promote learner's alert state behavior and to encourage communication (modify the physical and social environment)

The Use of Communicative Modes

There are many children who may not have developed conventional forms of communication (words, gestures). Thus, educators and clinicians need to be sensitive in both observing and responding to the unique signals that these early communicators display. The early communicator should be viewed as an active participant in communication exchanges; if carefully observed, he or she will be found to possess many communication behaviors and signals that can be further expanded and developed.

Early Forms of Communication   Any body movement or response can be a potential communicative signal if it is produced under circumstances that are interpretable to communicative partners. These movements may be conventional, idiosyncratic, or even unplanned. For instance, a child may signal interest in an activity by reaching towards the event (conventional), making tongue clicks (idiosyncratic), or changing muscle tone or breathing patterns (unplanned). Partners need to be sensitive to subtle and fewer movements in early communicators. For example, an individual's increased muscle tone might signal to his or her partner the need for a position change. Some forms of communication require specific action or the partner's responding to communicative signals. Conventional forms of aided AAC–

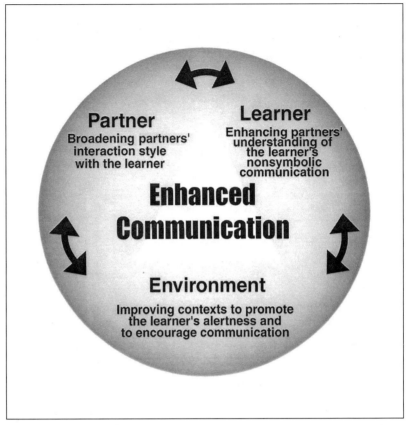

Figure 2.2. Considerations to help partners plan assessment areas and related interventions. (*Note:* Copyright © 2001 Ellin B. Siegel.)

including graphic symbols, gestures and signs, and VOCAs–can be incorporated as models for linguistic behaviors.

Partner Use of a Communicative Signal Inventory   As early communicators may use unique forms to produce communication, it is important to monitor their communicative signals and to respond consistently across situations. A number of terms describe methods to define elements of an existing communication repertoire–including a communicative signal inventory (e.g., Communication Signal Inventory [CSI], Blackstone, 1991), a gesture dictionary (Beukelman & Mirenda, 1998), or communication dictionary (Siegel & Wetherby, 2000)–all of which help partners recognize communication and respond consistently. Such strategies list what the user communicates, how the family and staff interpret each signal, and how a partner should react when that signal occurs. The communicator may not necessarily produce the signals intentionally, but they are recognized as being meaningful in the environment. Some signals, such as a look or a vocalization, may have alternative interpretations depending on context, and these differences should be reflected in the communication signal inventory. An example of a communicative signal inventory is included in Figure 2.3.

Whether one uses a communicative signal inventory or other strategy, the order of entries should allow partners to easily find a signal and interpret it appropriately. Communicative signals may be grouped on the inventory by communicative function (e.g., rejecting, requesting) or communicative form (e.g., movement of head, trunk, or hand) to make it easier for partners to quickly interpret the individual's behaviors. It is important for all communication partners to have easy access to these lists (e.g., in the form of posters, notebooks, or wallets) and add items to document new signals or new functions accomplished by existing signals. Because different signals may be observed in different contexts, it is important that all partners share their observations and agree on the types of alterations to make to the current signals.

The Use of Communicative Functions

Recognizing an early communicator's expressions is the starting point for effective communication interactions. Successful interactions with an early communicator require the partner to interpret or assign meaning to the message (signal) and then respond in a manner that presumes communication has occurred (communicative function).

Inventories of Communicative Behaviors and Functions   Wetherby and Prizant (1992) noted three primary early communicative functions: 1) behavior regulation (getting others to do or stop doing something), 2) social interaction (drawing attention to oneself or to social routines), and 3) joint attention (drawing others' attention to objects or events, commenting, or requesting information). Most early communication can be classified into these three groups based on the outcome that the communicator is presumed to want. Each of these functions can be expressed by a variety of communicative forms, and a given communicative form may be used to express more than one function. For instance, giving an object to a partner may express behavior regulation (e.g., "Make it go") or joint attention (e.g., "Look at this!").

Figure 2.4 provides a checklist to assess the communicative forms that a child may use to express different communicative functions. This checklist of communicative functions and nonsymbolic forms can be used as an ongoing record of the different forms that an individual uses to express communicative functions, and it can be routinely updated. The checklist describes the current level of communication, a tool for tracking progress, and a basis for planning possible intervention targets to expand the number or frequency of

Communication Signal Inventory

Child's name: _____ Date: _____

Signal What the communicator does	What it means What the partner thinks the signal means	What do you do/say? How the partners should consistently react

Figure 2.3. Communication signal inventory.

communicative forms and functions. A space is provided to list specific signals from the inventory that reflect unique communicative forms. It is important to include challenging behaviors in the assessment of communicative signals, as considerable research suggests that many challenging behaviors serve communicative functions for children with disabilities (Carr & Durand, 1985; Carr et al., 1994; Reichle & Wacker, 1993; see also Chapter 4). Communicative functions of challenging behaviors that correspond to the checklist's function categories include requesting, rejecting, gaining a desired item, escaping or avoiding situations (behavior regulation), commenting (joint attention), or obtaining attention (social interaction) (Brady & Halle, 1997; Carr et al., 1994; Durand & Crimmins, 1992; O'Neill et al., 1997; see also Chapter 4).

Intentionality of Communicative Functions   Not all signals in an individual's inventory that partners perceive as meaningful are produced intentionally. Consequently, it is important to examine observable characteristics that are typically associated with intentional communication. The more characteristics of intentionality observed (e.g., directing a signal toward the listener, watching expectantly in anticipation of a partner response), the more likely it is that the individual is intentionally communicating. It is important to distinguish between intentional behaviors, by which a person directly affects an object or event, and intentional communication, by which a person directs signals about an object or an event to a listener (Wetherby & Prizant, 1992).

Intentionality tends to emerge along with increasing ability to manage attention among the triad of speaker, listener, and object/event (Bakeman & Adamson, 1984). Gradually, communicators may display some of the behaviors associated with intentionality. For instance, a communicator may produce few intentional behaviors in object-based interactions but clearly direct vocalizations to a listener and anticipate responses in social situations. Recognizing the production of intentional communication does not necessarily imply that listeners can also determine the function of the communicator's specific intended message, as communicators may at times accept an alternative function if listeners misinterpret their intent. For example, a child gesturing for a glass of milk accepts a cookie that the listener offers. In this case, the listener correctly determined the intentionality of the child's behavior but incorrectly interpreted the precise message. A number of investigators (Bates, 1979; Bruner, 1978; Harding & Golinkoff, 1979; Wetherby & Prizant, 1992; Wilcox et al., 1995) have suggested that intentionality of communicative behavior can be inferred from a combination of the following criteria:

1. Directing a signal toward a listener through gaze, gesture, or other behaviors, deliberately soliciting partner attention
2. Alternating gaze between the goal and the listener
3. Conveying a particular goal or message, although not necessarily symbolically represented

Checklist of Communicative Functions and Nonsymbolic Forms

Child's name: _____ Date: _____ Setting: _____

Context: _____ Observer: _____

Communicative functions	Generalized movements or tone changes	Facial expressions	Orientation	Touching or manipulating objects	Acting on objects or using objects	Pause	Assuming positions or mobility	Conventional gestures	Depictive actions	Aggressive or self-injurious behavior	Withdrawal	Other: ___	Other: ___	Other: ___	Other: ___
Behavior regulation															
Request object/action															
Protect object/action															
Social interaction															
Request social routine															
Request comfort															
Greet															
Call															
Showing off															
Request permission															
Joint attention															
Comment on object/action															
Request information															
Other functions															

Figure 2.4. Checklist of communicative functions and nonsymbolic forms. (From Siegel, E., & Wetherby, A. [2000]. Nonsymbolic communication. In M. Snell & F. Brown [Eds.], *Instruction of students with severe disabilities* [5th ed., p. 426]. Upper Saddle River, NJ: Prentice Hall; reprinted by permission.)

40

4. Persistent signaling until the goal is accomplished or failure is indicated
5. Changing the signal quality until the goal has been met
6. Ritualizing or conventionalizing the signal form within specific communicative contexts
7. Awaiting a response from the listener
8. Terminating the signal when the goal is met
9. Showing satisfaction when a goal is attained or dissatisfaction when it is not

As individuals convey more intentional communication acts and recognize their impact on listeners, they must also develop skills at monitoring and evaluating the success of their communicative acts. When intentional communicators recognize that a communicative act has not resulted in a desired response, they must develop strategies for recognizing and repairing those communication breakdowns.

Competence with Communicative Functions and Communicative Breakdowns Communicative breakdowns occur when the individual initiates a communicative behavior and the listener fails to respond or responds in a manner that does not match the individual's intention. Skill at repairing breakdowns contribute to an early communicator's perceived communicative competence (Kublin, Wetherby, Crais, & Prizant, 1998; Prizant & Wetherby, 1990).

An approximate progression of skills for resolving communication breakdowns includes the following: 1) no response to the breakdown, 2) repeating the same signal that preceded the breakdown, and 3) modifying the original signal. Modifying a signal in response to a breakdown tends to increase successful social interaction by promoting reciprocity and supplying additional information for the listener to interpret (see Chapter 10 for an extensive discussion of communicative repair strategies). Frequent communication breakdowns may increase the probability that a challenging behavior may be used as a repair strategy. If individuals can successfully use conventional behaviors to resolve breakdowns, challenging behaviors tend to decrease (e.g., Mirenda, 1997; O'Neill & Reichle, 1993).

Challenging Behaviors and Functions of Communication   Numerous authors have emphasized that challenging behaviors should be considered communicative forms of behavior and responded to as a means of conveying communicative information (Carr et al., 1994; Mirenda, 1997; O'Neill et al., 1997; Reichle & Wacker, 1993; Siegel-Causey & Bashinski, 1997). A wide range of challenging behaviors may be viewed as being inappropriate for the interactive context, including patterns of stereotypy, agitation, aggression, or self-injurious behavior. Challenging behaviors as well as appropriate behaviors should be included on a communicative signal inventory or other format describing the child's communication, the assumed meaning, and the actions that one should take to respond consistently. A clear description of the form and function of a challenging behavior is essential to understanding contextual variables that influence an individual's behavior (see Carr et al., 1994; O'Neill, Vaughn, & Dunlap, 1998; Reichle & Wacker, 1993). Chapter 4 provides an extensive discussion of functional assessment and intervention strategies that are designed to replace challenging behaviors with socially accepted communicative alternatives.

Social Influences of Partners

The tri-focus framework, a primary basis for this chapter, emphasizes the premise that communication interactions are experienced mutually by the early communicator and his or her partner and that *both* are reciprocally affected. Therefore, communication assessment and intervention should focus on enhancing skills of the early communicator *and* understanding the influence of those skills on his or her partner. Determining the early communicator's preferences is important. Given the key role of the partners in assigning meaning and interpreting signals, it is essential that preference assessment also includes assessment of the partner's influences on the early communicator's skills (e.g., how long the partner waits for a response or all-verbal input might affect whether the communicator can process the input and relay preferences).

Determining the Preferences of Early Communicators and Their Partners   For all individuals who require AAC interventions, particularly for early communicators, it is important to establish and reinforce communication behaviors that reflect the individual's own preferences and interests. One of the primary intervention strategies for partner-perceived communicators is finding activities or situations that routinely elicit communicative signals that indicate preference. Most preference assessments for partner-perceived communicators involve caregiver interviews, environmental observations, and systematic offering of possible activities to observe the responses elicited (Lohrmann-O'Rourke & Browder, 1998). Several types of preference assessment strategies or inventories are available for people who already have intentional behavior signals (Dattilo, 1986; Houghton, Bronicki, & Guess, 1987; Mason & Egel, 1995; Wacker, Berg, Wiggins, Muldoon, & Cavanaugh, 1985).

Family members and partners also express preferences for their role in interactions with early AAC communicators (Calculator, 1997). In some cases, family members may express preferences for interacting in particular communicative modes (e.g., speech, VOCA) or environments (e.g., home, school). For a more detailed discussion of communicator preferences, see Chapter 5.

To have a clear understanding of how the person's signals may convey current preferences, it is important to use a variety of assessment techniques routinely (see Chapter 5). Early communicators rely on their partners to facilitate their interactions; thus, the assessment process should include discovering the partner's influences on the early communicator. Because communication is a transactional process in which the speaker and listener influence each other's behavior by their responses, any discussion of an individual's communication skills must also involve the skills of communication partners. Partners can influence the success of a child's interactions not only by their behavior during the interaction but also by the expectations and social support they bring to that interaction.

Opportunities Provided by Partners to Increase Participation   Enhancing an individual's communication means should coincide with providing opportunities to interact and respond to meaningful activities. Children who do not speak frequently have limited opportunities to express themselves; therefore, a "full participation" model has been advocated. Removing opportunity barriers increases an early communicator's participation and independence and, ultimately, his or her effective communication. As Beukelman and Mirenda noted, "Without participation, there is no one to talk to, nothing to talk about, and no reason to communicate" (1998, p. 269).

For early communicators, using many of their communication strategies relies on the opportunities presented by partners. For instance, children who use eye gaze or other partner-perceived communication modes require presentation of visible or auditory choices to which they can respond in order to communicate. Augmenting the input that the early communicator receives may enhance his or her comprehension (Wood, Lasker, Siegel-Causey, Beukelman, & Ball, 1998). This may include a range of strategies that minimize the physical and cognitive load on the communicator but depend on communicative options that are presented by the partner. For example, augmenting the message involves the partner's enhancing the meaning and salience of messages by elaborating on the primary message form with objects, pictures, gestures, and/or other forms of communication. The partner typically uses communicative strategies that are available to the early communicator to demonstrate functional alternatives for accomplishing a communicative goal or expanding an individual's communicative repertoire.

Key factors that determine the degree of social support that the partner provides are familiarity and responsiveness to the communicator. Familiar partners often recognize communicative signals and patterns of expected responses because they are "in tune" with the communicator's behaviors. If a partner's behavior is anticipated and familiar, the early communicator may insert communicative behaviors into the interaction. For instance, if the partner usually touches the communicator's shoulder before lifting him or her out of a chair, the communicator can display a number of signals (e.g., posture change, facial expression, gestures) that can be interpreted as an initiation or a request to be lifted out of the chair. Partners may interrupt a familiar activity to provide opportunities for signaling, as in interrupted behavior chains

(Goetz, Gee, & Sailor, 1985). Similarly, partner cues can provide support for behaviors that function as responses. For instance, many individuals' early signals for MORE depend on the partner's first presenting an activity, to which the individual signals acceptance or rejection with facial expressions or signal behaviors (Beukelman & Mirenda, 1998).

Interaction Styles of Communication Partners   Guidelines for communicating with people who are early intentional communicators include 1) waiting for the early communicator to initiate communication by pausing and looking expectantly, 2) recognizing the early communicator's behavior as communication by interpreting the communicative function that it serves, and 3) responding to the early communicator's behavior in a manner that is consistent with the individual's communicative intent and communicative level (MacDonald, 1989; MacDonald & Carroll, 1992). Many AAC strategies describe specific roles for the partner to actively promote the individual's signals as a natural part of the interaction. For instance, Jacob and his mother, Arlene, are playing with a ball. In order to promote Jacob's successful eye pointing, Arlene must wait for Jacob's attention to be directed towards an aspect of their activity (e.g., Arlene, the ball), verbally interpret the direction of his eye gaze and respond to Jacob's apparent intent to have the ball rolled toward him. Variations in Arlene's and Jacob's communication styles, including how quickly and actively they influence each others' behaviors, will influence the success of their interactions.

Considerable research has suggested that a partner who uses speech tends to have more turns in an interaction than a partner who relies on AAC (e.g., Light, 1988). This effect is probably related to the disproportionately long time that is required to communicate through most AAC modalities, even for skilled communicators, compared with verbal communication. For early communicators who rely on behavioral strategies, evidence suggests that other familiar partners also tend to take a dominant role in the interaction. For instance, parents of young children with Down syndrome (e.g., Crawley & Spiker, 1983) or physical impairments (Hanzlik & Stevenson, 1986; Wasserman & Allen, 1990) tend to be more directive and take more communicative turns than parents of developmental peers. Nevertheless, these results are complicated by the nature of early AAC communication, in which much of recognized communication is either situationally or directly prompted by the listener. In free play that is spontaneously initiated by parents of young children who rely on AAC, the children apparently anticipated their communicative role and required no more parent directiveness to be successful than typically developing children (Cress, Moskal, & Benal, 1999). Cress and colleagues found that parents of children with cerebral palsy were no more directive than parents of typically developing children if they were allowed to freely construct social or object play interactions, and they were significantly less directive than parents of children with physical impairments who were prompted to use object play (Hanzlik, 1990).

When partners maintain a responsive environment and increase communication opportunities, partner-perceived communicators are more likely to discover that their behaviors can control others and that they can initiate communication (Yoder & Warren, 1998). For more intentional communicators, structured programs can provide additional information on simple interaction strategies for promoting participatory interaction (e.g., Girolametto, Greenberg, & Manolson, 1986; Tannock, Girolametto, & Siegel, 1992).

Clinical implications of these research results provide additional factors to consider for promoting successful early AAC:

- Partners may vary in their ability to recognize early communication behaviors
- Individuals who rely on early AAC may need more time to respond or initiate communication
- Partners may be directive in prompting an individual's communication signals but are most effective if their prompts match and are responsive to the individual's signals

Interaction Between Behavior State and Environmental Influences on the Early Communicator

An early communicator's alertness and responsiveness (behavior state) can significantly influence patterns of learning and development and overall quality of life (e.g., Guess, Roberts, Siegel-Causey, & Rues, 1995). Behavior state observations may include assessment of an individual's sleep, drowsiness, behavior while awake (e.g., orienting, interacting), agitation, and stereotypic behavior. High incidence of drowsiness, sleep, or stereotypic behaviors, as well as low incidence of overt responsiveness, can limit an individual's response repertoire within communicative interactions. Guess and colleagues (1990) found that people with severe disabilities spent less time in alert responsive states (alert 58% of the time) than typically developing children at the preschool through secondary levels (alert 75% or more of the time). Other behavior state risk factors included low rates of overt responses and limited response repertoires.

Ault and colleagues (1995) and Guess, Roberts, and Guy (1999) applied an assessment strategy, the ABLE (Analyzing Behavior State and Learning Environments) Model, to document students' alertness patterns throughout the day. One premise for these assessments is that behavior state is a function of multiple aspects of the environment and not a specifically learned response. Factors that have been found to influence alertness include an individual's social contact, static body position, activity type, access to materials, and activity level in the immediate environment (Ault et al., 1995; Guess et al., 1990). Positioning and access to materials had the most effect on behavior state (alertness) and, given their influence on interaction, need to be considered in assessing a child's communication skills.

Positioning and Access to Materials   Communicative behaviors can be affected significantly by an individual's positioning and access to materials. Poor seating posture can limit an individual's control of the hand or head position that is involved in initiating communicative behaviors and/or deciphering a partner's communicative acts. Positions that require significant energy expenditure to stay upright or stabilize body position may result in the communicator's allocating inadequate cognitive and physical resources to communicating. Providing adapted materials or seating supports can decrease these interferences. Factors that have been shown to enhance communicative interactions (Ault et al., 1995) include the extent to which the individual is supported in a stable position that promotes interaction, the individual's interest in the referent activity (i.e., novelty), and the accessibility of materials. Of course, a variety of environmental factors can influence an individual's ability to attend to the relevant activity or interaction (e.g., noise, competing activities). Although addressing some variables may be challenging, interventionists can incorporate a variety of environmental changes that are likely to influence the individual's level of alertness.

INTERPRETATION OF COMMUNICATIVE BEHAVIORS

Interpretation of communicative behaviors demonstrates to learners that they can affect people and events and can gradually initiate, maintain, and terminate communication exchanges. Early intervention for individuals who may not produce intentional communicative acts focuses on partners noticing the expressions of learners.

A communication dictionary or inventory helps communication partners consistently respond to idiosyncratic gestures. An inventory provides communicative partners with a uniform means to list and describe the learner's nonsymbolic and symbolic behavior for familiar and unfamiliar partners. By using the inventory, partners can develop consistent responses that more clearly connect idiosyncratic signals to the communicative outcome. Figure 2.5 presents a completed communicative signal inventory, which can be used both to assess a communicator's present skills and to document changes in partner responses and individual behaviors over time. Using this instrument, a partner can examine a particular routine or activity and determine if changing responses to a particular signal might improve the communicator's consistent use of this signal.

Communication Signal Inventory

Child's name: _Maria_   Date: _April 24, 2001_

Signal What the communicator does	What it means What the partner thinks the signal means	What do you do/say? How the partners should consistently react
Vocalizes /ah/	I want attention. I need help.	Figure out what she means and respond accordingly with an action.
Wrinkles forehead or tries to spit out food	I don't like this food. (If I'm very agitated, I tense my whole body.)	Change the food if possible, model a "no" facial expression, and touch her face.
Watches intently	I am interested in this activity. I want _____ (action/object at hand).	Tell her you're watching her eyes, and give her more of the activity or access to the action/object.
Moves hand toward an object (e.g., switch)	I want to touch this. I want more.	Respond by touching her hand, saying "You want more," and continuing the activity.
Vocalizes a loud extended /ah/ while turning her body	I am getting ready to use my hand. This takes hard work.	Wait for her to get moving, give her feedback ("I see your hand moving"), and look expectantly toward her so she knows that you will wait for her.
Bats away partner or claws with arms; may make a fussy vocalization	I am angry. (I am more angry if I increase my arm lift.)	Help her calm down, and resolve the situation.
Vocalizes a soft /ne/ and/or whines	I am tired. I am going to cry soon.	Model a sad facial expression and touch her face. Change the situation or give her a break if possible.

Figure 2.5. Example of a completed communication signal inventory.

47

One powerful communication intervention strategy is for the partner to enhance his or her response to communicative signals. Particular qualities for doing so include heightening sensitivity to the communicator's behavioral acts. An increase in partner sensitivity will likely ensure a contingent reaction to a behavioral overture (a contextually related and timely response to potentially communicative behavior). Finally, it is important that contingent responses be situationally consistent, responding to the same behavior in the same ways over time (Wilcox et al., 1995). Other ways that partners can adapt their behaviors to enhance communication include recognizing levels of alertness and increasing communication opportunities by adapting the activities and materials that are available in the environment (Siegel & Wetherby, 2000).

Role of Dynamic Assessment in Establishing an Initial Communicative Repertoire

Most assessments rely on static measurements of an individual's present demonstration of skills. These only reflect an individual's independent performance at a particular time. In dynamic assessment, however, an individual's independent skills are compared with the skills that he or she demonstrates with partner support. The support is then systematically decreased to the minimal threshold of success. Systematic sampling of what an individual can perform with support provides a zone of proximal development, which highlights skills that an individual will likely perform independently with experience. (Vygotsky, 1986). Sampling skills with dynamic assessment also provides information about a person's rate of learning, which can help with decisions such as how quickly to introduce new communicative forms or new tasks that use previously established communicative behavior. AAC assessment commonly uses a dynamic perspective, in which multiple modes and contexts of communication are sampled. Across opportunities, supports are modified until the communicator is successful. Next, intervention plans from these assessments focus on strategies for systematically reducing necessary support and increasing independence. Continued information gathering from dynamic assessment is also useful to monitor ongoing intervention.

IMPLICATIONS FOR EARLY AAC INTERVENTION

Siegel-Causey and Guess (1989) and Siegel-Causey and Bashinski (1997) outlined general guidelines that can influence an individual's early communication expression. These have been revised to include the following: increase opportunities, sequence routines, enhance sensitivity, augment input, and modify the environment. The guidelines are not sequential but, instead, are equally relevant during any individual communicative interaction. When the intervention team, including the communicator's family, uses these guidelines, it may recognize a wide range of targets for instruction and develop additional targets for generalizing to other typically occurring activities. It is essential to prioritize the communicative targets that are most functional across people, events, and environments. Figure 2.6 provides a graphic representation: The outer, shaded circle contains these communication guidelines; the inner, white circle contains elements of best practice that should be included in any intervention for early communicators (Snell & Brown, 2000).

Communication intervention is best viewed as a reciprocal process between a partner and a communicator. The strategies to enhance the communicator's expression should include augmenting the partner's instruction and

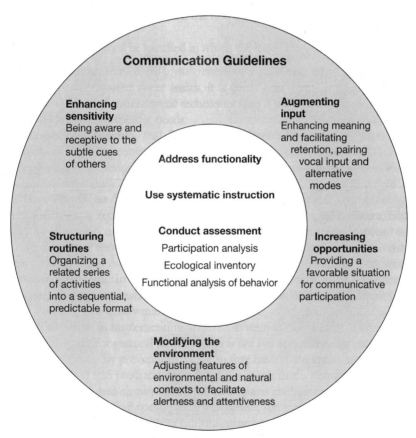

Figure 2.6. Guidelines to prioritize the communicative targets that are most functional across people, events, and environments. (*Note:* Copyright © 2001 Ellin B. Siegel.)

strengthening the communicator's communication repertoire. The most pertinent interventions account for the influences of both partners rather than assume that either partner has deficits to remediate. The previously outlined behavior description procedures provide a basis for understanding the behaviors of all communication partners and, thus, specifically guide aspects of the early AAC process. For more information on detailed early augmented behavior intervention strategies, see Chapter 8.

MATCHING INSTRUCTIONAL
STRATEGIES TO EARLY COMMUNICATION SKILLS

To be most effective, communication intervention should occur within the routines of natural home, school, or community environments so that individuals not only communicate more but also recognize that their communication can serve many purposes. Communication intervention strategies do not apply equally well to all individuals at all developmental ages. For instance, Warren and Yoder (1997) discussed matching early communication intervention strategies to different developmental theories that account for children's communicative behaviors. A responsive communication style has been demonstrated to improve communication for early communicators who do not yet demonstrate intentional communication (Yoder & Warren, 1999; Yoder et al., 1998). Individuals who initiate communicative acts can benefit from milieu and other prompted communication intervention strategies (e.g., Kaiser, Yoder, & Keetz, 1992).

Marvin (1996) presented strategies for matching intervention to children's observable communicative behaviors. Table 2.4 is an expansion of these strategies. The far-left column describes communicative characteristics of children (whose language ranges from typically developing to delayed) that correspond to intervention approaches. The next column associates these vocal expressive characteristics with developmental characteristics of early communicators. The third column describes common early intervention strategies, and the last column highlights additional AAC approaches. For early communicators who are infrequent initiators without symbolic skills, the adult primarily has the responsibility of managing the communication exchange through partner-perceived communication. Several researchers (e.g., Wilcox et al., 1995; Yoder & Warren, 1999) confirmed that parent responsivity is the best justified intervention strategy for children who do not yet demonstrate intentional communication. Types of AAC approaches that reflect an interactional focus include joint play, prompt-free strategies (Mirenda & Santogrossi, 1985), and expanded communication signal inventories. As children demonstrate some intentional communication but limited symbolic skills (mean length of utterance [MLU] of 1.0 to 1.5), interventionists might use prelinguistic

Table 2.4. Matching early intervention and AAC approaches to early communicator skills

Child's communicative characteristics	Early communicator skills	Early intervention approach	Additional AAC approaches
Nonsymbolic Infrequent initiator Not intentional	Partner-perceived communicators	RESPONSIVE Follow child's lead Mirror self-talk Use joint action routines	Communicative signal inventory Joint play Prompt-free strategies
Infrequent talker Infrequent initiator MLU = 1.0 to 1.5	Intentional communicator Limited range of one-concept signals Might not use formal symbols	MILIEU Expect child to take turns Use routine scripts Provide incidental teaching (e.g., mand-model, time delay)	Enhanced routines Communication temptations Choice making
Frequent talker Receptive language age > 2.5 years MLU = 1.6 to 3.0+	Symbolic communicators Can fast-map new gestures and symbols Uses signals for multiple purposes Combines two+ symbols/gestures	LANGUAGE IMMERSION Child not expected to take a turn or produce a symbol immediately Use modeling, expansion, and elaboration	Aided Language Stimulation Engineering the environment for communication Augmented input Topic-based and multifunction communication boards
High initiator Higher cognitive skills Articulation/grammar problems MLU > 3.6+	Independent communicator Uses memory or level-based systems Creatively constructs intended messages	DIDACTIC Provide one-to-one or group training Structure teacher-directed instruction Provide opportunities for social interaction within instruction	Procedural competence with strategies and/or devices Memory or message construction practice Communicator's modification of or influence on the content or organization of own system Frequent modification of system to meet situational demands

From Marvin, C. (1996). *Communication intervention strategies* (p. 1). Unpublished manuscript, University of Nebraska–Lincoln; adapted by permission.
MLU = mean length of utterance.

milieu strategies as well as AAC-specific strategies such as enhanced routines, communicative temptations, and choice making. As children become more frequent and symbolic communicators, they are better able to benefit from language-rich or broadly stimulating strategies as a primary intervention strategy, such as Aided Language Stimulation or Augmented Input, including programs such as the System for Augmenting Language (SAL; Romski & Sevcik, 1996; see also Chapter 14). Only when children are both symbolic and frequent initiators is a strictly didactic approach for teaching specific language skills likely to be a successful primary strategy.

CONCLUSION

Many children and youth with disabilities are early communicators. This chapter has presented a developmental framework to guide interventionists to focus on what an individual is communicating. We have provided a broadened view of AAC strategies to help enhance the intervention that team members provide for early communicators. Using the tri-focus framework expands the emphasis of intervention beyond the individual with disabilities to encompass the communication partner and the environment. It is our hope that the reader has gained a better understanding of early communication, can use this understanding to anticipate future levels of communication development, and can modify AAC interventions to produce results for early communicators. It is our belief that this broader view of early AAC will move early communicators toward symbolic communication. We are reminded of a young boy's mother who talked to one of this chapter's authors after attending a workshop presentation on nonsymbolic communication. The mother said, "I realized my son is not talking, but now I see how much he is communicating. I wonder if anyone is listening?"

REFERENCES

American Speech-Language-Hearing Association (ASHA). (1991). Report: Augmentative and alternative communication. *Asha, 33*(Suppl. 5), 9–12.

Ault, M.M., Guy, B., Guess, D., Bashinski, S., & Roberts, S. (1995). Analyzing behavior state and learning environments: Application in instructional settings. *Mental Retardation, 33,* 304–316.

Bakeman, R., & Adamson, L.B. (1984). Coordinating attention to people and objects in mother–infant and peer–infant interaction. *Child Development, 55,* 1279–1289.

Bates, E. (1979). *The emergence of symbols: Cognition and communication in infancy.* San Diego: Academic Press.

Beukelman, D.R., & Mirenda, P. (1998). *Augmentative and alternative communication: Management of severe communication disorders in children and adults* (2nd ed.). Baltimore: Paul H. Brookes Publishing Co.

Blackstone, S. (1991). Intervention framework. In *Technology in the classroom: Communication module* (pp. 37, J-1, J-2). Rockville, MD: American Speech-Language-Hearing Association Publications.

Brady, N.C., & Halle, J.W. (1997). Functional analysis of communicative behaviors. *Focus on Autism and Other Developmental Disabilities, 12*(2), 95–104.

Bruner, J. (1978). From communication to language: A psychological perspective. In I. Markova (Ed.), *The social context of language* (pp. 17–48). New York: John Wiley & Sons.

Calculator, S.N. (1997). Fostering early language acquisition and AAC use: Exploring reciprocal influences between children and their environments. *Augmentative and Alternative Communication, 13,* 149–157.

Carr, E.G., & Durand, V.M. (1985). Reducing behavior problems through functional communication training. *Journal of Applied Behavior Analysis, 18,* 111–126.

Carr, E.G., Levin, L., McConnachie, G., Carlson, J.I., Kemp, D.C., & Smith, C.E. (1994). *Communication-based intervention for problem behavior: A user's guide for producing positive change.* Baltimore: Paul H. Brookes Publishing Co.

Chapman, R.S., & Miller, J.F. (1980). Analyzing language and communication in the child. In R.L. Schiefelbusch (Ed.), *Nonspeech language and communication* (pp. 159–196). Baltimore: University Park Press.

Crawley, S.B., & Spiker, D. (1983). Mother–child interactions involving two-year-olds with Down syndrome: A look at individual differences. *Child Development, 54,* 1312–1323.

Cress, C., Havelka, S., Dietrich, C., & Linke, M. (1998, August). *Augmentative communication skill development checklist: Case examples for young children.* Paper presented at the International Society for Augmentative and Alternative Communication (ISAAC) International Conference, Dublin, Ireland.

Cress, C., Shapley, K., Linke, M., Havelka, S., Dietrich, C., Elliott, J., & Clark, J. (2000, August). *Characteristics of intentional communication in young children with physical impairments.* Paper presented at ISAAC Conference, Washington, DC.

Cress, C.J., Moskal, L., & Benal, A. (1999). *Parent directiveness in social and object play with their children with physical impairments.* Manuscript submitted for publication.

Dattilo, J. (1986). Computerized assessment of preference for severely handicapped individuals. *Journal of Applied Behavior Analysis, 19,* 445–448.

Dawson, G., & Osterling, J. (1997). Early intervention in autism. In M.J. Guralnick (Ed.), *The effectiveness of early intervention* (pp. 307–326). Baltimore: Paul H. Brookes Publishing Co.

Dore, J. (1986). The development of conversation competence. In R. Schiefelbusch (Ed.), *Language competence: Assessment and intervention* (pp. 3–60). San Diego: College-Hill Press.

Durand, V.M., & Crimmins, D.B. (1992). *The Motivation Assessment Scale (MAS) administration guide.* Topeka, KS: Monaco.

Girolametto, L.E., Greenberg, J., & Manolson, H.A. (1986). Developing dialogue skills: The Hanen Early Language Parent Program. *Seminars in Speech and Language, 7,* 367–382.

Goetz, L., Gee, K., & Sailor, W. (1985). Using a behavior chain interruption strategy to teach communication skills to students with severe disabilities. *Journal of The Association for Persons with Severe Handicaps, 10,* 21–30.

Goetz, L., & Sailor, W. (1988). New directions: Communication development in persons with severe disabilities. *Topics in Language Disorders, 8*(4), 41–54.

Guess, D., Roberts, S., & Guy, B. (1999). Implications of behavior state for the assessment and education of students with profound disabilities. In A. Repp & R. Horner

(Eds.), *Functional analysis of problem behavior: From effective assessment to effective support* (pp. 338–394). Belmont, CA: Wadsworth Publishing Co.

Guess, D., Roberts, S., Siegel-Causey, E., & Rues, J. (1995). Replication and extended analysis of behavior state, environmental events, and related variables in profound disabilities. *American Journal on Mental Retardation, 100*(1), 36–51.

Guess, D., Siegel-Causey, E., Roberts, S., Rues, J., Thompson, B., & Siegel-Causey, D. (1990). Assessment and analysis of behavior state and related variables among students with profoundly handicapping conditions. *The Journal of The Association for Persons with Severe Handicaps, 15*(4), 211–230.

Guralnick, M.J. (Ed.). (1997). *The effectiveness of early intervention.* Baltimore: Paul H. Brookes Publishing Co.

Hanzlik, J.R. (1990). Nonverbal interaction patterns of mothers and their infants with cerebral palsy. *Education and Training in Mental Retardation, 25,* 333–343.

Hanzlik, J.R., & Stevenson, M.B. (1986). Interaction of mothers with their infants who are mentally retarded, retarded with cerebral palsy, or nonretarded. *American Journal of Mental Deficiency, 90*(5) 513–520.

Harding, C., & Golinkoff, R. (1979). The origins of intentional vocalizations in prelinguistic infants. *Child Development, 50,* 33–40.

Harris, S.R. (1997). The effectiveness of early intervention for children with cerebral palsy and related motor disabilities. In M.J. Guralnick (Ed.), *The effectiveness of early intervention* (pp. 327–347). Baltimore: Paul H. Brookes Publishing Co.

Houghton, J., Bronicki, G.J., & Guess, D. (1987). Opportunities to express preferences and make choices among students with severe disabilities in classroom settings. *Journal of American Speech and Hearing, 12,* 18–27.

Kaiser, A.P., Yoder, P.J., & Keetz, A. (1992). Evaluating milieu teaching. In S.F. Warren & J. Reichle (Series Eds. & Vol. Eds.), *Communication and language intervention series: Vol. 1. Causes and effects in communication and language intervention* (pp. 9–47). Baltimore: Paul H. Brookes Publishing Co.

Kangas, K.A., & Lloyd, L.L. (1988). Early cognitive skills as prerequisites to augmentative and alternative communication use: What are we waiting for? *Augmentative and Alternative Communication, 4,* 211–221.

Kublin, K.S., Wetherby, A.M., Crais, E.R., & Prizant, B.M. (1998). Using dynamic assessment within collaborative contexts. The transition from intentional to symbolic communication. In S.F. Warren & J. Reichle (Series Eds.) & A.M. Wetherby, S.F. Warren, & J. Reichle (Vol. Eds.), *Communication and language intervention series: Vol. 7. Transitions in prelinguistic communication* (pp. 285–312). Baltimore: Paul H. Brookes Publishing Co.

Light, J. (1988). Interaction involving individuals using augmentative and alternative communication systems: State of the art and future directions. *Augmentative and Alternative Communication, 4*(2) 66–82.

Lohrmann-O'Rourke, S., & Browder, D.M. (1998). Empirically based methods to assess the preferences of individuals with severe disabilities. *American Journal on Mental Retardation, 103*(2) 146–161.

MacDonald, J.D. (1989). *Becoming partners with children: From play to conversation.* Itasca, IL: Riverside Publishing Co.

MacDonald, J., & Carroll, J. (1992). Communicating with young children: An ecological model for clinicians, parents, and collaborative professionals. *American Journal of Speech-Language Pathology, 1,* 39–48.

Marvin, C. (1996). *Communication intervention strategies.* Unpublished manuscript, University of Nebraska–Lincoln.

Mason, S.A., & Egel, A.L. (1995). What does Amy like? Using a mini-reinforcer assessment to increase student participation in instructional activities. *Teaching Exceptional Children, 28,*(1), 42–45.

McDonald, E.T. (1980). Early identification and treatment of children at risk for speech development. In R.L. Schiefelbusch, *Nonspeech language and communication: Analysis and Intervention* (pp. 49–80). Baltimore: University Park Press.

McLean, J., & Snyder-McLean, S. (1987). Form and function of communicative behaviour among persons with severe developmental disabilities. *Australia and New Zealand Journal of Developmental Disabilities, 13*(2) 83–98.

McLean, L.K., & Cripe, J.W. (1997). The effectiveness of early intervention for children with communication disorders. In M.J. Guralnick (Ed.), *The effectiveness of early intervention* (pp. 349–428). Baltimore: Paul H. Brookes Publishing Co.

McLean, L.K., & McLean, J.E. (1993). Communication intervention for adults with severe mental retardation. *Topics in Language Disorders, 13*(3), 47–60.

Miles, B. (2000). Conversation: The essence of communication. In B. Miles & M. Riggio (Eds.), *Remarkable conversations* (pp. 54–62). Watertown, MA: Perkins School for the Blind.

Mirenda, P. (1997). Supporting individuals with challenging behavior through functional communication training and AAC: A research review. *Augmentative and Alternative Communication, 13,* 207–225.

Mirenda, P., Iacono, T., & Williams, R. (1990). Communication options for persons with severe and profound disabiltities: State of the art and future directions. *Journal of The Association for Persons with Severe Handicaps, 16,* 3–21.

Mirenda, P., & Santogrossi, J. (1985). A prompt-free strategy to teach pictorial communication system use. *Augmentative and Alternative Communication, 1*(4) 143–150.

National Joint Committee for the Communication Needs of Persons with Severe Disabilities. (1992). Guidelines for meeting the communication needs of persons with severe disabilities. *Asha, 34*(Suppl. 7), 1–8.

O'Neill, R., & Reichle, J. (1993). Addressing socially motivated challenging behaviors by establishing communicative alternatives: Basics of a general-case approach. In S.F. Warren & J. Reichle (Series Eds.) & J. Reichle & D.P. Wacker (Vol. Eds.), *Communcation and language intervention series: Vol. 3. Communicative alternatives to challenging behavior: Integrating functional assessment and intervention strategies* (pp. 205–235). Baltimore: Paul H. Brookes Publishing Co.

O'Neill, R., Vaughn, B.J., & Dunlap, G. (1998). Comprehensive behavioral support: Assessment issues and strategies. In S.F. Warren & J. Reichle (Series Eds.) & A.M. Wetherby, S.F. Warren, & J. Reichle (Vol. Eds.), *Communication and language intervention series: Vol. 7. Transitions in prelinguistic communication* (pp. 313–341). Baltimore: Paul H. Brookes Publishing Co.

O'Neill, R.E., Horner, R.H., Albin, R.W., Sprague, J.R., Storey, K., & Newton, J.S. (1997). *Functional assessment and program development for problem behavior: A practical handbook* (2nd ed.). Pacific Grove, CA: Brookes/Cole Thompson Learning.

Owens, R.E., Jr., & House, L.I. (1984). Decision-making processes in augmentative communication. *Journal of Speech and Hearing Disorders, 49,* 18–25.

Prizant, B., & Wetherby, A. (1990). Assessing the communication of infants and toddlers: Integrating a socioemotional perspective. *Zero to Three, 11,* 1–12.

Reichle, J., & Karlan, G. (1985). The selection of an augmentative system in communication intervention: A critique of decision rules. *Journal of The Association for Persons with Severe Handicaps, 10,* 146–156.

Reichle, J., & Wacker, D.P. (Vol. Eds.). (1993). *Communication and language intervention series: Vol. 3. Communicative alternatives to challenging behavior: Integrating functional assessment and intervention strategies.* Baltimore: Paul H. Brookes Publishing Co.

Romski, M.A., & Sevcik, R.A. (1996). *Breaking the speech barrier: Language development through augmented means.* Baltimore: Paul H. Brookes Publishing Co.

Siegel, E., & Wetherby, A. (2000). Nonsymbolic communication. In M. Snell & F. Brown (Eds.), *Instruction of students with severe disabilities* (5th ed., pp. 409–451). Upper Saddle River, NJ: Prentice Hall.

Siegel-Causey, E., & Bashinski, S. (1997). Enhancing initial communication and responsiveness of learners with multiple disabilities: A tri-focus framework for partners. *Focus on Autism and Other Developmental Disabilities, 12*(2), 105–120.

Siegel-Causey, E., & Guess, D. (1989). *Enhancing nonsymbolic communication interactions among learners with severe disabilities.* Baltimore: Paul H. Brookes Publishing Co.

Sigafoos, J., Woodyat, G., Keen, D., Tait, K., Tucker, M., Roberts-Pennell, D., & Pittendreigh, N. (2000). Identifying potential communicative acts in children with developmental and physical disabilities. *Communication Disorders Quarterly, 22*(2), 77–86.

Silverman, F.H. (1995). *Communication for the speechless* (3rd ed.). Needham Heights, MA: Allyn & Bacon.

Snell, M., & Brown, F. (Eds.). (2000). *Instruction of students with severe disabilities* (5th ed.). Upper Saddle River, NJ: Prentice Hall.

Spiker, D., & Hopmann, M.R., (1997). The effectiveness of early intervention for children with Down syndrome. In M.J. Guralnick (Ed.), *The effectiveness of early intervention* (pp. 271–305). Baltimore: Paul H. Brookes Publishing Co.

Tannock, R., Girolametto, L., & Siegel, L.S. (1992). Language intervention with children who have developmental delays: Effects of an interactive approach. *American Journal on Mental Retardation, 97,* 145–160.

Vygotsky, L. (1986). *Thought and language.* Cambridge, MA: The MIT Press.

Wacker, D.P., Berg, W.K., Wiggins, B., Muldoon, M., & Cavanaugh, J. (1985). Evaluation of reinforcer preferences for profoundly handicapped students. *Journal of Applied Behavior Analysis, 18,* 173–178.

Warren, S.F., & Yoder, P.J. (1997). Emerging model of communication and language intervention. *Mental Retardation and Developmental Disabilities Research, 3,* 358–362.

Wasserman, G.A., & Allen, R. (1990). Aspects of communicative development in physically handicapped toddlers. *Annals of the New York Academy of Sciences, 583,* 129–142.

Wetherby, A.M., & Prizant, B.M. (1992). Profiling young children's communicative competence. In S.F. Warren & J. Reichle (Series Eds. & Vol. Eds.), *Communication and language intervention series: Vol. 1. Causes and effects in language assessment and intervention* (pp. 217–253). Baltimore: Paul H. Brookes Publishing Co.

Wetherby, A.M., & Prizant, B. (1993). *Communication and Symbolic Behavior Scales (CSBS).* Baltimore: Paul H. Brookes Publishing Co.

Wilcox, M.J., Bacon, C.K., & Shannon, M.S. (1995, November). *Prelinguistic intervention: Procedures for young children with disabilities.* Paper presented at the ASHA Annual Convention, Orlando, FL.

Wood, L., Lasker, J., Siegel-Causey, E., Beukelman, D., & Ball, L. (1998). Using an augmented comprehension framework: Concepts and practices. *Augmentative and Alternative Communication, 14,* 261–267.

Yoder, P.J., & Warren, S.F. (1993). Can developmentally delayed children's language development be enhanced through prelinguistic intervention? In S.F. Warren & J. Reichle (Series Eds.) & A.P. Kaiser & D.B. Gray (Vol. Eds.), *Communication and language intervention series: Vol. 2. Enhancing children's communication: Research foundations for intervention* (pp. 35–61). Baltimore: Paul H. Brookes Publishing Co.

Yoder, P.J., & Warren, S.F. (1998). Maternal responsivity predicts the prelinguistic communication intervention that facilitates generalized intentional communication. *Journal of Speech, Language, and Hearing Research, 41,* 1207–1219.

Yoder, P.J., & Warren, S.F. (1999). Maternal responsivity mediates the relationship between prelinguistic intentional communication and later language. *Journal of Early Intervention, 22*(2), 126–136.

Yoder, P.J., Warren, S.F., McCathren, R., & Leew, S.V. (1998). Does adult responsivity to child behavior facilitate communication development? In S.F. Warren & J. Reichle (Series Eds.) & A.M. Wetherby, S.F. Warren, & J. Reichle (Vol. Eds.), *Communication and language intervention series: Vol. 7. Transitions in prelinguistic communication* (pp. 39–58). Baltimore: Paul H. Brookes Publishing Co.

3

The Importance of
Responsivity in Developing Contingent
Exchanges with Beginning Communicators

Kerri Harwood, Steven F. Warren, and Paul Yoder

The quantity and quality of linguistic input that typically developing children experience before their third birthday has a significant and lasting effect on language and communication development. Highly responsive adult input to preintentional child behaviors can help facilitate the child's transition to intentional communication. In addition, children who receive more frequent, responsive linguistic input from their parents are more likely to develop vocabulary at a faster rate than children who receive less frequent, more directive linguistic input (Yoder, Warren, McCathren, & Leew, 1998). The rate of early vocabulary growth predicts later cognitive and language performance on standardized tests (Hart & Risley, 1995).

Researchers and clinicians have proposed that individuals with severe communication disorders may be at risk for receiving less frequent exposure to the types of responsive linguistic input from communication partners that facilitate communication and language development (Blackstone, 1997). Many of these individuals display low rates of communication, even when an augmentative and alternative communication (AAC) system is available (Basil, 1992; Light, Collier, & Parnes, 1985). They are also more likely to communicate using behaviors that partners do not always recognize as being communicative (Houghton, Bronicki, & Guess, 1987; Rowland, 1990). Individuals who communicate infrequently or who rely on idiosyncratic behaviors to communicate may miss opportunities to receive the types of responsive input that best facilitate language development.

Many individuals who have severe communication disorders use AAC systems to communicate. An AAC user is someone with a severe communication disorder who uses nonsymbolic means (e.g., gestures, vocalizations) and/or symbolic means (e.g., objects, photographs, line drawings, manual signs, written words) to enhance communication (Beukelman & Mirenda, 1998). The AAC literature has long recognized the importance of teaching facilitators, or people who assume responsibility for supporting the AAC user's communicative attempts, to identify and respond to nonsymbolic and symbolic acts to teach functional communication skills or to support communicative competence in social interactions (Beukelman & Mirenda, 1998; Calculator & Luchko, 1983; Culp & Carlisle, 1988; Houghton et al., 1987; Light, Dattilo, English, Gutierrez, & Hartz, 1992; McNaughton & Light, 1989; Rowland, 1990; Rowland & Schweigert, 1993; Siegel-Causey & Guess, 1989). Yet, the influence of facilitator responsivity on particular aspects of language development that underlie functional communication skills or communicative competence has yet to be examined. In general, very little is known about the language development of AAC users, and there is not much guidance concerning how to design interventions that facilitate language development as well as functional communication (Beukelman & Mirenda, 1998).

Typically, interventions that target the acquisition of functional communication skills and communicative competence have included recommendations for a variety of facilitator strategies (see Light & Binger, 1998; Light et al., 1992; Light, McNaughton, & Parnes, 1994; McNaughton & Light, 1989; Reichle, York, & Sigafoos, 1991; Romski & Sevcik, 1996; Rowland & Schweigert, 1993; and Siegel-Causey & Guess, 1989, for examples). One subset of these strategies includes recommendations for responding to AAC users because their application is contingent on the AAC user's communicative and noncommunicative acts. Examples of recommended facilitator strategies that function as responses include 1) immediately fulfilling the intent communicated; 2) labeling the object, activity, or event to which the AAC user is attending; 3) simultaneously modeling the AAC user's expressive mode when providing verbal labels; 4) verbally confirming the AAC user's intended message; 5) asking for clarification of nonverbal communicative acts; 6) using open-ended questions to continue the AAC user's topic; and 7) following the AAC user's lead.

Although authors have indicated that this subset of responsive strategies was taken from the literature on the communication and language development of typically developing children, it is unclear how these different types of responsivity might affect the AAC user's communication and language development. Nor is it clear which specific aspects of language development are being affected. Knowing more about the relationship between different types of responsivity and the various aspects of language development that they affect might help interventionists fine-tune the delivery of their responses to better facilitate particular language and communication skills. As beginning communicators make the transition from using nonsymbolic forms (e.g., gestures, vocalizations) for intentional communication to using symbolic communication (e.g., graphic symbols, manual signs), some types of responses may become more important than others.

For example, learners who are just beginning to understand and use graphic symbols or manual signs to communicate may continue to rely on a limited number of familiar nonsymbolic communicative forms (e.g., focusing attention on an object, gesturing, pointing, vocalizing). To expand and strengthen their ability to comprehend and use symbolic forms, facilitator responses should 1) verbally label the beginning communicator's nonsymbolic communication attempts or even their focus of attention and 2) model the appropriate manual sign or graphic symbol selection. Verbal responses that label the child's focus of attention have been associated with the comprehension and production of labels for objects by both typically and atypically developing children (see Yoder et al., 1998, for a review of this research). In addition, there is evidence that both typically and atypically developing children acquire object labels more readily when adults verbally label the children's nonsymbolic communicative acts (Tomasello & Farrar, 1986; Yoder, Kaiser, Alpert, & Fischer, 1993). Alternatively, learners who can already communicate well through the production of single signs or the selection of single graphic symbols are more likely to benefit from facilitator responses, which expand or recast their message both verbally and physically. Verbal expansions and recasts are most clearly associated with the development of semantic relations in typically and atypically developing children (see Yoder et al., 1998, for a review of this research).

Clearly, facilitator responsivity is an important component of any intervention that targets the development of communication and language. This chapter has four goals. First, we define and classify the various types of adult responsivity and review the empirical support for its influence on communication and language development. Second, we describe ways to increase adult responsivity. Third, we discuss the relative importance of adult responsivity as a component of language and communication intervention for children with developmental disabilities who are expected to learn to speak. Finally, we consider the clinical implications of this research for providing optimal contingent exchanges for beginning communicators who use nonsymbolic and symbolic forms of AAC to communicate.

DEFINITION AND
CLASSIFICATION OF ADULT RESPONSIVITY

Any discussion of the facilitative effects of adult responsivity on language and communication development must eventually refer to the extensive literature on interactions between mothers and their young children (with and without disabilities) during the prelinguistic period. A review of this literature by Yoder and colleagues (1998) defined adult responses as those which occur immediately after the child's behavior and are semantically or topographically related to the child's behavior. Adult contingent responsivity has been further categorized into three classes or types: 1) nonlinguistic contingent responses, 2) linguistic contingent responses to the child's focus of attention, and 3) linguistic contingent responses to the child's communicative act. These three types of responsivity have been shown to influence later child communication and language development in different ways. Moreover, different types of listener responses are likely to be most effective when matched to a child's developmental level.

Nonlinguistic Contingent Responses

The first type of responsivity, *nonlinguistic contingent responses,* are listener responses that acknowledge the child's behavior but contain little linguistic information. Nonlinguistic contingent responses include any of the following adult behaviors:

- Simply complying with the presumed meaning of the child's communicative act
- Imitating the child's facial expression, play, and/or vocalizations
- Engaging in nonimitative vocal turn taking
- Engaging in nonimitative turn taking in play with a complementary action
- Verbally acknowledging a change in the child's focus of attention without adding linguistic information to the child's act (e.g., "Uh-huh")
- Soothing a distressed child

Theoretically, nonlinguistic responsivity has been conceptualized as facilitating the emergence of certain "mediating variables" that are empirically related to later communication and language development. These include contingency learning (learning that one's behavior has an effect on the world), secure attachment to the mother, exploratory behavior, and the mother and the infant's joint attentional focus on the same object (see Yoder et al., 1998, for further explanation of the relationship between each of these variables and language development). Empirical support for the generalized effects of nonlinguistic responsivity can be found in studies in which maternal levels of nonlinguistic responses to children's prelinguistic behaviors were measured and associated with later child outcomes, such as contingency learning, exploratory play, symbolic play, language comprehension, or intelligence. Because these outcomes were measured months later in testing or observation sessions at which the mother was not present, any increase suggests that the effects of maternal levels of nonlinguistic responsivity can generalize outside of highly responsive mother–child interactions. Higher levels of maternal nonlinguistic responsivity have predicted higher levels of contingency learning, exploratory play, symbolic play, language comprehension, or intelligence in typically developing children (Bornstein & Tamis-LeMonda, 1989; Riksen-Walraven, 1978; van den Boom, 1994). Although not all of the studies specified which particular types of nonlinguistic responsivity were used by the mothers, they suggest that the following were observed most frequently: complying with the presumed meaning of the child's communicative act; imitating the child's facial expression, play, and/or vocalizations; and nonimitative vocal turn taking.

Based on the evidence, Yoder and colleagues (1998) concluded that nonlinguistic contingent responsivity may be most important to children who are at a preintentional developmental stage (developmental ages birth to 9 months) because of its indirect influence on later communication. This type of responsivity may result in increased contingency learning, exploratory behavior, and more frequent preintentional and intentional communication with responsive partners. Learning that one's behavior has an effect on the world may be the first step in the development of intentional communication, because it motivates children to explore their environment in search of other environmental responses. Realizing that adults can produce desired effects might encourage children to begin directing their behaviors toward the listener (Golinkoff, 1983; White, 1959).

Linguistic Contingent Responses to the Child's Focus of Attention

The second type of responsivity, *linguistic contingent responses to the child's focus of attention,* includes comments and directives about the child's focus of attention. Theoretically, linguistic contingent responses to the child's focus of attention may provide the child with labels for those objects or actions to which he or she is already attending, thereby making the associations between labels and their referents more salient (MacDonald, 1989; Tomasello, 1988).

Harris's (1994) review of the literature found that maternal linguistic contingent responses to the child's focus of attention predicted later language scores in children who were typically developing (developmentally 14 months of age) and in children with Down syndrome (developmentally 16 months of age). Specifically, the number of times the mother labeled objects to which her child was attending was positively associated with the child's receptive and expressive language performance on language tests 13 months later. Maternal labeling of objects to which the child was not attending was not associated with language performance, underscoring the importance of joint attention.

Yoder and colleagues (1998) hypothesized that linguistic contingent responses to the child's focus of attention may be most important for children who are beginning to intentionally communicate (developmentally 9–10 months of age). During this period, children demonstrate intentionality and an understanding of words by showing and giving objects to adults. Talking about their focus of attention may provide the child with labels for objects and actions, playing an important role in receptive language development. Yet, the existing research, which supports a facilitative effect for linguistic contingent responses to the child's focus of attention on language development, has evaluated joint attention's effectiveness on developmentally older children who have already started speaking (developmentally 12–18 months of age). This research found that linguistic input in joint attentional focus is most likely to facilitate object name acquisition (Akhtar, Dunham, & Dunham, 1991; Harris, 1994; Tomasello & Farrar, 1986). The absence of studies that evaluate this type of responsivity with developmentally younger children makes it prudent to hypothesize that linguistic contingent responses to the child's focus of attention may facilitate object name vocabulary in a child who has begun to use symbols to communicate (Yoder et al., 1998).

Linguistic Contingent Responses to the Child's Communicative Act

The third type of responsivity, *linguistic contingent responses to the child's communicative act,* adds linguistic information to the child's nonverbal or verbal communicative acts. These responses include both adult linguistic mapping of nonverbal communicative acts and topic-continuing adult utterances that follow verbal communication, such as expansions and recasts. *Linguistic mapping* has been defined as verbally stating the core meaning of what the child is trying to communicate nonverbally (Warren, Yoder, Gazdag, Kim, & Jones, 1993). *Expansions* and *recasts* are adult topic-continuing utterances that repeat part of the child's utterance but add semantic and syntactic information (Nelson, 1989). Both types of linguistic contingent responses may facilitate vocabulary development because the temporal proximity and semantic overlap between the child's communication act and the adult's response allows the child to compare the two and note the novel information in the adult's utterance (Nelson, 1989; Yoder et al., 1998).

Support for the facilitative effects of linguistic contingent responsivity to child communicative acts comes from studies with both typically developing children and children with developmental disabilities. All of the children used speech as their primary mode of communication. Linguistic mapping is associated with the subsequent acquisition of vocabulary, particularly object labels, by children with and without disabilities who are in the prelinguistic period of language development (Masur, 1982; Tomasello & Farrar, 1986; Yoder et al., 1993). Developmentally, linguistic mapping is most important when children begin acquiring their first spoken words during a stage that usually begins at 12–13 months of age. Although the acquisition of these words indicates the child's ability to use symbols to communicate, it does not represent the acquisition of a fully linguistic system. This system is marked by the combination of two or more words, which signals the child's acquisition of grammar (Wetherby, Reichle, & Pierce, 1998; Wilcox & Shannon, 1998).

Once children are at least at the single word stage and have acquired about 50 different words (developmentally 16–22 months of age), recasts and expansions facilitate the development of semantic relations. The frequency of maternal recasts was positively related to individual differences in mean length of utterance (MLU) and other specific aspects of grammar in typically developing children (Farrar, 1990; Nelson, Denninger, Bonvillian, Kaplan, & Baker, 1984). In addition, when adults other than mothers use expansions in response to the single word utterances of children with developmental disabilities, there are subsequent increases in early multiword combinations (Scherer & Olswang, 1989; Yoder, Spruytenburg, Edwards, & Davies, 1995). Continuing the child's topic when responding may also be important. Harris (1994) found that maternal use of topic-continuing utterances was positively related to later receptive language scores in children with and without disabilities. This investigation also reported that maternal use of topic redirections was negatively related to later receptive language scores.

INCREASING RESPONSIVITY

There is evidence that adult responsivity can be increased in two ways. One way is to directly teach adults to respond to a greater number of child communicative acts with language-facilitating responses (Girolametto, 1988; Girolametto, Pearce, & Weitzman, 1996; Wilcox, 1992; Wilcox & Shannon, 1998). The other way is to increase the frequency and clarity with which children use intentional communication, which may indirectly cause a natural increase in facilitative adult responses. The latter represents an attempt to capitalize on the transactional effects of language development observed in parents and their children. Transactional effects involve a change in the child which triggers a change in the parent. This change, in turn, affects the child, and so on (Warren & Yoder, 1998).

Directly Increasing Responsivity

In the 1980s, several responsivity-training programs were developed to teach caregivers to use various strategies that facilitate children's language development (Giralometto, 1988; MacDonald, 1989; Manolson, 1985). These programs were known as *responsive interaction programs,* or programs that incorporated the interactive model of language intervention. The goal of responsive interaction programs was to increase the frequency of children's social interaction by enhancing the quality of interaction between the caregiver and the child. A distinguishing characteristic of these programs was that they avoided eliciting particular language targets through prompting. In addition to techniques that established joint attentional episodes and promoted balanced turn taking, these programs attempted to teach the caregiver to time his or her verbal input so that it corresponded precisely to the child's attentional focus. Finally, adult utterances were delivered in a manner that matched the child's developmental level. Using various types of contingent responsivity as verbal input was encouraged (Tannock & Girolametto, 1992).

There is some evidence that these programs had an immediate impact on caregiver responsivity. Reported increases in caregiver behaviors included following the child's lead, using the child's focus of attention when initiating an interaction, and using communication modes and content that match the child's developmental level. Equally encouraging was the evidence that these programs decreased the number of caregiver directives and turns taken. These variables were hypothesized to contribute to more balanced, responsive interactions. Nonetheless, although their effects on caregiver responsivity were noteworthy, there was no strong evidence that these programs helped children acquire new communication skills. Rather, they appeared to help them increase their use of existing skills (Tannock & Girolametto, 1992).

In an attempt to strengthen child outcomes, an updated version of responsive interaction emerged in the 1990s. This version, known as *focused stimulation,* trains caregivers to frequently model preselected language targets when following the child's attentional lead (Fey, 1986). The targeted language forms may be presented within caregiver models, expansions, or recasts. As in the older responsive interaction programs, direct elicitation of specific child responses is discouraged (Wilcox & Shannon, 1998). Focused stimulation programs have proven effective in teaching vocabulary to children with expressive language delays (Girolametto, Pearce, & Weitzman, 1995, 1996) and in facilitating both intentional communication and later word use in children with developmental delays (Wilcox, Shannon, & Bacon, 1992, 1996). Like their predecessors, these newer responsive interaction programs successfully train caregivers to increase their use of the responsive behaviors and focused input in response to child behavior.

Indirectly Increasing Adult Responsivity

It may also be possible to indirectly increase adult responsivity to communicative acts, which are nonsymbolic in form, by increasing the frequency and clarity of the child's intentional communication. There is evidence that linguistic mapping (the type of responsivity that is most facilitative of early vocabulary for children in the prelinguistic period) is triggered by the production of clear, frequent intentional communication that is nonsymbolic in form. It appears that both clarity and frequency of communication are necessary for this transactional effect to occur. Frequent intentional communication elicits more responses from adults, which helps children refine their communication acts (Wilcox, 1992; Yoder & Warren, 1999b). Mothers of children with and without developmental delays respond more often to clear intentional communicative acts in which coordinated attention is combined with gestures and/or vocalizations than to gestures and/or vocalizations without coordinated attention (Kim, 1996; Yoder & Munson, 1995; Yoder, Warren, Kim, & Gazdag, 1994).

Yoder and Warren's (1999a, 1999b) findings from a longitudinal correlational study of 58 children with disabilities and their mothers provides support for this relationship among frequency of child communicative acts, adult responsivity, and later language development. The children were between 17 and 32 months of age, with an average mental age of 15 months. All participants had normal vision and hearing, and none had any significant physical disabilities. All of the children showed evidence of intentional communication, as demonstrated by coordinated attention to a person and an object or vocalization with attention to an adult. Only 6 of the 58 children used any words or manual signs to communicate. Of these 6, none used more than five different words or manual signs.

The frequency of children's intentional communicative acts—defined as gestures, vocalizations, manual signs, or word approximations with coordinated attention to the caregiver and object—was measured at the beginning of the study by observing the children in semistructured play sessions with their mothers. The play session was repeated 6 months later, and mothers' nonlinguistic and linguistic responses to their children's preintentional and intentional acts were measured. Twelve months after the beginning of the study, child expressive and receptive language level was determined with the Reynell Developmental Language Scales–Third Edition (Edwards et al., 1997). Results showed that children who produced more intentional communicative acts in semistructured play sessions with their mothers at the beginning of the study had 1) mothers who demonstrated higher levels of nonlinguistic and linguistic contingent responsivity in identical semistructured play sessions 6 months later and 2) higher expressive and receptive language scores 12 months later.

Although these results are preliminary, they suggest that intentional communication may be related to later language development, in part, because it is more salient and interpretable to mothers than is preintentional communication. Therefore, it elicits the types of maternal responsivity that are so facilitative to language development. Directly increasing clear, intentional communication may lead some adults to use the types of responses that have been shown to facilitate language development, even though they have not been trained directly to do so.

COMBINING RESPONSIVITY AND MILIEU
TEACHING TECHNIQUES IN EARLY INTERVENTION

Adult contingent responsivity is a powerful facilitator of both intentional communication and symbolic communication in children with disabilities who are expected to learn to speak. Most early language intervention approaches reflect an understanding of this power and incorporate various types of responsivity that are contingent on the child's focus of interest and/or communicative behavior. Nevertheless, two of the most commonly used interventions for facilitating early vocabulary and multiword utterances, responsive interaction and milieu teaching, differ on the issue of how to elicit child communicative behavior so that language-facilitating adult responses can be delivered. Although the responsive interaction approach uses techniques to indirectly solicit child communicative behavior (e.g., following the child's attentional lead, environmental arrangement), the milieu teaching approach advocates the use of additional strategies that function to directly elicit child communication (Wilcox & Shannon, 1998).

Similar to the responsive interaction approach, milieu teaching emphasizes 1) teaching to the child's attentional focus, 2) manipulating the physical environment to create opportunities for communication, and 3) providing natural consequences to the child's communicative attempts (Wilcox & Shannon, 1998). Yet, milieu teaching incorporates some additional strategies such as the mand-model technique (Halle, 1982), incidental teaching (Warren & Kaiser, 1986), and time delays (Halle, Marshall, & Spradlin, 1979). Each of these strategies prescribes a particular sequence of prompts to get the child to produce a certain communicative act or target form.

There is evidence that milieu teaching strategies can facilitate the transition from presymbolic to symbolic communication in children with disabilities (for a review, see Kaiser, Yoder, & Keetz, 1992). Nonetheless, because intervention that is designed to facilitate the transition from preintentional to intentional communication is still new, there is relatively little data on the power of milieu techniques to facilitate intentional communication. Three studies have attempted to facilitate prelinguistic intentional communication in children with developmental disabilities (Warren et al., 1993; Yoder & Warren, 1998; Yoder et al., 1994). Similar to many of the symbolic communication interventions, these studies have combined adult responsivity with milieu techniques.

Facilitating Intentional Communication

For very young children who are expected to use speech as their primary mode of communication, the rate at which they intentionally communicate indicates their readiness for linguistic communication. As their rates of prelinguistic intentional communication acts approach 1.0 act per minute, children begin to use spoken words to communicate (Wetherby, Yonclas, & Bryan, 1989). Apparently, early nonverbal intentional communication forms the basis for the acquisition of an initial vocabulary. There is evidence that children who show delays in the emergence of basic communicative functions and the onset of coordinated attention (the ability to shift attention between the object or activity about which they want to communicate and the communication partner) are at risk for language development at a later age (McCathren, Warren, & Yoder, 1996).

Intervention to strengthen children's intentional communication skills was designed in response to evidence that children who intentionally communicated less than once per minute were less likely to benefit from intervention targeting linguistic skills (Tannock & Girolametto, 1992; Wilcox, 1993). This type of intervention targets the production of gestures and vocalizations combined with attention to the listener. The goal is to give prelinguistic children who are not ready for symbolic communication an effective, nonsymbolic means to control their environment. Increasing the frequency and clarity of children's intentional communication may also increase the probability that responsive caregivers will reinforce their own nonsymbolic efforts with the types of linguistic responsivity that are most facilitative of the development of symbolic communication skills (Warren & Yoder, 1998).

Yoder and Warren developed Prelinguistic Milieu Teaching (PMT; 1993) to directly facilitate clear, frequent intentional communication in children with developmental delays who were intentionally, nonverbally communicating less than once per minute. PMT combined nonlinguistic and linguistic contingent responsivity with procedures from the milieu teaching model to increase the frequency and clarity of self-initiated proto-imperatives and proto-declaratives. *Proto-imperatives* and *proto-declaratives* are gestures and vocalizations that, when combined with coordinated attention, function respectively as 1) requests for adult assistance in obtaining desired objects or activities or 2) as comments to gain another's attention to share an affective state.

Proto-imperatives and proto-declaratives were selected as targets for several reasons. First, they are the two most frequently produced communicative functions during the prelinguistic period (Wetherby, Cain, Yonclas, & Walker, 1988). Second, they function as powerful tools for controlling any environment that the child is likely to inhabit. Third, they are most likely to elicit some kind of response from adults, making adults more aware of the child's communication efforts in general and possibly eliciting the types of adult responsivity that promote language development (e.g., linguistic mapping) (Warren & Yoder, 1998).

In PMT sessions, adult trainers followed the child's attentional lead by playing with toys or engaging in activities that were of interest to the child. Nonlinguistic contingent responsivity was provided in the form of compliance with the presumed meaning of the child's communicative act and contingent motor and vocal imitation. Contingent imitation—characterized by the adult's exact, reduced, or slightly expanded imitation of the child's vocal or motor production—was used to increase child initiations and establish turn taking. Contingent imitation may be particularly suited to increasing child initiations (thereby balancing turn taking) because the child can control the amount of stimulation received from the adult by initiating vocal or motor acts that are already within his or her repertoire.

Once play routines were established, proto-imperatives were targeted. The adult created opportunities to request objects, assistance, or continuation of an activity through environmental arrangement and time delays. Verbal prompts to elicit proto-imperatives were delivered when necessary, and if a particular component of the targeted intentional communicative act was missing (i.e., eye contact with the adult or a gesture), then a demonstration of that particular component was prompted either verbally or nonverbally. To prompt eye contact, for example, the adult intersected the child's gaze or asked the child to look at him or her. To prompt a gesture, vocalization, sign, or word approximation, the adult modeled the targeted form. Proto-declaratives were targeted once the child developed a positive relationship with the adult and was motivated to recruit the adult's attention. Situations that would elicit proto-declaratives (e.g., introducing novel objects or events, sabotaging routines) were provided during which the adult modeled proto-declarative use with the forms targeted for that particular child.

Other forms of contingent responsivity in PMT included 1) linguistic responses to the child's focus of attention, 2) linguistic mapping of the child's nonverbal communication acts, and 3) specific acknowledgment that the child did something that the trainer was targeting (e.g., "You looked at me," "I heard you") when the child was acquiring a new behavior. Linguistic mapping was used in response to intentional communication attempts to facilitate vocabulary development.

To test the efficacy of PMT, Yoder and Warren (1998, 1999a) designed a randomized study involving the 58 children with developmental delays who were described previously in this chapter. Twenty-eight children received individualized, clinic-based PMT from a trainer for 20 minutes per day, 3 or 4 days per week, for 6 months. The other 30 children were assigned to a contrast treatment group, the Responsive Small Group (RSG). The RSG was a playgroup in which three children engaged in parallel play with a highly responsive trainer who was instructed to respond to child communication but not to prompt communication in any way. Frequency of self-initiated proto-imperatives and proto-declaratives was measured 1) prior to intervention, 2) immediately following the intervention period, and 3) 6 months after intervention, with the child's mother and with a staff member who was not the child's trainer, to determine whether the acquired intentional communication generalized outside the training context and whether the effects of the intervention were maintained over time. Interactions with the staff member and the parent took place in clinic-based settings that were not used during intervention and with materials that were not used during intervention.

The results showed that PMT facilitated an increase in self-initiated child proto-imperatives and proto-declaratives immediately following the intervention period. This increase remained intact 6 months following treatment. Yet, the effectiveness of PMT varied by pretreatment levels of maternal responsivity. Children whose mothers were relatively responsive before treatment benefited more from PMT than from RSG, showing increases in the generalized use of self-initiated proto-imperatives and proto-declaratives at the post-treatment and the 6-month follow-up evaluations. Children whose mothers were relatively unresponsive prior to intervention appeared to benefit more from RSG, showing increases in the generalized use of self-initiated proto-imperatives at the post-treatment and the 6-month follow-up evaluations. Nevertheless, evidence that RSG had a similar effect on self-initiated proto-declaratives 6 months after intervention was somewhat weaker.

Maternal responsivity was measured while observing mother–child interaction in a semistructured play session. The proportion of child communication acts that were immediately followed by maternal linguistic and nonlinguistic responses served as the index of maternal responsivity, with responsive mothers acting on more than 60% of child communication acts and relatively unresponsive mothers responding to fewer than 40% of child communication acts prior to intervention. This study measured maternal responsivity both pre- and postintervention, and found that, although the number of maternal responses changed after intervention, the proportion of maternal responses did not change.

Maternal responsivity may influence which prelinguistc interventions are most beneficial because children may develop generalized expectations concerning interactions with adults (including interventionists) through their interactions with their mothers. For example, children of responsive mothers may come into intervention expecting adults to respond to their immature communication attempts. These children may be more likely to persist in their efforts to communicate, even when the adult response is in the form of a prompt, as it often is in PMT. Because they are motivated to continue the interaction even when faced with prompts, they are more likely to learn from the information contained in those prompts. Alternatively, children of unresponsive mothers may learn not to expect an adult response. A prompt to communicate, such as that used in PMT, may result in their withdrawal from the interaction or resistance to the adult's demand, causing the children to miss the information embedded in the adult prompt. Such children may better process the input from an adult who complies with and linguistically maps their communicative acts, as the RSG trainers did (see Yoder & Warren, 1998, for more on hypotheses concerning the influence of maternal responsivity on the development of child expectations).

In summary, there is strong evidence that PMT facilitates intentional communication in children whose parents are relatively responsive. For the children of relatively unresponsive parents, the evidence is weaker. Future research is needed to determine whether teaching this latter group to be more responsive can enhance the efficacy of PMT. In this way, both caregivers and children may be able to take full advantage of the transactional effects that promote language development (Yoder & Warren, 1998; 1999a).

Facilitating Symbolic Communication

The most optimal intervention for learners who are making the transition from presymbolic to symbolic communication targets increasing the linguistic contingent responsivity of adults to the learner's communicative attempts. In addition, optimal intervention strategies attempt to directly teach symbolic forms through specific elicitation or prompting techniques (Warren & Yoder, 1997; Wilcox & Shannon, 1998; Yoder et al., 1998). Comparisons have been made between the efficacy of responsive interaction and milieu teaching for children with mild to severe disabilities who were able to speak. These comparisons have shown that milieu teaching was more efficient than the responsive interaction approach in teaching basic vocabulary and initial two- and three-term semantic relationships to children who were at the single word stage of language learning and had receptive vocabulary levels of approximately 24 months of age. In contrast, children who were at the simple sentence stage and receptive vocabulary levels at or above 36 months of age made greater gains with the responsive interaction approach (Kouri & Wilcox, 1996; Yoder, Kaiser, et al., 1995).

Several reasons have been suggested for the superiority of milieu teaching for children at the single word stage of language development. First, the milieu approach is not as dependent on how often the child communicates to respond with the types of input that are most facilitative of language learning (Yoder et al., 1998). Requests for imitation, asking topic-continuing questions, or requests for specific communicative behavior all function as ways to get the child to use his or her existing communication. By contrast, the responsive interactive approach may use descriptive talk about the child's focus of attention as a model for the child's attention, but it has no specific strategy for getting the child to use his or her existing communication.

A second reason that milieu teaching may be superior to responsive interaction for children at the single word stage of development is that milieu's direct elicitation techniques may help the child attend more closely to the linguistic information in the adult's utterance. For some children who are struggling with the acquisition of first words, simply responding to their focus of attention or communicative acts with linguistic mapping, recasts, or expansions may not draw their attention to the novel linguistic information contained within (Yoder et al., 1998; Warren & Yoder, 1997). Children with MLUs under 2.0 may lack the attentional and memory resources necessary to efficiently learn from recasts that require them to compare their own utterance with the following adult utterance (Yoder, Kaiser, et al., 1995).

As children move past the acquisition of the first 10–15 words, however, the differential effectiveness of milieu versus responsive interaction diminishes (Wilcox & Shannon, 1998). In fact, Yoder, Kaiser, and colleagues (1995) found that the responsive interaction approach was more effective than milieu teaching with children who had MLUs above 2.5, possibly because this approach uses more expansions and recasts of child-initiated utterances than does milieu teaching. Presumably, adult responses that repeat part of the child's utterance are more salient to children at this developmental level because they have the attentional and memory resources necessary to compare their own utterance with the adult utterance that follows and to learn from this comparison.

In summary, the research on early language intervention with children with disabilities who are expected to learn to speak suggests that exposure to highly responsive adults may be a necessary but not all-sufficient component of an optimally effective intervention program (Warren & Yoder, 1997). Milieu teaching procedures can provide an effective way to elicit child communicative behavior so that language-facilitating adult responses can be delivered. There is evidence that combining milieu techniques and adult contingent responsivity can facilitate clearer, more frequent prelinguistic intentional communication, particularly if the children have caregivers who are already relatively responsive. In addition, direct elicitation techniques appear to be important for learners who are making the transition to symbolic communication. There is some evidence that these techniques are particularly effective when teaching an initial vocabulary and early multiword combinations to beginning communicators. Nevertheless, direct elicitation techniques may be less effective when targeting higher level morphological and syntactic skills with children who are already at the simple sentence stage of language development. Combining high levels of responsivity with an intervention strategy that is appropriate to the child's developmental level is likely to improve child outcomes.

DEVELOPING CONTINGENT EXCHANGES WITH BEGINNING COMMUNICATORS WHO USE AAC

Evidence of the beneficial effects of all three types of adult contingent responsivity was acquired by studying children who were expected to eventually develop speech as their primary form of communication; however, it is reasonable to conclude that each type may be similarly effective at facilitating the communication and language development of AAC users who must learn to rely on gestures and/or graphic symbols to communicate. Nonlinguistic contingent responsivity may be particularly appropriate for the transition from preintentional to intentional communication because it helps the individual understand that his or her behavior can be directed toward a listener to achieve a desired effect. Linguistic contingent responsivity may have special relevance for those who are making the transition from using nonsymbolic forms of intentional communication to using manual signs and/or graphic symbols, as it facilitates the development of vocabulary and semantic relations. Learners who are making the transition to the use of symbols often are learning a referent's verbal label at the same time they are learning the manual sign or graphic symbol that represents that label. Therefore, simultaneously supplementing verbal responses to learner communicative acts with visual cues (e.g., modeling the manual sign, pointing to the graphic symbol) can augment the auditory information that the learner receives. This may make it easier for the learner to attach meaning to these visual forms of language as well as provide a model for the expressive use of manual signs and symbols. Finally, it is important to remember that facilitator responsivity is only one piece of communication intervention. Combining adult responsivity with milieu teaching procedures is an effective way of teaching individuals with cognitive impairments to use both nonsymbolic and symbolic forms to express communicative functions.

Developmental versus Functional Approaches in AAC

Some experts in the AAC field have suggested using a developmental approach when choosing between intervention that targets nonsymbolic or symbolic communication. This approach, which is based on clinical experience, suggests that learners who show little evidence of intentional communication should learn the basic elements of communication before symbolic communication systems involving manual signs or graphic symbols are introduced. Turn taking and the ability to coordinate attention between an object of interest and a communication partner are some examples of skills that underlie successful communicative exchanges. The use of natural gestures and vocalizations to seek attention, to indicate acceptance and rejection, to protest, and to comment are additional skills that would build a foundation on which new symbolic forms could be integrated (Beukelman & Mirenda, 1998). Some researchers in language intervention for children with developmental delays who are expected to learn to speak have advocated a similar sequence (Warren & Yoder, 1998; Wilcox & Shannon, 1998). Building a broad base of prelinguistic communication skills may be more important and realistic than linguistic communication for children who are expected to learn to speak but who demonstrate low rates of intentional communication. It is interesting to note that some preliminary research has indicated that prelinguistic children with low rates of intentional communication (less than once per minute) did not appear to benefit much from intervention that targeted spoken words as the primary goal (Tannock & Girolametto, 1992; Wilcox, 1992).

Alternatively, a developmental approach may not be appropriate for all learners with disabilities. For example, some learners with autism or severe mental retardation are not socially motivated to communicate. Not only do they lack the curiosity to explore and respond to novel stimuli, but they also are not reinforced by the social reactions of communication partners. They are unlikely to initiate social contacts with others, participate in turn-taking activities, alternate eye gaze between the communication partner and the focus of attention, or imitate vocalizations and gestures (Bondy & Frost, 1994; Reichle, Halle, & Drasgow, 1998). For these learners, intervention that is focused on the development of these behaviors may be slow and lengthy. The decision concerning whether to continue to focus on nonsymbolic communication becomes even more relevant with older learners who are preparing to make the transition to more community-based settings that contain unfamiliar communication partners. Although many nonsymbolic acts (e.g., pointing, gesturing while looking at the referent) are readily interpretable by unfamiliar communication partners, others are only interpretable by those who are familiar and/or particularly responsive. In these situations, intervention that develops the functional use of symbols while simultaneously developing intentional communication may be appropriate.

An example of such an intervention is Bondy and Frost's Picture Exchange Communication System (PECS; 1994), a functional communication training program that teaches the learner to request and comment by giving picture cards to a communication partner. Prerequisite behaviors such as the recognition of picture symbols or the ability to communicate intentionally through clear, nonsymbolic means are not required of participants in PECS training. This intervention approach has been advocated as a means to establish functional communication and possibly speech for learners who are not responsive to socially mediated reinforcement. For these learners, the length of time it would take to establish a particular set of prelinguistic behaviors (e.g., joint attention, motor and verbal imitation skills) as prerequisites to symbolic communication training is seen as prohibitive (Bondy & Frost, 1994).

A close examination of the initial phases of PECS training reveals how a learner who previously did not demonstrate intentional communication can be taught to spontaneously select the appropriate picture symbol, obtain the communication partner's attention, meet the partner's gaze, and initiate a request by handing him or her the picture symbol. Following a preference probe to identify particular objects that the learner finds reinforcing, the PECS teacher places one desired object within reach of the learner. When the learner reaches for the object, the teacher interrupts the reach by placing the picture symbol that depicts that object into the learner's hand. The teacher then immediately opens his or her other hand and guides the learner to release the picture symbol. At this point, linguistic mapping of the physically prompted picture exchange is delivered, (e.g., "You want the tape player. Here it is."). At no point is the learner verbally prompted to either initiate or perform the picture exchange, (e.g., "What do you want?"). Teacher prompts to initiate or produce communicative acts are seen as unlikely to be motivating for these individuals, as they are primarily rewarded by social responses. In addition, they may lead to the learner's dependence on the communication partner's verbal prompting (Bondy & Frost, 1994).

Eventually, the learner must learn to pick up a single picture symbol off of the table and give it to the teacher, who fades the open-hand cue over time. Once the learner is reliably able to request this single reinforcer, proximity to both the teacher and to the picture symbol is altered so that the learner must actively initiate an exchange by seeking the picture symbol and then approaching the communication partner. Persistence in attempting to gain the teacher's attention is taught by a second teacher physically prompting the learner to touch the first teacher's shoulder. The first teacher deliberately looks away from the learner until this attempt is made and subsequently meets the learner's gaze before the picture symbol exchange can take place. In this way, eye contact with the communication partner becomes a part of the requesting routine. Once the learner can spontaneously obtain the picture symbol, approach the communication partner, gain his or her attention, and initiate a picture exchange, the number of pictures are gradually increased so that the learner must discriminate among them to request different reinforcers. Communication partners, contexts, and reinforcers are varied to promote generalization (Bondy & Frost, 1994). In these beginning phases of PECS, a learner who has not previously demonstrated intentional communication can be taught to produce what is essentially a gesture (i.e., giving the communication partner a picture symbol) combined with attention to the communication partner in order to request.

PECS has been used primarily with nonspeaking children younger than 5 years of age who have autism (Bondy & Frost, 1994; Schwartz, Garfinkle, & Bauer, 1998). Yet, it has been used with young, nonspeaking children with other severe developmental disabilities as well (Schwartz et al., 1998). Although experimental data on PECS are still unavailable, anecdotal reports and program evaluation data have been positive (Bondy & Frost, 1994; Schwartz et al., 1998). In addition to the establishment of self-initiated requesting and labeling in response to a question by constructing messages with one or more graphic symbols, many of the PECS training participants have been reported to subsequently develop speech. Bondy and Peterson (1990) reported that 59% of the nonverbal children with autism who used PECS acquired speech as their only means of communication to make requests and label items after 1 year of training, and an additional 30% used a combination of speech and picture symbols. Schwartz and colleagues (1998) reported that 44% of their sample of nonverbal children with autism and other severe developmental disabilities acquired speech as their sole means of communication. Although neither report is based on experimental data, both are particularly encouraging given the estimate that 50% of individuals with autism do not develop speech as a result of social-cognitive and/or oral-motor impairments (Prizant, 1996).

The mechanism by which PECS may influence the development of speech is unknown. The picture symbols themselves may make it easier for some individuals with autism to learn the meaning behind spoken words, enabling them to build a receptive vocabulary in preparation for the emergence of expressive language. Several authors have hypothesized that some learners with autism may have trouble comprehending spoken language because of the transient, sequential nature of speech (Mirenda & Schuler, 1988; Peterson, Bondy, Vincent, & Finnegan, 1995; Quill, 1995). A case study by Peterson and colleagues found that two nonspeaking students with autism and severe mental retardation performed better on tasks when the spoken instructions were either replaced or supplemented with pictorial cues in the form of line drawings. In addition, Quill reviewed research that suggested that some children with autism process visuospatial information much better than auditory-temporal information, suggesting that the amount of time the stimulus remains available to the children influences their ability to process it.

Although typically developing children learn new vocabulary as a result of the adult's linguistic contingent responses to their focus of attention or the adult's linguistic mapping of their communicative acts, children with autism may have difficulty attaching meaning to the new word simply as a result of hearing the adult's verbal input. With PECS, the learner may initially understand the teacher's verbal response to be triggered by the physical gesture of giving the picture symbol. Eventually, however, the learner must attend to the picture symbol itself when discriminating between pictures in order to request the desired reinforcer. Attending to a static, visual representation of language (e.g., the picture symbol) that remains available for processing while initiating a request and then subsequently hearing the teacher's linguistic mapping of the picture exchange may help some learners extract the relevant information from the communicative interaction.

The resulting increase in speech comprehension may also facilitate an increase in productive language. The ability to understand some spoken language is a developmental precursor to the development of first words in typically developing children (see Wetherby, Reichle, & Pierce, 1998, for a review). In addition, research involving learners with severe mental retardation showed that learners who could comprehend spoken language at the outset of AAC intervention had an advantage in learning to produce language, even when their mode of production was the selection of graphic symbols (Romski & Sevcik, 1996; Sevcik & Romski, 1997). With PECS, the use of picture symbols to supplement the communication partner's linguistic mapping may help the learner acquire enough receptive vocabulary to facilitate the development of productive language.

Another reason PECS may be associated with the development of speech is that the picture symbols themselves may function as prompts for expressive communication (Quill, 1995). Having a visual representation of words available for recognition and use precludes the need to recall a new word from memory. The picture symbols may serve as a scaffold for the learner's emergent linguistic attempts.

PECS is one example of communication intervention that can be characterized as incorporating more of a functional approach than a developmental one. Because the research on adult contingent responsivity has been linked to specific aspects of early language development as opposed to specific aspects of functional communication, the remainder of this chapter reflects a more developmental approach to AAC intervention in that suggestions for facilitating nonsymbolic intentional communication and symbolic communication are offered separately. Nevertheless, we believe that these implications are applicable to both AAC intervention approaches.

Clinical Implications for Facilitating Nonsymbolic Intentional Communication

The AAC literature already reflects a good understanding of the power of adult contingent responsivity to facilitate the development of intentional communication (see Beukelman & Mirenda, 1998; Oregon Research Institute, 1989; Rowland & Schweigert, 1991, 1992; and Siegel-Causey & Guess, 1989). Because there is evidence that nonsymbolic communicators are particularly at risk for not having facilitators recognize, interpret, and respond to their communicative attempts, facilitator training is critical for adults who work with these learners (Houghton et al., 1987; Light & Binger, 1998; Rowland, 1990). Siegel-Causey and Guess's text on nonsymbolic communication interactions contained a variety of strategies for facilitators of AAC users who are just beginning the transition to intentional communication. So that interactions can better elicit and support nonsymbolic communication attempts, strategies were illustrated to 1) develop nurturing relationships, 2) enhance sensitivity to nonsymbolic behaviors, 3) increase opportunities for communication, 4) create social routines, and 5) create movement "dialogues."

For learners who already show some intentional communication, intervention should focus on increasing the frequency and clarity of nonsymbolic intentional acts as well as on facilitator responsivity. Although the AAC literature contains several examples of interventions that are designed to teach choice making and requesting through the use of nonsymbolic forms (Baumgart, Johnson, & Helmstetter, 1990; Beukelman & Mirenda, 1998; Reichle et al., 1991), relatively little attention has been given to the importance of increasing the clarity of nonsymbolic communication by requiring attention to the adult as well as to the object or event that is the focus of the communication. Specific behaviors that would add clarity to the learner's communicative acts can be elicited through prompts or models. For example, eye gaze can be elicited by intersecting the learner's gaze or, if necessary, verbally prompting the learner to look at the facilitator. Vocalizations can be modeled while imitating the learner's gesture. Clearer nonsymbolic communication may be more likely to trigger language-facilitating responses in facilitators, especially those who are naturally responsive (Yoder & Warren, 1999b).

Facilitator training programs for people who already have some intentional communication should include training on the provision of linguistic contingent responses. Recommendations for the specific form that these linguistic responses might take as well as the rationale for using them might assist facilitators in matching their input to the AAC user's developmental level. Adult contingent linguistic responses to the individual's focus of attention and linguistic mapping of intentional communication acts are likely to facilitate the development of receptive vocabulary at this developmental stage. These types of responses imply that the facilitator should 1) follow the learner's attentional lead as much as possible, 2) arrange the environment to increase communication opportunities, and 3) build social routines to elicit communication attempts (Warren & Yoder, 1998). Although these responses are vocal, simultaneously supplementing them with visual cues (e.g., modeling the manual sign, pointing to the graphic symbol) can augment the auditory information that the learner receives.

Facilitator behaviors play a large part in intervention with nonsymbolic communicators. For interventionists who want a structured approach to facilitator training, Light and Binger (1998) developed instructional procedures that can be used when training facilitators to use a variety of strategies to support AAC. Light and Binger reviewed suggestions for teaching facilitators how to provide opportunities for the learner to practice targeted skills as well as strategies to support the acquisition, maintenance, and generalization of skills. These procedures would be similarly beneficial when training facilitators to use both the linguistic and nonlinguistic responsive behaviors discussed in this chapter.

Clinical Implications for Facilitating Symbolic Communication

The transition to symbolic communication is characterized by the acquisition of an initial lexicon followed by the emergence of multiword combinations. The adult responses that are most likely to facilitate these achievements are primarily linguistic responses. Linguistic contingent responsivity to the learner's focus of attention and communicative attempts promotes the acquisition of vocabulary; expansions and recasts promote multiword utterances. The mechanism by which linguistic contingent responses are hypothesized to work depends on semantic overlap and temporal proximity to the individual's communicative act. Presumably, an individual who is engaged in communication about something in which he or she is interested will hear the adult's topic-continuing response and compare the new linguistic information it contains to his or her own communicative act. Attending to the salient differences between the two acts may help the learner incorporate the new linguistic information into his or her own linguistic system (Nelson, 1989).

Yet, facilitators who work with individuals who use graphic symbols or manual signs to communicate may encounter at least four situations that reduce the effectiveness of their responses. These situations occur when the learner is unable to 1) repair a communication breakdown, 2) initiate communication due to lack of familiarity with a graphic symbol or manual sign system, 3) precisely represent messages because a particular sign or graphic symbol is unknown or unavailable, and 4) represent multiword combinations because a particular sign or graphic symbol is unknown or unavailable. The effect of each of these situations on the quality of the facilitator's response is discussed next, along with strategies that may reduce their occurrence.

Inability to Repair Communication Breakdowns   The first situation occurs when communication breaks down and the facilitator cannot continue responding to the AAC user's message. Many AAC users who use graphic symbols and/or gestural communication have some functional speech, even though it may be unintelligible to unfamiliar listeners. These individuals will use AAC primarily as a backup system to repair breakdowns in verbal communication. Others depend more on graphic symbol selections or manual signs to communicate. A responsive facilitator can provide linguistic contingent responses to an individual's verbal utterances, graphic symbol selections, or manual signs if the communication is sufficiently intelligible. When the message is unintelligible and communication breaks down, the facilitator is forced to respond to the communication breakdown itself rather than to the individual's focus of attention. Such a response violates the principles of semantic overlap and temporal proximity to the individual's message, impeding the acquisition of new vocabulary and grammatical structures.

For this reason, the development of repair strategies should be targeted early in intervention with individuals with speech-language impairments (Light & Binger, 1998; Reichle et al., 1991; Wetherby, Alexander, & Prizant, 1998). This intervention should reflect what is known about the developmental sequence with which the various strategies are acquired and used by both typically and atypically developing children (see Wetherby et al., 1998, for a review). For example, typically developing young children who are beginning to use words rely heavily on repeating or modifying gestures (e.g., giving, showing, pointing, miming) to repair their communication breakdowns, even after they develop the ability to use verbal repairs (Alexander, 1994). This has interesting implications for AAC users who are making the transition to symbolic communication but have nonexistent or weak repair strategies. Because the use of natural gestures to repair communication persists even among typically developing children who are learning to speak, it is reasonable to assume that gestures may be easier to learn than graphic symbols or manual signs when targeting beginning repair strategies.

Social routines in which the learner is motivated to request continuation of an interrupted activity provide good opportunities to develop early repairs. The facilitator can withhold a turn and look expectantly at the learner, feigning ignorance of the learner's request to continue the routine. The facilitator can use a verbal prompt (e.g., "What?") and model the appropriate gestural repair if necessary (Warren & Yoder, 1998). As the learner's competence with gestural repair increases, the facilitator can model additional modalities (e.g., the coordination of vocalizations with gestures, word approximations, the use of a particular symbol or sign). Optimally, the learner should acquire a variety of repair strategies that can be used to meet the demands of different listeners and environments. The ability to quickly repair a communication breakdown can increase the probability that the facilitator's linguistic response contains salient information.

Lack of Familiarity with a Graphic Symbol or Manual Sign System
Another situation that may compromise the effectiveness of facilitator contingent responsivity occurs when the learner does not communicate frequently enough for language-facilitating responses to be delivered. There are many reasons why AAC users might fail to initiate communicative acts. Learners who are making the transition to graphic symbols or manual signs may not have automatic recognition of the meaning behind some of the symbols on the symbol display, or they may not have fluent recall of the manual signs that have been taught thus far. Unable to quickly recognize or recall the symbols needed to communicate self-initiated messages, such an individual is unlikely to communicate frequently enough for contingent responsivity to have much of an effect on his or her language development.

Facilitators who work with learners who are just beginning to use symbolic communication often find that they must teach the meaning behind all but the most transparent symbols and signs to encourage their use. Selecting graphic symbols and manual signs that are identified as being functional and motivating to the user allows their meaning and use to be taught concurrently. Although a thorough review of intervention approaches that simultaneously teach the comprehension and production of graphic symbols or manual signs is beyond the scope of this chapter, two interventions involving graphic symbols are of particular interest. Both were designed to teach graphic symbol users the meanings of the symbols as they are prompted to use them within the context of everyday activities. Both share the unique feature of the facilitator's augmenting spoken language through facilitator use of symbols during interaction. Aided Language Stimulation (Elder & Goossens', 1994; Goossens', Crain, & Elder, 1992) and the System For Augmenting Language (SAL; Romski & Sevcik, 1992, 1993, 1996; see also Chapter 14) may be especially effective ways to augment the input that the AAC user receives from the graphic symbol display in order to teach symbol meanings and encourage the use of the symbols in interactions.

In Aided Language Stimulation, the facilitator teaches symbol meanings by augmenting his or her own verbal input to the AAC user. This is done by simultaneously selecting symbols on the graphic symbol display while speaking, either by pointing to symbols or by highlighting them with a penlight. Comprehension of the graphic symbol is promoted by combining the visual cue of the highlighted symbol with the symbol's spoken label. In addition, the facilitator's use of symbol selection to augment his or her own spoken language serves to model the use of symbols for communication. In addition to modeling production, learners are prompted to use symbols to communicate within the context of motivating, frequently occurring routines by the incorporation of time delays, the sabotage of routines, and/or the use of verbal cues. Prompts are faded as the AAC user gains proficiency (see Beukelman & Mirenda, 1998; Elder & Goossens', 1994; and Goossens' et al., 1992, for a more complete description of Aided Language Stimulation).

Although several case studies and anecdotal reports have verified that Aided Language Stimulation is an effective intervention that promotes the understanding and use of graphic symbols, there is no empirical evidence that it promotes language development in AAC users (Beukelman & Mirenda, 1998). Nevertheless, its use of techniques to elicit visual referencing of the graphic symbol and the simultaneous delivery of matched verbal input seem likely to facilitate symbol comprehension. The learner is provided with a carefully focused amount of visual and auditory input during communicative interactions so that the new form (i.e., the graphic symbol) is highlighted. In addition, if the graphic symbol is easily recognizable by the learner, the facilitator's spoken input may be augmented by highlighting the graphic symbol, thereby enabling the learner to comprehend a previously unfamiliar spoken word. Finally, it is reasonable to assume that the inclusion of milieu techniques (e.g., incidental teaching, time delay procedures, mand-model techniques) in Aided Language Stimulation will facilitate the use of graphic symbols. As reviewed previously in this chapter, milieu techniques have proven to be an efficient means for facilitating early vocabulary and multiword utterances in children with developmental delays who are expected to learn to speak.

The SAL is similar to Aided Language Stimulation in that it teaches comprehension and the use of graphic symbols within the context of daily activities. Nonetheless, a critical component of the SAL is a voice output device that "speaks" the graphic symbol's label as soon as it is selected (Romski & Sevcik, 1996). A study suggests that the auditory feedback from speech output may contribute to comprehension of graphic symbol meaning (Schlosser, Belfiore, Nigam, Blischak, & Hetzroni, 1995). As with Aided Language Stimulation, the facilitator who uses the SAL augments his or her own verbal input to the AAC user by simultaneously selecting symbols on the graphic symbol display that is affixed to the voice output communication aid (VOCA), which then provides the symbol's label. Yet, unlike Aided Language Stimulation, symbol use is not explicitly prompted but encouraged through exposure to facilitator modeling of symbol selection in naturally occurring interactions (see Romski & Sevcik, 1996, and Chapter 14 for a more complete description of the SAL).

A longitudinal, 2-year study of the SAL was implemented with 13 male children and youth with moderate and severe mental retardation who demonstrated significant delays in receptive and expressive language on standardized and informal language assessments prior to the study. All of the participants demonstrated intentional communication but had fewer than 10 intelligible word approximations at the onset of the study. By the end of the study, the participants demonstrated 1) successful and effective use of their VOCAs with both adults and peers (Romski, Sevcik, Robinson, & Bakeman, 1994; Romski, Sevcik & Wilkinson, 1994), 2) comprehension and production of a graphic symbol vocabulary (Adamson, Romski, Deffebach, & Sevcik, 1992; Romski & Sevcik, 1996), and 3) the emergence of the production of untaught symbol combinations (Wilkinson, Romski, & Sevcik, 1994).

These studies represented a first step in developing and implementing the SAL intervention, thereby generating further hypotheses about the language development of nonspeaking youth with severe mental retardation (Romski & Sevcik, 1996). Nevertheless, generalizability of the results is restricted due to the small number of participants. Consequently, it is not clear how the SAL participants would compare with other participants who did not experience the intervention or who had experienced a different intervention. In addition, because the SAL is composed of several components, (e.g., speech output, partner modeling of symbol selection), it is difficult to know which component may be responsible for the participants' performance or whether some combination of components is the critical factor in the SAL's success (Romski & Sevcik, 1996). Preliminary reports of student outcomes suggest that the SAL may hold promise for enhancing both receptive and expressive communication skills for nonspeaking learners with severe mental retardation who have acquired some spoken words but cannot communicate intelligibly.

Aided Language Stimulation and the SAL have potential for teaching the meanings behind graphic symbols while simultaneously promoting functional communication and language development. Both interventions help the learner visually reference the symbol (e.g., by pointing to, highlighting, or selecting a symbol paired with speech output). Both interventions also provide immediate auditory feedback, whether through natural speech or a VOCA, that helps the learner focus on the symbol's verbal label. If the graphic symbols on the learner's display are transparent enough, both interventions have the potential to help the learner understand the facilitator's verbal input because a static, visual representation of speech exists after the auditory signal has faded. Ideally, the resulting recognition of symbols will help increase the number of self-initiated communication acts, which, in turn, gives the facilitator more opportunities to respond linguistically in ways that will affect language development.

Inability to Represent Messages Precisely   Even when the AAC user has a fluent understanding of the meanings behind his or her graphic symbols or signs, the number of symbols depicted or signs learned may be insufficient when the AAC user is engaged in interactions that have the potential to promote language development. A third situation occurs when the AAC user fails to communicate the intended message because he or she does not have a particular graphic symbol on the symbol display or does not know the precise manual sign to use. The AAC user may compensate by using whatever graphic symbol or sign is available in an attempt to get the facilitator to guess the true message, causing the facilitator to respond to these compensatory symbols instead of the intended message. For example, a young graphic symbol user may select the symbols *play* and *red* in an attempt to request gain access to a red toy barn because the symbol for *barn* is not on his or her display. Because even a highly responsive facilitator often has no way of knowing whether the user's symbol selection is genuinely representative of his or her internal communicative message or whether it represents a strategy of using existing symbols to communicate a related message, the facilitator's linguistic response has the potential to map the wrong message (e.g., "You want the fire truck," "Yes, we played with that red barn yesterday"). This example is in no way unique to graphic symbol users. Users of manual signs may also resort to using known, related signs in an attempt to reference something for which they do not know the sign. In either situation, the facilitator is unlikely to have vocabulary that matches the AAC user's internal message, therefore violating the principle of semantic overlap.

It is virtually impossible for designers of picture-based symbol displays to anticipate and provide the necessary vocabulary for every communicative exchange. The graphic symbol user must filter self-generated communicative acts through the process of having to select symbols that have been chosen and organized by another person. Beginning manual sign users are similarly encumbered when attempting to express messages with a limited repertoire of signs that have been selected and taught by others. Therefore, the ability of a graphic symbol or gestural system to accurately represent the words and phrases that exist inside the user's mind is always suspect. However, organizing a beginning communicator's graphic symbol vocabulary into a collection of separate environmental or activity displays is a strategy worth considering when attempting to provide the user with as much relevant vocabulary as possible to promote language learning as well as functional communication. Providing the AAC user with multiple environmental or activity displays has the potential not only to increase the number of symbols available for selection throughout the day but also to expose the user to more vocabulary items (Goossens' et al., 1992). Having a variety of graphic symbol displays available for interaction across different daily activities can enable the user to gain experience with a richer variety of communicative functions as well because the space constraints that are imposed by one communication display are eliminated. Activity-specific vocabulary that enables the user to request, comment, provide information, ask questions, and otherwise initiate and maintain a topic can be generated by observing activities and identifying opportunities in which these communicative functions could be modeled or prompted to occur (see Elder & Goossens', 1994, and Goossens' et al., 1992, for instructions on vocabulary selection for activity displays).

These displays are small graphic symbol displays that contain vocabulary items that are specific to a particular environment or activity. They can function as overlays on VOCAs or as stand-alone, low-technology communication aids. A single-symbol display on a dedicated communication device is less likely to provide all of the symbols that an AAC user will need for participating in a variety of activities and environments throughout the day. In addition, when one display attempts to provide all of the symbols that may be needed, the result is that the user must take more time to visually scan the symbol array in order to find the needed symbol. In contrast, providing many smaller activity- or environment-based displays provides the user with more vocabulary that is easier to access (Elder & Goossens', 1994; Goossens' et al., 1992).

Inability to Represent Multiword Combinations A fourth situation that may prevent the graphic symbol or manual sign user from taking full advantage of facilitator linguistic responsivity involves vocabulary breadth. When a symbol display or sign repertoire inadequately represents vocabulary from different grammatical categories, the user has few opportunities to practice constructing multiword messages. Consequently, the facilitator has few opportunities to assess a beginning communicator's grasp of semantic relations and to tailor his or her expansions and recasts to model correct grammatical usage. When designing graphic symbol displays, several interventionists have recommended that symbols representing grammatical categories other than nouns be included and that symbol displays be organized according to spoken word order and usage (Beukelman & Mirenda, 1998; Elder & Goossens', 1994; Goossens' et al., 1992; McDonald & Schultz, 1973). By modeling or prompting combinations of symbols that represent multiword utterances, the facilitator can help the AAC user discover visually how words can be combined and recombined to express different meanings.

Whether to use a word-based or a sentence-based approach when designing graphic symbol displays is an important decision (see Beukelman & Mirenda, 1998; Elder & Goosens', 1994; and Goosens' et al., 1992). In word-based symbol displays, one symbol represents one word. In sentence-based symbol displays, one symbol may represent an entire sentence or phrase. From a language-learning standpoint, the advantage of word-based displays is their potential to provide the AAC user with vocabulary from a variety of grammatical categories, thereby encouraging the formulation of multiword combinations. The research on typically and atypically developing children who could speak that was previously presented in this chapter showed that adult use of expansions and recasts were associated with the development of early multiword combinations (Yoder et al., 1998). Because a sentence-based system already depicts grammatically correct multiword utterances, such a system may prevent a facilitator from knowing precisely how to expand or recast an AAC user's message. In contrast, a word-based symbol display would provide the facilitator with a way to see how the learner combines single words. The symbol display itself could serve as a visual representation of language on which the facilitator could verbally expand or recast the AAC user's message while physically modeling the combination of symbols (see Elder & Goossens', 1994, and Goossens' et al., 1992, for examples of this type of instruction).

Communicating through the selection of individual symbols to compose a single message may be laborious for many AAC users with significant physical disabilities who use scanning techniques as well as for some individuals who use direct selection. Word-by-word messaging may be unacceptably slow for particular communication partners or for specific environments. Several authors have provided some decision-making guidelines to use when determining which messages should be represented by word-based or sentence-based symbols (Beukelman & Mirenda, 1998; Elder & Goosens', 1994; Goosens' et al., 1992). If the primary goal is efficient, functional communication, as it might be for older learners with severe mental retardation for whom language development is less of a priority, then a sentence-based communication display is an appropriate choice. This will enable them to communicate essential messages independently and quickly, reducing the cognitive and motor challenges that come with combining symbols in order to produce multiword combinations. For younger children and learners who function at a higher cognitive level, a balance of sentences and individual words (e.g., nouns, verbs, adjectives, adverbs, prepositions) that can be combined to make a sentence will provide a means to develop vocabulary and syntax as well as a means to communicate essential messages quickly (Elder & Goosens', 1994; Goosens' et al., 1992). In addition, should a word-based system be chosen in support of vocabulary and language growth, Beukelman and Mirenda (1998) provided suggestions for "developmental vocabulary" based on Lahey and Bloom's (1977) recommendations concerning the selection of an initial lexicon that is conducive to the development of semantic relations.

For manual sign users, the choice of sign system is relevant to the facilitator's ability to provide expansions and recasts that will promote multiword combinations. The majority of interventions that have been used with people with disabilities other than hearing impairments have used Key-Word Signing (KWS; Beukelman & Mirenda, 1998). In KWS, manual signs are used for the most critical words in a sentence, and English word order is retained. The KWS user may speak the critical words while signing them. KWS differs from the American Sign Language (ASL) and the Signing Exact English (SEE-2) systems. ASL, which is primarily used by the Deaf community, does not follow English word order, nor is English spoken while signing. Like KWS, SEE-2 systems follow English word order and use spoken English while signing. Nevertheless, SEE-2 systems sign all of the words in a sentence, and contain special sign markers to indicate tense, word endings, and affixes (see Beukelman & Mirenda, 1998, or Reichle et al., 1991, for a discussion of the differences between manual sign systems).

Obviously, a sign system that supports English word order and the simultaneous use of spoken English would be critical for language learning for beginning communicators without hearing impairments for whom manual signs are the chosen communication mode. For these communicators, responding verbally with expansion or recasts in which the critical words are signed would help them learn semantic relations as well as the particular signs that express those relations. Responding by signing only the most critical words is likely to increase the saliency of those signs for learners who simultaneously have to learn vocabulary, semantic relations, and the manual signs that represent these words.

Making sure that the learner has access to vocabulary from different grammatical categories is crucial to the facilitation of multiword combinations through contingent responses. For graphic symbol users, the selection of symbol vocabulary should reflect a balance of the need for quick, functional communication with the need for practice at constructing multiword combinations through symbols that represent single words. When the learner attempts to construct a multiword combination through symbols, the facilitator can expand or recast the attempt by selecting the appropriate symbols to match his or her verbal response. With manual sign users, teaching a signing system that approximates English word order is important for the same reason. Facilitator contingent responses have the power to facilitate semantic relations only if the learner's symbolic language reflects vocabulary from different semantic categories.

CONCLUSION

The research on the early communication development of young children with and without disabilities who are expected to learn to speak has demonstrated that adult contingent responsivity plays an important role in facilitating intentional communication, the acquisition of an initial lexicon, and the emergence of multiword utterances. In addition, various adult responses appear to differentially affect these communication and language outcomes when they are appropriately matched with the child's developmental level (Yoder et al., 1998). Because no studies have examined the effects of caregiver responsivity on the communication and language development of AAC users or on older individuals who are at the beginning stages of language learning, the generalizability of these findings is unclear. Nonetheless, it is reasonable to conclude that adult responsivity may play an equally important role in the language development of such individuals.

For this reason, focusing on increasing the responsivity of caregivers to learners' communicative attempts may need to be an additional priority when considering intervention with beginning communicators. Studies of young children with developmental disabilities and their caregivers show that it is possible to successfully increase caregiver responsivity in at least two ways. Responsive interaction programs have shown that adults can be trained to increase their use of language-facilitating responses to children's communicative acts (Girolametto, 1988; Girolametto et al., 1995, 1996; Wilcox et al., 1992, 1996). Yoder and Warren's PMT intervention demonstrated that prelinguistic children can be trained to increase the frequency and clarity of their intentional communication, thereby increasing the probability of triggering a natural increase in caregiver responsivity (Yoder & Warren, 1999a; 1999b). Further research is needed before either of these results can be generalized outside of the mother–child context (Yoder et al., 1998). In addition, their generalizability for caregivers of individuals who are not expected to use speech as their primary expressive mode is also unclear, as few studies have looked at increasing the responsivity of AAC users' caregivers (e.g., Light et al., 1992; McNaughton & Light, 1989) and no studies have examined the transactional effects of increasing the clarity and frequency of intentional communicative behavior by individuals with severe expressive impairments. Yet, given the studies that have shown that some AAC users may be at risk for not experiencing frequent, high-quality responses from caregivers (Basil, 1992; Houghton et al., 1987; Light et al., 1985; Rowland, 1990), continued research on facilitator training is warranted.

Although caregiver responsivity is an important component of intervention, it is insufficient, by itself, when attempting to facilitate communication and language outcomes (Tannock & Girolametto, 1992). Combining responsivity with focused input (e.g., Wilcox et al., 1992; 1996) or with milieu teaching techniques (Kouri & Wilcox, 1996; Yoder et al., 1995; Yoder & Warren, 1999a) appears to be more effective for helping young children with developmental disabilities acquire intentional communication and symbolic language skills than intervention based solely on older responsive interaction principles. Again, because none of these intervention approaches have been compared in studies with participants who have severe expressive impairments, generalizability is limited.

In spite of the caveats concerning generalizability, it is possible to derive several clinical implications from the research on adult contingent responsivity for facilitators who work with AAC users. For individuals who do not yet show evidence of intentional communication, intervention should focus primarily on the responsivity of the facilitator. Facilitators should be encouraged to develop student-led, responsive social routines in which nonsymbolic behaviors are recognized and responded to as intentional communication. For individuals who are just beginning to show evidence of intentional communication, intervention should have a dual emphasis. Increasing the frequency and clarity of the AAC user's nonsymbolic communication may subsequently elicit more frequent responding from caregivers across many of the individual's daily environments. In addition, directly training caregivers to verbally respond to the AAC user's focus of attention and to linguistically map the individual's communicative acts may help facilitate the development of an initial vocabulary.

For individuals who are making the transition from nonsymbolic communication to the comprehension and use of graphic symbols and manual signs for communication, the ability of facilitators to provide enough of the kinds of linguistic responses that are most facilitative for an initial vocabulary and multiword combinations depends heavily on the learner's ability to perform certain activities. These are 1) repair communication breakdowns, 2) frequently initiate communication with the new symbol system, 3) represent messages precisely given the graphic symbols or signs available, and 4) produce multiword combinations given the graphic symbols or signs available. In addition to targeting repair strategies early in intervention, facilitators of individuals who heavily rely on graphic symbols or manual signs to communicate may want to consider using intervention strategies that attempt to teach the simultaneous understanding and use of graphic symbols. Prompting or modeling techniques that help the learner visually attend to the graphic symbol while its referent is spoken (e.g., pointing or shining a penlight on the symbol) may play an important role in helping beginning communicators learn the meanings behind graphic symbols. VOCAs may play a similarly important role in facilitating symbol comprehension and use. Multiple, smaller graphic symbol displays that contain word-based vocabulary that is specific to particular environments and representative of a variety of grammatical categories may be preferable to sentence-based or noun-only symbol displays when the goals are the development of vocabulary and semantic relations. Manually signing the key words when responding contingently to a beginning manual user's message may highlight new signed vocabulary as well as the combination of signs.

Facilitator contingent responsivity has the potential to facilitate the communication and language development of learners with severe expressive impairments, whether they are preintentional, intentional but nonsymbolic, or making the transition to symbolic communication. The challenge for interventionists is clear: to provide learners with a sufficient amount of developmentally appropriate, responsive input by carefully responding to communicative behaviors that are not always clear or reflect the learner's struggle with acquiring fluency in the use of an artificial symbolic system. This is especially challenging when the symbol system itself is unable to fully represent the learner's communicative intent. It is hoped that both researchers and clinicians will continue to explore ways to meet this challenge.

REFERENCES

Adamson, L.B., Romski, M.A., Deffebach, K.P., & Sevcik, R.A. (1992). Symbol vocabulary and the focus of conversations: Augmenting language development for youth with mental retardation. *Journal of Speech and Hearing Research, 35,* 1333–1343.

Akhtar, N., Dunham, F., & Dunham, J. (1991). Directive interactions and early vocabulary development: The role of joint attentional focus. *Journal of Child Language, 18,* 41–50.

Alexander, D. (1994). *The emergence of repair strategies in chronologically and developmentally young children.* Unpublished dissertation, Florida State University, Tallahassee.

Basil, C. (1992). Social interaction and learned helplessness in severely disabled children. *Augmentative and Alternative Communication, 8,* 188–199.

Baumgart, D., Johnson, J., & Helmstetter, E. (1990). *Augmentative and alternative communication systems for persons with moderate and severe disabilities.* Baltimore: Paul H. Brookes Publishing Co.

Beukelman, D.R., & Mirenda, P. (1998). *Augmentative and alternative communication: Management of severe communication disorders in children and adults* (2nd ed.). Baltimore: Paul H. Brookes Publishing Co.

Blackstone, S.W. (1997, January–February). The intake's connected to the input. *Augmentative Communication News, 10*(1), 1–6.

Bondy, A., & Frost, L. (1994). The Picture Exchange Communication System. *Focus on Autistic Behavior, 9*(3), 1–19.

Bondy, A., & Peterson, S. (1990, May). *The point is not to point: Picture Exchange Communication System with young students with autism.* Paper presented at the annual meeting of the Association for Behavioral Analysis, Nashville.

Bornstein, M.H., & Tamis-LeMonda, C. (1989). Maternal responsiveness and cognitive development. In M. Bornstein (Ed.), *Maternal responsiveness: Characteristics and consequences* (pp. 49–62). San Francisco: Jossey-Bass.

Calculator, S., & Luchko, C. (1983). Evaluating the effectiveness of a communication board training program. *Journal of Speech and Hearing Disorders, 48,* 185–191.

Culp, D., & Carlisle, M. (1988). *PACT: Partners in augmentative communication training.* Tucson, AZ: Communication Skill Builders.

Edwards, S., Fletcher, P., Garman, M., Hughes, A., Letts, C., & Sinka, A. (1997). *Reynell Developmental Language Scales–Third Edition*. Windsor, England: NFER-Nelson.

Elder, P., & Goossens', C. (1994). *Engineering training environments for interactive augmentative communication: Strategies for adolescents and adults who are moderately/severely developmentally delayed*. Birmingham, AL: Southeast Augmentative Communication Conference Publications.

Farrar, M.J. (1990). Discourse and the acquisition of grammatical morphemes. *Journal of Child Language, 17*, 607–624.

Fey, M.J. (1986). *Language intervention with young children*. Austin, TX: PRO-ED.

Girolametto, L.E. (1988). Improving the social-conversational skills of developmentally delayed children: An intervention study. *Journal of Speech and Hearing Disorders, 53*, 156–167.

Girolametto, L.E., Pearce, P.S., & Weitzman, E. (1995). The effects of focused stimulation for promoting vocabulary in young children with delays: A pilot study. *Journal of Childhood Communication Development, 17*(2), 39–49.

Girolametto, L.E., Pearce, P.S., & Weitzman, E. (1996). Interactive focused stimulation for toddlers with expressive vocabulary delays. *Journal of Speech and Hearing Research, 39*, 1274–1283.

Golinkoff, R.M. (1983). Infant social cognition: Self, people, and objects. In L. Liben (Ed.), *Piaget and the foundations of knowledge* (pp. 179–196). Mahwah, NJ: Lawrence Erlbaum Associates.

Goossens', C., Crain, S., & Elder, P. (1992). *Engineering the preschool environment for interactive, symbolic communication*. Birmingham, AL: Southeast Augmentative Communication Conference Publications.

Halle, J., Marshall, A., & Spradlin, J. (1979). Time delay: A technique to increase language use and facilitate generalization in retarded children. *Journal of Applied Behavior Analysis, 12*, 431–439.

Halle, J.W. (1982). Teaching functional language to the handicapped: An integrative model of natural environment teaching techniques. *Journal of The Association for Persons with Severe Handicaps, 7*, 29–37.

Harris, S. (1994). *The relation of maternal style to the language development of children with Down Syndrome*. Unpublished doctoral dissertation, University of California at Los Angeles.

Hart, B., & Risley, T.R. (1995). *Meaningful differences in the everyday experience of young American children*. Baltimore: Paul H. Brookes Publishing Co.

Houghton, J., Bronicki, B., & Guess, D. (1987). Opportunities to express preferences and make choices among students with severe disabilities in classroom settings. *Journal of The Association for Persons with Severe Handicaps, 11*, 255–265.

Kaiser, A.P., Yoder, P.J., & Keetz, A. (1992). Evaluating milieu teaching. In S.F. Warren & J. Reichle (Series Eds. & Vol. Eds.), *Communication and language intervention series: Vol. 1. Causes and effects in communication and language intervention* (pp. 9–47). Baltimore: Paul H. Brookes Publishing Co.

Kim, K. (1996). *Maternal behavior related to prelinguistic intentional communication in young children with developmental delays*. Unpublished doctoral dissertation, Vanderbilt University, Nashville.

Kouri, T., & Wilcox, M. (1996). *Initial lexical training in prelinguistic children with developmental delays: A comparison of two intervention approaches*. Unpublished manuscript, Arizona State University, Tempe.

Lahey, M., & Bloom, L. (1977). Planning a first lexicon: Which words to teach first. *Journal of Speech and Hearing Disorders, 42*, 340–349.

Light, J., Collier, B., & Parnes, P. (1985). Communication interaction between young nonspeaking physically disabled children and their primary caregivers. *Augmentative and Alternative Communication, 1,* 74–133.

Light, J., Dattilo, J., English, J., Gutierrez, L., & Hartz, J. (1992). Introducing facilitators to support the communication of people who use augmentative communication systems. *Journal of Speech and Hearing Research, 35,* 865–875.

Light, J., McNaughton, D., & Parnes, P. (1994). *A protocol for the assessment of the communication interaction skills of nonspeaking severely handicapped adults and their facilitators.* Toronto, Canada: Sharing to Learn, Hugh MacMillan Rehabilitation Center.

Light, J.C., & Binger, C. (1998). *Building communicative competence with individuals who use augmentative and alternative communication.* Baltimore: Paul H. Brookes Publishing Co.

MacDonald, J.D. (1989). *Becoming partners with children: From play to conversation.* San Antonio, TX: Special Press.

Manolson, H.A. (1985). *It takes two to talk: A Hanen early language parent guide-book.* Toronto, Canada: Hanen Early Language Resource Centre.

Masur, E.F. (1982). Mothers' responses to infants' object-related gestures: Influences on lexical development. *Journal of Child Language, 9,* 23–30.

McCathren, R.B., Warren, S.F., & Yoder, P.J. (1996). Prelinguistic predictors of later language development. In S.F. Warren & J. Reichle (Series Eds.) & K.N. Cole, P.S. Dale, & D.J. Thal (Vol. Eds.), *Communication and language intervention series: Vol. 6. Assessment of communication and language* (pp. 57–75). Baltimore: Paul H. Brookes Publishing Co.

McDonald, E., & Schultz, A. (1973). Communication boards for cerebral palsied children. *Journal of Speech and Hearing Disorders, 38,* 73–88.

McNaughton, D., & Light, J. (1989). Teaching facilitators to support the communication skills of an adult with severe cognitive disabilities: A case study. *Augmentative and Alternative Communication, 5,* 35–41.

Mirenda, P., & Schuler, A.L. (1988). Augmenting communication for persons with autism: Issues and strategies. *Topics in Language Disorders, 9,* 24–43.

Nelson, K.E. (1989). Strategies for first language teaching. In M.L. Rice & R.L. Schiefelbusch (Eds.), *The teachability of language* (pp. 263–310). Baltimore: Paul H. Brookes Publishing Co.

Nelson, K.E., Denninger, M., Bonvillian, J.D., Kaplan, B.J., & Baker, N. (1984). Maternal input adjustments and nonadjustments as related to children's linguistic advances and to language acquisition theories. In A.D. Pellegrini & T.D. Yawkey (Eds.), *The development of oral and written languages: Readings in developmental and applied linguistics* (pp. 31–56). Stamford, CT: Ablex Publishing Corp.

Oregon Research Institute. (1989). *Getting in touch: Communicating with a child who is deaf-blind.* [Film]. Champaign, IL: Research Press.

Peterson, S.L., Bondy, A.S., Vincent, Y., & Finnegan, C.S. (1995). Effects of altering communicative input for students with autism and no speech: Two case studies. *Augmentative and Alternative Communication, 11,* 93–100.

Prizant, B.M. (1996). Brief report: Communication, language, social, and emotional development. *Journal of Autism and Developmental Disorder, 26*(2), 173–178.

Quill, K.A., (1995). Visually cued instruction for children with autism and pervasive developmental disorders. *Focus on Autistic Behavior, 10*(3), 10–20.

Reichle, J., Halle, J.W., & Drasgow, E. (1998). Implementing augmentative communication systems. In S.F. Warren & J. Reichle (Series Eds.) & A.M. Wetherby, S.F. Warren, & J. Reichle (Vol. Eds.), *Communication and language intervention series: Vol. 7. Transitions in prelinguistic communication* (pp. 417–436). Baltimore: Paul H. Brookes Publishing Co.

Reichle, J., York, J., & Sigafoos, J. (Eds.). (1991). *Implementing augmentative and alternative communication: Strategies for learners with severe disabilities*. Baltimore: Paul H. Brookes Publishing Co.

Riksen-Walraven, J.M. (1978). Effects of caregiver behavior on habituation and self-efficacy in infants. *International Journal of Behavioral Development, 1,* 105–130.

Romski, M.A., & Sevcik, R.A. (1992). Developing augmented language in children with severe mental retardation. In S.F. Warren & J. Reichle (Series Eds. & Vol. Eds.), *Communication and language intervention series: Vol. 1. Causes and effects in communication and language intervention* (pp. 113–130). Baltimore: Paul H. Brookes Publishing Co.

Romski, M.A., & Sevcik, R.A. (1993). Language learning through augmented means: The process and its products. In S.F. Warren & J. Reichle (Series Eds.) & A.P. Kaiser & D.B. Gray (Vol. Eds.), *Communication and language intervention series: Vol. 2. Enhancing children's communication: Research foundations for intervention* (pp. 85–104). Baltimore: Paul H. Brookes Publishing Co.

Romski, M.A., & Sevcik, R.A. (1996). *Breaking the speech barrier: Language development through augmented means*. Baltimore: Paul H. Brookes Publishing Co.

Romski, M.A., Sevcik, R.A., Robinson, B.F., & Bakeman, R. (1994). Adult-directed communications of youth using the system for augmenting language. *Journal of Speech and Hearing Research, 37,* 617–628.

Romski, M.A., Sevcik, R.A., & Wilkinson, K.M. (1994). Peer-directed communicative interactions of augmented language learners with mental retardation. *American Journal on Mental Retardation, 98,* 527–538.

Rowland, C. (1990). Communication in the classroom for children with dual sensory impairments: Studies of teacher and child behavior. *Augmentative and Alternative Communication, 6,* 262–274.

Rowland, C., & Schweigert, P. (1991). *The early communication process using microswitch technology.* Tucson, AZ: Communication Skill Builders.

Rowland, C., & Schweigert, P. (1992). Early communication and microtechnology: Instructional sequence and case studies of children with severe multiple disabilities. *Augmentative and Alternative Communication, 8,* 273–286.

Rowland, C., & Schweigert, P. (1993). Analyzing the communication environment to increase functional communication. *Journal of The Association for Persons with Severe Handicaps, 18,* 161–176.

Scherer, N.J., & Olswang, L.B. (1989). Using structured discourse as a language intervention technique with autistic children. *Journal of Speech and Hearing Disorders, 54,* 383–394.

Schlosser, R., Belfiore, P., Nigam, R., Blischak, D., & Hetzroni, O. (1995). The effects of speech output technology on the learning of graphic symbols. *Journal of Applied Behavior Analysis, 28,* 537–549.

Schwartz, I.S., Garfinkle, A.N., & Bauer, J. (1998). The Picture Exchange Communication System: Communicative outcomes for young children with disabilities. *Topics in Early Childhood Education, 18*(3), 144–159.

Sevcik, R.A., & Romski, M.A. (1997). Comprehension and language acquisition: Evidence from youth with severe cognitive disabilities. In L.B. Adamson & M.A. Romski (Eds.), *Communication and language acquisition: Discoveries from atypical language development* (pp. 187–202). Baltimore: Paul H. Brookes Publishing Co.

Siegel-Causey, E., & Guess, D. (1989). *Enhancing nonsymbolic communication interactions among learners with severe disabilities.* Baltimore: Paul H. Brookes Publishing Co.

Tannock, R., & Girolametto, L. (1992). Reassessing parent-focused language intervention programs. In S.F. Warren & J. Reichle (Series Eds. & Vol. Eds.), *Communication and language intervention series: Vol. 1. Causes and effects in communication and language intervention* (pp. 49–79). Baltimore: Paul H. Brookes Publishing Co.

Tomasello, M. (1988). The role of joint attention in early language development. *Language Sciences, 11,* 69–88.

Tomasello, M., & Farrar, M.J. (1986). Joint attention and early language. *Child Development, 57,* 1454–1463.

van den Boom, D.C. (1994). The influence of temperament and mothering on attachment and exploration: An experimental manipulation of sensitive responsiveness among lower-class mothers with irritable infants. *Child Development, 65,* 1457–1477.

Warren, S.F., & Kaiser, A. (1986). Incidental language teaching: A critical review. *Journal of Speech and Hearing Disorders, 51,* 291–299.

Warren, S.F., & Yoder, P.J. (1997). Emerging model of communication and language intervention. *Mental Retardation and Developmental Disabilities Research Reviews, 3,* 358–362.

Warren. S.F., & Yoder, P.J. (1998). Facilitating the transition from preintentional to intentional communication. In S.F. Warren & J. Reichle (Series Eds.) & A.M. Wetherby, S.F. Warren, & J. Reichle (Vol. Eds.), *Communication and language intervention series: Vol. 7. Transitions in prelinguistic communication* (pp. 365–384). Baltimore: Paul H. Brookes Publishing Co.

Warren, S.F., Yoder, P.J., Gazdag, G.E., Kim, K., & Jones, H.A. (1993). Facilitating prelinguistic communication skills in young children with developmental delay. *Journal of Speech and Hearing Research, 36,* 83–97.

Wetherby, A.M., Alexander, D.G., & Prizant, B.M. (1998). The ontogeny and role of repair strategies. In S.F. Warren & J. Reichle (Series Eds.) & A.M. Wetherby, S.F. Warren, & J. Reichle (Vol. Eds.), *Communication and language intervention series: Vol. 7. Transitions in prelinguistic communication* (pp. 135–159). Baltimore: Paul H. Brookes Publishing Co.

Wetherby, A.M., Cain, D.H., Yonclas, D.G., & Walker, V.G. (1988). Analysis of intentional communication of normal children from prelinguistic to the multiword stage. *Journal of Speech and Hearing Research, 31,* 240–252.

Wetherby, A.M., Reichle, J., & Pierce, P.L. (1998). The transition to symbolic communication. In S.F. Warren & J. Reichle (Series Eds.) & A.M. Wetherby, S.F. Warren, & J. Reichle (Vol. Eds.), *Communication and language intervention series: Vol. 7. Transitions in prelinguistic communication* (pp. 197–230). Baltimore: Paul H. Brookes Publishing Co.

Wetherby, A.M., Yonclas, D.G., & Bryan, A.A. (1989). Communicative profiles of handicapped preschool children: Implications for early identification. *Journal of Speech and Hearing Disorders, 54,* 148–158.

White, R.W. (1959). Motivation reconsidered: The concept of competence. *Psychological Review, 66,* 297–323.

Wilcox, M. (1993, November). *Issues regarding language readiness in young children with developmental disabilities.* Paper presented to the American Speech-Language-Hearing Association Annual Convention, Anaheim, CA.

Wilcox, M., Shannon, M., & Bacon, C. (1992, December). *From prelinguistic to linguistic behavior: Outcomes for young children with developmental disability.* Paper presented to the International Early Childhood Conference on Children with Special Needs, Washington, DC.

Wilcox, M., Shannon, M., & Bacon, C. (1996). *Longer-term outcomes of prelinguistic intervention.* Unpublished manuscript, Arizona State University, Tempe.

Wilcox, M.J. (1992). Enhancing initial communication skills in young children with developmental disabilities through partner programming. *Seminars in Speech and Hearing, 13,* 194–212.

Wilcox, M.J., & Shannon, M.S. (1998). Facilitating the transition from prelinguistic to linguistic communication. In S.F. Warren & J. Reichle (Series Eds.) & A.M. Wetherby, S.F. Warren, & J. Reichle (Vol. Eds.), *Communication and language interven-*

tion series: Vol. 7. Transitions in prelinguistic communication (pp. 385–416). Baltimore: Paul H. Brookes Publishing Co.

Wilkinson, K.M., Romski, M.A., & Sevcik, R.A. (1994). Emergence of visual-graphic symbol combinations by youth with moderate or severe mental retardation. *Journal of Speech and Hearing Research, 37,* 883–895.

Yoder, P.J., Kaiser, A.P., Alpert, C., & Fischer, R. (1993). The effect of following the child's lead on the efficiency of teaching nouns with preschoolers with mental retardation. *Journal of Speech and Hearing Research, 35,* 1–35.

Yoder, P.J., Kaiser, A.P., Goldstein, H., Alpert, C., Mousetis, L., Kaczmarek, L., & Fischer, R. (1995). An exploratory comparison of milieu teaching and responsive interaction in classroom applications. *Journal of Early Intervention, 19,* 218–242.

Yoder, P.J., & Munson, L. (1995). The social correlates of coordinated attention to adult and objects in mother–infant interaction. *First Language, 15,* 219–230.

Yoder, P.J., Spruytenburg, H., Edwards, A., & Davies, B. (1995). Effect of verbal routine contexts and expansions on gains in the mean length of utterance in children with developmental delays. *Language, Speech, and Hearing Services in the Schools, 26,* 21–32.

Yoder, P.J., & Warren, S.F. (1993). Can developmentally delayed children's language development be enhanced through prelinguistic intervention? In S.F. Warren & J. Reichle (Series Eds.) & A.P. Kaiser & D.B. Gray (Vol. Eds.), *Communication and language intervention series: Vol. 2. Enhancing children's communication: Research foundations for intervention* (pp. 35–62). Baltimore: Paul H. Brookes Publishing Co.

Yoder, P.J., & Warren, S.F. (1998). Maternal responsivity predicts the prelinguistic communication intervention that facilitates generalized intentional communication. *Journal of Speech, Language, and Hearing Research, 41,* 1207–1219.

Yoder, P.J., & Warren, S.F. (1999a). Facilitating self-initiated proto-declaratives and proto-imperatives in prelinguistic children with developmental disabilities. *Journal of Early Intervention, 22*(4), 337–354.

Yoder, P.J., & Warren, S.F. (1999b). Maternal responsivity mediates the relationship between prelinguistic intentional communication and later language. *Journal of Early Intervention, 22*(2), 126–136.

Yoder, P.J., Warren, S.F., Kim, K., & Gazdag, G. (1994). Facilitating prelinguistic communication in very young children with developmental disabilities II: Systematic replication and extension. *Journal of Speech and Hearing Research, 37,* 841–851.

Yoder, P.J., Warren, S.F., McCathren, R., & Leew, S.V. (1998). Does adult responsivity to child behavior facilitate communication development? In S.F. Warren & J. Reichle (Series Eds.) & A.M. Wetherby, S.F. Warren, & J. Reichle (Vol. Eds.), *Communication and language intervention series: Vol. 7. Transitions in prelinguistic communication* (pp. 39–58). Baltimore: Paul H. Brookes Publishing Co.

4

Replacing Socially Unacceptable Behavior with Acceptable Communication Responses

David P. Wacker, Wendy K. Berg, and Jay W. Harding

This chapter provides an overview of how communication responses can be used as functional alternatives to socially unacceptable behaviors such as self-injury or aggression. We suggest evaluating all behavior, regardless of form, relative to its impact on the environment. Thus, to replace one behavior (e.g., self-injury, aggression) with a second behavior (e.g., a communicative response), one must first identify the function of the unacceptable behavior. We begin this chapter by considering functional equivalence, or how a communicative response might be equivalent to or compete effectively with unacceptable behavior. This is followed by discussion of selecting an appropriate communicative response, then a description of how to identify the function(s) of unacceptable behavior. Finally, we describe how functional communication training can be conducted in home environments using augmentative and alternative communication (AAC) responses.

FUNCTIONALLY EQUIVALENT RESPONSES

The goal for functional communication training (FCT; Carr & Durand, 1985) is to replace an unacceptable behavior with an acceptable communicative response, which is referred to as a *mand* in this chapter. The unacceptable behavior is commonly viewed as being an aberrant response that simply needs to be suppressed or reduced. It is easy to assume that any gain in communication will reduce unacceptable behavior. Parents and other caregivers often conclude that if they teach their child to communicate, unacceptable behavior will no longer occur. Unfortunately, this is often not the case. Instead, the interventionist must ensure that the newly trained mand serves the same function as the unacceptable behavior. Thus, the relation between mands and unacceptable behavior is the key variable for effective intervention.

Functional equivalence (Carr, 1988) refers to the relation between responses. If two responses serve the same function, they are said to be equivalent. Although this is usually a necessary component for effective replacement of one response with another, often it is not sufficient. In addition to being equivalent in function, the replacement response must be as efficient; that is, it cannot require increased effort (Horner & Day, 1991). It must also have a greater probability of being reinforced than the response it is replacing. Table 4.1 summarizes these three essential components and lists them as steps to consider in selecting a replacement response. These items are discussed in detail in the following section.

It is hoped that following the steps in Table 4.1 will increase the distribution of responses in favor of the communicative response (i.e., bias responding). *Bias* means that the child chooses or displays the response that is acceptable to the interventionist more often than the unacceptable behavior. As discussed by Mace and Roberts (1993), all behavior can be considered a choice response. The child chooses to produce one response instead of any other response in his or her repertoire. In this case, the interventionist hopes to bias the choice made by the child to strongly favor the communicative response over the unacceptable behavior.

Table 4.1.   Steps for selecting an acceptable communicative response

Step	Description	Rationale
1. Identify the function(s) of the unacceptable behavior.	Conduct a functional analysis of the unacceptable behavior.	If the function is known, then a communication response that is functionally equivalent can be used to obtain the same reinforcers.
2. Ensure the efficiency of the communicative responses that compete with unacceptable behavior.	Select a communication response that is at least as efficient as the unacceptable behavior regarding 1) physical effort, 2) amount of reinforcement, and 3) delay to reinforcement (Horner & Day, 1991).	If the communication response requires substantially more effort, results in less reinforcement, or results in a greater delay to reinforcement than the unacceptable behavior, then the child may be motivated to continue to display the unacceptable behavior.
3. Evaluate the reinforcers provided for unacceptable behavior and communicative responses.	Eliminate or substantially reduce reinforcement for the unacceptable behavior and increase reinforcement for the communicative response.	If both responses result in the same amount or same probability of reinforcement, then both will likely continue to occur.

SELECTING AN ACCEPTABLE COMMUNICATIVE RESPONSE

In the following subsections, each step of Table 4.1 is described briefly. In addition, a rationale for each step is provided.

Step 1: Identify the Function(s) of Unacceptable Behavior

In Step 1 of Table 4.1, the choice is biased by determining that the communicative response does, in fact, obtain the same reinforcers as the unacceptable behavior. The most valid way to accomplish this step is to conduct a functional analysis (Iwata, Dorsey, Slifer, Bauman, & Richman, 1982/1994) to identify the events that reinforce socially unacceptable behavior. If the function of the unacceptable behavior is known, then one can eliminate or substantially reduce reinforcement for unacceptable behavior and provide it differentially for the communicative response. If the function is not known, then one must hope that the arbitrary reinforcers that are provided for the communicative response will compete effectively with the unknown reinforcers that maintain unacceptable behavior. Thus, identifying the function of unacceptable behavior is a critical component of FCT and, as recommended by Durand and Carr (1985), should always be the first intervention step.

Knowing the function of the behavior also can give care providers increased confidence that their FCT program will be successful. FCT is a type of differential reinforcement program and, like any other differential reinforcement program, will seldom be smooth or steady (Wacker & Reichle, 1993). Instead, fluctuations in behavior will occur over time (see Parrish & Roberts, 1993, for a description of covariation), and one may be tempted to discontinue the program. If, via a functional analysis, an interventionist is confident that he or she has identified the reinforcers that maintain behavior, then he or she will be more likely to make the necessary adjustments to the intervention program. The interventionist will also persist through the crises that are likely to occur rather than giving up on the program. Behaviors such as self-injury and aggression may seem to occur randomly for no functional reason. Knowing the function can be an invaluable aid for persisting with long-term treatment.

Step 2: Ensure the Efficiency of Communicative Responses that Compete with Unacceptable Behavior

An often overlooked factor, listed as Step 2 in Table 4.1, is the efficiency or response effort of the communicative response. As discussed by Horner and Day (1991), the communicative response must be as efficient or more efficient than the unacceptable behavior. Horner and Day demonstrated the importance of this variable by considering three dimensions of response efficiency: 1) physical effort, 2) schedule of reinforcement, and 3) delay between the display of the appropriate response and the presentation of the reinforcer. They showed that alternative behaviors did not replace problem behavior unless they were at least as efficient as the problem behavior in each of the previously listed areas. This was true even if the same reinforcer was used for both responses. As an example of the effects of delay, a young woman with autism and severe mental retardation was taught to hand to a care provider a work card with *break* written on it. This communicative response was functionally equivalent to aggression in that both responses resulted in brief breaks from nonpreferred tasks. The word card competed successfully with (i.e., replaced) aggression if the delay between touching the word card and receiving a break was 1 second but not if the delay was 20 seconds.

Sometimes a program that is initially successful will develop difficulties because of response efficiency. It may then seem that the child is tired of the program or that the program worked only briefly when, instead, the interventionist altered the program in seemingly minor or subtle ways. In our experience, variables that are related to efficiency, especially to the delay dimension of efficiency, often cause problems that develop in initially successful programs.

On a practical level, the selection of the communication response must be based on both the effort required by the child and the ongoing availability of reinforcement. Table 4.2 provides a comparison of signing PLEASE, touching a word card, pressing a microswitch, and engaging in aggression along these two dimensions of efficiency. If one assumes that hitting the care provider serves the function of gaining attention, then this behavior will occur during situations in which the care provider is not interacting with the child. Given this function and context, signing PLEASE matches well (i.e., competes effectively) in terms of effort (i.e., similar topography). Yet, it may result in longer

Table 4.2. Comparison of unacceptable and acceptable responses based on efficiency

Behavior	Effort of response	Delay to reinforcement
Aggression (hitting the care provider)	The child must approach the care provider and move his or her hand to the care provider's arm.	Minimal
Signing PLEASE	Less than aggression	Longer than aggression (must be observed)
Touching a word card	Less than aggression	Longer than aggression (must be observed)
Pressing a microswitch	Less than aggression	Same as aggression (gives an auditory cue to the care provider)

delays because the care provider will not always see the sign, such as when the care provider's back is toward the child. Touching a word card may take less effort, but it also may result in longer delays if it is not observed immediately. Pressing a microswitch with a prerecorded message also appears to take less effort and, because of the auditory output, may result in shorter delays for receiving attention. Although many variables need to be considered in establishing an alternative communicative response, an evaluation of efficiency in this situation would lead to strong consideration of the microswitch.

Step 3: Evaluate the Reinforcers Provided for Unacceptable Behavior and Communicative Responses

Step 3 of Table 4.1 involves the reinforcers provided for unacceptable behavior as well as to communicative (i.e., acceptable) responses. Especially during the initial sessions but also intermittently throughout intervention, the unacceptable behavior will co-occur or occur intermittently with the new communication response that is being taught. As an example, assume that the unacceptable behavior is aggression and the communicative response is pressing a microswitch. Both behaviors occur to gain attention. How the interventionist responds to the unacceptable behavior is likely to influence the child's bias toward choosing to press the microswitch rather than to use aggression. Table 4.3 provides various response options, which are listed as a continuum of functional effects. As shown in the table, a number of options are available for responding to hitting, but not all of these options are therapeutic. Procedure 1 (reprimand, redirect, or discuss) provides attention that is contingent on

Table 4.3. Functional consequences for aggression maintained by attention

Procedure	Functional description	Functional effect
1. Reprimand, redirect, or discuss	Attention that is contingent on hitting is provided.	Hitting is reinforced.
2. Reduce amount/quality of attention	Brief neutral attention is provided for hitting. The attention given for hitting is lower in quality and quantity than that provided for pressing the microswitch.	Reinforcement occurs, but the relative value and amount of reinforcement weakens the behavior.
3. Planned ignoring (extinction)	Hitting is ignored.	Reinforcement of hitting is eliminated.
4. Time-out (nonexclusionary)	The care provider looks away for a brief period of time (e.g., 30 seconds) whenever hitting occurs.	Reinforcement of hitting is eliminated, and a mild punisher is provided.

hitting. If the amount or quality of this attention is comparable to what is received for pressing the microswitch, then hitting would perhaps persist indefinitely. Thus, if the function of hitting is to gain attention and the child receives extended attention (even in the form of a reprimand), then the alternative communicative response may never replace aggression. This is especially true if the communicative response is not as efficient as hitting.

Fisher and colleagues (1993) and Wacker and colleagues (1990) showed that either extinction or mild punishment is usually required for FCT to have optimal effects. Combining extinction or mild punishment for unacceptable behavior with high amounts of attention for pressing a microswitch provides an ideal motivational context for displaying communication and suppressing unacceptable behavior. All motivation (reinforcement) is provided for the communicative response and is eliminated for hitting. Therefore, both procedures should be effective if they are implemented as part of an ongoing FCT program. The choice between extinction and time-out is based on two factors. First, time-out will likely produce quicker effects because it is more discriminable to the child (the care provider looks away, which signals the child that attention is no longer available) and because it is mildly aversive. Everything else being equal, a procedure that is mildly aversive will reduce the probability of behavior more quickly than simply ignoring the unacceptable behavior. Second, the care provider's preference is an important consideration. When care providers strongly prefer one option over the other, they are usually encouraged to choose the preferred option.

Some care providers find neither extinction nor mild punishment to be acceptable; in addition, some responses (e.g., life-threatening behavior) cannot be ignored. When one is forced to provide at least some attention that is contingent on the unacceptable behavior, the amount or quality of attention is reduced (see Procedure 2 in Table 4.3). With this procedure, reinforcement (in this case, attention) is provided for both the unacceptable behavior and pressing the microswitch, but the quality and quantity of attention is substantially greater for the communicative response. Peck and colleagues (1996) provided an example of this approach with young children with disabilities, some of whom displayed life-threatening behaviors (e.g., pulling on a central line that was inserted to provide nourishment). Following a functional analysis in which attention was identified as the reinforcer for one child, Peck and colleagues provided either 1 minute of high-quality reinforcement (playing enthusiastically with preferred toys) for communication or 10 seconds of low-quality reinforcement (neutral redirection) for life-threatening behavior. This approach was highly effective in teaching the child to communicate using a microswitch and in suppressing self-injury to zero or near-zero levels.

These results show that the relation between the consequences provided for unacceptable behavior and for a communicative response is just as important as the relationship between the behaviors. If one emphasizes the quality and quantity of reinforcement provided for a communicative response and either substantially reduces (Table 4.3, Procedure 2) or eliminates (Table 4.3, Procedures 3 and 4) reinforcement for unacceptable behavior, then one can increase the probability of successful intervention.

In summary, the relationship between the unacceptable and the acceptable behaviors as well as the reinforcers that are associated with each response are key to developing replacement behaviors. One must first ensure that the behaviors serve the same function and then bias responding in favor of the communicative response by focusing on efficiency and on the amount and quality of reinforcement. Because the first critical step is ensuring functional equivalency, the following section discusses the specific procedures used for identifying the social-communicative functions of behaviors.

ASSESSING THE
SOCIAL-COMMUNICATIVE FUNCTIONS OF BEHAVIORS

Unacceptable behaviors such as self-injury, aggression, and property destruction often limit an individual's participation in community-based leisure, vocational, and educational activities. Yet, unacceptable behaviors may be functional for the individual because they result in desired changes in his or her immediate environment. For example, throwing a hairbrush may result in a break from grooming if the person is given time to calm down or the activity is terminated. If brushing one's hair is a nonpreferred activity, then throwing the hairbrush may be an effective means for ending that activity. As another example, head banging may result in a change from less preferred to more preferred activities. Head banging may serve as a signal to care providers that an individual is ready to change activities. In both of these examples, the behavior is socially unacceptable, but it is also functional because it results in a predictable reaction by care providers and leads to specific changes in the person's immediate environment. A problem behavior that is used to affect the actions of others is social even though the behavior is unacceptable. If one is able to understand why the behavior occurs, then it is also communicative.

Sometimes, unacceptable behavior occurs because something about the behavior or the sensation provided by the behavior is reinforcing. In these cases, the unacceptable behavior is not maintained by changes in the external environment but appears to be maintained by internal events. Behavior is said to serve an automatic function (Goh et al., 1995) in such instances. Fortunately, the majority of children display unacceptable behaviors that are social (Wacker et al., 1998), and these unacceptable behaviors can be replaced with acceptable communicative responses. In this chapter, therefore, we focus on behavior that serves a social-communicative function.

The goal of assessment is to identify the function of unacceptable behavior for a given individual. This is accomplished by identifying the environmental events that set the occasion for unacceptable behavior and the events that reinforce (i.e., increase) the occurrence of the behavior. Based on the results of the assessment, an alternative behavior (i.e., a mand) is selected that will have the same effects on the environment and that can serve as a replacement response for the unacceptable behavior. This goal is accomplished through a two-step process of assessment, which consists of descriptive assessment and functional analysis.

Descriptive Assessment

Descriptive assessment procedures are used to outline a child's specific behaviors of concern. During the descriptive assessment, the assessor attempts to identify the specific behaviors that are occurring, the frequency with which they occur, and the antecedents and consequences that are associated with each behavior. Three procedures are used to collect this information.

Parent Interview / Survey   The descriptive assessment typically begins with a detailed interview or survey with parents or other care providers who have extensive contact with the child. Within the interview/survey, parents are asked to describe the specific behaviors of concern and to indicate the severity of each behavior. They are then asked to describe the child's daily schedule during a typical week. Finally, parents are asked to describe any interventions that they have used in the past and to indicate each intervention's effectiveness in reducing the unacceptable behavior.

Daily Behavior Log   After the specific behaviors of concern have been clarified, parents are asked to keep track of each behavior occurrence on a daily behavior log for 1 week. The behavior log provides a space for each hour of the day to record any unacceptable behavior. By comparing the occurrence of unacceptable behavior on the daily behavior log with the child's daily schedule, one can often observe patterns of responding. For example, one may notice that most severe problem behavior occurred during the hour preceding each meal.

A-B-C Assessment   An antecedent-behavior-consequence (A-B-C) assessment (Bijou, Peterson, & Ault, 1968) provides information that is useful in developing hypotheses about the function of behavior. The A-B-C assessment is used to identify the environmental events that occur immediately prior to the behavior and the events that immediately follow the behavior. The events that occur immediately before or are concurrent with the unacceptable behavior may serve as establishing operations (Michael, 1982) for the unacceptable behavior. *Establishing operations* are events that temporarily increase or decrease the value of a reinforcer and affect the frequency of behaviors that are associated with obtaining the reinforcer. Using the example of problem behavior that occurs most frequently within the hour before meals, one might hypothesize that the child was hungry and that food deprivation served as an establishing operation for problem behavior. The A-B-C assessment can be used to gather information to either confirm or refute initial hypotheses. For example, if the assessment revealed that a parent was occupied with preparing the meal during the time that the problem behavior occurred, one might hypothesize that deprivation of parental attention, in addition to food deprivation, served as an establishing operation for problem behavior.

Events that occur immediately following the behavior are the consequences of the behavior, regardless of whether the events are intended as consequences, and may either reinforce or punish the behavior. In the previous example, the assessment might reveal that the problem behavior resulted in the parent bringing the child a small snack. In this situation, the consequence resulted in the child's receiving attention and food; thus, both hypotheses appeared to be logical interpretations of the effects of the environment on the child's behavior. In other words, the results of the A-B-C assessment suggested that problem behavior could have served an attention function (the child gains parent attention) or tangible function (the child gains food). Although this assessment is useful for developing hypotheses regarding the influence of environmental events on behavior, it does not provide a direct test of those hypotheses.

Functional Analysis

Conducting a functional behavior analysis is the most direct and effective method to test hypotheses regarding the function of behavior (Iwata et al., 1982/1994). A functional analysis consists of a series of analogue conditions in which the antecedent (i.e., establishing operations) and consequences to behavior are systematically manipulated, and the effect of both on behavior is compared across sessions. Functional analyses provide tests for four hypotheses: 1) The behavior occurs to escape an activity, situation, or person (negative reinforcement); 2) the behavior occurs to gain attention (positive reinforcement); 3) the behavior occurs to gain tangible items or activities (positive reinforcement); and 4) the behavior is not influenced by environmental events and occurs because something about the behavior itself is reinforcing (automatic reinforcement). Before any hypothesis is tested, however, a control condition must be established.

Control Condition   Typically, functional analyses begin with a control condition. None of the establishing operations that are often associated with problem behavior are present, and the events that are hypothesized to reinforce and maintain problem behavior are provided noncontingently. The control condition is most often a free-play situation and usually consists of noncontingent social attention, unlimited access to preferred play materials, and no task demands. No or minimal unacceptable behavior is expected to occur in the free-play condition because the establishing operations for the most likely functions (escape, attention, tangibles) for problem behavior are not present; thus, there is no motivation to engage in problem behavior that serves a social function. The free-play condition is interspersed with the remaining assessment conditions to bring behavior under control as needed and to demonstrate experimental control over the behavior during the evaluation. *Experimental control* refers to predicting when (under what assessment conditions) problem behavior will or will not occur. This type of control is needed for the assessor to have confidence in the assessment results.

Escape Condition   The contingent escape condition evaluates the effectiveness of escaping a nonpreferred activity or situation as a reinforcer for unacceptable behavior. During this condition, the care provider presents a series of task requests to the child (e.g., "Put the blocks into the container"). Any occurrence of unacceptable behavior results in the immediate removal of the task materials, and the child is told that he or she can take a brief break (e.g., 30 seconds) from the task. When the allotted break period has expired, the task requests are immediately presented.

Attention Condition   The contingent attention condition is conducted to evaluate the role of attention as a reinforcer for problem behavior. In this condition, the child is left alone on one side of the room while the care provider engages in an alternative activity in a separate area of the room. The care provider ignores the child until the child engages in the unacceptable behavior. Each time the child displays the unacceptable behavior, the care provider immediately approaches the child and provides brief social attention (e.g., "Blocks are for stacking, not throwing," "Use gentle touches"). The care provider then returns to his or her alternative activity until another instance of unacceptable behavior occurs.

Tangible Condition   During the tangible condition, a preferred item such as a blanket or a toy is removed from the play area and the child is given other items with which to play. If the child engages in the unacceptable behavior, the preferred item is returned to the child for a brief period (e.g., 30 seconds). After the time has elapsed, the preferred item is removed.

By comparing the frequency of occurrence of the unacceptable behavior across assessment conditions, the examiner can determine which consequences reinforced (i.e., increased) the frequency of the unacceptable behavior. After the consequences that reinforce the unacceptable behavior are identified, an alternative behavior can be taught that will result in the same consequence and can serve as a replacement for the unacceptable behavior.

Summary of Assessing the Social Functions of Behaviors

Durand and Carr (1985) described FCT as a two-step process: 1) assessing the function of unacceptable behaviors and 2) replacing those unacceptable behaviors with communicative responses. The blending of descriptive assessment and functional analysis provides a direct and efficient approach to identifying the reinforcers that maintain unacceptable behavior. Descriptive assessments help one to formulate hypotheses about the social functions of unacceptable behavior, and functional analyses provide a direct test of those hypotheses. As discussed previously, the information that is provided by assessment is necessary to design effective FCT programs. Knowing the function of unacceptable behavior permits one to eliminate the reinforcers for unacceptable behavior or to restrict the value or amount of reinforcement that is received relative to communicative responses. One reason some FCT programs fail is that the function of unacceptable behavior is not identified correctly. Although it is certainly tempting to skip the assessment and go directly to FCT, this may actually lead to a much longer intervention because one does not know why the unacceptable behavior occurs or how to reinforce the desired communicative responses.

In the next section, we describe the process of conducting FCT in home environments. We discuss the steps to completing the intervention and provide further reasons why augmentative communication procedures may help to foster generalization as well as initial positive outcomes. We end the section by describing FCT for a specific individual over a 2-year period.

IMPLEMENTING FUNCTIONAL COMMUNICATION TRAINING IN HOME ENVIRONMENTS

We have conducted two federally funded research projects (Wacker & Berg, 1992a, 1992b) that have evaluated the use of functional analysis and functional communication training in home and classroom environments. Participants in these studies were families with young children (ages 1–8 years) with developmental disabilities who engaged in severe problem behavior (e.g., self-injury, aggression). The children's primary care providers (usually parents) conducted all assessment and treatment procedures in the child's home or other community environment (e.g., school) with coaching from our staff during weekly visits. The children were diverse across multiple characteristics, including estimated cognitive functioning, communication skills, medical diagnoses, and topographies of unacceptable behavior (Wacker et al., 1998). Although the children represented a diverse group, they were similar in that it was necessary to identify the function of the unacceptable behavior before we could effectively implement a treatment program for each child.

Components of Functional Communication Training

For each child in the studies, the intervention process included an assessment of the social function of the unacceptable behavior, followed by FCT. Table 4.4 provides an outline of the FCT procedures. Assessing the social function of the unacceptable behavior (Step 1) enabled us to select an appropriate communicative response that could serve as a replacement response. The contingencies that had reinforced the unacceptable behavior then were provided contingent on the selected communicative response (Step 2) and were withheld when the unacceptable behavior occurred (Step 3). After the child began to display the communicative response and unacceptable behavior decreased, additional attention and preferred activities were provided to reinforce other appropriate behaviors that occurred along with the communicative response (Step 4). As the child's repertoire of alternative social behaviors expanded, the care provider had increased opportunities to reinforce the occurrence of these emerging appropriate behaviors (Step 4) across multiple situations (Step 5). The following section provides a description of how we implement these steps in home environments.

Step 1: Assess the Social Function of Unacceptable Behavior   Our approach to FCT in home environments is to provide the care provider with a very structured program that is based on the function of the problem behavior. As discussed in the previous section, the first step in this process is to

Table 4.4.   Components of functional communication training (FCT)

Component	Purpose
1. Assess the social function of unacceptable behavior.	Identify events that reinforce unacceptable behavior.
2. Provide the identified reinforcer contingent on a selected acceptable communicative response.	Replace unacceptable behavior with a functionally equivalent communicative response.
3. Reduce or eliminate reinforcement for unacceptable behavior.	Remove the motivation to engage in the unacceptable behavior and bias responding to the acceptable communicative response.
4. Reinforce associated prosocial behaviors (promote response generalization).	Increase the occurrence of other appropriate behaviors that may be functionally equivalent to the unacceptable behavior.
5. Promote stimulus generalization.	Increase the likelihood that the child will choose the communicative response across novel tasks, people, and environments.

identify the events that reinforce the occurrence of the unacceptable behavior. This is accomplished through the previously described descriptive assessment and functional analysis procedures.

Step 2: Provide Reinforcement for the Communicative Response

After we identify the events that reinforce the unacceptable behavior, delivery of the reinforcer can be made contingent on an acceptable communicative response. Thus, the second component of this program is to identify a mand that is at least as efficient as the problem behavior. In selecting an initial response for training, we must consider each child's current motor and sensory capabilities and his or her ability to discriminate when to perform the response. Stated simply, we want the parents to teach their child a system of what to do and when to do it. Given these objectives, we typically combine distinct auditory and visual cues during FCT to make the relationship between the new communication response and the delivery of reinforcement as clear as possible. For example, when teaching a child to say "play" to gain parent attention, we ask the parent to present a picture card along with a verbal prompt. In this situation, the card serves as an additional cue that attention is now available and will be provided when the child says "play." Thus, the card signals both what to say and when to say it.

The choice of which communicative system to use is based on a number of factors including the child's skills, parent preferences, and response efficiency. We have used a variety of communicative systems successfully and, when possible, defer to the judgment of the child's IEP team. Yet, we usually suggest that a visual cue such as a picture, word card, or microswitch be used in conjunction with signing or speaking to provide visual cues to the child and to make requests as clear as possible to the person responding to the request. For example, a child who engages in problem behavior to escape nonpreferred activities may need to learn how to appropriately ask for a break. In this case, we provide the parent with two picture cards that represent *work* or *play*. The work card is always paired with a designated task that the child needs to complete (e.g., picking up toys). The play card is always paired with preferred toys or activities. Initially, the child is given a choice between work and play and is physically guided to touch the card to indicate his or her selection. Initially, we often prefer to use a simple touch response because it usually requires less physical prompting. Even if the child speaks, we frequently use pictures because it is not possible to physically prompt a child to say "play." Nevertheless, children with vocal or signing repertoires often independently incorporate these responses and we, of course, enthusiastically provide reinforcement when they are displayed.

As the children become successful at indicating their choices (e.g., a desire to play), they are required to do a small amount of work before being given an opportunity to choose the play activity. At this time, the parent presents the play card and asks the child, "Do you want to do more work or play?" If the child selects the play card, he or she is allowed to take a break from the work activity. Following a brief play break, the child is given the work card and is required to complete another small amount of work. As the child demonstrates proficiency at completing work and requesting breaks appropriately, the amount of work that needs to be completed during each trial can be increased gradually until a desired criterion is reached. In this manner, the child learns both to complete parent requests in a timely fashion and to discriminate when the communication response will result in reinforcement (i.e., when a choice is offered).

A second option is to increase the delay between when a break is requested and when it is provided (i.e., develop increased tolerance for delays to reinforcement). We increase the delays by providing a visual signal (e.g., raising an index finger), saying that we will soon take a break, and then waiting to provide the break for increasing lengths of time. Usually, we begin with no delay or very quick delays and then increase those delays by 10–30 seconds after several sessions of appropriate waiting.

When increasing the amount of work and the length of delay, it is important to make increases very gradually over time. If increases are too large, unacceptable behaviors may occur because of inefficiency. Some children have difficulty increasing the amount of work they complete or the delay to reinforcement without displaying unacceptable behavior. In these cases, the use of extinction or mild punishment may be warranted to progress more quickly in the intervention. With mild punishment, for example, unacceptable behavior results in the loss of reinforcers and the return to the work task; thus, motivation to engage in the unacceptable behavior is reduced.

In general, a number of features make word/picture cards useful tools in FCT programs that are designed to reduce unacceptable behaviors. First, they can be individualized to maximize the child's recognition of the desired response. Modifications include the use of printed words, line-drawn symbols, or photographs. Second, for many children, they are a convenient and portable method of communicating simple requests. For instance, a child can simply point to a specific card or present the card to a care provider. Third, cards can be designed so that the message is easily recognizable to others, thus increasing the likelihood that the child will receive reinforcement for communicating appropriately across a variety of people in community environments. We have found that this form of communication is highly effective in community environments, such as restaurants, where listeners have limited experience with other AAC systems (Berg et al., 1990).

Although word/picture cards are often effective, an auditory signal for reinforcement may be needed or desired in some situations. For example, if the care provider is not looking at the child, then the delivery of attention for an appropriate visual signal may be delayed. Children with physical disabilities may experience difficulties in either manipulating or transporting cards to request reinforcement but may be able to use a microswitch effectively. Therefore, when the function of behavior is to gain attention and the child is not mobile, we often use microswitches rather than cards.

In our in-home FCT programs, we often incorporate a simple microswitch recording device. Our preferred device is one that can be programmed to replay a selected message each time it is touched. There are several advantages to using this type of microswitch. First, this message can be individualized and is easily changed across difference contexts (e.g., "Let's play," "Please come here"). Second, it provides auditory feedback to the child about the appropriate message that is needed to obtain reinforcement. Third, it can be used to signal a care provider who may not be in a position to receive a message visually.

Step 3: Reduce or Eliminate Reinforcement for Unacceptable Behavior   During the initial implementation of FCT, some children may display "bursts" of problem behavior instead of using the new communicative response (Lerman, Iwata, & Wallace, 1999). This is understandable if one considers that the unacceptable behavior, in comparison to newly trained communicative behaviors, has a longer history of reinforcement and have resulted in a richer schedule of reinforcement. Thus, the third basic component of FCT is for parents to either reduce or eliminate reinforcement for the occurrence of unacceptable behavior. This point is illustrated with Kristen, for whom a microswitch was used within an FCT program.

Kristen was a 3-year-old girl with mental retardation who engaged in self-injurious behaviors (e.g., hair pulling, face scratching). A functional analysis showed that these behaviors were maintained by her mother's attention. Kristen had minimal speech but could independently sign MOM. We wanted Kristen to continue to develop her sign language; yet, we also wanted to teach her an alternative response that was incompatible with her self-injurious behavior, easy to perform motorically, and effective in getting her mother's attention. Given these criteria, we selected a microswitch that, when pressed, played the message, "Mom, come play with me." During FCT, Kristen's mother presented the switch, prompted Kristen to touch the switch, and provided enthusiastic praise and attention as soon as Kristen activated the switch. In this case, the microswitch was a clearly discriminable cue that signaled the availability of attention. It required little motor effort and was an effective way for Kristen to gain her mother's attention, particularly in situations in which her mother might not have noticed Kristen signing (e.g., while preparing dinner).

In Kristen's program, her mother reduced reinforcement for self-injury by neutrally blocking Kristen's attempts to pull her hair or scratch her face without providing any additional attention (e.g., no discussion or eye contact). After Kristen stopped attempting to engage in self-injury for about 15 seconds, her mother prompted her to touch the microswitch and then played enthusi-astically with Kristen for 1–2 minutes. Thus, a delay between self-injury and a prompt to touch the microswitch was built into the intervention. This delay was necessary to prevent Kristen from pairing self-injury with pressing the mi-croswitch. This approach was successful in teaching Kristen to use the mi-croswitch instead of engaging in self-injury to gain her mother's attention.

Step 4: Reinforce Associated Prosocial Behaviors   Kristen's program illustrates the components of differential reinforcement that form the basis of FCT. For FCT to have lasting effects, however, it is important to expand the child's repertoire of prosocial behaviors beyond the performance of a single mand. *Response generalization* refers to increases in other behaviors that occur when a specific behavior is targeted for reinforcement. For example, provid-ing reinforcement for using a specific form of communication may occasion a variety of other prosocial behaviors, such as smiling, vocalizations, and ap-propriate play behavior. If these prosocial behaviors are also reinforced by the parent, then it is likely that they will continue to occur and provide opportu-nities for positive reciprocal interactions between the child and the parent (Derby et al., 1997). Thus, FCT can be used to increase a large variety of prosocial behaviors (i.e., produce response generalization) that are not speci-fically targeted during intervention. These behaviors are referred to as *collat-eral behaviors*.

Derby and colleagues (1997) evaluated the long-term effects of FCT on unacceptable behavior, manding, and collateral behavior (e.g., social and toy play) with 4 young children with developmental disabilities. A functional analysis was conducted and parents were taught to implement an FCT pro-gram in which the identified reinforcer for problem behavior was provided for a specific mand. The results of this study showed that long-term decreases in problem behavior were correlated with increases in both appropriate social and toy play behaviors. As discussed by Derby and colleagues, the ongoing suppression of problem behavior may occur because of the increased avail-ability for reinforcement across multiple social behaviors. The results of our re-search (Wacker et al., 1998) showed that most children displayed increases in appropriate collateral behavior in addition to reductions in aberrant behavior. Therefore, as problem behavior decreases, parents have more opportunities to interact in positive ways with their children. This as a distinct advantage of FCT.

Peck, Derby, Harding, Weddle, and Barretto (in press) used an example to describe this type of improvement. They studied changes in parent beha-vior during FCT with a 5-year-old boy named Cal. Cal had been diagnosed with pervasive developmental disorder and moderate mental retardation, and he engaged in aggression and property destruction. Cal displayed no vocal language but could sign a few words independently. The results of a functional analysis showed that Cal's problem behavior was maintained primarily by escape from his parents' requests. During FCT, Cal was required to follow his parents' instructions in completing a variety of academic tasks (e.g., sorting objects by color and shape). After Cal had completed several requests, he was prompted to touch a *done* card to receive a break from his work and to obtain his parents' attention and preferred toys. The results showed that decreases in Cal's problem behavior covaried inversely with increases in appropriate social behaviors such as laughing, toy play, and physical affection. With respect to parent behaviors, reductions in Cal's problem behaviors covaried directly with decreases in parent reprimands, response blocking, and guided compliance. Thus, as Cal's behavior improved, his parents spent less time managing problem behavior and more time engaging in mutually reinforcing interactions.

Step 5: Promote Stimulus Generalization   Another important component of FCT is promoting generalization of appropriate communication from an initial training context to other situations that are associated with problem behavior. Wacker and Berg (1996) assessed the occurrence of unacceptable behavior across multiple tasks (e.g., dressing, meals, academic activities), people (e.g., parents, teachers, respite providers), and environments (e.g., home, school, relatives' homes) in childrens' communities. Following a functional analysis, parents conducted FCT in a selected context, for example, picking up toys (task) with Mom (person) at home (environment). After their child demonstrated a reduction in unacceptable behavior of 80% of the time or more, the investigators observed the child's behavior across other contexts associated with unacceptable behavior. Overall, the children in the study displayed substantial reductions in unacceptable behavior across multiple problem situations following FCT.

The use of augmentative communication devices, such as picture cards or microswitches, may enhance generalization because their presence signals the availability of reinforcement across contexts. As mentioned previously, in FCT programs, the child needs to learn both how to communicate in an appropriate way and when (i.e., in which situations) to use the communication response. The presence of a picture card or microswitch provides the child with a signal that a trained response (e.g., touching the picture card) is likely to result in reinforcement. Thus, a child who learns to communicate with these types of devices may, with little or no additional training, continue to use the devices across a variety of untrained contexts.

Vignette: Rob

The following example (see Wacker, Berg, & Harding, 1999) provides an illustration of how each of these intervention steps can contribute to the successful long-term treatment of challenging behavior. Rob was 4 years old and had been diagnosed with fragile X syndrome, pervasive developmental disorder, and mental retardation. Problem behaviors included self-injury (e.g., head slapping, finger biting), aggression, and property destruction. Rob was able to say a few words but rarely used these words in a meaningful context. A functional analysis conducted in Rob's home indicated that both parent attention and escape from nonpreferred activities, depending on the context, maintained Rob's problem behaviors. Thus, Rob wanted his parents to watch him play but did not want them to place any demands on him.

Rob's parents conducted an FCT program on a daily basis. Components of this program included the following:

- Providing Rob with specific instructions on how to complete designated tasks
- Prompting Rob to touch a card that represents *help* if he needed assistance
- Providing praise for appropriate communication and task completion
- Providing access to preferred activities and parent attention contingent on task completion
- Using guided compliance if Rob refused to complete the task request

We used the help card as the mand because it resulted in both attention and reduced demands, the two functions that were maintaining the problem behaviors. This program was conducted across two activities. The first activity was Rob's working one to one with his mother on academic tasks such as identifying numbers, shapes, and letters. The second activity was picking up toys. Training sessions were also conducted across different home environments (e.g., kitchen, living room) and at different times of the day to further promote stimulus generalization. Thus, Rob received numerous opportunities to request assistance appropriately and to receive reinforcement (e.g., praise, access to attention and toys) contingent on appropriate communication and social collateral behaviors.

The results of Rob's FCT program with academic tasks are shown in Figure 4.1. This graph shows the percentage of 6-second intervals of problem, social, and manding behavior and the percentage of independent task completion that occurred during each training session over a 2-year period. A 6-second partial-interval recording system was used to record the occurrence of problem, social, and manding behavior during each session. In this procedure, each session was divided into 6-second intervals. A behavior was scored if it occurred at any time within a 6-second interval. The percentage of occurrence for each behavior was calculated by dividing the number of intervals in which the behavior occurred by the total number of intervals within a session. The percentage of independent task completion for each session was evaluated via an event-recording system. In this procedure, task completion for each parent request was scored as being completed independently if guided compliance was not required. The percentage of independent task completion was calculated by dividing the number of task requests that were completed independently by the total number of task requests that were made within the session.

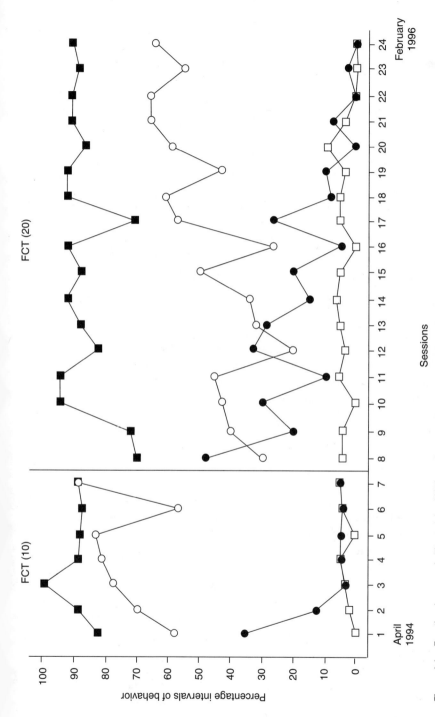

Figure 4.1. Functional communication training (FCT) conducted for Rob over a 2-year period on academic demands. Percentage of intervals of social behavior, problem behavior, targeted mand, and percentage of independent task completion during treatment probes. (Key: ■ = the percentage of independent task completion; ○ = the percentage of intervals of social behavior; ● = the percentage of intervals of problem behavior; □ = the percentage of intervals of the targeted mand ["help"].)

During the initial phase of treatment (see the left panel of Figure 4.1), Rob was required to complete 10 parent requests to identify letters, shapes, or numbers. During initial training sessions, Rob displayed high percentages of problem behavior. Yet, the occurrence of problem behavior quickly decreased and covaried with increases in appropriate social behavior. He also displayed high levels of independent task completion. Rob's success led us to increase the amount of work (e.g., identifying 20 letters; see right panel of Figure 4.1) to approximate the academic demands that were required in his preschool. With these increased demands, problem behaviors reoccurred but decreased over time and covaried with increases in both appropriate social behaviors and in independent task completion. These results are typical of the outcomes we have observed with FCT that is conducted in home environments (Wacker et al., 1998).

In summary, Rob's training program exemplifies how multiple components may contribute to intervention success. First, Rob's communicative response ("help") addressed both of the functions (attention and escape) that were identified as maintaining unacceptable behavior (i.e., they were functionally equivalent). The word *help* enabled Rob to gain parent attention and assistance in completing a nonpreferred task, thereby reducing his demands. Second, Rob's parents gave him attention for appropriate behaviors (e.g., talking, task completion); thus, Rob received reinforcement for a variety of prosocial behaviors (i.e., response generalization) in addition to receiving reinforcement for the mand. Finally, Rob's parents conducted FCT across contexts (e.g., two tasks, two environments) so that Rob learned how to request assistance in different situations (i.e., stimulus generalization).

Overall, the FCT program that was used with Rob and other children in our projects follow a general set of rules:

1. Do not continue to reinforce unacceptable behavior.
2. Make sure that the alternative communicative response (i.e., the mand) is more efficient than the unacceptable behavior.
3. Specifically train the child to use the desired mand with prompting and differential reinforcement procedures.
4. Train communication responses that will be understood and reinforced by others.
5. Reinforce prosocial behaviors that are correlated with the mand.
6. Increase the amount of work or the length of delay before reinforcement.

IMPLICATIONS FOR FUTURE RESEARCH

As discussed previously, FCT is a two-step process; the first step involves assessment of the function of unacceptable behavior and the second step involves the replacement of unacceptable responses with mands. The first generation of studies published in the literature documented the merits of this two-step approach to intervention (e.g., Carr & Durand, 1985; Wacker et al., 1990). In considering the types of studies that are needed in the future, we might be best served by categorizing these studies based on the steps listed above. Thus, studies that refine or extend the assessment procedures are categorized separately from those that extend the training techniques as part of intervention procedures.

Assessment Procedures

The majority of functional analyses that have been conducted to date have focused specifically on the effect of the presentation of a single contingency on the display of a specific response. This approach to assessment was needed in order to show how mands might replace socially unacceptable behavior. That relationship has been established, and now assessment of more complex relationships is needed. For example, the evaluation of response hierarchies (Lalli, Mace, Wohn, & Livezey, 1995) has received recent attention by applied behavior analysts. *Response hierarchies* refers to the sequences in which behavior occurs. If, for example, screaming always preceded aggression, that would be an important relationship to note in a functional analysis. To demonstrate this relationship, the functional analysis would need to provide reinforcement differentially to screaming only (aggression should not occur) and then to aggression only (both screaming and aggression should occur, because screaming always occurs before aggression). If reinforcement was provided for the display of either response, then only screaming would occur, and one might not identify that screaming and aggression occurred in a two-step sequence.

Substantial work is being conducted on assessing the antecedents, in addition to the consequences, that are related to unacceptable behavior (Luiselli & Cameron, 1998). As part of this research, biological variables such as sleep (Kennedy & Meyer, 1996; O'Reilly, 1995) are being studied. To more precisely match intervention to the results of assessment, greater emphasis on antecedents as well as on consequences is now necessary.

Research is particularly needed in the area of establishing operations (Michael, 1982). As noted by Iwata, Pace, and colleagues (1994), the results of a functional analysis can be influenced by events that immediately precede any given assessment condition. When preceding events alter the value or effectiveness of the reinforcer being tested, this is referred to as an *establishing operation*. As one example, assume that when 5 minutes of free play precedes the functional analysis attention condition, the child is willing to play alone. Yet, if the child is ignored for several minutes just prior to the attention condition, he or she will engage in unacceptable behavior to gain attention. In this case, the presence of continuous attention (free play) decreased the reinforcing value of attention because of satiation. Thus, if a free-play condition always preceded the attention condition in a functional analysis, then one would fail to identify that attention was a reinforcer for unacceptable responses.

Intervention Procedures

The majority of studies have evaluated FCT when a single social function has been identified. For cases in which two social functions have been identified, the most common procedures has been to train two different mands to be used in different social contexts. Therefore, if unacceptable behavior is shown to be maintained by both attention and escape from demands, it is most common to teach the child to request some version of *play* when ignored and *break* when provided with demands. The efficacy of this approach is depicted in figures that show occurrences of *play* in ignore contexts, *break* in demand contexts, and unacceptable behavior in both.

Future studies need to take an additional step and show the conditional probability that the child will emit the relevant mand in the relevant context. Thus, in addition to the previously described data, the *irrelevant* mand should also be depicted. Brown and colleagues (2000) provided an example of the approach to analyzing intervention programs. For every child in their study, Brown and colleagues showed graphs depicting the occurrence of both relevant and irrelevant mands across social contexts. Showing the results in this manner clarified that the children not only had replaced unacceptable responses with mands but also had discriminated when (i.e., in which contexts) to display those mands.

Very few studies have evaluated how to select the mand that is used to replace unacceptable behavior. As discussed previously in this chapter, Horner and Day (1991) showed that the efficiency of the mand in relation to unacceptable behavior is an important variable. It is reasonable to infer that other variables that are related to the mand may be just as important. For example, the use of preexisting versus novel mands might be studied. Assume that a child often shakes his or her head "no" when engaging in aggression to escape a demand. On the one hand, it makes sense to reinforce this mand because the child obviously knows how and when to display this response. On the other hand, "no" may have a very long history of being paired and being reinforced with aggression. Thus, the child may have difficulty discriminating "no" from aggression.

These two examples of future research in both assessment and intervention are simply that: examples. Although the results of FCT have been very impressive, the exact procedures for assessing and training replacement behavior are not yet known.

CONCLUSION

Identifying the events that reinforce unacceptable behavior is the first step in replacing unacceptable behavior with an appropriate communicative response. When one knows the reinforcer for unacceptable behavior, one can arrange the contingencies in the child's environment so that the relevant reinforcer is made available only when the child displays the desired behaviors and the reinforcer is withheld when unacceptable behavior occurs. To further ensure that the child selects the appropriate communication response rather than engages in unacceptable behavior, one biases responding by selecting a communication response that will result in 1) a larger amount of the reinforcer, 2) a qualitatively better variation of the reinforcer, or 3) more immediate access to the reinforcer than what was achieved through engagement in unacceptable behavior. By providing reinforcement for socially desirable behaviors that occur within the context of the acceptable communicative response, one strengthens a broad repertoire of appropriate behaviors that can serve as additional replacement responses. Finally, one can further increase the likelihood that the child will select the appropriate communicative response by conducting FCT across a variety of contexts and with different care providers.

REFERENCES

Berg, W.K., Wacker, D.P., McMahon, C., Ebbers, B., Henryson, K., & Clyde, C. (1990). Visual cues as a means to direct the behavior of others in community settings. *National Forum of Special Education, 1,* 26–43.

Bijou, S.W., Peterson, R.F., & Ault, M.H. (1968). A method to integrate descriptive and experimental field studies at the level of data and empirical concepts. *Journal of Applied Behavior Analysis, 1,* 175–191.

Brown, K.A., Wacker, D.P., Derby, K.M., Peck, S.M., Richman, D.M., Sasso, G.M., Knutson, C.L., & Harding, J.W. (2000). Evaluating the effects of functional communication training in the presence and absence of establishing operations. *Journal of Applied Behavior Analysis, 33,* 53–71.

Carr, E.G. (1988). Functional equivalence as a mechanism of response generalization. In R.H. Horner, G. Dunlap, & R.L. Koegel (Eds.), *Generalization and maintenance: Lifestyle changes in applied settings* (pp. 221–241). Baltimore: Paul H. Brookes Publishing Co.

Carr, E.G., & Durand, V.M. (1985). Reducing behavior problems through functional communication training. *Journal of Applied Behavior Analysis, 18,* 111–126.

Derby, K.M., Wacker, D.P., Berg, W., DeRaad, A., Ulrich, S., Asmus, J., Harding, J., Prouty, A., & Laffey, P. (1997). The long-term effects of functional communication training in a home setting. *Journal of Applied Behavior Analysis, 30,* 507–531.

Durand, V.M., & Carr, E.G. (1985). Self-injurious behavior: Motivating conditions and guidelines for treatment. *School Psychology Review, 14,* 171–176.

Fisher, W., Piazza, C., Cataldo, M., Harrell, R., Jefferson, G., & Conner, R. (1993). Functional communication training with and without extinction and punishment. *Journal of Applied Behavior Analysis, 26,* 23–36.

Goh, H.L., Iwata, B.A., DeLeon, I.G., Lerman, D.C., Ulrich, S.M., & Smith, R.G. (1995). An analysis of the reinforcing properties of hand mouthing. *Journal of Applied Behavior Analysis, 28,* 269–283.

Horner, R., & Day, M. (1991). The effects of response efficiency on functionally equivalent competing behaviors. *Journal of Applied Behavior Analysis, 24,* 719–732.

Iwata, B.A., Dorsey, M.F., Slifer, K.J., Bauman, K.E., & Richman, G.S. (1982/1994).

Toward a functional analysis of self-injury. *Journal of Applied Behavior Analysis, 27,* 197–209.

Iwata, B.A., Pace, G.M., Dorsey, M.F., Zarcone, J.R., Vollmer, T.R., Smith, R.G., Rodgers, T.A., Lerman, D.C., Shore, B.A., Mazaleski, J.L., Goh, H.-L., Cowdery, G.E., Kalsher, M.J., McCosh, K.C., & Willis, K.D. (1994). The functions of self-injurious behavior: An experimental-epidemiological analysis. *Journal of Applied Behavior Analysis, 27,* 215–240.

Kennedy, C.H., & Meyer, K.A. (1996). Sleep deprivation, allergy symptoms, and negatively reinforced problem behavior. *Journal of Applied Behavior Analysis, 29,* 133–135.

Lalli, J.S., Mace, F.C., Wohn, T., & Livezey, K. (1995). Identification and modification of a response-class hierarchy. *Journal of Applied Behavior Analysis, 28,* 551–559.

Lerman, D.C., Iwata, B.A., & Wallace, M.D. (1999). Side effects of extinction: Prevalence of bursting and aggression during the treatment of self-injurious behavior. *Journal of Applied Behavior Analysis, 32,* 1–8.

Luiselli, J.K., & Cameron, M.J. (Eds.). (1998). *Antecedent control: Innovative approaches to behavioral support.* Baltimore: Paul H. Brookes Publishing Co.

Mace, F.C., & Roberts, M.L. (1993). Factors affecting selection of behavioral interventions. In S.F. Warren & J. Reichle (Series Eds.) & J. Reichle & D.P. Wacker (Vol. Eds.), *Communication and language intervention series: Vol. 3. Communicative alternatives to challenging behavior: Integrating functional assessment and intervention strategies* (pp. 113–133). Baltimore: Paul H. Brookes Publishing Co.

Michael, J. (1982). Distinguishing between the discriminative and motivational functions of stimuli. *Journal of Experimental Analysis of Behavior, 37,* 149–155.

O'Reilly, M.F. (1995). Functional analysis and treatment of escape-maintained aggression correlated with sleep deprivation. *Journal of Applied Behavior Analysis, 28,* 225–226.

Parrish, J.M., & Roberts, M.L. (1993). Interventions based on covariation of desired and inappropriate behavior. In S.F. Warren & J. Reichle (Series Eds.) & J. Reichle & D.P. Wacker (Vol. Eds.), *Communication and language intervention series: Vol. 3. Communicative alternatives to challenging behavior: Integrating functional assessment and intervention strategies* (pp. 135–173). Baltimore: Paul H. Brookes Publishing Co.

Peck, S.M., Derby, K.M., Harding, J., Weddle, T., & Barretto, A. (in press). Behavioral support with parents of school-aged children with developmental disabilities and problem behavior. In J. Lucyshyn, G. Dunlap, & R. Albin (Eds.), *Families and positive behavioral support: Addressing the challenge of problem behavior in family contexts.*

Peck, S.M., Wacker, D.P., Berg, W.K., Cooper, L.J., Brown, K.A., Richman, D., McComas, J.J., Frischmeyer, P., & Millard, T. (1996). Choice-making treatment of young children's severe behavior problems. *Journal of Applied Behavior Analysis, 29,* 263–290.

Wacker, D.P., & Berg, W.K. (1992a). *Functional analysis of feeding and interaction disorders with young children who are profoundly disabled.* Washington, DC: Department of Education, National Institute on Disability and Rehabilitation Research.

Wacker, D.P., & Berg, W.K. (1992b). *Inducing reciprocal parent/child interactions.* Washington, DC: Department of Health and Human Services, National Institute of Child Health and Human Development.

Wacker, D.P., & Berg, W.K. (1996). *Promoting stimulus generalization with young children.* Washington, DC: Department of Health and Human Services, National Institute of Child Health and Human Development.

Wacker, D.P., Berg, W.K., & Harding, J. (1999). Mental retardation. In R.T. Ammerman, M. Hersen, & C.G. Last (Eds.), *Handbook of prescriptive treatments for children and adolescents* (2nd ed., pp. 31–47). Needham Heights, MA: Allyn & Bacon.

Wacker, D.P., Berg, W.K., Harding, J.W., Derby, K.M., Asmus, J.M., & Healy, A. (1998). Evaluation and long-term treatment of aberrant behavior displayed by young children with disabilities. *Journal of Developmental and Behavioral Pediatrics, 19,* 26–32.

Wacker, D.P., & Reichle, J. (1993). Functional communication training as an intervention for problem behavior: An overview and introduction to our edited volume. In S.F. Warren & J. Reichle (Series Eds.) & J. Reichle & D.P. Wacker (Vol. Eds.), *Communication and language intervention series: Vol. 3. Communicative alternatives to challenging behavior: Integrating functional assessment and intervention strategies* (pp. 1–8). Baltimore: Paul H. Brookes Publishing Co.

Wacker, D.P., Steege, M.W., Northup, J., Sasso, G., Berg, W., Reimers, T., Cooper, L., Cigrand, K., & Donn, L. (1990). A component analysis of functional communication training across three topographies of severe behavior problems. *Journal of Applied Behavior Analysis, 23,* 417–429.

5

Strengthening Communicative Behaviors for Gaining Access to Desired Items and Activities

Jeff Sigafoos and Pat Mirenda

The purpose of this chapter is to describe exemplary strategies for strengthening communication skills that enable individuals to gain and maintain access to desired objects and activities—that is, to make choices among or request access to preferred items or activities. We acknowledge that requesting can also be used to escape and avoid, as occurs when someone requests a break from a nonpreferred task (see Chapter 6). In addition, requesting skills are often used to gain information, such as when a person asks for the time of day or asks whether an approaching bus is going downtown. This chapter describes strategies to identify and strengthen existing, acceptable behaviors that individuals may already use to gain access to desired objects and activities, as well as procedures for teaching new symbolic communication skills. When attempting to strengthen existing behaviors and teach communicative behaviors, it is important to ensure that an individual's communication behaviors are contextually and pragmatically appropriate. Therefore, this chapter includes a discussion of strategies that can be used to select initial communication behaviors for instruction and promote appropriate use of communication skills across a range of typical environments and activities. This chapter primarily focuses on strategies that are relevant to individuals with severe communication impairments who are at the beginning stages of augmentative and alternative communication (AAC) intervention.

REQUESTING AS A PRIORITY IN EARLY AAC INTERVENTION

This chapter presents the view that requesting is an important instructional priority for many beginning communicators during the early stages of AAC intervention. Effective requesting skills provide a means to gain and maintain access to preferred items and activities. Some individuals may not have socially acceptable ways to gain access to preferred items or activities, and they may learn to engage in challenging behaviors such as aggression or self-injury in order to do so (Durand, 1993b). Thus, individuals with severe communication impairments often require systematic instruction to strengthen appropriate forms of requesting. In this context, *systematic instruction* refers to arranging a history of experiences in which beginning communicators are successful in gaining access to desired objects and activities by using appropriate communication. Systematic instruction does not imply highly structured environments or materials. Instead, exemplary practice incorporates systematic instructional strategies into typical daily routines so that communication skills are acquired in real-life situations with a variety of communicative partners (Sigafoos, Kerr, Roberts, & Couzens, 1994).

What Is Requesting?

The term *requesting* refers to a range of communicative acts. Some types function primarily to enable individuals to gain or maintain access to desired items and activities. These types of responses can be viewed as examples of requests (Skinner, 1957), which are communicative responses that specify their reinforcement. In pragmatic terms, requests serve an important communicative function in their own right. Yet, this pragmatic conceptualization is complicated by the fact that requests can function in many ways. For example, a request may be used to indicate rejection, such as when a person requests an alternative item in order to avoid or reject a nonpreferred item. As noted previously, requests can also be used to escape or avoid events or to gain information. Nonetheless, when the goal of intervention is to teach skills that enable the individual to gain and maintain access to desired items and activities, the term *requesting* captures the function or purpose of the communicative act.

In this chapter, requesting is viewed as a reciprocal social-communicative interaction. A request occurs or recurs because, in the past, it has been followed by access to desired objects and activities and, for whatever reason, an individual is motivated to gain access to an object or activity. Thus, a typical requesting interaction involves at least two components. First, there must be an individual who is motivated to gain access to a particular object or activity but who cannot do so without the assistance or mediation of another. Second, there must be a second person (the communicative partner) who is inclined to mediate the request and assist the individual to gain access to the requested item or activity. Consider a few examples of requesting that are relevant to individuals with severe communication impairments who are at the beginning stages of AAC interventions:

1. Tom is a young adult with multiple disabilities who uses a wheelchair and is learning to use a spelling board. Each week Tom and his support worker

go shopping for groceries. During these trips, Tom often needs to indicate his choices to the support worker. For example, as the pair enters the fruits and vegetables aisle, Tom stops his motorized wheelchair, scans the array of produce, and gestures towards a stack of apples. Upon seeing this, the support worker assists Tom to open his communication board and spell APPLES. The support worker then asks, "How many?" Tom responds by spelling out FOUR. By using his spelling board, Tom was able to clarify the precise meaning of his initial gesture.

2. Four-year-old Sara, who has a developmental delay and has not yet begun to speak, is struggling to open a backpack that contains her coloring book and crayons. After she has made several attempts to unzip the bag, her father approaches and waits to see if Sara will request help by using one of the manual signs that she is being taught at preschool. After waiting about 15 seconds, her father thinks Sara may need a prompt and so he asks, "Do you need help?" Sara proceeds to make a reasonably good approximation of the manual sign OPEN. Delighted that Sara has made an attempt to sign, her father acknowledges the sign by saying, "Okay, you want it open," physically guides her hands and arms to repeat the sign with proper articulation, and opens the bag for Sara.

3. During a school physical education class, a small group of students is playing basketball. Molly, an 11-year-old girl with autism, stands on the sidelines and begins to vocalize. One of the students asks his peers whether they think Molly wants to join the fun. They all agree that she does, so the first student approaches Molly, invites her to join the game, and passes her the ball. Molly catches the ball, smiles, and laughs, then passes the ball to another student.

Each of these three examples illustrates strategies that may function to strengthen communication skills. As shown in the examples, some strategies focus on making use of the individual's existing behaviors whereas others focus on replacing, augmenting, or expanding an individual's communicative repertoire to develop more effective and efficient ways to gain and maintain access to desired objects and activities. For example, Tom currently relies on pointing and reaching to indicate what he wants. Although these actions generally serve him well, there are some situations—such as when numerous items are present—when it is difficult to determine the referent of Tom's gestures. Thus, together with his support workers, Tom has decided to learn to use a spelling board to clarify his initial requests when necessary. In the second example, Sara is learning to use manual signs because she has not developed speech. Although efforts to teach her speech are continuing, manual signs are being taught as well to provide Sara with an augmentative mode of functional communication. In the final vignette, Molly has never acquired speech, but she often vocalizes when she wants something. People who know Molly well, in-

Table 5.1. Examples of beginning communication skills that are related to requesting

Communicative function	Example
Request an object	Sign I WANT A DRINK
Request access to an activity	Point to the swing while on the playground
Give affirmation	Sign ME when offered a turn
Request more	Ask for more when given a small piece of cake
Request continuation	Ask for another turn at the video game
Request alternative	Select symbol for *cracker* when offered a cookie
Request action or assistance	Request help in opening a package of snacks

cluding her peers at school, can usually figure out from the context exactly what she wants. Nevertheless, Molly's parents and teachers are beginning to realize that Molly needs to supplement her existing vocalizations with gestures or pictures so that she can make specific requests that will allow her to communicate more effectively with unfamiliar people. As these vignettes illustrate, there are various types of requests and various modes of requesting. Some of these are outlined in Table 5.1.

A Continuum of Requesting

A number of elements are essential to the success of interventions designed to teach individuals to gain and maintain access to preferred items or activities. *Success,* of course, is a relative term when it comes to teaching communication skills and may depend on the type of requesting skill targeted for instruction. Requesting behavior can be conceptualized as occurring on a continuum that is defined by the necessary amount of partner support and the task's memory requirements. Table 5.2 summarizes one version of this continuum, which arranges formats for requesting from those that are easier to those that are more difficult in terms of the demands that are placed on the beginning communicator.

In attempting to apply the continuum shown in Table 5.2, it may be difficult to assess the necessary amount of partner support. Some partners may consistently provide verbal and gestural cues to prompt requests from beginning communicators, but this does not necessarily imply that such supports are required. In some cases, it may be the partner, rather than the beginning communicator, who is prompt dependent.

In addition, it may be difficult to assess the memory requirements of the task. To gain some understanding of the individual's short-term memory, interventionists could complete an assessment by using a delayed match-to-sample task (Brady & McLean, 1996; Lane & Critchfield, 1998). This involves presenting a sample stimulus (e.g., a cup), then presenting corresponding choices (e.g., pictures of a cup, spoon, and fork). When the individual is able to consistently select the picture that matches the sample, short-term memory

Table 5.2. Continuum of formats for requesting

Type of choice/ request	Necessary amount of partner support	Memory requirements		Initiation/ knowledge demands
		Array	Example	
Elicited (offered) choice	Partner initiates ("What do you want?") and offers two or more explicit choice options	Array of two or more explicit options	Alfred's teacher offers him a red crayon and a blue crayon; asks "Which one do you want?"	No demands for either initiation or independent knowledge of available options
Elicited request	Partner initiates ("What do you want?") and AAC user makes request	No explicit array available	Ronnie's classmate asks him what he wants to do at recess; Ronnie signs for SWING.	No demands for initiation; demands independent knowledge of available options
User-initiated request, offered choice	AAC user initiates generic request ("want") and partner offers two or more explicit choice options	Array of two or more explicit options	Jordan approaches his mother with a *want* symbol; she offers a cracker and an apple; asks, "Which one do you want?"	Demands initiation but access to array is supported and requires no memory of the available options
User-initiated request, independent choice from array	AAC user initiates and makes choice without partner support	Array of two or more explicit options	Alisha scans a catalog, selects the blouse she wants to order, and points it out to her roommate.	Demands initiation and the ability to independently gain access to information about available options from array
User-initiated request	AAC user initiates and makes request without partner support	No explicit array available	Jared approaches a clerk and points to his *help* symbol to ask for assistance in getting a desired item from a high shelf.	Demands initiation and memory of available options

is assessed by inserting a delay between the sample and the availability of the picture choices. For example, the sample may be presented for 3 seconds and then removed. The picture choices are then brought into view after 5-, 10-, 20-, 30-, and 60-second delays. In this way, interventionists might gain some insight into the type of requesting task that best matches the individual's ability to remember the sample.

Furthermore, it must be emphasized that there is no direct empirical evidence in support of the continuum that is outlined in Table 5.2. Yet, there is considerable research that supports the logic underlying it. For example, both elicited (i.e., offered) choices and elicited requests, which do not require initiation on the part of beginning communicators, appear first on the continuum. This placement is based on research that suggests that learning to initiate communication is quite difficult for many beginning communicators (Carter, Hotchkis, & Cassar, 1996; Halle, 1987). The remaining three formats are arranged according to the extent to which the available options require independent performance and place demands on short-term memory (Light & Lindsay, 1991). There appears to be a strong relationship between short-term memory and intellectual disability such that the more profound the intellectual disability, the more limited the short-term memory capacity (e.g., Evans & Bilsky, 1979; Siegel & Linder, 1984). Hence, requests that simply require an individual to choose an item from an array (e.g., make an offered choice or an independent choice from an array; see Table 5.2) can be thought of as having lower memory requirements than those that require the individual to retrieve a symbol from memory (e.g., a user-initiated request with no array; see Table 5.2). We emphasize that an individual's ability to make one type of request in a specific context does not guarantee his or her ability to make a different type of request in a different context. Thus, exemplary strategies for teaching requesting must consider a number of important variables, depending on the type of request and context. These are reviewed in detail in the next section of this chapter.

Using General-Case Instruction to Promote Appropriate Requesting

Strategies to ensure the appropriate use of newly acquired communication skills can be integrated into the early stages of intervention by using general-case instructional strategies (DePaepe, Reichle, & O'Neill, 1993). In the general-case approach, the instructional universe—that is, the full range of teaching contexts—is described and teaching opportunities are identified to systematically sample the range of variation within the instructional universe. Consider the communication skill of requesting access to preferred leisure activities. In this case, the instructional universe might consist of all environments in which leisure activities typically occur. Thus, the specific environments and conditions that are identified for teaching purposes might include the school playground during recess, the backyard at home in the afternoon, the local gymnasium in the evenings, and the local park on the weekends. An intervention that is designed to teach an individual to request preferred leisure activities in each of these four environments is more likely to promote generalized use of the newly acquired communication skill than an intervention that is implemented in only one of these environments.

Teaching Self-Initiation General-case instruction can also be used to facilitate generalization across interpersonal contexts. As is the case for environments and conditions, there are a number of interpersonal contexts under which a particular communication skill may be appropriate, and instructional opportunities should systematically sample the range of such contexts. For example, an adolescent may be taught to request access to preferred activities when offered a number of activity-related items (e.g., a swimsuit, a Frisbee) and asked, "Which one do you want?" Nevertheless, teaching the individual to make a choice in this context may not ensure that he or she will be able to make a choice when asked "What do you want to do?" without the accompanying items. In addition, the individual may not learn to initiate choices if instruction only occurs when his or her teacher provides a discrete and explicit opportunity. When a partner always initiates opportunities, a beginning communicator is placed in the role of respondent and, as a consequence, may not learn how to self-initiate communication. Thus, instruction may need to occur in a variety of contexts that are selected to encourage both elicited and self-initiated communication. For example, a child could be taught to initiate a request to gain access to a desired leisure activity when other children are playing or when play items are inaccessible, not just when the teacher asks, "What do you want to play with?"

Sigafoos (1995) examined whether individuals who had been taught to respond to partner-provided opportunities would begin to initiate communicative requests in the absence of specific cues. The study involved Jim and Fred, two adults with severe disabilities who were taught to gain access to preferred objects by producing the corresponding manual signs. During the initial intervention phase, a communicative partner initiated all instructional opportunities by removing a preferred item from a container and offering it to the adult. Within this interpersonal context, both of the beginning communicators quickly learned to request preferred items. Subsequently, probes were conducted to determine if Jim and Fred initiated requests when the partner did not offer a preferred item. Results from the probes revealed that Jim initiated requests in this condition but Fred did not. Thus, additional strategies were implemented in an attempt to promote more self-initiated use of Fred's request response. Before offering an item, the partner progressed through a sequence of increasingly explicit cues (e.g., place the container in view, open the container, and remove an item). Over time, Fred began to initiate requests as the partner began to remove an item from the container rather than only when the item was offered directly to him. These data suggest that some individuals (such as Jim) who are taught to respond to opportunities initiated by a communicative partner may learn to produce more self-initiated requests when given opportunities to do so. Yet, other individuals (such as Fred) may require additional interventions to promote such self-initiated requesting.

Requesting versus Helping Oneself   Another issue that fits within the discussion of general-case instruction is the distinction between using communication to mediate access to preferred items or activities versus independently gaining access to items or activities. Because of the reciprocal interaction involved, communicative requesting is a more indirect way of gaining and maintaining access to desired items and activities. Requesting is different from helping oneself. There are many times and occasions when getting what one wants requires intervention by another person, such as when a desired item is out of reach or otherwise inaccessible. Nonetheless, there are other times when it is more appropriate and acceptable to help oneself, such as when a desired item is within easy reach. The environment and the context often dictate the most efficient strategy. Lim, Browder, and Sigafoos (1998) explored this issue in a study involving three students with severe disabilities. Each child was observed when trying to gain access to preferred snack items. Sometimes the snack items were in easy-to-open packages and the children simply helped themselves. In terms of effort, this was the most efficient way of gaining access to the preferred items. At other times, however, the packages were closed with twist ties that the children could not undo without assistance. The children quickly learned to request help in opening the tied packages by using various AAC techniques.

Assessment of conditional use of newly acquired communication skills may enable interventionists to identify individuals who will need explicit instruction to learn to help themselves and use a communicative request discriminatively. In Sigafoos (1998), 6-year-old Larry, who had autism and a severe communication impairment, was taught to request access to preferred objects (e.g., picture books, toys, snacks) by pointing to the graphic symbol for *want*. As is typical of interventions that aim to establish an initial requesting skill, instruction occurred only when the desired items were inaccessible. In this case, the items were visible but placed out of reach. After Larry learned to point to the *want* symbol to request the items, an assessment was conducted to determine what he would do when these same items were within easy reach. Even though the items were easily within his grasp, Larry continued to request the items during about 40% of the opportunities. Additional intervention strategies were implemented to teach Larry the discrimination between when to request and when to help himself. Specifically, opportunities in which the items were out of reach were alternated with opportunities in which items were within reach. Larry was prompted to request in the former condition but to simply reach out and take the desired item under the latter condition. In this way, Larry learned when to request and when to help himself.

This example illustrates the value of conducting assessments during intervention to assess the appropriate use of the targeted communication skills. Assessments have rarely been incorporated into AAC interventions. As a result, it is often unclear whether interventions have resulted in the appropriate conditional use of newly acquired communication skills. When such assessment data indicate problems with conditional use, as was the case with Larry, efforts to teach conditional discriminations may be required.

What Motivates Individuals to Make Requests?

A number of variables are likely to motivate individuals to request objects, activities, or specific actions from others. One of these variables is deprivation. For the purposes of this chapter, *deprivation* refers to the increased reinforcement value of items or activities that have not been available for some period of time. For example, if a person has not had anything to eat or drink for 3 hours, that person would most likely be considered somewhat deprived and, thus, highly motivated to request food and drink. Of course, deprivation is a relative condition that, no doubt, is influenced by context and preference. Although a person may not be especially thirsty or hungry, he or she might nonetheless indulge when offered food or drink at a party.

Another variable that may motivate an individual to request is the presentation of an aversive stimulus. In this context, an aversive stimulus is simply an item or activity that the individual does not prefer. A person may be motivated to request an alternative when confronted with a nonpreferred object or activity. For example, when offered a bunch of green bananas at the produce stand, most people would be motivated to request an alternative (e.g., "Do you have any ripe bananas?"). Communication skills that enable individuals to escape or avoid objects, attention, or activities are considered separately in Chapter 6.

Preference is a third variable that may motivate an individual to communicate in an attempt to gain and maintain access to items or activities. Along with context, deprivation also interacts with preference to influence the motivation to request. For example, if an item is not preferred, an individual is unlikely to be motivated to request that item even when deprived. Yet, a severe state of deprivation (e.g., extreme thirst) may motivate the individual to accept a beverage that is ordinarily nonpreferred, especially if that beverage happens to be the only option available. In contrast, when an object is highly preferred, an individual may remain highly motivated to request even when deprivation is low (e.g., there always seems to be room for one more potato chip, no matter how many have just been consumed).

When beginning to teach communication behaviors that result in access to desired objects or activities, it is important to ensure that the individual is motivated to make the request. The motivation to request can be created by arranging for a relative state of deprivation and by offering preferred objects and activities. To do so effectively obviously requires that some initial effort be devoted to identifying individual preferences and arranging the environment to create the need for communication. Both of these issues deserve further discussion.

Identifying Individual Preferences   A number of effective procedures have been developed to identify preferences in people who are unable to communicate their wants and needs symbolically (Lohrmann-O'Rourke & Browder, 1998). For individuals who can directly indicate a choice in some way (e.g., reaching for or looking at one of two available items), preferences can be assessed in the context of a choice-making activity. Parsons and Reid (1990) described a typical preference assessment. Their study focused on assessing preferences for foods and beverages among adolescents and adults with developmental disabilities and pervasive support needs. The individuals were presented with pairs of food items (e.g., applesauce and pudding, a banana and corn chips) and asked to select one of the two items. In most cases, and usually after only 20–30 such pairings, individual preferences for one of the items in each pair tended to emerge. *Preference* in this case was defined as consistent selection of one item over the other. Similar arrangements have been used to assess choice making and to identify preferences among children who have developmental and physical disabilities and are in the beginning stages of communication (Sigafoos, Laurie, & Pennell, 1995; Windsor, Piché, & Locke, 1994).

In assessments such as those described previously, it is assumed that items that are selected more frequently are preferred over items that are selected less frequently. Additional evidence shows that this assumption is often correct. Items that are selected more frequently from a pair tend to act as reinforcers for that individual (Paclawskyj & Vollmer, 1995; Piazza, Fisher, Hagopian, Bowman, & Toole, 1996). This means that frequently selected items can often be assumed to be preferred and will represent items that the individual is likely to be motivated to request. Because choice and preference may be influenced by numerous other factors and may change over time, however, it is also important to systematically reassess preferences on a regular basis (Fisher, Piazza, Bowman, & Amari, 1996). Indeed, we have found it useful to incorporate "mini" preference assessments prior to and even during communication intervention. From our experiences, shifting and fleeting preferences are more the rule than the exception. It is therefore critical to incorporate regular preference assessments into interventions that aim to strengthen communicative behaviors for gaining access to desired item and activities. If an item or activity is not desired or preferred, then it is unlikely that an individual will be motivated to request it unless the need for requesting is created in some other way.

Arranging the Environment to Create the Need for Requesting
Creating the need for requesting is often an important component when implementing AAC with beginning communicators (Sigafoos, 1999). The goal in creating the need for communication is to ensure the availability of an adequate number of motivating instructional opportunities. Opportunities should be created in ways that are relevant to the individual and that occur as naturally as possible. A number of empirically validated naturalistic strategies, which are designed to enhance motivation by creating the need for requesting, have been developed under the rubric of incidental teaching procedures (Beukelman & Mirenda, 1998). These strategies are summarized in Table 5.3.

The strategies outlined in Table 5.3 have been used as the context for teaching new forms of communication that enable the individual to gain and

Table 5.3. Description of naturalistic strategies to create the need for communication

Strategy	Description
Time delay	Preferred items or activities are present but access is delayed until a request occurs. For example, a toy is placed on the table but access to it is delayed for 10 seconds. This delay creates an opportunity for the individual to request the toy (Halle, Baer, & Spradlin, 1981).
Missing item	An item needed for a preferred activity is missing. For example, a child may be given a coloring book but not crayons, thereby creating a need for the child to request the missing crayons (Cipani, 1988).
Blocked response/ interrupted behavior chain	Momentarily blocking a response or interrupting an ongoing activity. For example, the child is blocked from reaching for a toy, creating a need for the child to request (Goetz, Gee, & Sailor, 1985). Another example is removing an item that is needed to engage in an ongoing activity. This creates the need for the child to request the object to reinstate the activity.
Incomplete presentation	The initial request is followed by an incomplete presentation of the requested item. For example, after requesting a toy that has several parts, the child is given only half of the parts. This creates a need for the child to request the remaining parts (Duker, Kraaykamp, & Visser, 1994).
Delayed assistance	Required assistance is delayed until a request occurs. For example, if the person needs help to open a jar of pickles, then the communicative partner waits for the person to ask for help (Reichle, Anderson, & Schermer, 1986).
Wrong-item format	Individual is given a nonmatching referent. For example, the individual requests a bottle of sparkling water but is "mistakenly" given a bottle of regular water. This creates a need for the person to clarify the initial request (e.g., "No thanks—I wanted sparkling water") (Duker, Dortmans, & Lodder, 1993; Sigafoos & Roberts-Pennell, 1999).

maintain access to preferred items. For example, Roberts-Pennell and Sigafoos (1999) used the blocked response/interrupted behavior chain strategy to teach three preschool children with developmental disabilities to gain access to preferred leisure items or activities. Three preferred activities (e.g., using the playground slide, playing with an electronic keyboard, listening to music) were identified for each child. Prior to intervention, when the children were blocked from gaining access to their preferred activities, none of them used the targeted communication responses (e.g., saying "more," signing MORE, pointing to a black-and-white line drawing that represented *more*). When interrupted, the children typically attempted to gain access to the preferred activity directly by reaching for the item. During intervention, the children were prompted to produce the targeted communication response. As the prompts were faded using a progressive time delay procedure (i.e., waiting 3, then 5, then 10 seconds before prompting), two of the three children showed acquisition of the new communication response within 24 teaching sessions. The third child did not reach the criterion (i.e., 80% correct or better over 3 successive sessions) within the time limits of the study, which was restricted to 38 sessions. In this study, the blocked response/interrupted behavior chain strategy was used to teach new communicative forms to enable the children to gain access to preferred activities.

A second focus of use for the strategies described in Table 5.3 is to increase the frequency of existing communication skills. This focus is appropriate when the individual's repertoire includes the desired communicative response but the response occurs inconsistently or at too low a frequency. In these cases, it may be sufficient to simply create the need for communication by using one of the procedures described in Table 5.3.

Supporting Partners' Use of Instructional Strategies Based on Incidental Teaching Procedures

Each of the strategies outlined in Table 5.3 has proven to be effective for teaching beginning communicators to gain and maintain access to desired items and activities. An important extension of this work involves documenting application of these strategies by typical partners. Along these lines, Sigafoos and colleagues (1994) developed an intervention program that focused on supporting teachers to increase the number of opportunities to make requests that they provided for students with developmental disabilities.

As part of the intervention, teachers received descriptions of three strategies that could be used to create opportunities for requesting during typical classroom routines and activities. Specifically, the teachers were informed on the use of the missing item format, behavior chain interruption, and delayed assistance procedure (see Table 5.3). This information was provided in a 1-hour in-service consultation. During the in-service, teachers were given a one-page description of each strategy. In addition, each strategy was explained to the teachers by a consultant. The innovative aspect of this study was that the teachers generated their own ideas on how to incorporate these strategies in the typical routines and activities of their classrooms. The consultant facilitated the discussion by asking questions such as, "How might the missing item format be used with Jane?" and "Do you think the delayed assistance strategy could be used during toy play?" In most cases, teachers needed little prompting to generate ideas for using each of the three strategies. Subsequent observations revealed that the strategies were incorporated into a variety of typical classroom routines, including leisure and play (e.g., playing with toys; swimming; using puzzles, clay, and books), meal preparation and lunchtime, academic instruction, and self-care training activities. For example, one teacher used the delayed assistance strategy during an outdoor swimming activity. To enter the swimming pool, children needed assistance in opening the gate. When a child attempted to open the gate, the teacher waited for the child to make a request for help before providing the needed assistance. If the child did not make a request within 10 seconds, the teacher prompted the child to request help before opening the gate. The child was then able to go swimming, which was the preferred activity. Another teacher used the missing item format during lunch by giving a child a carton of pudding but not the needed spoon. Behavior chain interruption was often used during play routines by momentarily interrupting the child during ongoing play. As a result of the intervention program, the teachers provided more opportunities for requesting across a range of classroom activities, and the students responded in kind with increased requesting.

Comparing the Relative Effectiveness of Instructional Strategies

Sigafoos and Meikle (1995) compared the missing item format and the interrupted behavior chain strategy. The study involved three 5- to 8-year-old boys with autism who were learning to request preferred items. The missing item format involved giving the child only one of two needed items (e.g., a puzzle board but not the pieces, a carton of juice but not the accompanying straw) and allowing the child 10 seconds to make a request for the missing item. The interrupted behavior chain strategy involved giving the child both items initially, then removing them after a few seconds; to reinstate the activity, the child had to request the items. Although the underlying rationale for these two strategies is similar (e.g., both are designed to create the need for a request), the procedures involved different operations (i.e., withholding versus removing needed items). Despite these differences, both procedures were equally effective in strengthening requests to gain (missing item format) and maintain (interrupted behavior chain) access to desired objects and activities. Based on these comparable results, Sigafoos and Meikle concluded that interventionists might be able to choose among several equally effective procedures to create opportunities for requesting, depending on the context and the preferred items to be requested. Conversely, the relative effectiveness of these two interventions may depend on certain yet-to-be-determined variables. For example, if an individual is likely to become agitated and escalate to challenging behavior when a preferred item is removed, then the interrupted behavior chain strategy may be contraindicated. Similarly, the effectiveness of the missing item format may depend on the extent to which an individual is familiar with the functional relationship between the given item and the missing item. For example, if an individual does not readily select a straw when given a carton of juice, withholding the straw may not provide an effective context for teaching that individual to make the corresponding request. On a more general level, it is clear that additional research is needed to identify specific variables that might make each of the strategies outlined in Table 5.3 more or less effective.

Roles and Abilities of Communication Partners in Requesting

Successful communicative exchanges that are related to gaining and maintaining access to desired items and activities require communicative partners who are willing and able to honor requests. Potential partners may not always be skilled in this role, especially when they interact with beginning communicators. There is growing recognition that intervention must focus as much on communicative partners as on beginning communicators (Bruno & Dribbon, 1998; Butterfield, Arthur, & Sigafoos, 1995). Several simple strategies can assist partners in this regard.

Teach Recognizable Communication Forms   One strategy for facilitating partner responsiveness to requests is to teach beginning communicators to produce easily recognized and readily interpreted forms of communication. Consider Molly's vocalizations. This form of requesting works quite well with familiar partners and in situations when the context provides sufficient cues about the object being requested. Yet, undifferentiated vocalizations are less effective with unfamiliar communicative partners or in situations in which few contextual cues are available. Thus, it might be advisable to encourage Molly to try vocalizing to get what she wants, then to try a back-up strategy (e.g., pointing to a symbol, producing a manual sign) if her initial message is not understood (e.g., Reichle & Ward, 1985).

Provide Partner Instruction and Support   A second strategy is to provide additional instruction and support to ensure that others have the skills to be responsive partners. This might be especially important when partners have little or no experience with beginning communicators who use AAC. Carter and Maxwell (1998) described an intervention to teach peers to be effective communicative partners to four children who had cerebral palsy and used AAC. The study was conducted in a primary school that included children with and without disabilities. Peers without disabilities were taught to 1) establish eye contact, 2) ask questions, 3) wait for a response, and 4) respond to communicative overtures. After they had mastered these four simple strategies, the quantity and quality of the social-communicative interactions between the peers and their schoolmates who used AAC increased. It remains unclear, however, if all four components were important to the effectiveness of the intervention. It is possible, for example, that similar results would have been obtained if the peers had been taught simply to make eye contact and wait or to ask questions and wait. This empirical question could be addressed in future research in which the importance of each component of the "package" is determined. Nevertheless, from a practical perspective, it seems unnecessary to be concerned with this issue because the package of four strategies seems simple and natural.

In a larger-scale study with a similar aim, Arthur, Butterfield, and McKinnon (1998) described a professional development program that was designed, in part, to teach professionals and paraprofessionals how to be more effective communicative partners to people with severe disabilities. The participants were involved in an in-service program that focused on developing knowledge and skills related to communication assessment, program development, and systematic instruction. As part of the training, participants learned how to create opportunities for communication to increase the participation of individuals with severe disabilities in meaningful communicative exchanges throughout the day. Following the program, participants reported greater knowledge about and skills related to their roles as communicative partners to people with severe disabilities. A significant limitation of the study was the lack of direct observation to determine if the in-service training actually led to positive changes in social interaction between the participants and the beginning communicators to whom they provided support. Nonetheless, the data provide some evidence for the potential utility of large-scale in-service training to disseminate information that might assist individuals in becoming more responsive partners to beginning communicators.

Teach Partners to Respond to Prelinguistic Behaviors and Requests

A third strategy that is related to improving interpersonal communication is to teach partners to identify and respond appropriately to existing behaviors that individuals already use to gain and maintain access to desired objects or activities. Beginning communicators often use a variety of informal and idiosyncratic behaviors in their attempts to gain and maintain access to desired items and activities. Examples include vocalizations, body movements, facial expressions (see Chapter 2), breathing patterns, and even challenging behaviors, such as aggression and self-injury (Durand, 1993b; Siegel-Causey & Guess, 1989; see also Chapter 4). For example, when a desired item is present, a beginning communicator may reach for, move toward, or simply stare at the desired item (Sigafoos et al., 1995). Similarly, if a preferred activity is momentarily interrupted, an individual may protest by crying or screaming in an apparent attempt to reinstate the activity. Because such actions can represent effective, albeit informal and not always socially acceptable, means of communication, it seems important to ensure that partners are able to identify the communicative functions of nonsymbolic communicative acts and react appropriately when these behaviors are observed. Exemplary strategies to identify and react appropriately to nonsymbolic behaviors are described on pages 142–143. The partner's actions in this regard will often function either to strengthen or weaken future communication interactions. With beginning communicators, it is important to react positively to approximations of appropriate requests during the early stages of intervention. Over time, partners can wait for closer and closer approximations and, in this way, gradually shape the initial attempts into the final desired form of communication.

The instructional benefit of a communicative exchange is increased when a communicative partner is responsive to the beginning communicator's attempts to gain and maintain access to a desired item or activity. To shape these initial attempts into more sophisticated forms of communication, partners need to acknowledge and expand the individual's communicative attempts (Hart & Risley, 1975). For example, a beginning communicator might attempt to gain access to a preferred toy by reaching for it. At this point, the partner could maximize the instructional benefit of this naturally arising opportunity by following three steps:

1. Acknowledge the presumed intent of the action (e.g., "Oh, I see you want the puzzle").
2. Expand the response by prompting the child to point to a symbol that represents the desired activity (e.g., "Use your symbol to ask for the puzzle").
3. React to the expanded response both verbally (e.g., "That's right, you told me you want the puzzle") and nonverbally by delivering the requesting item or by explaining why the request cannot be honored (e.g., "Sorry, your sister has the puzzle—you have to wait your turn").

It is important to emphasize that this strategy is appropriate *only* if a beginning communicator's initial nonsymbolic request behavior is well established as part of his or her communicative repertoire. The goal is to extend the old function (i.e., the well-established request function) to include a new form—in the previous case, the use of a symbol for *puzzle*. If the request function is not firmly established in the communicator's repertoire, expanding the response in this way may be premature and may result in loss of the function altogether (Wetherby & Prizant, 1992).

Teach Attention Getting Prior to Requesting   A fourth strategy is related to preventing communication breakdowns that may occur because communication partners fail to attend to requests that beginning communicators make. A typical scenario for this problem often starts with a beginning communicator's attempting to gain access to a desired item by signing or by pointing to a picture on a communication board. Yet, because the communicative partner does not happen to be watching at the precise moment that the individual produces the sign or points to the picture, the request goes unnoticed. If this happens often enough, requesting may occur less and less frequently because of a lack of partner response.

Of course, partners should learn to be "on the lookout" for initiations from beginning communicators. In addition, it is important to consider teaching beginning communicators to recruit the attention of their partners. Interventions to establish initial requesting skills in beginning communicators have tended to ignore this issue. Instead, in most interventions that are designed to teach requesting, the partner is already present and attending when the opportunity to request occurs. Instruction under these conditions may not equip beginning communicators with the skills needed to communicate effectively when their partners are not present and attending. Furthermore, there is considerable evidence that some beginning communicators, especially those with autism, may have particular difficulty establishing joint attention with communicative partners (Mundy & Gomes, 1997; Sarria, Gomez, & Tamarit, 1996). For instance, a child may make a request even though his or her communicative partner is turned away or preoccupied with another activity. Thus, some beginning communicators will require interventions to teach them how to first recruit the attention of their partners (Sobsey & Reichle, 1989).

One way to do this is to establish a chain of two responses. First, the individual recruits the attention of a partner, then the individual makes the request. Cipani (1990) used such an approach with two children with severe disabilities. Both children could make requests when they were in the presence of an adult, but neither had the skills needed to recruit the adult's attention. The children were first taught to walk over to the adult to gain attention and to then make a request.

Although the preceding strategy has been effective (Cipani, 1990), its efficiency when compared with a strategy in which attention getting and requesting are taught simultaneously has not been examined empirically. With the use of technology, it may be possible to select one or more communication modes that combine attention getting with requesting. For example, an individual may be taught to use a voice output communication aid (VOCA) so that whenever a request is made, it can be heard by nearby communicative partners. Of course, voice output will not be effective if communicative partners are hearing impaired, if the environment is too noisy, or if no listener is nearby to receive the message. Thus, even when VOCAs are used, it is still important that users learn to seek a listener and that partners are skilled in recognizing attempts by beginning communicators to initiate communication.

Issues Involved in Honoring Initial Communicative Requests   When a beginning communicator makes an appropriate attempt to request under the right conditions, the partner should be quick to honor the request by providing the desired item or activity. Consistent, predictable, and immediate reinforcement facilitate the acquisition of requesting. Yet, it is also important for a beginning communicator to learn that not all requests can be honored each and every time. For example, an individual may request a particular beverage. If that beverage is not available, then the request cannot be honored and will go unfulfilled. In this instance, one might teach the individual to make a request for a specific item only when it is likely to be available and to request an alternative if the item is not available. In other situations, it may not be acceptable to honor the request. A parent may not wish to allow a child to go outside to play if the request occurs at night. In this situation, the parent may have to deny the child's request. The parent might respond by explaining, "Yes I know that you want to go outside, but this isn't possible because it's dark. Would you like to stay inside and play a game with me instead?"

When a request is honored, it can be viewed as a positive teaching exemplar in that the response leads to reinforcement and, therefore, will become more likely under similar conditions in the future. When a request is not honored, it can instead be viewed as a negative exemplar in that the request is not reinforced. In this context, a *positive exemplar* is a discriminative stimulus that indicates when a request will be honored. A *negative exemplar* is associated with nonreinforcement. DePaepe and colleagues (1993) proposed that positive and negative exemplars should be included from the beginning of intervention to ensure the appropriate use of requests.

Generally speaking, it is important to ensure consistent, predictable, and immediate reinforcement during the early stages of intervention, and several issues remain unresolved concerning when and how often partners honor requests. For example, it is unclear whether all requests should be honored during acquisition or whether negative exemplars should be included from the very beginning of intervention. It is also unclear whether an optimal ratio of positive to negative exemplars exists. It is likely that the answers to such questions will vary with the nature of the request being taught and from one individual to another. Interventionists must carefully balance the need to facilitate acquisition with the equally important need to ensure that learning is not disrupted when initial attempts to request are not honored.

EXEMPLARY STRATEGIES FOR TEACHING COMMUNICATIVE FUNCTIONS TO ACHIEVE ACCESS TO DESIRED OBJECTS AND ACTIVITIES

A number of strategies have been developed for teaching beginning communicators to gain and maintain access to desired objects and activities. When implementing instruction to achieve this goal, various options exist in terms of the *what, where,* and *how* of instruction. This section considers specific instructional issues that arise in attempting to strengthen existing nonsymbolic behaviors as well as teaching more symbolic forms of requesting behavior. A first consideration, however, is determination of when and whether beginning communicators are ready to participate in these types of exemplary strategies for teaching communicative functions that achieve access to desired objects and activities.

Prerequisites for Requesting

Many beginning communicators, especially those with limited cognitive abilities, were once required to show evidence of various prerequisite cognitive abilities prior to participating in interventions designed to teach requesting. In this context, the prerequisites were often stated in terms of showing evidence of formal underlying cognitive abilities based on the developmental stages of Piagetian theory (see Reichle & Karlan, 1985, for a review). These abilities included components such as attending skills, object permanence, and an underlying intentionality to communicate as evidenced by using a parent as an indirect means to an end. As a result, past practice often focused on trying to develop attending skills, or waiting for the concepts of object permanence and intentionality to emerge, before starting intervention. In addition, when intervention did begin, it often focused on teaching receptive language skills, such as pointing to objects that were named by a partner rather than teaching expressive communication (e.g., requesting a preferred object) (Reichle, Sigafoos, & Remington, 1991).

In the early 1990s, however, practice began to move away from the notion that beginning communicators should be required to achieve these types of cognitive prerequisites before starting an AAC intervention. Instead, Reichle, York, and Sigafoos (1991) suggested that interventions to teach requesting could begin once two very different types of conditions had been met. First, the communicative partner must be able to identify at least one item or activity that an individual will be motivated to request. An individual is often highly motivated to request preferred items, so it is often useful to conduct an initial assessment to identify preferences. A variety of strategies, some of which were described previously in this chapter, can be used to identify preferences. In addition to identifying preferences, the communicative partner must be able to define an acceptable form of behavior that the individual is capable of learning to produce reliably, such as pointing to a symbol or gesturing. This behavior will serve as the communicative request. One might think of these two conditions as being functional, rather than cognitive, prerequisites. Following the suggestions of Reichle, York, and Sigafoos, it is clear that almost all beginning communicators will be appropriate candidates for interventions that are designed to teach requesting.

Strengthening Nonsymbolic Behaviors for Requesting

As noted previously, some beginning communicators may have limited means by which they can indicate to others their desire to gain or maintain access to items or activities. As a result, initial interventions often focus on teaching use of symbolic communication modes for requesting, such as manual signs, tangible symbols, or line drawings. Yet, there is also growing recognition of the importance of strengthening nonsymbolic (i.e., informal, prelinguistic) behaviors—such as facial expressions, eye contact, and body movements—for this purpose, as many beginning communicators already have such behaviors in their repertoires (Siegel-Causey & Guess, 1989). For example, a beginning communicator might reach for or look at one of two items to make a choice. Not only do such actions reveal the individual's motivation to communicate, they might also function as legitimate forms of communication in their own right. Indeed, nonsymbolic acts might themselves be the focus of assessment and intervention (Wetherby, Warren, & Reichle, 1998).

It is often difficult to determine whether nonsymbolic actions are intentional acts of communication or are merely interpreted by others as if they were intentional (Iacono, Carter, & Hook, 1998). One way to decide is to look for collateral behaviors that may indicate an intent to communicate. Wetherby and Prizant (1992) discussed behaviors that may be associated with intentionality:

- Alternating eye gaze between the goal (e.g., a desired object) and the communicative partner
- Persistently signaling until either the goal is accomplished or failure is indicated
- Changing the signal quality until the goal has been met
- Ritualizing or conventionalizing the form of the signal within specific communicative contexts
- Awaiting a response from the partner
- Terminating the signal when the goal is met
- Displaying satisfaction when the goal is attained or dissatisfaction when it is not

Sigafoos and colleagues (2000) suggested that intentionality can be difficult to judge in some beginning communicators. This is because many of these individuals have a limited repertoire of conventional signals such as those delineated by Wetherby and Prizant (1992). In these cases, any existing nonsymbolic behaviors may best be viewed as potential communicative acts until their communicative intent can be verified through direct observation. Regardless, intervention may be necessary to ensure that the communicative potential of these behaviors is realized, especially when they are socially acceptable but are used either inconsistently or unintentionally. The goal of such intervention would be to produce more consistent and fluent use of socially acceptable nonsymbolic behaviors and/or to develop intentionality.

Structured Overinterpretation   An example of one such intervention strategy, referred to as *structured overinterpretation*, was described by von Tetzchner (1997). This strategy involves teaching communicative partners to recognize potential communicative acts in the repertoires of beginning communicators and to provide consistent interpretations of the presumed communicative intent of these actions. Interpretation of intent is based on the contexts in which the actions are observed. By reacting in ways that are consistent with the presumed intent of the prelinguistic actions, partners may shape such actions into effective forms of communication. For example, a child may be observed to jump up and down as she approaches the sandbox on the playground. Using structured overinterpretation, the teacher would recognize this behavior as a potential communicative act and interpret it to mean *I want to play in the sand.* She might then respond to the interpreted intent by saying, "Oh, I see you are jumping. I guess you must want to play in the sand," and then assisting the child in doing so. If the teacher behaves similarly in a variety of contexts when the child engages in her jumping behavior, the child is likely to learn over time that jumping means *I get what I want.*

Effective application of structured overinterpretation may benefit from an initial inventory of the idiosyncratic and often subtle communication signals that a beginning communicator uses. Unless this is done systematically, it may be difficult to ensure that different partners will recognize, interpret, and react consistently to these potential communicative acts. Beukelman and Mirenda (1998) suggested that caregivers develop gesture dictionaries for individual beginning communicators to document their nonsymbolic behaviors and their presumed meanings, thereby possibly facilitating response consistency across communicative partners.

Teaching Replacement Behaviors for Requesting   Developing fluent and intentional use of idiosyncratic nonsymbolic behaviors for requesting is not always appropriate. For example, if a beginning communicator relies on screaming and crying to gain access to preferred items, one would not want to strengthen or encourage such behaviors (see Chapter 4). In this instance, replacing screaming and crying with a more socially acceptable form of requesting is the preferred strategy (e.g., Durand, 1993a). Similarly, nonsymbolic behaviors that are highly idiosyncratic or very subtle may be difficult for communicative partners to recognize and interpret (Houghton, Bronicki, & Guess, 1987; Rowland, 1990). For instance, a child who flaps her hands when offered food items may be either indicating a request or rejecting the offer. Again, there may be value in replacing such nonsymbolic or prelinguistic acts with those that are more transparent.

Keen, Sigafoos, and Woodyatt (in press) described an intervention that focused on replacing nonsymbolic behaviors with other communication modalities for requesting. The study involved four young children with autism. The first step of the intervention was to identify the existing nonsymbolic behaviors that the children used to achieve various communicative functions (e.g., making choices, gaining access to objects, maintaining activities). This identification process involved interviews with teachers and direct observations in the classroom. The children were often observed to initiate requesting behaviors such as reaching for preferred foods at morning snack time and reaching for toys during small-group playtime. Next, interventionists identified replacement forms that constituted more recognizable and symbolic communication to achieve the same functions. Instead of reaching for a toy, a child might be encouraged to point to a photograph of the desired item.

The unique aspect of this study was that intervention was directed at the teachers rather than at the children. The teachers participated in an in-service program during which they learned how to encourage, acknowledge, and respond to the replacement communicative forms that were selected for each child. Specifically, they were given information on how to create requesting opportunities for the children and how to acknowledge communicative attempts and prompt replacement behaviors when necessary. To illustrate, a request opportunity for one child involved having the teacher present a photo of an activity, look at the child, and ask if he wanted a turn. Once the opportunity was provided, the teacher acknowledged the child's attempt to move toward the activity (e.g., "Oh, you want a turn") and prompted him to point to the photo (i.e., the replacement behavior). If the prelinguistic behavior occurred, the child was prompted to perform the replacement response. The same approach was used when the child made an incorrect response or engaged in challenging behavior. Over time, the teachers began to use these strategies in the context of typical classroom routines, and there was a substantial increase in the children's use of the replacement communicative forms for requesting. In most cases, collateral decreases in nonsymbolic requesting behaviors also occurred.

Use of Natural Contexts

During the initial stage of AAC interventions that are related to requesting, it is often helpful to distribute numerous teaching opportunities throughout the day and to incorporate them into a range of real-life activities (Beukelman & Mirenda, 1998; Sigafoos, 1999). Goldstein, Kaczmarek, and Hepting (1994) argued that much of the interventionist's work involves providing training to change the interaction styles of communicative partners (e.g., parents, teachers, peers). Such training focuses on increasing the number of opportunities for teaching and learning as well as on ensuring that partners consistently attend to, comment on, and acknowledge attempts to communicate (Goldstein,

Kaczmarek, Pennington, & Shafer, 1992). Increased opportunities, along with consistent reactions from typical partners across a variety of everyday contexts, can help to increase and strengthen communicative interaction and facilitate generalization (Halle, 1988). The implication for beginning communicators is that partners should provide intervention in natural contexts across the day (Goldstein et al., 1994). Table 5.4 gives some examples of such real-life opportunities. As noted in the table, during breakfast, an individual may need to request assistance so that he or she can gain access to jam to spread on toast. Or, after having one glass of orange juice, the person might want to request another. The situations illustrated in Table 5.4 can serve as natural contexts for instruction to strengthen communication skills that are related to gaining and maintaining access to desired items and activities. For example, by waiting for the individual to make a request before opening a jar of jam, the communicative partner will help to strengthen communication skills that are related to requesting help.

Brown and colleagues (1988) presented several criteria for prioritizing instructional goals that, when applied to interventions that are designed to teach requesting, may help ensure that they will be of real benefit to beginning communicators across a range of typical environments and communicative partners. Table 5.5 summarizes these features. For instance, a communication skill that would be readily interpreted by unfamiliar partners and useful across a va-

Table 5.4. Examples of communication opportunities for gaining and maintaining access to preferred items and activities in the context of typical daily routines and activities

Daily routine/activity	Examples of opportunities
Breakfast	Request help to open the jar of jam for toast Request more orange juice Ask partner to pass the marmalade
Choosing an activity	Indicate a desire to go to the beach, a museum, shopping, or a baseball game
Lunch	Order from a menu Request sugar for coffee Ask for change to play the jukebox
Free time at home	Indicate which CD to listen to Select a TV program, magazine, or book Request leisure materials
Dinner	Choose what to eat Request help with opening a package of a preferred food item Ask for a second serving of vegetables Ask for desert
Evening	Request a number from directory assistance to call a friend Indicate a desire to go to an exercise class Request a turn to play a computer game

Table 5.5.   Criteria for identifying requesting skills for beginning communicators

Criterion	Description
Increase access to a greater number of typical environments.	A requesting skill can be considered of more benefit and of higher priority if it enables the individual to gain access to and participate in a greater range of typical environments.
Make the skill functional.	A request should be functional in the sense that it is necessary. If a desired item is readily accessible, a request is not needed. Learning to request inaccessible items would be considered more functional and a higher priority.
Make the skill age appropriate.	Requesting skills that enable the individual to gain access to desired, age-appropriate items and activities are considered higher priorities so as to promote peer acceptance and meet social expectations. A 6-year-old and a 16-year-old might both be taught to request access to leisure activities, but the 6-year-old is taught to request toy trucks and dolls, whereas the 16-year-old is taught to request access to golf and tennis.
Ensure opportunities for use.	Skills for which there is ample opportunity for use throughout the day are of more potential benefit than skills with few or no opportunities for use. Making a choice between two work tasks would be of benefit only if the job allowed such discretion.
Select skills with long-term usefulness.	The acquisition process for beginning communicators may be rather lengthy. If valuable time and effort is required to teach a communication skill, then it would make sense to target skills with long-term benefit.
Ensure that the skills reflect individual preferences.	Most people have fairly strong preferences for some things but not for others. One person might never consider drinking tea over coffee but would drink either Coke or Pepsi. For this individual, the ability to request coffee over tea would be more beneficial than the ability to specify Coke or Pepsi.

Source: Brown et al. (1988).

riety of environments, such as ordering preferred items from a menu, might be a high priority because it would facilitate eating at a range of restaurants.

Instructional Techniques for the Acquisition of Graphic Mode Requesting

A graphic communication mode involves the use of line drawings, photographs, miniature objects, and other tangible symbols. The act of selecting a graphic symbol (e.g., pointing to a line drawing of a spoon) is considered equivalent to speaking the word. Because the selection response is identical across vocabulary and because the symbols provide a permanent display, graphic mode systems may be relatively easy for beginning communicators to learn. This section reviews instructional techniques for teaching graphic mode requesting to beginning communicators.

Selecting and Offering Two-Dimensional Symbols   Several studies have taught beginning communicators to use graphic mode AAC to gain and maintain access to a variety of preferred objects and activities (e.g., Duker & van Lent, 1991; Reichle & Brown, 1986; Romski, Sevcik, & Pate, 1988; Turnell & Carter, 1994). Sigafoos, Couzens, Roberts, Phillips, and Goodison (1996) taught requesting to two young girls (ages 5 and 6) with cerebral palsy and severe cognitive delay. The children were unable to speak and were initially taught to point to line drawings of *food* and *drink* to request a variety of preferred foods and beverages during morning snack time in the classroom. Intervention involved offering a preferred food or drink item, prompting a child to point to the corresponding line drawing, and then providing the requested item. Prompts included the systematic use of verbal cues, gestures, modeling, and physical assistance, arranged in a least-to-most hierarchy (see Sigafoos, Mustonen, DePaepe, Reichle, & York, 1991). Over successive instructional opportunities, the prompts were faded using a 10-second time delay. After only five or six teaching sessions, both children were consistently and independently pointing to the food or drink symbol when offered a preferred food or beverage.

Kozleski (1991) taught four children (7–13 years old) with autism who had no speech to request preferred foods, beverages, and leisure activities. A request consisted of pointing to the correct graphic symbol on a communication board. First, preferred items were placed near a participant, and the partner asked, "What do you want?" If a participant reached for a desired item, it was not provided. Instead, the partner presented symbols that corresponded to all of the items in the array and again asked, "What do you want?" A request was considered correct if the participant pointed to the symbol that corresponded to the previously indicated item. If the participant did not make a correct request, then the partner pointed to the correct symbol and physically guided the participant's finger to it. To ensure initial success, intervention began with just one symbol. Over time, discrimination training was introduced to maintain correct requesting when two and finally three symbols were presented on the communication board. Overall, the results suggested that the intervention procedures were effective in teaching the children to point to graphic symbols to gain access to preferred objects; in addition, the more iconic (i.e., "guessable") symbols were easier for them to learn.

Another instructional method that can be used to teach requesting is the Picture Exchange Communication System (PECS; Bondy & Frost, 1995). PECS is unique in that it is designed to teach self-initiated requesting as the very first skill in a person's communicative repertoire. Although PECS was originally designed for preschoolers with autism, it has also been used successfully with individuals of various ages who have other developmental disabilities (Bondy & Frost, 1993).

Instruction in PECS begins after an assessment of potential reinforcers for the individual. In the first phase of PECS, the person is taught to pick up a single symbol (e.g., a photograph, a line drawing), place it into the teacher's open hand, and receive the corresponding preferred item (e.g., food, drink, toy). Physical and gestural prompts—but no verbal prompts (e.g., "What do you want?" "Give me the picture")—are used to teach this sequence of behaviors. In the next phase, the teacher gradually moves away from the preferred item while extending an open palm so that the communicator must select the symbol and walk to the teacher to exchange it for the desired item. Gradually, the number of symbols is increased by introducing distracter symbols; symbols of lower preference; and, finally, additional symbols of equal preference. Comprehension checks are done by having the individual select the requested item from an array after offering the symbol and by providing natural consequences and/or corrective feedback as appropriate.

Once basic requesting has been mastered, the PECS approach can be extended to build sentence structures (e.g., teaching the person to chain an I WANT symbol and a specific referent symbol), answer yes/no questions in a request context, and label items. Outcome data for 66 children with autism ages 5 and younger who were taught PECS over a 5-year-period were quite encouraging. Bondy and Frost (1995) reported that 34 of the children acquired functional speech and no longer required any AAC supports, 14 used a combination of words and pictures or written words, and the remaining 18 children continued to use aided symbols for communication in functional contexts.

Tangible Symbols   Systematic instructional strategies have also been applied to teaching the use of tangible symbols for requesting (Locke & Mirenda, 1988; Turnell & Carter, 1994). For example, Locke and Mirenda worked with an 11-year-old boy who was blind, did not speak, and had severe mental retardation. He was given an AAC device that included six textured squares that were used to represent preferred snacks (e.g., mesh = potato chips, velvet = juice). He was taught to request preferred snacks by selecting these tangible symbols, which were affixed to a computer keyboard overlay. When a texture was selected, the name of the corresponding snack item was produced via synthesized speech. During intervention, the teacher first oriented the child to the device by placing his hand on each texture to activate the speech synthesizer. Initially, the teacher physically prompted the child to touch textures by nudging his arm towards the keyboard; these prompts were faded over 16 sessions. The child received a corresponding snack item any time he independently touched a texture on the overlay. In addition, he received verbal feedback for each independent request (e.g., "Oh, you want a potato chip"). The number of textures on the overlay was gradually increased from 3 to 6. The results showed that the boy acquired the use of the device for requesting and demonstrated generalized use of the device to make independent requests during snack time. Thus, although instruction occurred in a structured environment away from the classroom, he was able to use his newly acquired requesting responses under appropriate natural conditions.

Eye Gaze Selection of Two-Dimensional Symbols   Prompting and reinforcement procedures have also been used to develop initial requesting skills in communication modes other than those requiring a pointing response. For example, Sigafoos and Couzens (1995) reported an intervention to teach a 6-year-old boy with multiple disabilities to use an eye pointing chart to make requests. The chart consisted of a clear, rectangular Plexiglas board with space for one photograph in each corner. The child was taught to look at the photograph that represented an item needed to gain access to a preferred activity. The preferred activity was listening to music, which required a cassette tape, a tape player, and headphones. Initially, the child was given only two of the three required items and was offered the chart by his teacher. The chart contained photographs of all three required items, plus a fourth distracter photograph. The teacher waited 10 seconds for the child to request the missing item by gazing at the correct photograph for a full 3 seconds. If the child did not make a correct request within 10 seconds, the teacher asked, "What do you need?" and tapped on the correct photograph. Both correct and prompted requests were reinforced by giving the child the missing item and allowing him to listen to his preferred music. When the child gave an incorrect response or no response, an error correction procedure was implemented. This involved showing the missing item; asking, "What is this?"; and tapping on the correct photograph. These procedures were effective in teaching the child to use the chart to request whichever item was missing. Thus, the child was able to gain access to the materials that were needed for this preferred activity.

Summary   Studies such as those described in this section suggest that several features facilitate the acquisition of AAC skills related to gaining and maintaining access to desired items and activities. Specifically, the following conditions appear to enhance AAC interventions that focus on teaching requesting skills to beginning communicators:

1. *Intervention opportunities occur in the context of familiar routines when the individual is clearly motivated to make a request.* Drasgow, Halle, Ostrosky, and Harbers (1996) referred to this as *behavioral indication*. If a child reaches toward an item, for example, this may be an indication that he or she is highly motivated to gain access to that item. This would be considered an ideal time to teach the child to request the desired item.

2. *The request behavior is easy for the individual to produce.* For instance, it appears that manual signs that are more complicated motorically or require more response effort take longer to learn (Duker, 1988; Reichle & Karlan, 1985).

3. *Initially, requests lead to consistent, predictable reinforcement.* That is, when the individual makes a request under the right conditions, there is a high probability that the communicative partner will quickly honor that request by supplying the requested item or activity.

4. *A range of prompts is used to ensure that each instructional opportunity ends with a successful communicative exchange.* A successful communicative exchange occurs when a beginning communicator uses an appropriate form of communication to gain or maintain access to the desired item or activity. The availability of effective prompts ensures that there will be a high rate of initial success, which is likely to facilitate acquisition. Communicative partners should be careful not to rely too heavily on partner-delivered prompts, however, because some individuals may become overly dependent on them (Mirenda & Santogrossi, 1985). In general, it is wise to use the least intrusive type of prompt and fade the prompt as quickly as possible.

5. *Strategies are introduced to minimize errors during the early stages of intervention.* This is an important instructional consideration because errors that occur during the early stages of intervention may persist and, thus, interfere with the acquisition of communication behavior as well as inhibit the fluent use of newly acquired communication skills. Fortunately, a variety of strategies can be used during the early stages of communication intervention to prevent and minimize errors (McIlvane, Dube, Green, & Serna, 1993).

6. *Discriminative stimuli are present, which make it clear that a request is required.* When communicative partners create opportunities for requesting, it may be important to ensure that the initial opportunities include clear signals that a communicative response is expected. For some individuals, it may also be important to implement strategies to ensure attention to the relevant discriminative stimuli.

Instructional Techniques to Build Fluency

An important but often neglected instructional concern relates to fluency of use. *Fluency* can be conceived in terms of rate of response or how quickly and efficiently an individual can convey the intended communicative message. With speech, communication is typically quick and effortless. When an individual must rely on AAC, however, communicative exchanges can be slow and cumbersome. Indeed, one of the biggest problems in AAC has been the lack of fluency among beginning communicators who are using aided communication devices (Calculator & Dollaghan, 1982).

Although there has been little research on the specific effects of limited fluency, it is conceivable that a lack of fluency may result in considerable problems in using communication to gain or maintain access to desired items and activities. For example, if a beginning communicator is too slow in making a request for a preferred item, his or her partner may lose patience and ignore the individual's communicative attempts. The partner may also override the individual as he or she attempts to communicate and deliver the item before a request has been made, thereby preempting communication (Halle, 1984). In turn, a beginning communicator may bypass his or her AAC system in favor of nonsymbolic communicative acts, which may be more efficient initially, but are perhaps open to greater misinterpretation. Over time, familiar communicative partners are likely to simply "jump in" and speak for the beginning communicator (e.g., "He wants some juice"), rather than waiting for appropriate request behaviors. Such dysfunctional patterns of interaction may stem in part from a lack of fluency on the part of beginning communicators (Light, Collier, & Parnes, 1985). Thus, lack of fluency may seriously hinder the extent to which beginning communicators actively participate in social-communicative exchanges, even if they have acquired the necessary communication skills.

Fluency may need to be developed through direct instruction, although it has rarely been an explicit goal in AAC interventions. Instead, AAC interventions often end following acquisition, with few opportunities for beginning communicators to practice their newly acquired skills and become fluent. McCook, Cipani, Madigan, and LaCampagne (1988) presented data suggesting that acquisition and fluent use of verbal requesting were independent aspects of performance for two women with moderate intellectual disabilities. Yet, fluency was improved using the same naturalistic mand-model procedure that resulted in acquisition. The results from this study provide some support for the conclusion that fluency may need to be the focus of direct intervention. Nevertheless, this remains a largely uncharted area, and it clearly requires additional research.

CONCLUSION

This chapter has illustrated some of the conceptual and practical issues that arise when designing interventions that enable beginning communicators to gain and maintain access to desired items and activities. Our aim was to provide an overview of some of the exemplary strategies that can be used in this regard. The overriding theme of the chapter has been that although many beginning communicators will require systematic instruction to acquire functional communication, exemplary interventions should be conducted in the context of typical routines to be maximally effective. In addition, they should emphasize the development of partner skills to ensure that communicative attempts are recognized, acknowledged, and reinforced.

We have also argued that it is critical for beginning communicators to learn to exert control over their environments and the people with whom they interact. Participation in communicative exchanges in which beginning communicators can influence others to "deliver" preferred goods and services provides an excellent introduction to both the power and the promise of interpersonal communication. In the absence of interventions that focus on strengthening socially acceptable and effective communication skills at this most basic level, beginning communicators are likely to either become extremely passive or develop unacceptable ways of indicating their wants and needs. Thus, exemplary strategies to strengthen the type of skills described in this chapter should be introduced as early as possible.

REFERENCES

Arthur, M., Butterfield, N., & McKinnon, D.H. (1998). Communication intervention for students with severe disability: Results of a partner training program. *International Journal of Disability, Development and Education, 45,* 97–115.

Beukelman, D.R., & Mirenda, P. (1998). *Augmentative and alternative communication: Management of severe communication disorders in children and adults* (2nd ed.). Baltimore: Paul H. Brookes Publishing Co.

Bondy, A., & Frost, L. (1993). Mands across the water: A report on the application of the Picture Exchange Communication System in Peru. *The Behavior Analyst, 16,* 123–128.

Bondy, A., & Frost, L. (1995). Educational approaches in preschool: Behavior techniques in a public school setting. In E. Schopler & G. Mesibov (Eds.), *Learning and cognition in autism* (pp. 311–333). New York: Kluwer Academic/Plenum Publishers.

Brady, N.C., & McLean, L.K. (1996). Arbitrary symbol learning by adults with severe mental retardation: Comparison of lexigrams and printed words. *American Journal on Mental Retardation, 100,* 423–427.

Brown, L., Shiraga, B., Rogan, P., York, J., Albright, K.Z., McCarthy, E., Loomis, R., & VanDeventer, P. (1988). The "why" question in programs for people who are severely intellectually disabled. In S.N. Calculator & J.L. Bedrosian (Eds.), *Communication assessment and intervention for adults with mental retardation* (pp. 139–153). San Diego: College-Hill Press.

Bruno, J., & Dribbon, M. (1998). Outcomes in AAC: Evaluating the effectiveness of a parent training program. *Augmentative and Alternative Communication, 14,* 59–70.

Butterfield, N., Arthur, M., & Sigafoos, J. (1995). *Partners in everyday communicative exchanges.* Sydney, Australia: MacLennan & Petty Pty Limited.

Calculator, S., & Dollaghan, C. (1982). The use of communication boards in a residential setting: An evaluation. *Journal of Speech and Hearing Disorders, 47,* 281–287.

Carter, M., Hotchkis, G.D., & Cassar, M.C. (1996). Spontaneity of augmentative and alternative communication in persons with intellectual disabilities: Critical review. *Augmentative and Alternative Communication, 12,* 97–109.

Carter, M., & Maxwell, K. (1998). Promoting interaction with children using augmentative communication through a peer-directed intervention. *International Journal of Disability, Development and Education, 45,* 75–96.

Cipani, E. (1988). The missing item format. *Teaching Exceptional Children, 21,* 25–27.

Cipani, E. (1990). "Excuse me: I'll have . . .": Teaching appropriate attention-getting behavior to young children with severe handicaps. *Mental Retardation, 28,* 29–33.

DePaepe, P., Reichle, J., & O'Neill, R. (1993). Applying general-case instructional strategies when teaching communicative alternatives to challenging behavior. In

J. Reichle & D.P. Wacker (Eds.), *Communicative alternatives to challenging behavior: Integrating functional assessment and intervention strategies* (pp. 237–262). Baltimore: Paul H. Brookes Publishing Co.

Drasgow, E., Halle, J.W., Ostrosky, M.M., & Harbers, H.M. (1996). Using behavioral indication and functional communication training to establish an initial sign repertoire with a young child with severe disabilities. *Topics in Early Childhood Special Education, 16,* 500–521.

Duker, P.C. (1988). *Teaching the developmentally handicapped communicative gesturing: A how-to-do book.* Lisse, Netherlands: Swets & Zeitlinger.

Duker, P.C., Dortmans, A., & Lodder, E. (1993). Establishing the manding function of communicative gestures with individuals with severe/profound mental retardation. *Research in Developmental Disabilities, 14,* 39–49.

Duker, P.C., Kraaykamp, M., & Visser, E. (1994). A stimulus control procedure to increase requesting with individuals who are severely/profoundly intellectually disabled. *Journal of Intellectual Disability Research, 38,* 177–186.

Duker, P.C., & van Lent, C. (1991). Inducing variability in communicative gestures used by severely retarded individuals. *Journal of Applied Behavior Analysis, 24,* 379–386.

Durand, V.M. (1993a). Functional communication training using assistive devices: Effects on challenging behavior. *Augmentative and Alternative Communication, 9,* 168–176.

Durand, V.M. (1993b). Problem behavior as communication. *Behaviour Change, 10,* 197–207.

Evans, R., & Bilsky, L. (1979). Clustering and categorical list retention in the mentally retarded. In N. Ellis (Ed.), *Handbook of mental deficiency: Psychological research and theory.* Mahwah, NJ: Lawrence Erlbaum Associates.

Fisher, W.W., Piazza, C.C., Bowman, L.G., & Amari, A. (1996). Integrating caregiver report with a systematic choice assessment. *American Journal on Mental Retardation, 101,* 15–25.

Goetz, L., Gee, K., & Sailor, W. (1985). Using a behavior chain interruption strategy to teach communication skills to students with severe disabilities. *Journal of The Association for Persons with Severe Handicaps, 10,* 21–30.

Goldstein, H., Kaczmarek, L., & Hepting, N. (1994). Communication interventions: The challenges of across-the-day implementation. In R. Gardner, III, D.M. Sainato, J.O. Copper, T.E. Heron, W.L. Heward, J. Eshleman, & T.A. Gross (Eds.), *Behavior analysis in education: Focus on measurable superior instruction* (pp. 101–113). Pacific Grove, CA: Brooks/Cole Thomson Learning.

Goldstein, H., Kaczmarek, L., Pennington, R., & Shafer, K. (1992). Peer-mediated intervention: Attending to, commenting on, and acknowledging the behavior of preschoolers with autism. *Journal of Applied Behavior Analysis, 25,* 289–305.

Halle, J. (1988). Adopting the natural environment as the context for training. In S.N. Calculator & J.L. Bedrosian (Eds.), *Communication assessment and intervention for adults with mental retardation* (pp. 155–185). San Diego: College-Hill Press.

Halle, J.W. (1984). Arranging the natural environment to occasion language: Giving severely language-delayed children reasons to communicate. *Seminars in Speech and Language, 5,* 185–197.

Halle, J.W. (1987). Teaching language in the natural environment: An analysis of spontaneity. *Journal of The Association for Persons with Severe Handicaps, 12,* 28–37.

Halle, J.W., Baer, D.M., & Spradlin, J.E. (1981). An analysis of teachers' generalized use of delay in helping children: A stimulus control procedure to increase language use in handicapped children. *Journal of Applied Behavior Analysis, 14,* 389–409.

Hart, B., & Risley, T.R. (1975). Incidental teaching of language in the preschool. *Journal of Applied Behavior Analysis, 8,* 411–420.

Houghton, J., Bronicki, B., & Guess, D. (1987). Opportunities to express preferences and make choices among students with severe disabilities in classroom settings. *Journal of The Association for Persons with Severe Handicaps, 11*, 255–265.

Iacono, T.A., Carter, M., & Hook, J. (1998). The identification of intentional communication in students with severe and multiple disabilities. *Augmentative and Alternative Communication, 14*, 102–114.

Keen, D., Sigafoos, J., & Woodyatt, G. (in press). Replacing prelinguistic behaviors with functional communication. *Journal of Autism and Developmental Disorders.*

Kozleski, E.B. (1991). Visual symbol acquisition by students with autism. *Exceptionality, 2*, 173–194.

Lane, S.D., & Critchfield, T.S. (1998). Classification of vowels and consonants by individuals with moderate mental retardation: Development of arbitrary relations via match-to-sample training with compound stimuli. *Journal of Applied Behavior Analysis, 31*, 21–41.

Light, J., Collier, B., & Parnes, P. (1985). Communicative interaction between young nonspeaking physically disabled children and their primary caregivers: I. Discourse patterns. *Augmentative and Alternative Communication, 1*, 74–83.

Light, J., & Lindsay, P. (1991). Cognitive science and augmentative and alternative communication. *Augmentative and Alternative Communication, 7*, 186–203.

Lim, L., Browder, D.M., & Sigafoos, J. (1998). The role of response effort and motion study in functionally equivalent task designs and alternatives. *Journal of Behavioral Education, 8*, 81–102.

Locke, P., & Mirenda, P. (1988). A computer-supported communication approach for a child with severe communication, visual, and cognitive impairments: A case study. *Augmentative and Alternative Communication, 4*, 15–22.

Lohrmann-O'Rourke, S., & Browder, D.M. (1998). Empirically-validated methods to assess the preferences of individuals with severe disabilities. *American Journal on Mental Retardation, 103*, 146–161.

McCook, B., Cipani, E., Madigan, K., & LaCampagne, J. (1988). Developing requesting behavior: Acquisition, fluency, and generality. *Mental Retardation, 26*, 137–143.

McIlvane, W.J., Dube, W.V., Green, G., & Serna, R.W. (1993). Programming conceptual and communication skill development: A methodological stimulus-class analysis. In S.F. Warren & J. Reichle (Series Eds.) & A.P. Kaiser & D.B. Gray (Vol. Eds.), *Communication and language intervention series: Vol. 2. Enhancing children's communication: Research foundations for intervention* (pp. 243–285). Baltimore: Paul H. Brookes Publishing Co.

Mirenda, P., & Santogrossi, J. (1985). A prompt-free strategy to teach pictorial communication system use. *Augmentative and Alternative Communication, 1*, 143–150.

Mundy, P., & Gomes, A. (1997). A skills approach to early language development: Lessons from research on developmental disabilities. In L.B. Adamson & M.A. Romski (Eds.), *Communication and language acquisition: Discoveries from atypical development* (pp. 107–133). Baltimore: Paul H. Brookes Publishing Co.

Paclawskyj, T.R., & Vollmer, T.R. (1995). Reinforcer assessment for children with developmental disabilities and visual impairment. *Journal of Applied Behavior Analysis, 28*, 219–224.

Parsons, M.B., & Reid, D.H. (1990). Assessing food preferences among persons with profound mental retardation: Providing opportunities to make choices. *Journal of Applied Behavior Analysis, 23*, 183–195.

Piazza, C.C., Fisher, W.W., Hagopian, L.P., Bowman, L.G., & Toole, L. (1996). Using a choice assessment to predict reinforcer effectiveness. *Journal of Applied Behavior Analysis, 29*, 1–9.

Reichle, J., Anderson, H., & Schermer, G. (1986). *Establishing the discrimination between re-*

questing objects, requesting assistance, and "helping yourself." Unpublished manuscript, University of Minnesota, Minneapolis.

Reichle, J., & Brown, L. (1986). Teaching the use of a multi-page direct selection communication board to an adult with autism. *Journal of The Association for Persons with Severe Handicaps, 11,* 68–73.

Reichle, J., & Karlan, G. (1985). The selection of an augmentative system in communication intervention: A critique of decision rules. *Journal of The Association for Persons with Severe Handicaps, 10,* 146–156.

Reichle, J., Sigafoos, J., & Remington, B. (1991). Beginning an augmentative communication system with individuals who have severe handicaps. In B. Remington (Ed.), *The challenge of severe mental handicap: A behavior analytic approach* (pp. 189–213). New York: John Wiley & Sons.

Reichle, J., York, J., & Sigafoos, J. (Eds.). (1991). *Implementing augmentative and alternative communication: Strategies for learners with severe disabilities.* Baltimore: Paul H. Brookes Publishing Co.

Reichle, J., & Ward, M. (1985). Teaching the discriminative use of an encoding electronic communication device and Signing Exact English to a moderately handicapped child. *Language, Speech, and Hearing Services in Schools, 16,* 58–63.

Roberts-Pennell, D., & Sigafoos, J. (1999). Teaching young children with developmental disabilities to request more play using the behaviour chain interruption strategy. *Journal of Applied Research in Intellectual Disabilities, 12,* 100–112.

Romski, M.A., Sevcik, R.A., & Pate, J.L. (1988). Establishment of symbolic communication in persons with severe mental retardation. *Journal of Speech and Hearing Disorders, 53,* 94–107.

Rowland, C. (1990). Communication in the classroom for children with dual sensory impairments: Studies of teacher and child behavior. *Augmentative and Alternative Communication, 6,* 262–274.

Sarria, E., Gomez, J.C., & Tamarit, J. (1996). Joint attention and alternative language intervention in autism: Implications of theory for practice. In S. von Tetzchner & M.H. Jensen (Eds.), *Augmentative and alternative communication: European perspectives* (pp. 49–64). London: Whurr Publishers.

Siegel, L., & Linder, B. (1984). Short term memory processes in children with reading and arithmetic disabilities. *Developmental Psychology, 20,* 200–207.

Siegel-Causey, E., & Guess, D. (1989). *Enhancing nonsymbolic communication interactions among learners with severe disabilities.* Baltimore: Paul H. Brookes Publishing Co.

Sigafoos, J. (1995). Testing for spontaneous use of requests after sign language training with two severely handicapped adults. *Behavioral Interventions, 10,* 1–16.

Sigafoos, J. (1998). Assessing conditional use of graphic mode requesting in a young boy with autism. *Journal of Developmental and Physical Disabilities, 10,* 133–151.

Sigafoos, J. (1999). Creating opportunities for augmentative and alternative communication: Strategies for involving people with developmental disabilities. *Augmentative and Alternative Communication, 15,* 183–190.

Sigafoos, J., & Couzens, D. (1995). Teaching functional use of an eye gaze communication board to a child with multiple disabilities. *British Journal of Developmental Disabilities, XLI,* 114–125.

Sigafoos, J., Couzens, D., Roberts, D., Phillips, C., & Goodison, K. (1996). Teaching requests for food and drink to children with multiple disabilities in a graphic communication mode. *Journal of Developmental and Physical Disabilities, 8,* 247–262.

Sigafoos, J., Kerr, M., Roberts, D., & Couzens, D. (1994). Increasing opportunities for requesting in classrooms serving children with developmental disabilities. *Journal of Autism and Developmental Disorders, 24,* 631–645.

Sigafoos, J., Laurie, S., & Pennell, D. (1995). Preliminary assessment of choice making among children with Rett syndrome. *Journal of The Association for Persons with Severe Handicaps, 20*, 175–184.

Sigafoos, J., & Meikle, B. (1995). A comparison of two procedures for increasing spontaneous requests in children with autism. *European Journal on Mental Disability, 2*(6), 11–24.

Sigafoos, J., Mustonen, T., DePaepe, P., Reichle, J., & York, J. (1991). Defining the array of instructional prompts for teaching communication skills. In J. Reichle, J. York, & J. Sigafoos (Eds.), *Implementing augmentative and alternative communication: Strategies for learners with severe disabilities* (pp. 173–192). Baltimore: Paul H. Brookes Publishing Co.

Sigafoos, J., & Roberts-Pennell, D. (1999). Wrong-item format: A promising intervention for teaching socially appropriate forms of rejecting to children with developmental disabilities? *Augmentative and Alternative Communication, 15*, 135–140.

Sigafoos, J., Woodyatt, G., Keen, D., Tait, K., Tucker, M., Roberts-Pennell, D., & Pittendreigh, N. (2000). Identifying potential communicative acts in children with developmental and physical disabilities. *Communication Disorders Quarterly, 21*, 77–86.

Skinner, B.F. (1957). *Verbal behavior.* Upper Saddle River, NJ: Prentice Hall.

Sobsey, D., & Reichle, J. (1989). Components of reinforcement for attention signal switch activation. *Mental Retardation and Learning Disabilities Bulletin, 17*(2), 46–59.

Turnell, R., & Carter, M. (1994). Establishing a repertoire of requesting for a student with severe and multiple disabilities using tangible symbols and naturalistic time delay. *Australia and New Zealand Journal of Developmental Disability, 19*, 193–207.

von Tetzchner, S. (1997). Communication skills among females with Rett syndrome. *European Child & Adolescent Psychiatry, 6*(Suppl. 1), 33–37.

Wetherby, A.M., & Prizant, B.M. (1992). Profiling young children's communicative competence. In S.F. Warren & J. Reichle (Series Eds. & Vol. Eds.), *Communication and language intervention series: Vol. 1. Causes and effects in communication and language intervention* (pp. 217–251). Baltimore: Paul H. Brookes Publishing Co.

Wetherby, A.M., Warren, S.F., & Reichle, J. (Vol. Eds.). (1998). *Communication and language intervetion series: Vol. 7. Transitions in prelinguistic communication.* Baltimore: Paul H. Brookes Publishing Co.

Windsor, J., Piché, L.M., & Locke, P.A. (1994). Preference testing: A comparison of two presentation methods. *Research in Developmental Disabilities, 15*, 439–455.

6

Strategies to Achieve Socially Acceptable Escape and Avoidance

Jeff Sigafoos, Mark F. O'Reilly, Erik Drasgow, and Joe Reichle

This chapter focuses on strategies to achieve socially acceptable escape and avoidance. The acquisition of socially acceptable forms of escape and avoidance is an important instructional priority for beginning communicators. Communication repertoires that include a range of socially appropriate responses to achieve escape and avoidance under a variety of conditions should enable the individual to: 1) indicate preferences, 2) escape and avoid nonpreferred objects and activities, 3) exert some degree of control over the environment, and 4) make their wishes and needs more generally known to others (Reichle, York, & Sigafoos, 1991).

Socially acceptable escape and avoidance is defined as the use of appropriate forms of communication to escape from or avoid objects, activities, or interactions that are nonpreferred, difficult, or otherwise not wanted, needed, or desired by the individual at that point in time. In the absence of readily interpreted and socially acceptable forms of communication, many beginning communicators may rely on idiosyncratic gestures and body movements to achieve escape and avoidance. Although some idiosyncratic forms may be socially acceptable, they are nonetheless limiting in that they may be difficult for an unfamiliar communicative partner to interpret (Iacono, Carter, & Hook, 1998). Other individuals may learn to use socially unacceptable behaviors, such as aggression, self-injury, and property destruction, to indicate escape and avoidance (Carr et al., 1994). In the first case, intervention is directed toward developing more conventional and symbolic forms of communication. In the second case, intervention is focused on replacing unacceptable behavior with socially acceptable forms of communication. Along these lines, socially acceptable escape and avoidance can be achieved through the use of vocalizations, speech, manual signs, natural gestures, or graphic mode communication systems (e.g., picture-based communication boards, electronic communication aids). The information in this chapter is applicable to people who may already be using idiosyncratic but socially acceptable forms of communication to indicate escape and avoidance as well as individuals who have acquired socially unacceptable behaviors to achieve escape and avoidance.

It is important to emphasize that escape and avoidance are not exclusively associated with items or events that are nonpreferred. An individual may prefer coffee, for example, but after two cups, the individual may want to reject any more offers. Sigafoos, Pennell, and Versluis (1996) worked with a young boy who initially appeared to enjoy playing with a certain doll. After about 3 minutes, however, he often become satiated with this particular toy, as evidenced by his tossing the doll to the side and engaging in self-injurious head banging. When given a different toy, he would cease self-injury and play appropriately with the new toy. In this situation, a potentially effective intervention would have been to teach the child to request an alternative toy when he became bored with a particular toy. As another example, a child might offer to show a parent that she can tie her own shoes. If the child is unsuccessful, however, she may become upset and throw the shoe. In this situation, intervention could focus in teaching the child to request help with difficult tasks.

As these examples illustrate, it is sometimes difficult to distinguish clearly between communication functions that are used to gain or maintain access to desired items and activities (see Chapter 5) from communication functions to escape and avoid objects and activities. This is because the distinction may be somewhat arbitrary (Michael, 1975). A hungry child who receives food is an example of gaining access to a preferred item, but it could also be viewed as escaping from hunger. Similarly, one could request silence or reject noise. The characteristic consequence maintaining both responses would be identical (i.e., no noise and silence). Another difficulty stems from the lack of one-to-one correspondence between communicative functions and social functions. For example, a request for assistance can be used to gain access to a preferred item (e.g., help in operating a vending machine) or to more quickly escape undesired activity (e.g., help in completing a complex or boring task). Although it can be difficult at times to distinguish between communicative and social functions that are related to gaining access to preferred items and escaping from nonpreferred items, there does appear to be some value in describing a class of communication skills that appear to function primarily to achieve escape and avoidance. This is because in everyday experiences there are numerous opportunities in which the primary goal of communication is to escape and avoid objects or activities.

Under the many everyday conditions associated with escape, an appropriate response (e.g., saying, "Stop" or "Take it away") enables the individual to escape from a nonpreferred object or situation. *Avoidance,* in contrast, refers to situations in which a nonpreferred, unwanted, disliked, or unneeded object, activity, or interaction is about to be experienced but is not currently impinging on the individual. In this situation, an appropriate response enables the individual to avoid contact with the object, activity, or interaction. Although the conditions associated with escape and avoidance are often similar, there may be some practical reasons for distinguishing between the two. Unlike escape, the individual who is taught appropriate avoidance learns how to indicate rejection prior to experiencing the nonpreferred object or activity. This could be advantageous when the object or activity is difficult to present or when its presentation is likely to occasion unacceptable escape behaviors, such as tantrums or aggression. In addition, unacceptable escape behaviors could occur when the nonpreferred object or activity is experienced, and these behaviors may interfere with teaching. Alternatively, the presence of the nonpreferred item or activity may help to ensure that the learner is highly motivated to escape, which may facilitate acquisition of appropriate responses. An important question is whether an individual would more readily learn an escape response or an avoidance response. This is an empirical question that has not been studied in relation to beginning a communication intervention. From an applied perspective, however, many beginning communicators will still need to be taught how to escape some situations and avoid others.

Communicative acts that are used to convey escape and avoidance include rejecting and protesting, as well as some types of requesting skills. The terms *protesting* and *rejecting* typically describe behaviors that occur in the presence of objects or activities that the individual is motivated to escape or avoid. Because the two terms may describe behaviors that could occur under similar situations to achieve similar outcomes, they are often synonymous. Consider this example: For dinner, a young child is given a plate that includes broccoli, and the child responds by crying and pushing the broccoli onto the floor. The child's behavior could be described as rejecting or protesting. In many pragmatic classification schemes, rejecting and protesting are defined in ways that appear to describe a single class of communicative behavior. Wetherby and Prizant (1989), for example, defined *protesting* as acts that are used to refuse an undesired object or to command another person to cease an undesired action. McLean and Snyder-McLean (1987) classified these same types of behaviors as *request for cessation* and *reject/avoid*.

Yet, there may be situations when it could be helpful to distinguish a reject from a protest. For example, a child who has learned to say "no" to reject the offer of an nonpreferred item may not use this response to protest when her sibling takes her favorite toy from her. In these two different contexts, the situations (offer of nonpreferred item, removal of preferred item) and reinforcing consequences (withdrawal of nonpreferred item, return of preferred item) are operationally distinct. Although it would make sense to reject by saying "no," a better form of protesting might be to call attention to the matter by "telling Mom." The important distinction for intervention planning is not in the term used to describe the communicative behavior but in the context surrounding the response and in the vocabulary or form of response that would best fit the context.

Beginning communicators will often need explicit instruction to learn socially acceptable forms of communication for escape and avoidance. To acquire a comprehensive repertoire of communicative behavior that will enable escape and avoidance across the range of everyday contexts, beginning communicators will often need to participate in interventions to teach rejecting or protesting as well as interventions to teach a variety of related communicative functions—specifically, 1) requesting an alternative when offered a nonpreferred item, 2) requesting cessation of an activity or another's action (e.g., "Stop, please"), 3) requesting a break after a period of sustained work, and 4) requesting assistance with a difficult task. Table 6.1 lists examples of some beginning communication skills to achieve escape and avoidance.

Table 6.2 shows the emergence of escape and avoidance responses in typical language development. As illustrated in the table, rejecting or protesting, along with requesting, may be among the earliest classes of communication to emerge in language development (Carpenter, Mastergeorge, & Coggins, 1983; Yamamoto & Mochizuki, 1988). During a child's first 6 months, most infants cry in response to hunger, discomfort, or pain. Each of these acts could be interpreted by a listener as an early escape response, even though these responses are more physiological than communicative. Between 4 and 10 months of age, infants acquire a number of gestures and vocalizations that are also often interpreted as the child's informal or idiosyncratic way of rejecting or protesting (Bates, Camaioni, & Volterra, 1975; Carpenter et al., 1983). Parental acknowledgment and reinforcement of these early prelinguistic signals may help to shape these actions into effective forms of communication sometime during the second half of the infant's first year (Ogletree, Wetherby, & Westling, 1992). By 18 months of age, more conventional gestures (e.g., pointing, shaking one's head for "yes" and "no") and spoken words (Bates, Benigni, Bretherton, Camaioni, & Volterra, 1979) have typically emerged that enable

Table 6.1.   Examples of communication skills that are related to escape and avoidance

Communicative action	Example
Reject object	Push away a nonpreferred or an incorrect item
Protest action or event	Cry when placed in bed for a nap
Indicate "no"	Shake head "no" in response to a question
Terminate/leave taking	Wave goodbye to the teacher at the end of the school day
Request cessation	Ask others to stop making noise
Request alternative	Select the symbol for *cracker* when offered a cookie
Request a break	Point to the staff room to ask for a short break at work
Request assistance	Request help to avoid a difficult task

Table 6.2. Emergence of escape and avoidance responses in typical language development

Age/stage (in months)	Example
Birth–6/Birth cry	After feeding, 3-month-old Sara begins to cry. Her father says, "Oh, Sara, are you telling me that you have a wet diaper? Yes, nasty wet diaper. Let's change it." Sara stops crying after diaper is changed. Her father ends with "Happy now?"
4–10/Perlocutionary	Surrounded by toys, 6-month-old Jason is playing contently on the floor. His father starts to pick up Jason, but Jason begins to cry and struggle. His father says, "Don't you want a cuddle? Just want to play? Okay, here you go back to the toys." After Jason is returned to the toys, he continues to cry for another minute or so.
9–18/Illocutionary	After eating several mouthfuls of applesauce, 10-month-old Billy reacts to the next presentation of the spoon by turning his head away and frowning. His mother says, "Are you telling me you don't want any more? Okay, no more," and she withdraws the spoon.
12+/Locutionary	At 14 months of age, Rita consistently says "no" when offered certain (nonpreferred) foods or beverages. She is also beginning to say "no" to the direct action of others. For example, in the evening when her mother tries to put Rita into her pajamas, Rita playfully says "no" and runs away.

the child to achieve escape and avoidance through socially appropriate communication.

Some individuals with developmental disabilities and severe communication impairments use informal gestures, facial expressions, body movements, and vocalizations to communicate (Butterfield, 1994; Cirrin & Rowland, 1985; Drasgow & Halle, 1995; McLean, McLean, Brady, & Etter, 1991; Ogletree et al., 1992; Wetherby & Prutting, 1984; Wetherby, Yonclas, & Bryan, 1989; Woodyatt & Ozanne, 1994). Some of these informal and idiosyncratic behaviors appear to be used to escape and avoid (e.g., Iacono, Waring, & Chan, 1996; Sigafoos, Woodyatt, Tucker, Roberts-Pennell, & Pittendreigh, 2000). As part of beginning an intervention, it seems useful to systematically identify and describe the range of communicative forms and functions that are related to escape and avoidance and may be expressed by a beginning communicator.

IDENTIFYING AND DESCRIBING COMMUNICATIVE FORMS THAT FUNCTION TO ACHIEVE ESCAPE AND AVOIDANCE

Numerous pragmatic functions have been proposed to classify and describe beginning communication function (see Reichle, Halle, & Johnston, 1993, for a summary). One potential difficulty in classifying pragmatic functions of early communicative acts is that it may require a considerable degree of inference and speculation as to the individual's presumed intent. For example, one of the chapter authors was involved in educating a 4-year-old boy with autism. The boy engaged in extreme tantrums whenever he was asked to sit in a chair to participate in instructional activities. It was hypothesized that tantrums were attempts to escape the activity, so an extinction procedure was implemented. With this procedure, tantrums no longer enabled the boy to escape from the task. Instead, the instructors persisted with the activity and the tantrums were rapidly extinguished. As his tantrums decreased, however, a new behavior emerged. At first, the new behavior was thought to be a request for attention because the form of the behavior involved approaching the instructor to give her hugs and kisses. Yet, it soon became evident that this attention seeking was in fact an alternative means of escaping instruction. This example illustrates that it is often difficult to identify the communicative function of a behavior from its form alone. From a behavioral point of view, communicative functions such as requesting or rejecting an object are observable, whereas the communicative intent is not. Wetherby and colleagues (e.g., Wetherby et al., 1998) suggested that a behavior's function may or may not correspond with the communicator's intent. A child may show a cup to a parent with the intention of gaining access to a preferred beverage, whereas the parent may respond to this as if the child was commenting (e.g., by saying to the child, "Oh, yes, look at the nice red cup"). Interventions that will enable a beginning communicator to achieve escape and avoidance in socially acceptable ways need to specify precisely the antecedent conditions under which the communicative behavior is to occur and the consequence that will function as reinforcement.

A better understanding of the antecedent conditions and maintaining consequences may result from systematic documentation of an individual's prelinguistic acts and the conditions under which these occur. Table 6.3 provides example of behaviors reportedly used by Peter, a 2-year-old child with cerebral palsy and severe communicative impairment, to indicate rejecting and protesting. The information in Table 6.3 was obtained from Peter's mother during a structured interview as part of a larger study involving 20 children with developmental and physical disabilities (Sigafoos, Woodyatt, Keen, et al., 2000). To identify potential communicative acts for rejecting and protesting, parents and teachers were asked five questions based on the Motivation Assessment Scale (Durand & Crimmins, 1988). Specifically, what does the child do if

1. His or her routine is interrupted?
2. He or she is required to do something that he or she does not want to do?
3. He or she does not like something?
4. His or her favorite toy or food is taken away?
5. An adult stops interacting with him or her (e.g., stops playing)?

Table 6.3. Examples of behaviors used by Peter to reject and protest

Questions What does the child do if	Behaviors	Examples of occurrences
His or her routine is disrupted?	Whines, rolls over, gets upset	When his meal time is changed
He or she is required to do something that he or she does not want to do?	Pushes away with hands, feet, or whole body; rolls over and tries to get away	When an adult bends down to pick him up and he knows that it is time for his bath
He or she does not like something?	Cries and whines, gets upset, gets stiff and angry looking	At bath time
His or her favorite toy or food is taken away?	Cries, searches for the object, kicks and screams, jerks head back and forth	When his favorite bunny toy is taken away
An adult stops interacting with him or her?	Follows the adult or whines, rolls toward the adult	When the adult gets up from sitting on the floor or leaves the room

Parents and teachers were also asked to provide examples of typical daily routines in which the behaviors were observed to occur consistently. Table 6.3 includes examples that were provided by Peter's mother.

A complete description of potential communicative acts that are related to escape and avoidance must include more information than that provided in Table 6.3. Analysis of existing or needed communication skills to achieve escape and avoidance should consider three variables: 1) the contexts or situations under which the communicative form should occur, 2) the range of forms that would be acceptable and effective in those situations, and 3) the reactions from communicative partners that would represent reinforcement of the communication behavior. These three variables are described in detail in the following sections. (For the purposes of this chapter, a communicative act is said to exist when there is a functional relation among context, form, and partner reaction.)

Describing the Context of Instruction

Part of designing a communication intervention is to identify appropriate contexts for instruction. Best practice makes use of typical daily routines that include the need and opportunity for communication (Sigafoos, 1999; Ylvisaker & Feeney, 1994). To guide the provision of instruction, interventionists need to describe the natural cues within typical daily routines that create the need (i.e., establishing operations) and set the occasion (i.e., discriminative stimuli) for communication. Generalization and spontaneous use of newly acquired skills often represent significant challenges for beginning communicators. Nevertheless, problems with generalization and spontaneity can be circumvented when instruction occurs in the context of typical routines that include the natural cues for communication. The routines that are used in teaching should systemically sample the range of natural cues for communication (Chadsey-Rusch, Drasgow, Reinoehl, Halle, & Collet-Klingenberg, 1993).

Within the various routines typical of the home, school, and community, there are numerous natural cues that may function to create the need and opportunity for communication to achieve escape and avoidance. Table 6.4 provides examples of such natural cues that were identified in a preschool program that included young children with autism.

When considering a specific communication skill, such as rejecting a nonpreferred object, it is clear that numerous natural cues should control the response. Consequently, to promote generalized rejecting of nonpreferred objects, instruction may need to focus on teaching the beginning communicator to indicate rejection in all of the following contexts:

1. When the communicator is offered a nonpreferred object
2. When a nonpreferred item is likely to be offered (e.g., the communicator can see that someone is cooking a nonpreferred food item)
3. When the communicator is asked if he or she wants a nonpreferred item
4. When the communicator is satiated with a preferred item
5. When the communicator is offered a preferred item but an even more preferred item is available
6. When a normally preferred object is unappealing (e.g., preferred fruit is overly ripe)
7. When there is a need for self-control (e.g., refusing a second piece of cake because others have not yet had a piece)

It is also important to realize that *preference* and *nonpreference* are relative concepts that can be viewed in terms of a continuum. Therefore, an ordinarily preferred item may receive a rejecting response should a more preferred item become available. Initially, one might order apple pie but then reject this in favor of cheesecake upon seeing the two on the dessert trolley. The varying nature of preferences for objects and activities may complicate intervention. If preferences change, the interventionist may not be able to predict whether, at any given time, a particular item or activity is preferred or nonpreferred. Thus, an ordinarily nonpreferred item might be offered to create an opportunity for teaching rejecting. If the item is no longer sufficiently nonpreferred, however, then the individual will not be motivated to reject the offer and the teaching opportunity will be ineffective.

In addition to changing preferences, other variables may make it more difficult to determine whether the beginning communicator is motivated to reject or protest at any given time. As a simple example, if an individual is known to dislike pizza, opportunities for rejecting might arise by merely suggesting a trip to the local pizza restaurant for dinner. Yet, if the person were very hun-

Table 6.4.   Examples of natural cues for teaching communication skills to achieve escape and avoidance in a preschool program

Activity/routine	Natural cue	Communication skill
Arrival/departure	After meeting the teacher at the door and interacting briefly, there is a pause. This is the cue to terminate the interaction, to put away belongings (at arrival), or to exit the building to go home (at departure).	In the presence of a natural cue, the child is taught to hold out his or her backpack and say "Got to go" (at arrival) or wave good-bye and exit the building (at departure).
Group instruction	During group instruction, the teacher asks if everyone has had a turn. If a child has not had a turn, there is a natural opportunity for that child to indicate "no" and request a turn.	In response to the teacher's question, the child is taught to reach out to the teacher and shake his or head "no" if he or she has not had a turn.
Snack/lunch	During snack or lunch, the child is offered various food and beverages, some of which the child indicates are nonpreferred by refusing the items (e.g., turning away, pushing items away).	When the child indicates refusal, the teacher accepts this as a rejection but also prompts the child to indicate rejection in a more conventional manner by pointing to the symbol for *yuck.*
Toy play	Play is interrupted when a toy is broken or stops working. The child may indicate a protest by crying or engaging in a tantrum.	The child is taught to approach the teacher, point to the toy, and sign FIX.
Outdoor play	The temperature may affect playing outdoors on a cold or hot day.	When the child gets too cold or too hot, he or she spontaneously indicates a desire to return to the building by pointing to the symbol for *go back.*
One-to-one teaching	At various times during the teaching session, the child is offered a choice of activities to complete. Sometimes, the teacher mistakenly offers the wrong one. This creates a natural cue for the child to reject the wrong activity and request the other activity.	When he or she is offered the wrong item, the child uses his or her communication device to say, NO, THANKS. I WANT TO WORK ON THE OTHER ONE.

gry or if the restaurant happens to be the trendy place to be seen, then the person may not reject the suggestion.

To better predict whether a particular context will provide a good opportunity to teach rejecting, the interventionist might look for collateral behaviors that indicate when the individual is motivated to escape and avoid. Collateral behaviors—such as pushing away an object, engaging in tantrums when presented with task demands, and moving away from an offered item—most likely indicate that the individual is motivated to escape and avoid. For example, a beginning communicator may turn his or her head away as a spoonful of yogurt is offered. This behavior suggests that the item is not highly preferred. Therefore, offering the item provides an effective context for teaching the individual to indicate rejection by using more symbolic forms of communication, such as shaking his or her head "no." Similarly, if the individual is given a choice between two items, it is reasonable to assume that the item selected on any occasion is the more preferred. Consequently, offering the item that was not selected should represent an effective context for teaching rejecting (Sigafoos & Roberts-Pennell, 1999).

Natural cues for indicating escape may be distinguished from those to avoid. As mentioned previously, an escape response can occur once one has engaged in an activity from which he or she would now like to be extricated. An avoidance response occurs prior to experiencing a specific object or activity. Learning to escape may not necessarily equip one with the skills to avoid an activity in the first place. Similarly, the cues in the natural environment that create the need or set the occasion to reject a nonpreferred object may not exert control over responses to reject additional offers of a normally preferred item of which one has grown tired or satiated. Even if generalized rejecting responses are taught that would be appropriate across a range of contexts (e.g., "no," "stop"), beginning communicators may not use these responses in a variety of situations unless instruction includes a range of contexts and natural cues.

Explicit intervention may be necessary to obtain transfer from escape to avoidance functions. Unfortunately, there appears to be no research on this issue that is relevant to teaching communication skills to achieve escape and avoidance to beginning communicators. Nonetheless, based on available evidence from studies on teaching communicative requesting, transfer from escape to avoidance might be obtained by the careful application of stimulus control strategies (Billingsley & Romer, 1983; Cipani, 1988). Initially, the beginning communicator might be taught to reject the offer of a nonpreferred object when it is offered directly. Because the item is offered, producing a rejecting communicative act would function as an escape response. Yet, it would be desirable to transfer stimulus control to an earlier component in the chain (i.e., before the nonpreferred item is offered). To achieve this type of transfer, the individual might be prompted to produce a rejecting response as the communicative partner removes the item from its package or prepares to offer the item. Transfer could be established by using a time delay procedure in which the offer of the item is delayed for increasingly greater intervals as the learner becomes increasingly successful.

There are advantages to rejecting an item before it is actually experienced. First, it can speed up the communicative exchange with the resulting increase in efficiency for both the speaker and the listener. For example, suppose that the interventionist is teaching an individual to escape from an activity such as swimming. Sometimes the activity is preferred and sometimes it is not. Instruction to teach rejecting might occur initially when the individual is taken to the swimming pool. Nonetheless, it would be desirable to transfer stimulus control to an earlier component in the chain, such as when the person is at home and is invited to join peers in a trip to the swimming pool. In this situation, common stimuli, such as a photograph of the swimming pool, might be used in the presence of the activity and at home as a way of promoting transfer. At home, the individual could be shown the photograph and asked if he or she would like to do the corresponding activity. Use of the rejecting response in this situation would enable the individual to avoid going all the way to the swimming pool only to declare that he or she did not want to go swimming. To transfer stimulus control from the location of the activity to the home, the photograph would probably have to be paired with the actual activity a number of times. In addition, the person would have to experience differential outcomes for rejecting versus not rejecting when shown the photograph. That is, the intervention would have to ensure that an appropriate rejecting response in the presence of the photograph resulted in no access to the activity, whereas if the rejecting response did not occur, then the activity would proceed. Over time, presentation of the photograph or some other relevant symbol may come to function as a vicarious offer of the actual item or activity, thereby helping bridge the gap between escape and avoidance responding.

An additional distinction involves cues that signal when a response is obligatory and when it is nonobligatory (Davis, Reichle, Southard, & Johnston, 1998). For example, if an individual likes black coffee and a host offers cream, the recipient is obliged to reject the cream (e.g., "No, thanks"). In other instances, there may be no explicit requirement or obligation to communicate a reject. If one orders coffee in a cafe and receives a container of cream on the side, there is no obligation to reject, but one may do so nonetheless as a social courtesy (e.g., "Oh, thanks, but you can have this back—I don't use cream"). When acceptance means that the item must be used (e.g., the host is about to pour dressing directly onto your salad), then avoidance of the nonpreferred item requires the use of a communicative rejecting response. Another example involves using communication to terminate activities. Some activities have a very clear end point, such as the buzzer signaling the end of a basketball game. At a basketball game, there may be no obligation or need to indicate a desire to leave the event. Instead, one can just leave without appearing rude. Other situations may impose more of a social obligation to indicate the desire to exit by using appropriate communication. When visiting friends for dinner, there is the always difficult decision as to when to bid farewell. In these types of situations, there is an implied social obligation to indicate the desire to escape using appropriate (and tactful) communication. Ensuring that beginning communicators have the skills to participate in social-communicative interactions requires that learners act on both obligatory and nonobligatory cues for communicating escape and avoidance.

With beginning communicators, instruction often occurs in the presence of cues that require a response (e.g., the interventionist offers a nonpreferred item and asks, "Want this?"). Nonetheless, it is unclear whether socially appropriate forms of communicative rejecting that are acquired in the presence of these types of obligatory cues would generalize to nonobligatory situations in which a response is not required. As with generalization from escape to avoidance functions, this type of generalization may need to be explicitly programmed. Unfortunately, there appears to be no research that demonstrates effective procedures for promoting this type of generalization. Based on general-case instructional principles, generalization of this type might be achieved by including exemplars that sample a range of both obligatory and nonobligatory cues during the initial stages of intervention (Halle, Chadsey-Rusch, & Collet-Klingenberg, 1993). Transfer of stimulus control procedures would also be indicated for developing the generalized use of rejecting across obligatory and nonobligatory cues. If the beginning communicator reliably indicates rejection as the communication partner is about to pour salad dressing onto the person's bowl of salad, for example, control can be transferred to other stimuli, such as the partner's offering the bottle, placing the bottle near the beginning communicator, or giving the communicator an expectant look with an alternating shift of gaze to the bottle of salad dressing. In summary, it appears useful to use teaching exemplars that include both types of cues—that is, cues signaling that a response is required and cues signaling that a response would be socially appropriate but is not required. Of course, because the response is not required for these latter types of cues, it seems more critical to ensure the desired response occurs consistently when it is required.

Identifying Contexts for Teaching Escape and Avoidance

As noted previously, at the outset of intervention, beginning communicators have informal and idiosyncratic ways to indicate escape and avoidance. Intervention for these individuals could begin by identifying these existing behaviors (Sigafoos, Woodyatt, Keen, et al., 2000). Information on existing potential communicative acts can be useful in at least three ways when developing intervention programs that aim to establish socially acceptable forms of communication to achieve escape and avoidance. Specifically, these items are as follows:

1. *Existing behaviors may indicate the motivation to communicate.* For example, if the beginning communicator consistently turns away, frowns, and produces a negative vocalization when he or she is offered certain objects, it is reasonable to conclude that these behaviors indicate rejection. Behavioral indications of this type may suggest an optimal time to teach a more conventional form of communicative rejecting such as signing NO (Drasgow, Halle, Ostrosky, & Harbers, 1996).

2. *Analysis of the contexts in which potential communicative acts occur may also provide information on the natural cues that control the individual's responses.* Intervention may then focus on expanding the range of natural cues that control responding and on bringing more conventional or sophisticated forms of communication under the control of these same natural cues. In some cases, the natural cues for rejecting will be internal, private events (e.g., satiation). For instance, it may be observed that after drinking two cups of coffee, the individual is likely to refuse an offer for a third cup. Offers of a third cup of coffee thus provide a natural opportunity to teach the individual to refuse the offer by using a socially acceptable form of communication (e.g., signing NO MORE).

3. *Analysis of contexts may also provide information on the objects or activities that a person dislikes and, therefore, should be taught to reject.* It is important to note that preferred or neutral objects may only be disliked after the person has become satiated with these objects or activities or when a more appealing alternative becomes available. In these instances, behavioral indication may reveal when the person has had enough and is thus motivated to reject the object, protest continuation, terminate participation, or request an alternative.

Determining When to Honor Communicative Attempts to Escape and Avoid   A side issue that arises once communicative forms have been identified is determining when to honor communicative attempts to escape and avoid. There is a need to consider whether it is appropriate to provide the functional consequence for each and every protest or reject. If the individual uses an existing idiosyncratic form to protest a situation that cannot be avoided (e.g., taking seizure medication), then it would not be appropriate to honor the protest by allowing the individual to avoid the medication. Yet, the idiosyncratic form of protesting used in this situation may be encouraged and reinforced on other occasions, such as when the individual is given the opportunity to participate in a leisure activity. In this latter situation, the idiosyncratic protest could be honored by allowing the individual to escape from the activity.

In developing a comprehensive intervention program, it is important to consider a longitudinal direction for communication development. Part of this development requires considering whether existing forms are acceptable or whether these need to be replaced or expanded with more acceptable, conventional, or symbolic forms of communication. Along these lines, several options might be considered. These options are explored next.

Strengthen Existing Forms if Acceptable   If existing forms are socially acceptable but occur inconsistently, intervention might focus on strengthening these forms so that they occur more consistently (Warren & Yoder, 1998; Warren, Yoder, Gazdag, Kim, & Jones, 1993; Yoder & Warren, 1998). Accepting existing forms provides the individual with an immediately useful communication skill. The form is already within the individual's repertoire and can be reinforced when it occurs under appropriate conditions. Existing forms are strengthened when the communicative partner learns to recognize the communicative potential of existing forms and reacts to these in ways that are consistent with their presumed communicative function. For example, one of the chapter authors worked with a beginning communicator who had multiple disabilities. The child would turn her head to one side when offered certain food items. When this behavior occurred in the mealtime context, it was interpreted as a form of communication (i.e., "I don't want this"), and the item was withdrawn.

Expand Existing Forms / Teach New Forms   In the long term, prelinguistic forms may limit the individual's communicative effectiveness. Reliance on prelinguistic forms may be especially problematic for individuals with subtle or highly idiosyncratic forms of communication. Subtle and idiosyncratic forms of communication are often difficult to recognize and interpret (Sigafoos, Woodyatt, Tucker, et al., 2000). Even if existing forms are clearly recognized and provide a consistent communicative signal, there is still considerable long-term value in teaching more conventional and symbolic forms of communication to replace or supplant existing forms (Reichle et al., 1993). In the previous example, the child would turn away when offered certain foods, and this was accepted as a reject. This occasion was also used to prompt a more conventional head-shake gesture, thereby expanding her existing form of rejecting into a more conventional and readily interpreted gesture. Doing so may help ensure that the individual's communication ability continues to expand and develop to correspond with the demands of new and changing roles, responsibilities, and communicative partners.

A relevant intervention strategy involves chaining a new form to an existing idiosyncratic form. This strategy was used to develop socially acceptable forms of greeting skills in a young child with autism (Keen, Sigafoos, &

Woodyatt, in press). The child's existing greeting behavior consisted of look-ing at the other person. Intervention focused on teaching the child to also wave whenever the child looked at a person in a greeting context (e.g., upon encountering someone for the first time each day, when another person initi-ated a greeting). A similar chaining strategy might be used to expand existing forms of rejecting. For example, if the individual currently pushes away un-wanted items, intervention might focus on chaining to this action the more sophisticated head-shake gesture for "no."

Replace Unacceptable Forms   In some instances, existing behaviors may be unacceptable and will need to be replaced by teaching socially acceptable forms that serve the same purpose. For example, a beginning communicator might engage in tantrum behavior to escape from nonpreferred activities. Al-though the tantrum may have a clear communicative function, it is not socially acceptable. In this instance, intervention might focus on replacing tantrums by teaching a functionally equivalent and more socially acceptable way for the child to achieve escape from nonpreferred tasks, such as by pointing to the printed word *stop* on a communication board (Carr et al., 1994). A consider-able amount of literature has developed in reference to replacing challenging behavior by teaching functionally equivalent forms of communication (see Chapter 4). Generally, this literature has demonstrated the effectiveness of functional communication training (FCT) as a treatment for challenging be-haviors that have a social-communicative basis. FCT is indicated when a prior functional assessment reveals that the challenging behavior is maintained by either positive social reinforcement (e.g., attention, access to tangible items) or negative social reinforcement (e.g., escape from task demands). Socially moti-vated challenging behaviors can be replaced by teaching socially acceptable forms of communication, including the use of AAC, that serve the same func-tion or purpose as the challenging behavior (Mirenda, 1997). Successful re-placement occurs when the alternative is more efficient than the challenging behavior—that is, when the alternative is easier to perform and results in more immediate and consistent reinforcement and provided that challenging beha-vior is no longer reinforced.

Establish Conditional Use   It may not always be possible or desirable for an individual to achieve escape and avoidance, even through acceptable com-munication. For example, it would not be in the individual's best interest to avoid taking necessary medications or avoid going to work if the long-term consequences were increased risk of illness and unemployment. As a result, intervention may need to include strategies to establish conditional use of newly acquired communication skills to achieve escape and avoidance (Sigafoos, 1998). If an individual is taught to request a break from work but uses this escape response too often (e.g., every 5 minutes), then it will be nec-essary to teach the individual that requesting a break will only be honored at certain times of the day. When a break is requested at other times, the individual may be informed that although the message has been received, it is not yet break time. Similar limits on the use of escape and avoidance responses may be necessary in other situations such as when the individual refuses to participate in necessary activities (e.g., dressing, feeding, self-care routines).

Because nearly all communicative interactions have some conditional aspect, there will almost always be the need for multi-element intervention strategies to ensure appropriate conditional use of newly acquired communication skills. This is an area that has yet to be fully explored in interventions for beginning communicators, especially in interventions to develop communication skills that achieve socially acceptable escape and avoidance. Nevertheless, it is clear that strategies often need to be implemented to teach beginning communicators when to use a newly acquired reject or protest and when to refrain from using a rejecting or protesting response. Part of the interventionist's task, therefore, is to gain stimulus control over rejecting and protesting. One way to achieve this is to ensure different outcomes under different conditions. For instance, it is necessary to ensure that the reject or protest is only successful (i.e., leads to escape and avoidance) in situations when it is acceptable to escape and avoid. In addition, it is necessary to ensure the reject or protest is not honored when escape and avoidance is not acceptable. By implementing a program of differential outcomes, the appropriate conditional discriminations should emerge over time.

Summary   The previously described intervention options are not mutually exclusive. In many instances, intervention programs will include concurrent implementation of multiple strategies. In all cases, however, it may be necessary to ensure that the targeted communication skills have the desired effect on the communicative partner. Beginning communication skills are often taught in the presence of attentive and highly responsive communicative partners. Individuals who are taught to communicate under these conditions may not learn how to recruit a partner when one is needed but no one is currently attending. Therefore, intervention may need to enhance the responsiveness of social partners in recognizing and reacting to beginning communicators' indications of escape and avoidance.

Reactions of Communicative Partners

Responsivity of communicative partners is critical to the success of communication intervention with beginning communicators (Yoder & Warren, 1998). Unfortunately, communicative overtures often are ignored by people in the environment (Houghton, Bronicki, & Guess, 1987). Thus, it is important that communicative partners provide sufficient opportunities for communication and react in ways that function as reinforcement for the individual's communication. If the partner does not provide the need and opportunity for communication and does not reinforce consistently and often enough, then the individual's communicative attempts may decrease and ultimately be extinguished (Reichle, Halle, & Drasgow, 1998). Yet, it may be difficult for partners to know how to create the need and opportunity for communication or to determine in advance what reaction would serve as reinforcement, especially when the beginning communicator's form of the response is less than conventional.

At times, it may be difficult to react to a beginning communicator's presumed communicative function. Say that a child who is a beginning communicator protests having to attend a family gathering. Although the parent might recognize that the child is protesting, it may be an unavoidable event. In this situation, the parent would acknowledge that a communicative attempt has occurred (e.g., "Yes, I know that you don't want to go") but would not reinforce the behavior (e.g., "But you have to go, so let's make the most of it"). During the early stages of intervention, it may be important to acknowledge the beginning communicator's protest, but that does not mean that each and every protest or reject can be reinforced.

In 1997, von Tetzchner described *structured overinterpretation* as a potentially useful intervention approach. Structured overinterpretation involves learning to recognize an individual's communicative attempts, providing a consistent interpretation of the presumed function or purpose of these attempts based on context, and then reacting in a manner consistent with that presumed function. The process can be illustrated by considering how partners might be taught to react to the informal communication of Tina, a young girl with multiple disabilities. One of the communicative behaviors that Tina emitted was closing her eyes. It was assumed that the function of this behavior was to terminate activities of which she had grown tired and to request an alternative activity. For example, if Tina closed her eyes after 20 minutes of a classroom activity, the teacher recognized this as a potential communicative act (e.g., "Oh, I see that you are closing your eyes. Are you bored with this?") and introduced a new activity. Although structured overinterpretation seems promising, there appears to be no systematic evaluations of this strategy's effectiveness.

There is growing recognition that intervention for beginning communicators should focus as much on the communicative partner as on the beginning communicator (Butterfield, Arthur, & Sigafoos, 1995). In particular, partners may need support in learning to recognize and react appropriately to the beginning communicator's behavioral indications of escape and avoidance as well as to promote the development of new and more conventional, communication skills to achieve escape and avoidance. The next section reviews empirically validated instructional strategies that have been used to teach beginning communicators socially acceptable communication skills that achieve escape and avoidance. In these studies, the communicative partner plays a central role in creating the need and opportunity for communication and in reacting in ways that reinforce communication behaviors.

EXEMPLARY STRATEGIES FOR TEACHING
SOCIALLY ACCEPTABLE ESCAPE AND AVOIDANCE

Since the 1990s, there has been an increase in empirically validated instructional strategies for teaching beginning communicators (Shafer, 1995). The forms of communication responses that have been targeted for instruction include speech, manual signs, and graphic mode communication (e.g., pictureboards, electronic communication devices). Yet, most of the published studies have concentrated on teaching requesting (Shafer, 1995). Fewer studies have sought to teach rejecting, protesting, and other skills to achieve socially acceptable escape and avoidance.

Sigafoos and Reichle (1991) outlined prototypic instructional paradigms for teaching rejecting to beginning communicators. Figure 6.1 outlines basic instructional paradigms for teaching general and explicit rejecting. A general rejecting response enables the individual to escape or avoid a variety of nonpreferred objects or activities by using a single response form. This may be an advantage for beginning communication, as it provides an immediately useful communication skill prior to the acquisition of multiple response forms. In addition, a general strategy may be most helpful when the referent of the reject has been established—that is, when it is clear what the person is trying to escape or avoid. One disadvantage, however, is that communicative partners may have difficulty interpreting exactly what the individual is trying to reject because the form of the response (e.g., the manual sign NO) is not precise. An explicit reject is obviously more specific, and this makes it easier for communicative partners to respond appropriately and consistently to the individual's communication. Using the example given in Figure 6.1, if the communicator selects line drawings that represent "no sugar," then the partner has a better idea of the intended message. Of course, before explicit rejecting can be used to reject a variety of objects or activities, the individual has to acquire multiple response forms (e.g., "no sugar," "no butter," "no music"). One possible intervention sequence is to begin by teaching general response forms and to introduce strategies subsequently or concurrently that teach more explicit forms (Reichle et al., 1991).

Some conditions exist for the use of general rejecting and explicit rejecting as outlined by Sigafoos and Reichle (1991). Briefly, when a beginning communicator has been taught a general reject (e.g., "no"), more dependence on context is needed to ascertain the object or activity that is the focus of the reject. That is, the beginning communicator may need to wait for the referent to

Natural cue (Discriminative stimulus)	Generalized rejecting response	Partner reaction (Consequence)
The partner offers nonpreferred items. More than one nonpreferred item may be offered, or the specific item that is offered may vary across opportunities.	The learner is prompted to indicate "no" in a socially acceptable manner that is vocal, graphic, or gestural. Prompts are faded over successive opportunities.	The nonpreferred item is removed by the partner.

Natural cue (Discriminative stimulus)	Explicit rejecting response	Partner reaction (Consequence)
The partner offers a specific nonpreferred item (e.g., the learner is offered sugar for his or her coffee).	The learner is prompted to indicate "no sugar" in a socially acceptable manner that is vocal, graphic, or gestural. Prompts are faded over successive opportunities.	The nonpreferred item (i.e., sugar) is withdrawn by the partner.

Figure 6.1. Prototypic instructional paradigms for teaching generalized and explicit rejecting.

be presented if the reject is to be successful. In an explicit reject (e.g., "no milk"), however, the partner would know immediately what the beginning communicator is rejecting. Sigafoos and Reichle recommended teaching a general reject (e.g., "no") initially to provide the beginning communicator with the means to reject a variety of items or activities. On one hand, a general reject makes sense: During a rejecting opportunity, the referent is often present and it is therefore clear what is being rejected. Thus, there may be many more opportunities to use a general reject. On the other hand, if a person is presented with coffee and sugar and indicates a general reject, it may be unclear whether the coffee or the sugar is being rejected. In this situation, an explicit reject would enable the individual to specify the unwanted referent. Intervention can then focus on teaching the person a chain of two responses (e.g., "no" + "milk," "no" + "music") to make explicit rejects. Of course, there are also many instances in which a person can simply walk away from an undesired object or activity. In these situations, a communicative reject of any type may not be necessary unless the issue is forced (e.g., someone makes an explicit offer or prompts the individual to make contact with the object or activity). This means that intervention will need to teach the conditional discriminations of when to reject versus when to simply not act and when to use a general versus an explicit reject. In either case, teaching general or explicit rejecting as a beginning communication skill involves five steps. Table 6.5 outlines these steps.

A study by Reichle, Rogers, and Barrett (1984) demonstrated the effectiveness of the instructional strategies outlined in Table 6.5. They taught a 15-year-old girl with severe disabilities to use a manual sign to indicate NO when offered an array of nonpreferred objects. To teach the sign, the individual was offered an array of nonpreferred items and the teacher asked, "Want one?" If the girl produced the sign for NO, then the array was removed. If the response did not occur, then the teacher offered one of the nonpreferred items. When the communicator showed behavioral indications of resistance (e.g., turning away from item), the teacher used physical guidance to prompt the sign for NO. Over successive teaching opportunities, prompts were faded by using graduated guidance. Under these conditions, the sign for NO was readily acquired and appeared to be controlled by the presentation of nonpreferred items and maintained by the withdrawal of these items contingent on the child signing NO. Signing NO could therefore be viewed as a rejecting response that was controlled by aversive stimulation (i.e., the offer of nonpreferred items)

Table 6.5 Instructional steps for teaching general or explicit rejecting as a beginning communication skill

Instructional step	Description
1. Define the response form.	Define the response form (generalized or explicit) that the person will be taught to indicate rejection. This could be the use of a particular vocalization, speech act, informal gesture, manual sign, or graphic-mode communication.
2. Identify non-preferences.	Identify nonpreferred objects or activities. Nonpreferred objects, activities, or events are things that the individual does not select or will make some effort to escape from or avoid. Identify these systematically by recording items that the person does not select when offered a choice of two or more items and by noting activities or events that the person refuses to participate in or even approach (Fisher et al., 1992).
3. Create the need for rejecting.	Offer or present nonpreferred objects or activities to teach the rejecting response. This creates the context for the individual to indicate rejection. When the person produces the response, remove the nonpreferred item or stop the nonpreferred activity.
4. Prompt the desired response.	Prompt the desired response if the individual does not produce the targeted rejecting response within a reasonable period of time following the offer (e.g., 10 seconds). Use verbal, model, or gestural prompts or physical assistance as necessary. Over successive opportunities, fade these prompts to promote independence.
5. Provide negative reinforcement.	Provide negative reinforcement for the rejecting response. Remove the nonpreferred object or stop the nonpreferred activity when the communicator uses the targeted rejecting response.

and maintained by negative reinforcement (i.e., the removal of nonpreferred items). Yet, following opportunities to reject nonpreferred items, the girl was also given the opportunity to request preferred items. It is possible that the opportunity to request partially maintained the learner's rejecting behavior. In addition, because the communicator was offered an array of only nonpreferred items during initial teaching opportunities, it is unclear if the acquired rejecting response was controlled by any specific nonpreferred item or, rather, by the more general context and materials associated with the task. It should be noted, however, that subsequent generalization probes revealed highly discriminated use of both the newly acquired rejecting response and a previously acquired requesting response.

Although the Reichle and colleagues (1984) study was limited to a single individual, the strategies were effective in teaching the targeted response and, therefore, provided support for the five instructional steps outlined previously. Additional evidence suggests these teaching strategies are appropriate for younger children as well. Specifically, Drasgow and colleagues (1996) used similar prompting procedures to teach a 4-year-old child with a developmental disability to reject nonpreferred objects (e.g., foods, beverages). In this study, however, there was no generalization to nonpreferred activities (e.g., large group activities, fine motor activities), possibly because such activities were not included as teaching exemplars during intervention.

Along with strategies to teach socially acceptable escape and avoidance responses, it is often necessary to establish the discriminated use of newly acquired communication skills. Hung (1980) described procedures to teach a discrimination between two types of responses. The two responses were 1) saying "yes" to request preferred food items and 2) saying "no" to reject nonpreferred food items. Preferred and nonpreferred food items were identified for a 8-year-old boy and a 10-year-old girl, both of whom had autism. To establish discrimination, the teacher would offer an item and ask, "Do you want (name of food item)?" The offered item was given to the child when he or she said "yes" and was removed when the child said "no." The intervention included the use of modeling, error correction, and differential reinforcement. Both children learned to produce "yes" or "no" depending on whether the offered item was preferred or nonpreferred, respectively.

Duker and Jutten (1997) also evaluated procedures for teaching yes/no responding to beginning communicators. The beginning communicators in this study were three adults with mental retardation and pervasive support needs who were taught to use communicative gestures rather than speech. The study began with the identification of preferred and nonpreferred objects and activities for each participant. The researchers then taught one gesture at a time to each participant by using prompting, repetition of the correct response, and reinforcement. That is, for two of the participants, teaching the request ("yes" response) preceded teaching the reject ("no" response). The third participant learned to reject first, and only when the "no" response was acquired did the intervention shift to teaching the "yes" gesture. Results indicated that all three participants rapidly increased correct responding when the first gesture was being taught, decreased correct responding when training to teach the second gesture was introduced, and then, over time, increased correct discriminated responding of both target responses. Generalization probes revealed a lack of generalization of yes/no responding from the training room to the classroom; thus, training was implemented in the classroom.

The procedures that Hung (1980) and Duker and Jutten (1997) used were effective in teaching a discrimination between requesting and rejecting. Both studies involved the presentation of highly preferred or nonpreferred objects or activities. Therefore, it is unclear whether beginning communicators would use newly acquired "yes" and "no" responses in other situations in which it would be useful to request versus to reject, such as when a child is asked if he or she needs help with a difficult (yes) versus an easy (no) task or when he or she is deprived from (yes) versus satiated with (no) a particular item or activity. Nonetheless, Duker and Jutten's results suggest that this type of discrimination would need to be taught explicitly.

Beginning communicators can be taught to request preferred items and reject nonpreferred items as initial intervention priorities (Reichle et al., 1991). It is often assumed that newly acquired requesting and rejecting responses function as valid communication in the sense that they are functionally related to a characteristic consequence. Yet, this is not always the case. Yamamoto and Mochizuki (1988) designed a study that is relevant to this issue. In this study, three children with autism were taught to request objects by speaking sentences such as "Give me a pencil," "Give me a cup," and so forth. To determine if the responses were in fact functioning as requests for the specific items (e.g., pencil, cup), sometimes the children were given the wrong item. For example, if the child asked for a cup, he or she was given the pencil. Because the children often accepted the wrong item, Yamamoto and Mochizuki concluded that the responses were not always requests for specific item, which made the responses less functional for the children. To overcome this problem, an additional intervention was implemented. Specifically, when the children were offered the wrong item, they were taught to say, "That's not it, give me (name of correct object)." Use of the repair strategy resulted in the children receiving the object that they originally requested.

In a study with a similar aim, Duker, Dortmans, and Lodder (1993) observed one adolescent and five young adults with mental retardation and substantial support needs. All six participants had been taught to request preferred items using manual signs (e.g., I WANT DRINK, I WANT EAT). Following a request, however, these learners would often accept a nonmatching referent. For example, if the student signed I WANT EAT but was given a drink, the person would often accept the wrong item. This observation suggested that the responses were not requests in that they were not under the functional control of a corresponding consequence. The solution was to teach these beginning communicators a repetition strategy. This involved teaching them to repeat the original sign when presented with the wrong item. The intervention was effective in that the participant would no longer accept the wrong item but would instead repeat his or her initial request. The potential for individuals to accept items that were not requested highlights the importance of offering both correct and wrong items, as well as collecting data on acceptance and refusal of offered items, to ensure that any intervention to teach requesting or rejecting does in fact lead to a correspondence between response and consequence (Reichle, Sigafoos, & Piché, 1989).

Sigafoos and Dempsey (1992) made further use of the wrong-item format to assess the validity of choice making among three children with multiple disabilities. Specifically, each child was presented with repeated opportunities to choose between foods and beverages. In one condition, the children were given the item that they had reached for (i.e., the correct item), but in another condition the wrong item was delivered. The results indicated that all three children were more likely to accept the correct item and refuse the wrong item. Refusals consisted primarily of informal and direct acts, such as dropping or turning away from the item. Yet, there were also a few instances in which the children used communicative behaviors to reject (e.g., shaking head "no," saying "no"). Based on these results, the wrong-item format would seem to offer a potential means by which to create effective contexts for teaching communication skills to reject objects.

Along these lines, Sigafoos and Roberts-Pennell (1999) described an intervention to teach children to reject wrong items as an initial communication objective. The study involved two 6-year-old boys with developmental disabilities and substantial support needs. Opportunities were provided for the children to choose between two items. After a child reached for an item, the instructor presented the child with either the item that he had reached for (i.e., the correct item) or the other unchosen item (i.e., the wrong item). Investigators assumed that the item reached for on any given opportunity was preferred over the item that was not reached for and, thus, provision of the wrong item created a need for the child to reject. When presented with the wrong item during baseline, the children showed little tendency to reject with socially appropriate communication. Intervention procedures were designed to teach one child to reject the wrong item by using the head-shake gesture "no." The other child was taught to use a voice output communication aid. His response consisted of pressing a switch to activate the recorded message NO, THANKS. I WANT THE OTHER ONE. Teaching involved presenting the wrong item, prompting the child to produce the rejecting response, and then removing the wrong item (negative reinforcement). Prompts were faded using the system of least prompts and progressive time delay (Reichle et al., 1991). Both children acquired the rejecting response and maintained high levels of correct responding at a 3-month follow-up. In addition, there was evidence of generalization to a new instructor and across one or two additional pairs of items that were not included as exemplars during intervention. The results are promising because they suggest that communication intervention can begin with the initial communication objective of teaching responses that are related to escape and avoidance.

The acquisition of communication skills to achieve escape and avoidance should be a high priority when designing interventions for beginning communicators. Yet, these types of communication skills appear to be somewhat overlooked in programs for beginning communicators (Sigafoos, 1997). This may reflect the fact that there is relatively little published literature on teaching rejecting and protesting. As the next section shows, much remains to be learned about teaching beginning communicators the skills to achieve socially acceptable escape and avoidance.

FUTURE DIRECTIONS

Contextual influences, such as internal states of satiation or deprivation, can alter the reinforcing effectiveness of consequence stimuli and the evocative effectiveness of discriminative stimuli. In other words, a particular food item could produce a request if presented when the person is hungry but a reject when the person is satiated from a large meal. Historically, researchers have placed great emphasis on representing the stimulus characteristics of the objects being requested or rejected (e.g., Chadsey-Rusch et al., 1993; Hupp & Mervis, 1981; Stokes & Baer, 1977) rather than ensuring that motivation to avoid or escape the stimulus is operating during every instructional trial. Acquisition and generalization of a new rejecting response may depend more on motivation to avoid or escape the stimulus than on any intrinsic characteristics of the objects themselves. Research on establishing operations (Michael, 1993) and setting events (Wahler & Fox, 1981) provides an approach for manipulating and assessing motivational states and evaluating their relationship with the acquisition of communication skills.

Response competition also may interfere with the acquisition and generalization of any newly acquired response. This is because functionally equivalent competing responses already may be widely generalized and have a longer history of reinforcement than the new response (Drasgow, Halle, & Ostrosky, 1998). For example, interventionists may want to teach a learner to avoid or escape a task by touching a *stop* icon. Yet, the learner may already have a generalized way of rejecting the task by closing his or her eyes or turning away. Widely generalized competing forms, however, can be conceptualized within the general-case framework (Horner, Sprague, & Wilcox, 1982). That is, the learner's existing competing forms define the range of situations in which instruction must occur. This view of a learner-defined range of instructional situations could be a problem for generalization. It may be difficult, for instance, to select representative exemplars, then to teach in these few situations and expect generalization because the learner may continue to respond with existing forms in communicative interactions outside of the teaching examples. Thus, teaching must occur in enough situations in which competing forms occur to keep the learner from continuing to respond with competing forms. That is, an approach that includes teaching in situations in which competing forms occur may not successfully supplant competing forms unless the new form 1) is reinforced in more situations, 2) is reinforced more quickly in those situations, and 3) requires less effort than the competing form (Horner & Day, 1991; Mace & Roberts, 1993). Future research could be directed at determining the number of teaching exemplars that are necessary to supplant the competing forms. To summarize, an approach to teaching rejecting may need to define the range of situations in which the learner currently uses competing forms as well as to teach the new form in a sufficient number of situations; otherwise, the communicator will continue to use competing forms (Horner & Budd, 1985).

Another area of future research includes evaluating methods for teaching a learner to use repair strategies when the first communicative response is not successful. In a study of preverbal repairs of three typically developing young children, Golinkoff (1986) found that 62% of communicative episodes were either negotiated or missed—only 38% were immediately successful. Relative to typically developing children, however, those with severe communication disabilities who communicate with subtle and idiosyncratic forms have an even higher probability of encountering communicative breakdowns (Wetherby, Alexander, & Prizant, 1998). Therefore, it is important to teach multiple repair strategies that enable a learner to persist in emitting socially desirable escape and avoidance responses for two reasons. First, teaching a socially acceptable repertoire of repairs equips a learner with a number of communicative responses; thus encouraging persistence and preventing "learned helplessness" (Guess, Benson, & Siegel-Causey, 1985). Second, a socially acceptable repertoire lessens the possibility of a learner quickly becoming frustrated at the lack of reinforcement that is contingent on a single response, which may result in the learner escalating to problem behavior as a "spontaneous repair" (see Chapter 10 for a more extensive discussion of communicative repair strategies that are used by beginning communicators).

Finally, the influence that social partners have on existing and newly acquired communicative forms needs to be examined. That is, the effect any communicative form has on a listener determines the probability of future use. For example, if screaming has a better and more consistent effect in obtaining a desired outcome than a word or gesture that was taught to serve the same function, the beginning communicator will continue to use screaming. It may be necessary to develop interventions that focus on changing the environments and the social partners' behaviors as well as changing the beginning communicator's behavior.

CONCLUSION

There are compelling reasons for making escape and avoidance skills instructional priorities during the early stages of intervention with beginning communicators. Behaviors to achieve escape and avoidance emerge early among typically developing children, suggesting the developmental importance of these skills. In addition, a large repertoire of effective communication skills to achieve escape and avoidance enables the individual to indicate preferences and to escape and avoid nonpreferred, aversive, unwanted, or unneeded objects, activities, or interactions. More generally, these types of skills enable the individual to exert some degree of control over the environment and make his or her wishes and needs known to others (Reichle et al., 1991). Communication skills can represent functionally equivalent alternatives to problem behaviors that may be used to escape and avoid (Carr et al., 1994).

A number of communication skills are related to escape and avoidance. These include rejecting, protesting, indicating "no," indicating a desire to take leave, and requesting (e.g., requesting cessation, an alternative, a break, or assistance). This variety suggests the need to establish a large repertoire of communication skills that are related to escape and avoidance.

Beginning communicators have been observed to use informal and idiosyncratic behaviors to indicate the desire to escape and avoid. Intervention programs may therefore need to include strategies to 1) strengthen existing forms if they are socially acceptable, 2) teach new communication skills to ensure that the individual has the ability to escape and avoid across the full range of situations in which these skills may be required, 3) expand existing forms to ensure long-term usefulness, 4) replace unacceptable forms by teaching functionally equivalent communication skills, and 5) establish conditional and discriminated use of newly acquired communication skills.

Empirically validated instructional strategies have been developed for teaching socially acceptable escape and avoidance to beginning communicators. Nonetheless, much remains to be learned about how to best teach these types of communication skills to beginning communicators. We hope that this chapter will stimulate interest and further research into this important yet somewhat neglected area of communication intervention.

REFERENCES

Bates, E., Benigni, L., Bretherton, I., Camaioni, L., & Volterra, V. (1979). *The emergence of symbols: Cognition and communication in infancy.* San Diego: Academic Press.

Bates, E., Camaioni, L., & Volterra, V. (1975). The acquisition of performatives prior to speech. *Merrill-Palmer Quarterly, 21,* 205–226.

Billingsley, F.F., & Romer, L.T. (1983). Response prompting and the transfer of stimulus control: Methods, research, and a conceptual framework. *Journal of The Association for Persons with Severe Handicaps, 8*(2), 3–12.

Butterfield, N. (1994). Assessment of preverbal communicative abilities in students with severe intellectual disability. *Australia & New Zealand Journal of Developmental Disabilities, 17,* 347–364.

Butterfield, N., Arthur, M., & Sigafoos, J. (1995). *Partners in everyday communicative exchanges: A guide to promoting interaction opportunities for people with severe intellectual disability.* Sydney, Australia: MacLennan & Petty Pty Limited.

Carpenter, R.L., Mastergeorge, A.M., & Coggins, T.E. (1983). The acquisition of communicative intentions in infants eight to fifteen months of age. *Language and Speech, 26,* 101–116.

Carr, E.G., Levin, L., McConnachie, G., Carlson, J.I., Kemp, D.C., & Smith, C.E. (1994). *Communication-based intervention for problem behavior: A user's guide for producing positive change.* Baltimore: Paul H. Brookes Publishing Co.

Chadsey-Rusch, J., Drasgow, E., Reinoehl, B., Halle, J. & Collet-Klingenberg, L. (1993). Using general-case instruction to teach spontaneous and generalized requests for assistance to learners with severe disabilities. *Journal of The Association for Persons with Severe Handicaps, 18,* 177–187.

Cipani, E. (1988). *Behavior Analysis Language Program (BALP): Theory, assessment and training practices for personnel working with people with severe handicaps.* Bellevue, WA: Edmark.

Cirrin, F.M., & Rowland, C.M. (1985). Communicative assessment of nonverbal youths with severe/profound mental retardation. *Mental Retardation, 23,* 52–62.

Davis, C.A., Reichle, J., Southard, K., & Johnston, S. (1998). Teaching children with severe disabilities to utilize nonobligatory conversational opportunities: An application of high-probability requests. *Journal of The Association for Persons with Severe Handicaps, 23,* 57–68.

Drasgow, E., & Halle, J.W. (1995). Teaching social communication to young children with severe disabilities. *Topics in Early Childhood Special Education, 15,* 164–186.

Drasgow, E., Halle, J.W., & Ostrosky, M.M. (1998). Effects of differential reinforcement on the generalization of a replacement mand in three children with severe language delays. *Journal of Applied Behavior Analysis, 31,* 357–374.

Drasgow, E., Halle, J.W., Ostrosky, M.M., & Harbers, H.M. (1996). Using behavioral indication and functional communication training to establish an initial sign repertoire with a young child with severe disabilities. *Topics in Early Childhood Special Education, 16,* 500–521.

Duker, P.C., Dortmans, A., & Lodder, E. (1993). Establishing the manding function of communicative gestures with individuals with severe/profound mental retardation. *Research in Developmental Disabilities, 14,* 39–49.

Duker, P.C., & Jutten, W. (1997). Establishing gestural yes-no responding with individuals with profound mental retardation. *Education and Training in Mental Retardation and Developmental Disabilities, 32,* 59–67.

Durand, V.M., & Crimmins, D. (1988). Identifying the variables maintaining self-injurious behavior. *Journal of Autism and Developmental Disorders, 18,* 99–117.

Fisher, W., Piazza, C.C., Bowman, L.G., Hagopian, L.P., Owens, J.C., & Slevin, I. (1992). A comparison of two procedures for identifying reinforcers in persons with severe and profound disabilities. *Journal of Applied Behavior Analysis, 25,* 491–498.

Golinkoff, R.M. (1986). "I beg your pardon?": The preverbal negotiation of failed messages. *Journal of Child Language, 13,* 455–476.

Guess, D., Benson, H.A., & Siegel-Causey, E. (1985). Concepts and issues related to choice-making and autonomy among persons with severe disabilities. *Journal of The Association for Persons with Severe Handicaps, 10,* 79–86.

Halle, J.W., Chadsey-Rusch, J., & Collet-Klingenberg, L. (1993). Applying contextual features of general case instruction and interactive routines to enhance communication skills. In R.A. Gable & S.F. Warren (Eds.), *Strategies for teaching students with mild to severe mental retardation* (pp. 231–267). London: Jessica Kingsley Publishers.

Horner, R.H., & Budd, C.M. (1985). Acquisition of manual sign use: Collateral reduction of maladaptive behavior, and factors limiting generalization. *Education and Training of the Mentally Retarded, 20,* 39–47.

Horner, R.H., & Day, H.M. (1991). The effects of response efficiency on functionally equivalent competing behaviors. *Journal of Applied Behavior Analysis, 24,* 719–732.

Horner, R.H., Sprague, J.R., & Wilcox, B. (1982). General case programming for community activities. In B. Wilcox & G.T. Bellamy (Eds.), *Design of high school programs for severely handicapped students* (pp. 61–98). Baltimore: Paul H. Brookes Publishing Co.

Houghton, J., Bronicki, G.B., & Guess, D. (1987). Opportunities to express preferences and make choices among students with severe disabilities in classroom settings. *Journal of The Association for Persons with Severe Handicaps, 12,* 18–27.

Hung, D.W. (1980). Training and generalization of yes and no as mands in two autistic children. *Journal of Autism and Developmental Disorders, 10,* 139–152.

Hupp, S.C., & Mervis, C.B. (1981). Development of generalized concepts by severely handicapped students. *Journal of The Association for Persons with Severe Handicaps, 6,* 14–21.

Iacono, T., Carter, M., & Hook, J. (1998). Identification of intentional communication in students with severe and multiple disabilities. *Augmentative and Alternative Communication, 14,* 102–114.

Iacono, T., Waring, R., & Chan, J. (1996). Sampling communicative behaviours in children with intellectual disability in structured and unstructured situations. *European Journal of Disorders of Communication, 31,* 417–431.

Keen, D., Sigafoos, J., & Woodyatt, G. (in press). Replacing prelinguistic behaviors with functional communication. *Journal of Autism and Developmental Disorders.*

Mace, F.C., & Roberts, M.L. (1993). Factors affecting selection of behavioral interventions. In S.F. Warren & J. Reichle (Series Eds.) & J. Reichle & D.P. Wacker (Vol. Eds.), *Communication and language intervention series: Vol. 3. Communicative alternatives to challenging behavior: Integrating functional assessment and intervention strategies* (pp. 113–133). Baltimore: Paul H. Brookes Publishing Co.

McLean, J.E., McLean, L.K.S., Brady, N.C., & Etter, R. (1991). Communication profiles of two types of gesture using nonverbal persons with severe to profound mental retardation. *Journal of Speech and Hearing Research, 34,* 294–308.

McLean, J.E., & Snyder-McLean, L. (1987). Form and function of communicative behaviour among persons with severe developmental disabilities. *Australia and New Zealand Journal of Developmental Disabilities, 13,* 83–98.

Michael, J.L. (1975). Positive and negative reinforcement, a distinction that is no longer necessary; or a better way to talk about bad things. *Behaviorism, 3,* 33–44.

Michael, J.L. (1993). Establishing operations. *The Behavior Analyst, 16,* 191–206.

Mirenda, P. (1997). Supporting individuals with challenging behavior through functional communication training and AAC: Research review. *Augmentative and Alternative Communication, 13,* 207–225.

Ogletree, B.T., Wetherby, A.M., & Westling, D.L. (1992). Profile of the prelinguistic intentional communicative behaviors of children with profound mental retardation. *American Journal of Mental Retardation, 97,* 186–196.

Reichle, J., Halle, J., & Johnston, S. (1993). Developing an initial communicative repertoire: Application and issues for persons with severe disabilities. In S.F. Warren & J. Reichle (Series Eds.) & A.P. Kaiser & D.P. Gray (Vol. Eds.), *Communication and language intervention series: Vol. 2. Enhancing children's communication: Research foundations for intervention* (pp. 105–136). Baltimore: Paul H. Brookes Publishing Co.

Reichle, J., Halle, J.W., & Drasgow, E. (1998). Implementing augmentative communication systems. In S.F. Warren & J. Reichle (Series Eds.) & A.M. Wetherby, S.F. Warren, & J. Reichle (Vol. Eds.), *Communication and language intervention series: Vol. 7. Transitions in prelinguistic communication* (pp. 417–436). Baltimore: Paul H. Brookes Publishing Co.

Reichle, J., Rogers, N., & Barrett, C. (1984). Establishing pragmatic discriminations among the communicative functions of requesting, rejecting, and commenting in an adolescent. *Journal of The Association for Persons with Severe Handicaps, 9,* 31–36.

Reichle, J., Sigafoos, J., & Piché, L. (1989). Teaching an adolescent with blindness and severe disabilities: A correspondence between requesting and selecting preferred objects. *Journal of The Association for Persons with Severe Handicaps, 14,* 75–80.

Reichle, J., York, J., & Sigafoos, J. (Eds.). (1991). *Implementing augmentative and alternative communication: Strategies for learners with severe disabilities.* Baltimore: Paul H. Brookes Publishing Co.

Shafer, E. (1995). A review of interventions to teach a mand repertoire. *The Analysis of Verbal Behavior, 12,* 53–66.

Skinner, B.F. (1957). *Verbal behavior.* New York: Prentice Hall.

Sigafoos, J. (1997). A review of communication intervention programs for people with developmental disabilities. *Behaviour Change, 14,* 125–138.

Sigafoos, J. (1998). Assessing conditional use of graphic mode requesting in a young boy with autism. *Journal of Developmental and Physical Disabilities, 10,* 133–151.

Sigafoos, J. (1999). Creating opportunities for augmentative and alternative communication: Strategies for involving people with developmental disabilities. *Augmentative and Alternative Communication, 15,* 183–190.

Sigafoos, J., & Dempsey, R. (1992). Assessing choice-making among children with multiple disabilities. *Journal of Applied Behavior Analysis, 25,* 747–755.

Sigafoos, J., Pennell, D., & Versluis, J. (1996). Naturalistic assessment leading to effective treatment of self-injury in a young boy with multiple disabilities. *Education & Treatment of Children, 19,* 101–123.

Sigafoos, J., & Reichle, J. (1991). Establishing an initial repertoire of rejecting. In J. Reichle, J. York, & J. Sigafoos (Eds.), *Implementing augmentative and alternative communication: Strategies for learners with severe disabilities* (pp. 115–132). Baltimore: Paul H. Brookes Publishing Co.

Sigafoos, J., & Roberts-Pennell, D. (1999). Wrong-item format: A promising intervention for teaching socially appropriate forms of rejecting to children with developmental disabilities? *Augmentative and Alternative Communication, 15,* 135–140.

Sigafoos, J., Woodyatt, G., Keen, D., Tait, K., Tucker, M., Roberts-Pennell, D., & Pittendreigh, N. (2000). Identifying potential communicative acts in children with developmental and physical disabilities. *Communication Disorders Quarterly, 21,* 77–86.

Sigafoos, J., Woodyatt, G., Tucker, M., Roberts-Pennell, D., & Pittendreigh, N. (2000). Assessment of potential communicative acts in three individuals with Rett syndrome. *Journal of Developmental and Physical Disabilities, 12,* 203–216.

Stokes, T.F., & Baer, D.M. (1977). An implicit technology of generalization. *Journal of Applied Behavior Analysis, 10,* 349–367.

von Tetzchner, S. (1997). Communication skills among females with Rett syndrome. *European Child & Adolescent Psychiatry, 6*(Suppl. 1), 33–37.

Wahler, R.G., & Fox, J.J. (1981). Setting events in applied behavior analysis: Toward a conceptual and methodological expansion. *Journal of Applied Behavior Analysis, 14,* 327–338.

Warren, S.F., & Yoder, P.J. (1998). Facilitating the transition from preintentional to intentional communication. In S.F. Warren & J. Reichle (Series Eds.) & A.M. Wetherby, S.F. Warren, & J. Reichle (Vol. Eds.), *Communication and language intervention series: Vol. 7. Transitions in prelinguistic communication* (pp. 365–384). Baltimore: Paul H. Brookes Publishing Co.

Warren, S.F., Yoder, P.J., Gazdag, G.E., Kim, K., & Jones, H.A. (1993). Facilitating prelinguistic communication skills in young children with developmental delay. *Journal of Speech and Hearing Research, 36,* 83–97.

Wetherby, A.M., Alexander, D.G., & Prizant, B.M. (1998). The ontogeny and role of repair strategies. In S.F. Warren & J. Reichle (Series Eds.) & A.M. Wetherby, S.F. Warren, & J. Reichle (Vol. Eds.), *Communication and language intervention series: Vol. 7. Transitions in prelinguistic communication* (pp. 135–159). Baltimore: Paul H. Brookes Publishing Co.

Wetherby, A.M., & Prizant, B.M. (1989). The expression of communicative intent: Assessment guidelines. *Seminars in Speech and Language, 10,* 77–91.

Wetherby, A.M., & Prutting, C.A. (1984). Profiles of communicative and cognitive-social abilities in autistic children. *Journal of Speech and Hearing Research, 27,* 364–377.

Wetherby, A.M., Yonclas, D.G., & Bryan, A.A. (1989). Communicative profiles of preschool children with handicaps: Implications for early identification. *Journal of Speech and Hearing Disorders, 54,* 148–158.

Woodyatt, G., & Ozanne, A. (1994). Intentionality and communication in four children with Rett syndrome. *Australia and New Zealand Journal of Developmental Disabilities, 17,* 173–184.

Yamamoto, J., & Mochizuki, A. (1988). Acquisition and functional analysis of manding with autistic children. *Journal of Applied Behavior Analysis, 21,* 57–64.

Ylvisaker, M., & Feeney, T.J. (1994). Communication and behavior: Collaboration between speech-language pathologists and behavioral psychologists. *Topics in Language Disorders, 15*(1), 37–54.

Yoder, P.J., & Warren, S.F. (1998). Maternal responsivity predicts the prelinguistic communication intervention that facilitates generalized intentional communication. *Journal of Speech, Language, and Hearing Research, 41,* 1207–1219.

7

"There's More to Life than Cookies"

Developing Interactions for Social Closeness with Beginning Communicators Who Use AAC

Janice C. Light, Arielle R. Parsons, and Kathryn Drager

"There's more to life than cookies." These words were spoken by the mother of Brian, an 8-year-old child with multiple disabilities. They poignantly illustrate her concern that communication intervention for her son was focused on helping him learn to express needs and wants but neglected other communicative purposes. Brian's mother recognized that it was important for her son to learn to express needs and wants so that he could request preferred food items (like cookies), request favorite activities, ask to be repositioned, ask for assistance, indicate his dislike for certain activities, or express his need for a break. Yet, she also recognized that it was important for Brian to learn to interact effectively to establish and develop social relationships with others. She understood that communication was a critical channel to allow her son to connect with others—to touch the lives of others and to be touched by others. She was frustrated that Brian's communication program focused only on helping him learn to express his needs and wants.

Unfortunately, the experience of Brian and his mother is not unique. Most augmentative and alternative communication (AAC) interventions that are designed for beginning communicators tend to focus on providing the beginning communicator with the means to express needs and wants to the neglect of other communication goals, especially the goal of social closeness (Light, 1997). Given the lack of attention to strategies that promote social closeness interactions (i.e., interactions that establish, maintain, or develop personal relationships with others) for beginning communicators, this chapter has three main objectives: 1) to describe the different types of communication goals, especially as they relate to beginning communicators; 2) to review what is known about designing strategies to enhance interactions for social closeness with beginning communicators; and 3) to highlight what is *not* known and, thus, suggest directions for future research to advance the field.

PURPOSES OF COMMUNICATIVE INTERACTION

There are four main purposes of communicative interactions: 1) expressing needs and wants, 2) developing social closeness with others, 3) exchanging information, and 4) fulfilling social etiquette routines (Light, 1988, 1997). Table 7.1 provides a summary of these four communication goals, their characteristics, and examples of these types of interactions for children and adults who are beginning communicators.

Expressing Needs and Wants

One basic reason why people communicate is to express their needs and wants, specifically to regulate someone else's behavior as a means to obtain desired objects or actions or to reject undesirable objects or actions (Light, 1988). Interactions to express needs and wants include requests for snacks or other food items, requests for preferred activities (e.g., toys, music, swimming), requests for assistance (e.g., help completing an activity, requests for repositioning), requests for a break, and rejections of a nonpreferred object or activity.

Interactions to express needs and wants focus not on the partner but, rather, on the target object or action (Light, 1988). Once the object or action is attained (or removed or terminated if it is undesirable), the communication usually ends. These interactions are typically quite short. In order to express a basic need or want, the communicator must gain the attention of the partner (if it is not already secured) and indicate the desired object or action (or reject the undesirable object or action). These requests or rejections can be accomplished through nonsymbolic means (e.g., eye pointing to the desired item, taking the partner to the desired item, pushing away the undesirable item) or through symbolic means (e.g., saying the name of the object or action, touching a graphic symbol on a communication board, signing to request the item, activating a single switch to operate a recorded message that requests the item).

Interactions to express needs and wants, which are referred to in the developmental literature as *interactions for behavior regulation*, emerge at an early developmental stage, well before "first words" (Bruner, 1981; Wetherby & Prizant, 1993). The communicative demands of these interactions are limited. The consequences are usually obvious and reinforcing (e.g., getting the desired item, removal of the undesirable item). As a result, interventions to teach beginning communicators to express needs and wants are relatively straightforward to design and implement (see Reichle, York, & Sigafoos, 1991, for further details). Outcomes are relatively easy to measure (e.g., the number of spontaneous requests made in various naturally occurring contexts, the number of these requests that resulted in the communicator obtaining the desired item or action). For these reasons, interventions to build skills in expressing

Table 7.1. Characteristics of the four main communication goals

	Communication goals			
Characteristics	Expressing needs and wants	Developing social closeness	Exchanging information	Fulfilling social etiquette routines
Goal of the interaction	To regulate the behavior of others to fulfill needs/wants	To establish and develop personal relationships	To obtain information and/or impart information	To conform to social conventions of politeness
Focus of the interaction	Desired object or desired action	Personal bond or affiliation	Shared topic (object or event of interest)	Social convention
Partners	Familiar or unfamiliar	Usually familiar	Familiar or unfamiliar	Usually unfamiliar or acquaintances
Primary communication demands	Emphasis is on initiating the interaction and indicating the desired object or action	Emphasis is on maintaining the interaction and maintaining the engagement of both participants	Emphasis is on establishing a shared focus or topic and developing the topic	Emphasis is on fulfilling designated turns politely
Examples of interactions for communicators who are presymbolic	Crying when uncomfortable Reaching for a favorite toy Pushing away nonpreferred food	Participating in social routines (e.g., Peekaboo game, imitative routines, tickle game, "high-five" routine)	Showing off toys within a shared play situation Pointing to objects and vocalizing	Smiling when meeting unfamiliar people
Examples of interactions for communicators who are minimally symbolic	Signing HELP to request assistance Pointing to a line drawing to request a snack Selecting a message on a VOCA to request a break	Participating in social routines Taking turns in shared activities (e.g., story reading, play) in which the social focus is the relationship	Asking simple questions (e.g., "What's that?") Commenting on events, people, objects	Selecting a greeting on a VOCA

From Light, J. (1988). Interaction involving individuals using augmentative and alternative communication systems: State of the art and future directions. *Augmentative and Alternative Communication, 4,* 76; adapted by permission. (Key: VOCA = voice output communication aid.)

needs and wants have formed the centerpiece of AAC programs for people who are beginning communicators (see Chapters 5 and 6).

Developing Social Closeness

Despite the importance of communication in expressing needs and wants, there are a number of other reasons for communicating with others. A second reason that people communicate is for the purely social reason of establishing, maintaining, and developing relationships with others (Light, 1988; Stillman & Siegel-Causey, 1989). These social interactions allow people to establish an affiliation or connection with others. Interactions for social closeness contrast sharply with those to express needs and wants. In social closeness interactions, the focus is on the participants and their relationship (Light, 1988). The interaction itself is what is important (see Table 7.1). Interactions to build social closeness may take on various forms: They may involve extended conversation using sophisticated language forms (e.g., teenagers' conversations on the bus or on the telephone), involve social routines with minimal linguistic content (e.g., Pat-a-cake, a tickle game), or be accomplished through nonsymbolic means (e.g., a smile, an extended mutual gaze, a shared laugh). From a developmental perspective, interactions to establish and develop social bonds emerge early on. Infants communicate to connect with their caregivers and to direct their caregivers' attention to themselves well before their first words (Bruner, 1981; Wetherby & Prizant, 1993).[1]

The communicative demands of social closeness interactions differ from the demands of interactions to express needs and wants. In social closeness interactions, the participants must sustain the interaction through active engagement or involvement of both participants. Social closeness interactions may be difficult to develop with some beginning communicators because they may not find traditional forms of social interactions reinforcing. The conse-

---

[1] Wetherby and Prizant (1993) described three purposes of communicative interactions: 1) behavioral regulation, 2) joint attention, and 3) social interaction. The social closeness interactions described in this chapter have many features that are similar to the social interactions described by Wetherby and Prizant. For example, Wetherby and Prizant defined *social interaction communicative functions* as ones that are used to attract or maintain another's attention to oneself. The goal of beginning communicators in these interactions is to get their partners to look at or notice them. These types of communicative functions are important to the initiation and maintenance of the social closeness interactions that we describe in this chapter. Yet, our definition of social closeness interactions also focuses on the *responsiveness* of beginning communicators to their partners. We take the position that beginning communicators must learn not only the skills to attract their partners' social attention but also the skills to respond effectively to their partners' social overtures. If beginning communicators are to become competent in social closeness interactions, they must be responsive to others, and they must be able to act effectively to initiate and maintain social contact. The focus of social closeness interactions as defined in this chapter is on the development of a reciprocal interpersonal bond within the interaction.

quences of social closeness interactions are not as concrete or obvious as the consequences of expressing needs and wants. As a result, interventions to teach beginning communicators to establish and develop social closeness are more difficult to design and implement. Outcomes are harder to measure. For example, how does an observer determine if an affiliation or personal bond has been established or further developed? Typically, social closeness goals have been neglected in AAC interventions, perhaps because of these many difficulties (Light, 1997). Yet, these types of interactions are critical to socioemotional development and to the development of a sense of social belonging.

Exchanging Information

A third reason that people communicate is to acquire information from others or to share information with others (Light, 1988). In these interactions, the focus is on the information (see Table 7.1). These types of interactions are of central importance in educational and vocational environments as well as in more informal learning situations. In general, interactions to exchange information impose more complex linguistic demands on the participants. These interactions can be lengthy. The range of topics can be varied and, hence, the vocabulary needs are diverse. The content and accuracy of the communication is very important. As a result, there is a low tolerance for communication breakdown in these types of interactions; it is important for the participants to use effective repair strategies when breakdowns do occur (see Chapter 10 for further discussion of communication breakdown and repair in interactions involving beginning communicators).

Interactions to exchange information have their precursors in the joint attention interactions displayed by young children (Bruner, 1981; Wetherby & Prizant, 1993).[2] In these interactions, young children direct their partner's attention for the purpose of sharing the focus on an entity or event (Bruner, 1981; Wetherby & Prizant, 1993). Early emerging communication functions that occur within joint attention interactions include comments on objects or actions or basic requests for information (e.g., "What's that?"). The objects or

---

[2] *Joint attention,* as defined by Wetherby and Prizant (1993), refers to acts that are used to direct another's attention to an object, an event, or a topic. In joint attention interactions, as with the information transfer interactions described in this chapter, the participants focus on the object, event, or topic, rather than the personal relationship between the beginning communicator and the partner. Yet, it should be noted that not all interactions that involve objects are interactions for the purpose of information transfer. In some of these interactions, the participants may focus on the interpersonal relationship, rather than the object, event, or topic involved. In the former case, the object or activity merely forms a backdrop for the social closeness interaction that is the main focus of the participants. For example, a mother who is playing with her toddler may use a puppet as a prop in a "I'm-gonna-get-you" game, but the focus of the interaction is on building a bond between the mother and child (a social closeness interaction) rather than on the characteristics of the puppet.

events of shared interest in these joint attention routines form the precursors for shared topics of conversation in interactions to exchange information at later stages of development. Joint attention routines emerge early in development, prior to first words (Wetherby & Prizant, 1993) and can be accomplished through nonsymbolic means (e.g., holding up or showing off an object to direct the partner's attention to the object). Nevertheless, these interactions are greatly facilitated with the emergence of symbolic communication and the availability of a means to communicate in more complex ways about shared topics of interest, including those that are present and those that are not. Increased attention has been directed toward the role of joint attention routines with beginning communicators and toward intervention strategies to build joint attention skills (Wetherby & Prizant, 1993).

Fulfilling Social Etiquette Routines

The fourth reason that people communicate is to fulfill social etiquette expectations (see Table 7.1). These interactions include greeting a passerby (e.g., "Hi, how are you?") or chatting briefly to the cashier in a store (e.g., "Have a nice day"). According to Light (1988), these interactions are usually brief. They typically occur with acquaintances or strangers, partners with whom there is no motivation or interest in establishing a personal bond or affiliation. In these interactions, the focus is not on the interpersonal relationship or the information exchanged but, rather, on fulfilling the required turns to be polite (Light, 1988). These turns are often fulfilled automatically, without much thought or real communicative intent. In fact, participants may not even pay much attention to the communication partner's response. Because these interactions are so limited in scope and are often "automatic," they pose limited communicative demands.

Expectations to fulfill these types of interactions emerge later in typical development, once children enter school and begin to interact with a much wider range of partners. From a developmental perspective, these types of interactions may not be priorities for beginning communicators, especially for those who are young and interact with a limited circle of familiar partners. From a functional perspective, however, these types of interactions may be important for beginning communicators who are older and interact in a variety of environments with a wider range of partners. Because the communicative demands in these interactions are minimal, they may serve as a key entry point for some adolescents and adults with severe disabilities to facilitate their participation in the broader social community. For example, an adult with severe disabilities may learn to participate in appropriate greeting routines during a work placement at a fast-food restaurant. Interventions that focus on building social etiquette interactions with beginning communicators must ensure that these interactions are reinforcing for the beginning communicators.

Summary of Communication Goals

In summary, there are four main communication goals: 1) expressing needs and wants, 2) developing social closeness with others, 3) exchanging information, and 4) fulfilling social etiquette routines. The importance and the nature of these communication goals will vary across individuals depending on their skills, their lifestyles, their partners, and the demands of their environments.

The limited scope and concreteness of outcomes have made interventions to teach beginning communicators to express needs and wants relatively easy, whereas social closeness interactions, which are broad in scope with less obvious consequences, have received less attention. Although it seems clear that interactions to promote social closeness are critical for beginning communicators, there has been only limited research to develop, implement, and evaluate strategies to promote social closeness interactions with beginning communicators. The following sections provide a review of this research, discuss clinical and educational implications, and suggest directions for future research for two groups of beginning communicators: 1) individuals who are presymbolic (including those who are preintentional and those who are intentional but not symbolic) and 2) individuals who are minimally symbolic. Each of the sections starts with a brief summary of the development of social closeness interactions in typically developing children and then discusses the implications of these developmental foundations for individuals with significant disabilities.

ENHANCING SOCIAL CLOSENESS INTERACTIONS WITH INDIVIDUALS WHO ARE PRESYMBOLIC

In typical development, the foundations of social closeness interactions are found in the early caregiving interactions of infants and caregivers. Very early in the first year of life, typically developing infants begin to focus attention on a social stimulus, typically their mother or another primary caregiver during daily routines, especially feeding (Beckman & Lieber, 1992). During the first stages of development, these episodes of shared social attention occur when the infant maintains a state of quiet alertness within a social context that is structured by the mother or other caregiver (Adamson & Chance, 1998). In fact, during their first weeks, infants begin to synchronize their periods of quiet alertness with the times when their caregiver is holding them and talking to them (Adamson, 1995). The interactions are defined by periods of extended mutual gaze. At this early stage, the infant and the caregiver establish a basic connection; they open a channel of communication (Adamson, 1995).

As infants develop a wider repertoire of smiles, facial expressions, and vocalizations, these social interactions develop more depth. Infants begin to respond to their caregivers' social overtures so that by 3 months of age infants are participating in contingent, mutually rewarding social exchanges with their caregivers (Beckman & Lieber, 1992). These interactions consist largely of exchanges of affect between the infants and their caregivers (Bakeman & Adamson, 1984). Adamson (1995) noted the critical importance of these early social interactions, arguing that they allow a rapport and emotional depth of interaction for the infants that is not possible in play with inanimate objects or in joint attention routines. She concluded that infants are both "socialized" and "socializers" (Adamson, 1995, p. 11). They respond to social overtures from their primary caregivers and act in subtle ways that maintain the social contact.

At this stage, infants are preintentional. They do not yet fulfill communicative turns within these shared interactions, but they are receptive to social contact and social content (Adamson & Chance, 1998). They produce gross (rather than discrete) behaviors such as crying, gazing toward the caregiver, facial expressions, and vocalizing. These behaviors are assigned meaning by responsive caregivers who interpret these preintentional acts as communicative acts (Adamson, 1995; Yoder, Warren, McCathren, & Leew, 1998). In these early social interactions, caregivers continually monitor the infant's degree of attention and adjust their own behaviors so as to maintain the infant's engagement at optimal levels (Snow, 1977). Caregiver responses to an infant's behavior occur immediately after the behavior and are typically imitations of the behaviors or other semantically related acts (Yoder et al., 1998).

At this early stage of development, infants have difficulty coordinating their attention between their caregiver and an object or an event. Therefore, early interactions to establish social closeness tend to involve only the infant and caregiver; no other objects or events are involved that might distract from the interpersonal interaction or the bond between the infant and caregiver. These early social closeness interactions serve to foster the infant's attachment with the caregiver, thus providing a secure base from which to explore both the social and the physical environment.

As infants grow and mature, they learn that their behavior has an effect on others, marking the emergence of intentionality (see Chapter 2 for a discussion of the transition from nonintentional acts to intentional communicative acts). They develop a wider repertoire of behaviors to engage others and facilitate social interactions (e.g., vocalizing to attract social attention, crawling to approach others, pointing, reaching and touching to initiate contact with others) (Beckman & Lieber, 1992). They learn to use these behaviors to elicit and sustain episodes of turn taking in social interactions with others.

As infants develop, they also learn to coordinate interaction with a caregiver and an object. Initially, this engagement is relatively passive: The infant attends to the object and the caregiver facilitates this engagement (Bakeman & Adamson, 1984). Later, the infant learns to coordinate joint engagement: He or she engages with the object but regularly exchanges looks with the caregiver to maintain the social involvement (Bakeman & Adamson, 1984). At this stage, interactions for social closeness may begin to involve simple shared activities (e.g., I'm-gonna-get-you games with a stuffed animal, routines of trading or exchanging objects or toys, sharing books together). Unlike interactions for the purpose of information exchange, however, the emphasis of the interactions in these shared activities is the interpersonal bond between the partner and the beginning communicator, not the exchange of information or ideas per se. Coordinated joint attention emerges relatively slowly in typically developing infants (Bakeman & Adamson, 1984). Therefore, at this intentional but presymbolic stage of communication, social closeness interactions are still more apt to focus on the infant and caregiver alone. It is only once the child has firmly established symbolic communication skills that he or she begins to regularly use shared activities as a medium for developing social closeness with others.

The primary focus of social closeness interactions for typically developing children who are presymbolic is on parents and other familiar caregivers. Infants who are presymbolic may smile and touch their peers, especially when no toys are present (Adamson, 1995), but they are not able to sustain social interactions with their peers until they are older (Bakeman & Adamson, 1984).

Implications for Beginning Communicators Who Are Presymbolic

Social closeness interactions are of critical importance for beginning communicators who are presymbolic for many reasons: to establish a connection between the individual and facilitators[3], to open a basic channel of communication, and to foster secure attachment with facilitators. Yet, there are numerous challenges in developing social closeness interactions with infants and toddlers who have severe disabilities or with older individuals who are presymbolic. These challenges may reflect factors that are related to the individuals themselves, the facilitators, and the environment.

Parents may experience significant stress and emotional upheaval as a result of the birth of a child with severe disabilities (Siegel-Causey & Ernst, 1989). Research suggests that parents of infants with disabilities demonstrate less positive affect in their interactions with their infants and that they enjoy these interactions less than parents of typically developing children (Crnic, Ragozin, Greenberg, Robinson, & Basham, 1983). They may have difficulty structuring their interactions with their infants to foster social closeness (Greenspan, 1988; Prizant & Wetherby, 1990).

Infants with severe disabilities may show delays in attending socially to their primary caregivers (Richard, 1986); they may produce fewer social smiles

---

[3] The term *facilitator* is used in this chapter to refer to the significant others in the life of the beginning communicator (McNaughton & Light, 1989). Facilitators might include parents, teachers, paraprofessionals, siblings, or classmates. The term *facilitator* does not refer to the technique of Facilitated Communication (FC) as described by Biklen (1990).

and vocalize less frequently (Stone & Chesney, 1978); and many of their behaviors (e.g., facial expressions, movements) may be inconsistent, ambiguous,
or idiosyncratic (Crais & Calculator, 1998; Grove, Bunning, Porter, & Olsson,
1999). Caregivers may have difficulty noticing the infant's unusual or subtle
behaviors and interpreting these behaviors and affective responses accurately
(e.g., Cress et al., 1999; Walden, Blackford, & Carpenter, 1997; Wilcox, Bacon,
& Shannon, 1995). Social closeness interactions are inhibited when communication partners miss or misread communicative attempts (Ostrosky, Donegan, & Fowler, 1998). There are no data available on the extent to which partners miss or misread communicative attempts that are specifically focused on
establishing or maintaining social closeness. Yet, there are data indicating that
partners frequently miss or misread expressions of choice or preference that
are initiated by beginning communicators with severe disabilities. For example,
Houghton, Broniki, and Guess (1987) found that classroom staff responded
at extremely low rates (less than 16%) to attempts by beginning communicators to express choice or preference, regardless of the age of the beginning
communicator; the staff missed more than 84% of the student-initiated expressions of needs or wants. Given that the intent of beginning communicators in initiating social closeness interactions may be less obvious than their
intent in expressions of preference or choice, it might be expected that partners
might miss an even greater number of attempts to initiate social closeness.
When partners repeatedly fail to respond to beginning communicators' attempts to initiate social closeness, it is highly likely that the beginning communicators will stop initiating because they are seldom successful at eliciting
the desired social response.

Parents and other caregivers not only have difficulty recognizing social
overtures by beginning communicators, they also have difficulty knowing how
to interact with individuals who have severe disabilities. Many early communicative routines involve hand or vocal skills that may not be available to children with severe disabilities (Cress et al., 1999). Even when parents initiate social interactions with their children, it may be difficult for parents to sustain
these interactions because the children may not participate frequently. For example, Cress (1999) reported that toddlers with physical impairments tended
not to imitate the behaviors of others or to direct their caregivers' attention.
She argued that children with physical impairments may be less likely to engage in spontaneous imitation of others because of the low cost–benefit ratio
of these small talk behaviors. All of these factors may disrupt the development
of social closeness within early infant–caregiver interactions.

The barriers are even more complex for establishing social closeness interactions with school-age children or adults who are presymbolic. As with
infants, these older individuals often have a limited repertoire of behaviors;
these behaviors may be used inconsistently and may be difficult to interpret.
Unlike infants, however, beginning communicators who are older typically

interact with a much wider range of partners (e.g., teachers, teacher's aides, workshop staff, group home staff, multiple therapists, parents, siblings, classmates). Each of these partners may interpret the individual's behaviors differently, making it difficult for the individual to learn to use signals to communicate with others (Wilcox & Shannon, 1998).

Many of the partners interacting with school-age children or adults who are beginning communicators may fulfill teaching roles. Most of their interactions may be directive (Houghton et al., 1987; Siegel-Causey & Ernst, 1989); they may have minimal time or inclination to interact for purely social purposes. As a result, children and adults who are presymbolic may have access to only a few partners with whom they could establish or maintain social closeness.

Beginning communicators who are presymbolic may not initiate many social closeness interactions themselves. Furthermore, when they do initiate, their communicative attempts may typically be interpreted by partners as requests for objects or actions (i.e., behavior regulation). For example, Ogletree, Wetherby, and Westling (1992) found that 10 children with profound mental retardation communicated infrequently (i.e., less that once per minute) and that the vast majority of their communicative attempts were interpreted as attempts to regulate the partner's behavior. Ogletree and colleagues concluded that these results may reflect the effects of several factors, including exposure to a less-than-optimal communicative environment that offered few opportunities for a range of communicative intents and results of differential responsiveness by caregivers (i.e., caregivers who responded more consistently to expressions of needs and wants than to other types of communicative intents). It is especially problematic when there is a discrepancy between the communicative function of the beginning communicator's act (e.g., initiating a social closeness interaction) and the partner's interpretation of the communicative attempt (e.g., requesting an object) (Stillman & Siegel-Causey, 1989).

Facilitators may experience significant difficulties knowing how to structure appropriate contexts to promote social closeness interactions with older children and adults who are presymbolic. The snuggling routines that provide the contexts for early social interactions with infants no longer seem appropriate for older children and adults who are presymbolic and their partners, especially when partners are not close family members. Yet, it is difficult to adapt the social contexts that are used by typically developing older children and adults to promote social closeness with individuals who are presymbolic. Many of these contexts involve coordinated joint attention to another object or event as well as to the partner (e.g., school-age children interacting to develop social closeness with friends while playing computer games or trading sports cards). Many contexts also involve significant linguistic demands, including "displaced talk" (e.g., gossip by teenagers on the school bus, talking about weekend activities with friends at lunch). Obviously, beginning communicators who are presymbolic will not be able to participate in displaced talk because this requires well-established symbolic language. They may also have significant difficulty coordinating attention to a shared activity and the partner.

Contexts to Facilitate Social Closeness Interactions with Beginning Communicators Who Are Presymbolic

Ideally, social closeness interactions for beginning communicators who are presymbolic would meet the following criteria (Brown et al., 1991; Siegel-Causey & Ernst, 1989; Stillman & Siegel-Causey, 1989):

1. Be chronologically age appropriate
2. Occur within the natural environment
3. Involve only the beginning communicator and a partner with whom the beginning communicator wishes to develop a social relationship
4. Be of interest to the beginning communicator
5. Involve reciprocal turn taking by both participants
6. Be sustainable over multiple exchanges
7. Allow the beginning communicator to participate in multiple ways by using gross rather than discrete behaviors (e.g., smiles, eye gaze, body movements)
8. Have a clear, repetitive structure
9. Provide caregivers with support in interpreting the beginning communicator's behaviors consistently and responding appropriately

It is critical that interventions to promote social closeness involve partners with whom the beginning communicator wishes to develop a social relationship. Beginning communicators who are intentional, especially those who are symbolic, may be able to indicate partner preferences by communicating choices between two potential partners. For example, a teacher presents a choice of partners by holding up photographs of two potential partners or by presenting the people themselves to the beginning communicator; the beginning communicator then points to the preferred partner. When beginning communicators are preintentional, however, they will not be able to communicate such choices. In these cases, careful observation is required to determine the beginning communicator's preferred social partners. Data should be collected on variables such as the following to determine partner preference: 1) the frequency with which the beginning communicator displays positive affect in the presence of different partners, 2) the frequency with which the beginning communicator calms (i.e., terminates displays of negative affect) in the presence of different partners, and/or 3) the frequency with which the beginning communicator approaches or issues requests for attention that are directed toward different partners. Some beginning communicators may not demonstrate interest in establishing social contact with others. In these situations, it is critical to identify preferred activities and build social interactions around these preferred activities. For example, if the beginning communicator enjoys music, social closeness interactions can be built around music activities such as dancing.

If the goal is to build social closeness, then the contexts selected for intervention should be pleasurable and should allow the participants to focus on each other. In a longitudinal study of toddlers (ages 1–3) who had significant physical disabilities, Cress (1999) found that parents built social closeness by creating unique interactive routines with their children that capitalized on the actions and sounds that the children could produce. Cress noted that communication was much stronger within these interactive play contexts than during more traditional object play, a particularly difficult type of play for young children with physical disabilities due to the demands of object manipulation and gaze shifting (Cress et al., 1999). Within object play, parents tended to be much more directive and controlling (Cress, 1999). Within social interactions outside of object play, however, parents were much less directive. In fact, Cress and colleagues (1999) reported that toddlers with physical disabilities who were presymbolic demonstrated their best communication within social routines. Therefore, they recommended that social routines be used as contexts to introduce new communication strategies (see Chapter 8).

For older children and adults who are presymbolic, it is challenging to identify appropriate contexts to foster social interaction that are chronologically age appropriate and also appropriate for the skills of beginning communicators. An example of a social context that meets these criteria is a high-five routine such as that used by athletes to celebrate achievements. This routine is considered chronologically age appropriate for older children and adults; it is engaged in by familiar partners who have a personal bond (but not necessarily a familial bond); with some creativity, it can be sustained over numerous exchanges; it allows the beginning communicator to participate in numerous ways using gross behaviors (e.g., smile, hand movement, vocalization); and it provides caregivers with a predictable structure to support them in responding to the individual's behaviors appropriately. Table 7.2 gives further examples of contexts that might be used to build social closeness interactions with beginning communicators across different ages (infants, toddlers and preschoolers, school-age children, and adolescents and adults).

Interventions to Facilitate Social Closeness Interactions with Beginning Communicators Who Are Presymbolic

There has been only limited research to investigate the efficacy of interventions to promote social closeness interactions with beginning communicators who are presymbolic. In fact, there are only a few interventions that have even

Table 7.2.   Examples of contexts to promote social closeness with beginning communicators at different ages

	Individuals who are presymbolic	Individuals who are minimally symbolic
Infants	Playing Peekaboo	Not applicable
	Rocking	
	Engaging in snuggling routines	
Toddlers and preschoolers	Playing tickle games	Looking at books
	Engaging in snuggling routines	Reading stories
	Rolling balls	
	Exchanging objects	
School-age children	Engaging in imitative routines (e.g., making funny faces)	Playing computer or board games
	Playing clapping games	Exchanging trading cards
	Playing chase games	Sharing a "joke of the day"
Adolescents and adults	Engaging in the high-five routine	Engaging in interactions that involve photo albums of holidays
	Dancing	Looking at various magazines together

Note: In all of these interactions, the focus is on the participants and their relationship, not on the objects or shared activities.

been documented, let alone evaluated. One of the few documented approaches to promoting social closeness with communicators who are preintentional was initially described by Van Dijk (1966) and his colleagues and later adapted by Writer (1987) for use with individuals who had significant auditory and visual impairments. This program involved a sequence of levels: nurturance, resonance, and coactive movement. In the first stage, nurturance, the goal is to establish a warm, positive relationship between the beginning communicator and the partner or caregiver—in other words, to establish social closeness (Siegel-Causey, Battle, & Ernst, 1989). According to Writer (1987) and Siegel-Causey and colleagues (1989), the following strategies may facilitate the attainment of this goal:

1. Limit the number of partners interacting with the beginning communicator who is preintentional so that the individual and caregivers interact frequently and can get to know each other well.
2. Encourage the primary caregivers to establish predictable routines.
3. Ensure that the caregivers provide support, comfort, and affection to the individual.
4. Encourage caregivers to focus on the individual's interests.

5. Encourage the caregivers to expand on the behaviors initiated by the individual.

The second level of intervention proposed by Van Dijk is resonance. At this level, the goal is to shift the individual's attention from him- or herself to the external world of people and objects. Intervention strategies to promote social closeness at this level include the use of rhythmic movements in which the individual and the caregiver are in close physical contact (e.g., rocking, stroking, bouncing, hair brushing, tickling). Caregivers initiate these activities and continue until an ongoing rhythm is established. In the early stages of intervention, they then pause and wait expectantly for the individual to act in some way to continue the movement. The caregivers immediately treat this act as an intentional signal to sustain the interaction and re-initiate the movement. The individual's attention and engagement is sustained through the caregivers' sensitivity to the individual's interests and through their responsiveness to the individual's actions (Stillman & Battle, 1984). At this level, the caregivers do not teach specific communicative behaviors; rather, they interpret the individual's actions as if they were intentional and communicative (Stillman & Battle, 1984).

The third level of intervention proposed by Van Dijk (1966), coactive movement, is an extension of the previous stage (i.e., resonance). The primary difference is that the partner is positioned in close proximity but not touching. The goal is to develop a sense of sequence and anticipation by the individual to sustain familiar routines.

It should be noted that neither Van Dijk (1966) nor Writer (1987) differentiated between interactions to fulfill needs and wants and those to fulfill social closeness purposes. If the interventions described by Van Dijk and Writer are to be used to promote social closeness, they should be structured to ensure that 1) the partner is salient to the beginning communicator at all times (e.g., by positioning the caregiver to foster face to face contact); 2) the focus is on the social bond between the participants; and 3) the interaction is sustainable, as the goal of social closeness interactions is to maintain and develop the social bond.

A second approach to promoting social closeness interactions with beginning communicators who are presymbolic involves the caregivers' imitation and expansion of the individuals' behaviors (Siegel-Causey & Ernst, 1989; see also Chapter 2). These imitative routines are intended to establish a synchrony between caregivers and children. They are intended to serve as a forum for shared attention and provide caregivers with a structure to sustain the social interaction. Several researchers have explored the impact of imitative routines on social interactions with beginning communicators. For example, Dawson and colleagues (e.g., Dawson & Adams, 1984; Dawson & Galpert, 1990) conducted a series of studies to investigate outcomes when adult partners imitated the actions of young children with autism. Results suggested that the children who were beginning communicators were more socially responsive, demonstrated more eye contact, and were less perseverative when an adult partner imitated their behavior. Parents who implemented the intervention noted that it was easy to implement, enjoyable, and helpful for their children (Dawson & Galpert, 1990).

Warren and Yoder (1998) and Yoder and Warren (1998) also discussed the use of contingent imitation by caregivers as a strategy to build social turn taking at the very early stages of intervention. They noted the importance of teaching caregivers to correctly match their children's social affect in the early stages of building social interactions. Unfortunately, it may be difficult for caregivers to imitate children with severe disabilities and correctly match their affect because the children may have a very limited range of behaviors, may use behaviors that are atypical, and may initiate these behaviors at very low rates (Reichle, Halle, & Drasgow, 1998). In fact, Cress (1999) found that adults rarely imitated the unique movements of toddlers with physical disabilities, although they did sometimes expand on these movements. Cress recommended that social routines be established using the behaviors that are already within the repertoires of beginning communicators; later, new communicative behaviors can be introduced that offer the potential for more effective and more complex communication. Communication signal inventories should be developed and regularly updated to provide partners with a visual record of each of the beginning communicator's behaviors and the appropriate interpretation of each behavior (Cress, 1999).

Given the lack of research, it is clear that future research is urgently needed to identify effective interventions to promote social closeness with beginning communicators who are presymbolic. Future research directions are described in detail in the final section of this chapter.

ENHANCING SOCIAL CLOSENESS FOR
BEGINNING COMMUNICATORS WHO ARE SYMBOLIC

As typically developing children develop symbolic communication, they begin to use speech and conventional gestures as well as nonsymbolic modes (e.g., physical contact) to initiate and sustain social interactions with caregivers. Most children only gradually introduce symbolic modes, such as speech, into their social interactions (Adamson & Chance, 1998). In fact, Adamson (1995) argued that the structure of social interactions between young children and their caregivers does not change substantially with the introduction of symbolic communication. These interactions are still defined by turn-taking exchanges between the caregiver and the child, with significant adult scaffolding to structure and sustain the interaction. Many of the social closeness routines at this stage involve only the child and caregiver (e.g., Peekaboo games). As children develop their joint attention skills and their symbolic communication, their social closeness interactions may also begin to be structured around shared activities in which the primary focus is the personal bond between the participants rather than information exchange (e.g., social closeness interactions during book reading). Although young children's interactions are typically rooted in the immediate environment, as they mature, they begin to relate outside of the immediate here and now and can expand their topics of social interaction to include shared experiences and memories as well as imaginary entities (Adamson & Chance, 1998). As young children are able to make increased use of symbolic language, they are able to sustain longer interactions (Adamson, 1995). They require less scaffolding support from adults to maintain social exchanges.

As young children mature, they also begin to interact with a wider range of partners. Toddlers interact not only with parents but also with other familiar adults (e.g., child care staff, preschool teachers, neighbors, relatives). Most notable, they begin to establish social interactions with other children. Interactions with peers at this early stage are very rudimentary because they lack the scaffolding support that adults usually provide. As a result, toddlers between 12 and 30 months frequently rely on basic imitation to participate in social exchanges with peers (Beckman & Lieber, 1992). It is only once their symbolic communication and interaction skills are more firmly established that preschoolers are able to implement these strategies with their peers. Typically developing children who are 12–24 months old initiate social interactions with their peers infrequently (i.e., less than one initiation directed toward peers per every 30 minutes) (Holmberg, 1980). Between 24 and 42 months of age, however, the rate of initiations toward peers increases steadily (at least 2 initiations per every 30 minutes at 30 months, 4 initiations at 36 months, and approximately 6 at 42 months) (Holmberg, 1980).

Implications for Beginning Communicators Who Are Symbolic

Beginning communicators who use AAC have few opportunities to develop social closeness with anyone other than adult caregivers. They tend to be involved primarily in adult-directed activities (Harris, 1982). Typically, when adults have a great deal of control over activities, there are limited opportunities to interact with peers (Harris, 1982; Kaczmarek, Evans, & Stever, 1995). Peer interactions are quite different from those with adults: They involve greater reciprocity and balanced participation between partners (Beckman & Lieber, 1992). They provide a venue for testing communication skills and learning social interaction strategies. With limited access to peers, beginning communicators who use AAC have few opportunities to build friendships or to develop social skills.

When children with significant disabilities do have opportunities to be with peers, they tend to make few social bids toward their peers and show few positive responses to their peers' advances (Beckman & Lieber, 1992). In general, they engage in lower frequencies of social interaction and play with their peers (Guralnick, 1992). Odom, McConnell, and McEvoy (1992) concluded that the peer interaction skills of children with significant disabilities seem to be both quantitatively and qualitatively different from the peer interaction skills of typically developing children. Clearly, intervention is required to ensure opportunities for peer interactions and to maximize the participation of beginning communicators within these interactions (see the following section for further discussion of interventions to facilitate social closeness interactions between beginning communicators who are symbolic and their peers).

Beginning communicators who are learning to use symbolic modes of communication face significant challenges in their social closeness interactions not only with their peers, but also with familiar adults. Whereas typically developing children are able to map quite seamlessly newly acquired spoken words onto the existing structures of their social closeness interactions, children who use AAC (especially those who use aided AAC) cannot simply infuse AAC symbols onto the existing structures of their social interactions. At a minimum, use of aided AAC systems in social interactions requires beginning communicators to coordinate attention between the partner and the aided AAC system (e.g., to shift gaze between the system and the partner during social interactions). When social interactions are structured around shared activities such as story reading or object play, the task is even more complex. Beginning communicators must monitor their own actions and must also coordinate attention to at least three external foci (i.e., partner, AAC system, and shared activity). This coordination is a complex process, all the more so for beginning communicators with motor or visual impairments who may experience significant difficulty with gaze shifting. Reichle and colleagues (1998) suggested that individuals who use AAC may tend to shift their attention primarily between the referent (shared activity) and the aided AAC system, thus neglecting the communication partner. This approach may work when the focus of the interaction is information exchange and the referent is of central importance; however, it may be problematic when the focus of the interaction is social closeness, as the partner (the main focus of social closeness interactions) is relegated to the "back seat." One way to reduce the demands on beginning communicators who use aided AAC is to bring the system, the activity, and the partner into close proximity, thus reducing the gaze-shifting demands. This could be accomplished by infusing the AAC system into the shared activity (e.g., incorporating AAC symbols into the storybook or play activity) and by positioning the partner so that his or her face is in close proximity with both the AAC system and the activity.

Cress (1999) cautioned that communication tasks may become too difficult for beginning communicators when they necessitate the control of numerous tools such as the individual's own body, a toy, the partner's body, and the AAC system—including symbol representation, selection, and output. If a communication task is too difficult, reduction of the number of tools and of the complexity of the tools may facilitate successful participation (Beukelman, 1991; Cress, 1999).

Beginning communicators may also experience challenges in developing the skills that are necessary for social closeness interactions if partners fail to provide opportunities for these types of interactions and fail to respond appropriately to attempts by beginning communicators to initiate or sustain social closeness interactions. Communicative interactions are transactional processes in which the participants influence each other; the ultimate success of the interaction depends on both participants (McNaughton & Light, 1989). To enhance social closeness interactions, intervention may be required to 1) enhance the beginning communicator's communication skills, techniques, and strategies and 2) teach the communication partners strategies to facilitate social closeness interactions. The former intervention will ensure that the beginning communicator has the necessary means of communication and the required linguistic, operational, social, and strategic skills to interact effectively in social closeness interactions. Intervention with the facilitators will ensure that the beginning communicator has the opportunity to build social closeness with others and the necessary scaffolding support required to do so successfully (Beukelman & Mirenda, 1988, 1998). Next, we consider both of these intervention approaches.

Interventions for Beginning Communicators that Build Skills to Participate in Social Closeness Interactions

Only a few studies have evaluated the efficacy of interventions to build social interaction skills with individuals who use AAC. Light and colleagues implemented the intervention program described by Light and Binger (1998) to teach two different skills that were designed to enhance social closeness interactions for individuals who use AAC: 1) the use of nonobligatory turns to increase participation in social interactions (Light et al., 1997) and 2) the use of partner-focused questions to demonstrate an interest in others during social interactions (Light, Binger, Agate, & Ramsay, 1999).

Light and colleagues (1997) targeted the use of nonobligatory turns as a strategy to increase participation in social closeness interactions by beginning communicators. This particular skill was targeted on the basis of the argument that participants should be responsive to partners, actively engaged, and able to sustain interactions over repeated turn exchanges to interact effectively in social closeness interactions (Light, 1988, 1997). The literature suggests that many individuals who require AAC participate infrequently in social interactions, typically forfeiting their nonobligatory turns (Light, Collier, & Parnes, 1985a). This limited participation may be problematic in social closeness interactions. Light and colleagues (1997) found that professionals with previous experience in AAC and adults and adolescents without experience in AAC felt that the use of nonobligatory turns enhanced the perceived communicative competence of individuals who used AAC, provided the AAC users were able to produce the turns relatively efficiently. In general, however, interactions involving individuals who use AAC often lack the reciprocity that is critical to social closeness interactions (Light et al., 1985a). Increasing the use of nonobligatory turns (e.g., the social interjections "cool," "no way," "yeah," and "gross") by beginning communicators may be one way to enhance engagement in social closeness interactions without imposing complex linguistic demands.

To test this hypothesis, Light and colleagues (1997) targeted the use of nonobligatory turns with beginning communicators as a strategy to increase their participation in social closeness interactions. Six individuals participated in the study: 1) a 4-year-old girl with cerebral palsy, 2) a 9-year-old girl with a moderate developmental delay, 3) a 12-year-old girl with a moderate developmental delay, 4) a 14-year-old boy with autism, 5) a 21-year-old woman with severe mental retardation and cerebral palsy, and 6) a 5-year-old boy with cerebral palsy. The participants used a variety of means to communicate, including some speech approximations, gestures, signs, communication boards with line drawings, and simple voice output communication aids (VOCAs). All of the participants were symbolic. With the exception of Participant 3, they had expressive vocabularies of between 50 and 200 items. The third participant had a larger expressive vocabulary of several hundred spoken words, signs, and graphic symbols. All of the participants understood familiar one-step commands. All were able to respond appropriately to simple "wh-" questions related to the here and now (e.g., "What's that?" "What's the boy doing?" "Who's that?"). The participants performed best when language input was concrete and related to the immediate context. All of the participants except the third participant had difficulty with displaced talk. The third participant was able to engage in conversations that involved displaced talk about events outside the immediate context.

Prior to intervention, the participants fulfilled fewer than 30% of their nonobligatory turns in social interactions. Contexts to promote social closeness interactions were selected for each of these individuals on the basis of their interests and daily routines. These contexts typically involved familiar, motivating shared activities that could be sustained over numerous turns and that allowed the partner and the AAC user to be in close proximity (e.g., play activities, looking at photo albums and magazines). The interventions for the individuals who required AAC involved the use of a least to most prompting hierarchy to provide guided practice for the individual in using nonobligatory turns within these social contexts. The prompting hierarchy included 1) the occurrence of a natural cue (i.e., something that happens within the natural environment that signals the opportunity for a nonobligatory turn, in this case a pause in the interaction or a comment by the partner followed by a pause), 2) the use of an expectant delay (i.e., an extended pause during which the communication partner maintains eye contact and an expectant body posture and facial expression, 3) the use of a pointing prompt (i.e., pointing to the individual or the individual's aided communication system), and 4) modeling the target communication behavior by producing an appropriate nonobligatory turn using a mode within the individual's repertoire (Light & Binger, 1998).

Results of the study indicated that five of the six participants learned to fulfill nonobligatory turns and significantly increased the frequency of their participation in social interactions. The sixth participant did not complete the instructional program. He made good progress during the first eight sessions; then, his speech-language pathologist made significant changes to his AAC system (i.e., made the transition from one-symbol selection for access to vocabulary to two-symbol sequences for access to vocabulary). His use of nonobligatory turns decreased dramatically with the increased operational demands of the AAC system. His speech-language pathologist felt that the participant needed to focus on developing operational competence with the new system setup; as a result, he did not complete the instruction. This case clearly illustrates the importance of setting priorities in interventions with beginning communicators so that interventions to meet target goals do not impose competing demands.

The other five participants required approximately 4–6 hours of instruction to demonstrate significant gains in social participation (i.e., increasing their use of nonobligatory turns from less than 30% at baseline to greater than 80% after intervention). Four of the five participants generalized the use of nonobligatory turns to new partners and social contexts. Participant 4 successfully generalized to new social situations but had difficulty generalizing to new partners. In this case, additional instruction was required to facilitate generalization to new partners. Probes conducted up to 2 months after instruction showed that all of the participants maintained their use of nonobligatory turns in social interactions. Adults with no prior experience in AAC, who were not aware of the goals of the study or the experimental conditions, rated four of the five participants as being "more competent" communicators after intervention. They perceived no significant difference in the communication skills of the third participant when comparing pre- and post-intervention videotapes. Social validation interviews with facilitators indicated that the beginning communicators participated more frequently in social interactions post-intervention and that the quality of the interactions improved as a result.

In a second study, Light, Binger, and colleagues (1999) targeted the use of partner-focused questions to enhance social closeness interactions. Light

(1988, 1997) argued that a key component of social closeness interactions is the participants' ability to demonstrate interest in each other. Yet, many individuals who use AAC may have difficulties with sociorelational skills such as "other-orientation" (Warrick, 1988). Light and colleagues (1999) adapted the intervention designed by Light and Binger (1998) to teach individuals who use AAC to ask partner-focused questions (i.e., questions directed to the partner about the partner and/or his or her interests, experiences, or feelings) as a strategy to demonstrate other-orientation. Six participants were involved in the study: 1) a 44-year-old woman who had severe spastic cerebral palsy, 2) a 25-year-old man with severe cerebral palsy, 3) a 33-year-old man with moderate mental retardation, 4) a 35-year-old man who had sustained severe brain injury in a motor vehicle accident 15 years earlier, 5) a 13-year-old boy with a developmental disability that included moderate cognitive impairment, and 6) a 10-year-old girl who had cerebral palsy. The participants represented a range of skill levels. They all understood basic social conversation and were able to respond appropriately to simple "wh-" questions. They were able to engage in displaced talk about people, objects, and events outside of the immediate context. The second and fourth participants were able to generate novel partner-focused questions, although they also made use of preprogrammed questions to enhance their rate of communication. The other participants relied on a limited range of partner-focused questions, which were preprogrammed into their VOCAs. At baseline, the second participant asked partner-focused questions in fewer than 10% of the opportunities he had, the fourth participant did so in fewer than 30% of his opportunities, and the remaining participants never asked partner-focused questions. All of the participants learned to ask partner-focused questions successfully as a result of the intervention. They required approximately 3–11 hours of instruction. The sixth participant required some additional instruction 4 weeks after intervention to ensure long-term maintenance of the skill. All of the participants generalized use of partner-focused questions to new partners and new situations. Social validation interviews with the participants and facilitators indicated that the use of partner-focused questions significantly enhanced the participants' social interactions. The participants interacted with others more frequently after intervention and sustained these interactions longer. Partners reported that the interactions were much more enjoyable when the participants asked partner-focused questions.

Taking nonobligatory turns and asking partner-focused questions are just two of the skills that may further social closeness interactions for individuals who require AAC. Future research is necessary to identify other skills and strategies that will allow beginning communicators to successfully meet the demands of social closeness interactions. Of particular interest are skills and strategies that allow beginning communicators to initiate social interactions effectively, participate actively in these interactions, sustain the interactions over multiple turn exchanges, demonstrate an interest in their partner, be responsive to their partner, and put their partner at ease.

Interventions with Facilitators to Ensure Opportunities for Social Closeness Interactions for Beginning Communicators

Interventions must ensure that beginning communicators learn the skills that are required to interact effectively within social closeness interactions. In addition, interventions that target changes in facilitators' interaction strategies are also crucial to ensure that beginning communicators have *opportunities* to participate in social closeness interactions (Blackstone, 1999). Beginning communicators may encounter numerous barriers within their environments that limit their opportunities for social closeness interactions. These opportunity barriers may include 1) legislation, policies, or practices that restrict communication opportunities; 2) others' negative attitudes that limit communication opportunities or expectations; and 3) facilitators' lack of knowledge and skills in interacting effectively with individuals who require AAC (Beukelman & Mirenda, 1998). For example, beginning communicators may live, go to school, or work in segregated settings that provide few opportunities for social interactions with peers (Mirenda, 1993). Their partners may not be knowledgeable or skilled in providing the necessary scaffolding support to facilitate social closeness interactions. Several interventions to enhance facilitator skills that foster social closeness interactions with beginning communicators have been empirically validated. These interventions, which have focused on instructing both adult and peer partners, are described next.

Light, Johnson, and Manley (1999) employed a single subject multiple baseline across subjects design to evaluate the effectiveness of an instructional program designed to teach partners to facilitate social interactions with children who used AAC during story reading. Four dyads were involved in the study: 1) a 16-year-old girl with moderate mental retardation and her mother, 2) an 11-year-old boy with autism and his babysitter, 3) a 7-year-old girl with cerebral palsy and her 9-year-old sister, and 4) a 7-year-old boy with autism and his mother. The first two children had fairly well-established symbolic communication skills; the latter two children were beginning communicators. At baseline, the facilitators dominated the story-reading interactions; the children participated minimally. During intervention, the facilitators were taught to use an expectant delay to ensure that the children had the opportunity to participate in the story-reading interactions and also to model appropriate turns for the children using communication modes that were within the children's repertoires. They also learned to ask appropriate questions to promote the social interaction. The facilitators learned to use the strategies at a minimum of 80% accuracy within two instructional sessions; they maintained the use of these strategies postinstruction as well.

After the facilitator instruction, all of the children participated more frequently in the social interactions. Of particular note is the performance of the
two children who were beginning communicators. Both demonstrated significant gains in their participation in the social interactions during story reading. At baseline, the 7-year-old girl who had cerebral palsy took a mean of 1
turn during four 15-minute story-reading interactions; after the facilitator instruction with her sister, she took a mean of 31 turns (range 26–36). At baseline, the 7-year-old boy with autism took a mean of 0 turns; after facilitator instruction with his mother, he took a mean of 22 turns (range 21–23). The
facilitators' use of expectant delays created frequent pauses in the social interaction. These pauses clearly marked the opportunity for the children to participate and also provided the children with the necessary time to participate.
The partners' use of AAC to model appropriate turns provided the children
with examples of how they could participate effectively within the social interactions. Social validation interviews that were conducted with the children's
parents after intervention indicated that story-reading times had become
much more enjoyable for them and their children.

Light, Seligson, and Lund (1998) conducted a study using a similar methodology to evaluate the effectiveness of facilitator instruction to increase the
participation of beginning communicators in social play interactions with
peers. Three dyads participated: 1) a 6-year-old boy with autism and the 8-
year-old daughter of his after-school day care provider, 2) a 6-year-old girl with
cerebral palsy and her 8-year-old sister, and 3) a 4-year-old boy with cerebral
palsy and a 4-year-old classmate at his inclusive preschool. The peers were
taught to use an expectant delay and to model the use of AAC during the free
play interactions. The peers' use of these strategies resulted in significant increases in the participation of the three children who were beginning communicators. The 6-year-old boy took a mean of fewer than 7 turns in the 20
minute free-play interactions at baseline but increased his participation dramatically to a mean of 70–75 turns after peer instruction. The 6-year-old girl
took a mean of fewer than 12 turns in 20-minute interactions at baseline but
increased her participation to a mean of greater than 75 turns after peer instruction with her sister. The 4-year-old boy took a mean of only 1 turn at baseline during 15-minute play interactions but increased his participation to a
mean of approximately 15 turns after peer instruction with his classmate. Results generalized across a variety of play situations with the trained peers but
did not generalize to untrained peers, suggesting that intervention with a range
of communicative partners is critical to the success of social closeness interactions. The peers reported that it was "easier" and "more fun" to interact with the
beginning communicators after the instruction. Adults, unaware of the goals
and conditions of the study, rated the children who used AAC as "better" communicators in the play interactions that occurred after the peer instruction.

Hunt and colleagues (e.g., Hunt, Alwell, Farron-Davis, & Goetz, 1996;
Hunt, Farron-Davis, Wrenn, Hirose-Hatae, & Goetz, 1997) conducted a series

of studies to investigate the efficacy of intervention to enhance social closeness interactions between typically developing peers and beginning communicators. The intervention varied somewhat across studies, but in general it was a multicomponent intervention that included the following social support strategies: 1) identifying "buddies" or a "social club" that was composed of typical peers for each of the beginning communicators, 2) giving information to the peers on the ways that the beginning communicators expressed themselves and on ways to facilitate interaction with the beginning communicators, and 3) identifying appropriate shared activities as media to promote social closeness interactions (e.g., toys, games, conversation books of photographs). Educational staff provided prompting for the beginning communicators and typical peers as required to foster their participation in social interaction. Results of the studies (Hunt et al., 1996, 1997) suggested that the intervention had a positive effect on social interactions between beginning communicators and their peers: After intervention, the beginning communicators interacted more frequently with their peers, the resulting interactions were more reciprocal, the beginning communicators initiated social interactions more frequently with their peers, and the peers initiated social interactions more frequently with the beginning communicators. It should be noted that the interventions by Hunt and colleagues relied on not only intervention with the peers as facilitators but also on direct intervention with the beginning communicators to enhance their skills.

The previously described research supports the argument for two-pronged interventions to promote social closeness:

1. Intervention with beginning communicators is necessary to ensure that they have the means of communication and the skills (linguistic, operational, social, and strategic) to participate effectively in social closeness interactions.

2. Intervention with facilitators is necessary to ensure that beginning communicators have opportunities to develop social closeness with adults and peers and are given the necessary scaffolding support to do so effectively.

FUTURE RESEARCH DIRECTIONS TO ENHANCE SOCIAL CLOSENESS WITH BEGINNING COMMUNICATORS

Clearly, future research is urgently needed to advance the understanding of intervention techniques to promote social closeness interactions with beginning communicators. Specifically, future research is required to

- Identify contexts within which partners can promote social closeness interactions with individuals who are presymbolic, especially those who are older children or adults
- Identify contexts to promote social closeness with beginning communicators who are symbolic, with special attention to minimizing the demands

for attention shifting and tool use that are imposed on the beginning communicators

- Specify and empirically validate the types of scaffolding support that partners should provide within these interactions to best support beginning communicators (for individuals who are presymbolic and those who are symbolic) to develop their skills in social closeness interactions
- Develop instructional programs to teach these scaffolding strategies to various partners and evaluate the relative efficacy of the different approaches to facilitator instruction
- Specify skills (linguistic, operational, social, or strategic) and AAC systems that will enhance the participation of beginning communicators in social closeness interactions
- Determine effective instructional techniques to teach these skills to beginning communicators
- Evaluate the outcomes of these interventions to build social closeness with beginning communicators, including those who are preintentional, those who are intentional but presymbolic, and those who are symbolic

This research agenda will pose significant challenges to the field for a number of reasons. For the most part, research and practice in the AAC field has tended to focus on the structural and functional aspects of communicative interactions at a microanalytic level and has ignored the underlying purposes of interactions at a more macroanalytic level (Light, 1988). Attention has been directed toward analyzing the components of communicative interactions—initiations, responses, communicative turns, and expressions of specific communicative functions (e.g., requests for objects, protests). Interventions have focused on increasing or decreasing these behaviors. Less attention has been directed toward the underlying purposes of these interactions (e.g., understanding whether the participants' goal is to express a need or want, develop a friendship with someone, or exchange information). Understanding the underlying purposes of individuals' communicative interactions is key to designing effective clinical interventions and evaluating the outcomes of AAC interventions. It is the underlying purpose of the communicative interaction that ultimately defines which component acts are required and which should therefore be targeted for intervention within these contexts. Ignoring the underlying purposes of the interaction can result in a misplaced focus; component acts may be targeted for intervention even though they are not critical to the successful attainment of the participants' goals. Conversely, skills that are critical to attaining the desired goal may be ignored with potentially negative consequences. For example, if beginning communicators seek social attention but are not taught socially appropriate means to initiate and maintain social closeness interactions, they may engage in challenging behaviors to attain the desired goal of social contact instead (see Chapter 4 for further discussion).

Revisiting the study on communicative interactions between young children who use AAC and their primary caregivers (Light, Collier, & Parnes, 1985a, 1985b, 1985c) provides another illustration of this problem. In the original analysis by Light and colleagues, the play interactions between the young children and their primary caregivers were analyzed as if the goal of the participants was to exchange information. If this were the case, then it would be critical that the participants were able to establish and develop the topic of interest and exchange novel and relevant information about the topic. Thus, the original analysis by Light and colleagues emphasized the lack of information communicated by the children who required AAC and the lack of opportunities provided by caregivers for meaningful information exchanges. Suppose, however, that the participants' goal was not to exchange information but, rather, to develop social closeness. In this case, it is less critical that the participants convey novel information to each other and much more important that they are able to participate actively, demonstrate an interest in each other, and be at ease with each other. The lack of novel information exchange may have been one strategy used by the caregivers to enhance their comfort level in the interactions; when turns are predictable, it is easier to maintain the smooth flow of turn taking, which is a critical component of social closeness interactions.

If the goal of AAC interventions is to facilitate the successful attainment of communication goals, then future research must be driven by these goals. Future research must go beyond analyses of the surface structure of interactions (e.g., number of initiations, frequency of specific communicative functions). Future research must focus on the purposes that drive these interactions—the social goals of the interactions (Wolfberg et al., 1999). Unfortunately, the intents of communicative acts can not be directly observed; they can only be inferred. It is critical to ensure that any inferences drawn regarding the purposes of communicative interactions are valid (Grove et al., 1999).

The consequences of social closeness interactions are not as concrete or obvious as the consequences of expressing needs and wants. As a result, it is more difficult to determine valid measures to evaluate outcomes. Typically, AAC research has focused on the communication disability experienced by individuals who use AAC and has employed measures of functional communication to evaluate outcomes. Less attention has been directed toward evaluating the impact of intervention on the social handicap that individuals who use AAC experience. Future research to evaluate the effect of interventions to build social closeness should consider the following two areas (Calculator, 1999; Doss & Reichle, 1991; Guralnick, 1992; Light, 1999; Mirenda, 1997):

1. The effect on the communication disability experienced by beginning communicators (e.g., measures of functional communication, initiations of social bids, the purposes of these social bids, the immediacy of response

to these social bids, the quality of the responses, the frequency of challenging behaviors)

2. The effect on the social handicap experienced by beginning communicators (e.g., the frequency and length of social interactions with others, the number of communication partners, the types of communication partners, the number of invitations to peers' birthday parties, partners' perceptions of the individual's competence, measures of the social status of the beginning communicator by peers, partner satisfaction and comfort in interactions with the beginning communicator, demonstrations of positive affect by the beginning communicator)

Social closeness interactions are at the heart of an individual's development of interpersonal relationships and his or her membership in a larger social community. These interactions are strongly influenced by cultural values and preferences—more so than expressions of needs and wants or interactions to exchange information. The specific goals and structures of social closeness interactions may be markedly different across different ethnic and racial backgrounds (Hetzroni & Harris, 1996). There is a paucity of research to consider issues of cultural diversity among beginning communicators who use AAC. Future research must consider cultural norms and expectations within the context of interventions to build social closeness for beginning communicators.

CONCLUSION

The previously described research agenda is challenging. Yet, it is important to proceed with this agenda to advance understanding of how to foster social closeness interactions with beginning communicators. Social closeness goals have typically been neglected in AAC interventions, perhaps because of the difficulties in defining appropriate goals, determining effective interventions, and identifying valid outcome measures (Light, 1997). Yet as Brian's mother so poignantly indicated, there is more to life that being able to fulfill needs and wants—"There's more to life than cookies." Social closeness interactions are central to our existence as human beings; thus, they are critical to beginning communicators' developing a sense of social belonging and secure attachment.

REFERENCES

Adamson, L. (1995). *Communication development during infancy*. Madison, WI: Brown & Benchmark Publishers.

Adamson, L.B., & Chance, S.E. (1998). Coordinating attention to people, objects, and language. In S.F. Warren & J. Reichle (Series Eds.) & A.M. Wetherby, S.F. Warren, & J. Reichle (Vol. Eds.), *Communication and language intervention series: Vol. 7. Transitions in prelinguistic communication* (pp. 15–37). Baltimore: Paul H. Brookes Publishing Co.

Bakeman, R., & Adamson, L. (1984). Coordinating attention to people and objects in mother–infant and peer–infant interactions. *Child Development, 55*(4), 1278–1289.

Beckman, P.J., & Lieber, P. (1992). Parent–child social relationships and peer social competence of preschool children with disabilities. In S.L. Odom, S.R. McConnell, & M.A. McEvoy (Eds.), *Social competence of young children with disabilities: Issues and strategies for intervention* (pp. 65–92). Baltimore: Paul H. Brookes Publishing Co.

Beukelman, D.R. (1991). Magic and cost of communicative competence. *Augmentative and Alternative Communication, 7,* 2–10.

Beukelman, D.R., & Mirenda, P. (1988). Communication options for persons who cannot speak: Assessment and evaluation. In C.A. Coston (Ed.), *Proceedings of the National Planners Conference on Assistive Device Service Delivery* (pp. 151–165). Arlington, VA: Rehabilitation Engineering and Assistive Technology Association of North America (RESNA).

Beukelman, D.R., & Mirenda, P. (1998). *Augmentative and alternative communication: Management of severe communication disorders in children and adults* (2nd ed.). Baltimore: Paul H. Brookes Publishing Co.

Biklen, D. (1990). Communication unbound: Autism and praxis. *Harvard Educational Review, 60,* 291–314.

Blackstone, S. (1999). Communication partners. *Augmentative Communication News, 12*(1 & 2), 2–6.

Brown, L., Schwarz, P., Udvari-Solner, A., Kampschroer, E.F., Jorgensen, J., & Gruenwald, L. (1991). How much time should students with severe intellectual disabilities spend in regular education classrooms and elsewhere? *Journal of The Association for Persons with Severe Handicaps, 16,* 39–47.

Bruner, J. (1981). The social context of language acquisition. *Language and Communication, 1,* 155–178.

Calculator, S. (1999). AAC outcomes for children and youth with severe disabilities: When seeing is believing. *Augmentative and Alternative Communication, 15,* 4–12.

Crais, E.R., & Calculator, S.N. (1998). Role of caregivers in the assessment process. In S.F. Warren & J. Reichle (Series Eds.) & A.M. Wetherby, S.F. Warren, & J. Reichle (Vol. Eds.), *Communication and language intervention series: Vol. 7. Transitions in prelinguistic communication* (pp. 261–283). Baltimore: Paul H. Brookes Publishing Co.

Cress, C. (1999, November). *Augmenting play and communication for young children with physical impairments.* Paper presented at the American Speech-Language-Hearing Association (ASHA) Annual Convention, San Francisco.

Cress, C., Shapley, K., Linke, M., Havelka, S., Dietrich, C., & Elliott, J. (1999). *Intentional communication patterns in young children with physical impairments.* Paper presented at the ASHA Annual Convention, San Francisco.

Crnic, K., Ragozin, A., Greenberg, M., Robinson, N., & Basham, R. (1983). Social interaction and developmental competence of preterm and full-term infants during the first year of life. *Child Development, 54,* 1199–1210.

Dawson, G., & Adams, A. (1984). Imitation and social responsiveness in autistic children. *Journal of Abnormal Child Psychology, 12*(2), 209–226.

Dawson, G., & Galpert, L. (1990). Mothers' use of imitative play for facilitating social responsiveness and toy play in young autistic children. *Development and Psychopathology, 2,* 151–162.

Doss, L.S., & Reichle, J. (1991). Replacing excess behavior with an initial communicative repertoire. In J. Reichle, J. York, & J. Sigafoos (Eds.), *Implementing augmentative and alternative communication: Strategies for learners with severe disabilities* (pp. 215–237). Baltimore: Paul H. Brookes Publishing Co.

Greenspan, S. (1988). Emotional and developmental patterns in infancy. In C.J.

Kestenbaum & D.T. Williams (Eds.), *Handbook of clinical assessment of children and adolescents: Vol. 1* (pp. 154–179). New York: New York University Press.

Grove, N., Bunning, K., Porter, J., & Olsson, C. (1999). See what I mean: Interpreting the meaning of communication by people with severe and profound intellectual disabilities. *Journal of Applied Research in Intellectual Disabilities, 12,* 190–203.

Guralnick, M.J. (1992). A hierarchical model for understanding children's peer-related social competence. In S.L. Odom, S.R. McConnell, & M.A. McEvoy (Eds.), *Social competence of young children with disabilities: Issues and strategies for intervention* (pp. 37–64). Baltimore: Paul H. Brookes Publishing Co.

Harris, D. (1982). Communicative interaction processes involving nonvocal physically handicapped children. *Topics in Language Disorders, 2*(2), 21–37.

Hetzroni, R., & Harris, O. (1996). Cultural aspects in the development of AAC users. *Augmentative and Alternative Communication, 12,* 52–58.

Holmberg, M.C. (1980). The development of social interchange patterns from 12 to 42 months. *Child Development, 51,* 448–456.

Houghton, J., Bronicki, G.J., & Guess, D. (1987). Opportunities to express preferences and make choices among students with severe disabilities in classroom settings. *Journal of The Association for Persons with Severe Handicaps, 12,* 18–27.

Hunt, P., Alwell, M., Farron-Davis, F., & Goetz, L. (1996). Creating socially supportive environments for fully included students who experience multiple disabilities. *Journal of The Association for Persons with Severe Handicaps, 21*(2), 53–71.

Hunt, P., Farron-Davis, F., Wrenn, M., Hirose-Hatae, A., & Goetz, L. (1997). Promoting interactive partnerships in inclusive educational settings. *Journal of The Association for Persons with Severe Handicaps, 22*(3), 127–137.

Kaczmarek, L., Evans, B.C., & Stever, N. (1995). Initiating expressive communication: An analysis of the listener preparatory behaviors of preschoolers with developmental disabilities in center-based programs. *Journal of The Association for Persons with Severe Handicaps, 20*(1), 66–79.

Light, J. (1988). Interaction involving individuals using augmentative and alternative communication systems: State of the art and future directions. *Augmentative and Alternative Communication, 4,* 66–82.

Light, J. (1997). "Communication is the essence of human life": Reflections on communicative competence. *Augmentative and Alternative Communication, 13,* 61–70.

Light, J. (1999). Do augmentative and alternative communication interventions really make a difference?: The challenges of efficacy research. *Augmentative and Alternative Communication, 15,* 13–24.

Light, J., Binger, C., Agate, T. & Ramsay, K. (1999). Teaching partner-focused questions to individuals who use AAC to enhance their communicative competence. *Journal of Speech, Language, and Hearing Research, 42,* 241–255.

Light, J., Binger, C., Bailey, M., Gathercole, M., Greiner, N., & Millar, D. (1997, November). *Increasing turn taking by individuals who use AAC to enhance communicative competence.* Miniseminar presented at the ASHA Annual Convention, Boston.

Light, J., Collier, B., & Parnes, P. (1985a). Communicative interaction between young nonspeaking physically disabled children and their primary caregivers: Part I– Discourse patterns. *Augmentative and Alternative Communication, 1,* 74–83.

Light, J., Collier, B., & Parnes, P. (1985b). Communicative interaction between young nonspeaking physically disabled children and their primary caregivers: Part II– Communicative functions. *Augmentative and Alternative Communication, 1,* 98–107.

Light, J., Collier, B., & Parnes, P. (1985c). Communicative interaction between young nonspeaking physically disabled children and their primary caregivers: Part III– Modes of communication. *Augmentative and Alternative Communication, 1,* 125–133.

Light, J., Johnson, S., & Manley, M. (1999, November). *Increasing participation for children who use AAC during story reading.* Poster presented at the ASHA Annual Convention, San Francisco.

Light, J., Seligson, L., & Lund, S. (1998, August). *Teaching nondisabled peers to interact with children who use AAC.* Paper presented at the biennial conference of the International Society for Augmentative and Alternative Communication, Dublin, Ireland.

Light, J.C., & Binger, C. (1998). *Building communicative competence with individuals who use augmentative and alternative communication.* Baltimore: Paul H. Brookes Publishing Co.

McNaughton, D., & Light, J. (1989). Teaching facilitators to support the communication skills of an adult with severe cognitive disabilities: A case study. *Augmentative and Alternative Communication, 5,* 35–41.

Mirenda, P. (1993). Bonding the uncertain mosaic. *Augmentative and Alternative Communication, 9,* 3–9.

Mirenda, P. (1997). Supporting individuals with challenging behavior through functional communication training and AAC: Research review. *Augmentative and Alternative Communication, 13,* 207–225.

Odom, S.L., McConnell, S.R., & McEvoy, M.A. (1992). Peer-related social competence and its significance for young children with disabilities. In S.L. Odom, S.R. McConnell, & M.A. McEvoy (Eds.), *Social competence of young children with disabilities: Issues and strategies for intervention* (pp. 3–35). Baltimore: Paul H. Brookes Publishing Co.

Ogletree, B., Wetherby, A., & Westling, D. (1992). Profile of the prelinguistic intentional behaviors of children with profound mental retardation. *American Journal on Mental Retardation, 97,* 186–196.

Ostrosky, M.M., Donegan, M.M., & Fowler, S.A. (1998). Facilitating transitions across home, community, work, and school. In S.F. Warren & J. Reichle (Series Eds.) & A.M. Wetherby, S.F. Warren, & J. Reichle (Vol. Eds.), *Communication and language intervention series: Vol. 7. Transitions in prelinguistic communication* (pp. 437–460). Baltimore: Paul H. Brookes Publishing Co.

Prizant, B., & Wetherby, A. (1990). Communication in preschool autistic children. In E. Schopler, G. Mesibov, & M. Van Bourgondien (Eds.), *Preschool issues in autism and related developmental handicaps* (pp. 95–128). New York: Kluwer Academic/Plenum Publishers.

Reichle, J., Halle, J.W., & Drasgow, E. (1998). Implementing augmentative communication systems. In S.F. Warren & J. Reichle (Series Eds.) & A.M. Wetherby, S.F. Warren, & J. Reichle (Vol. Eds.), *Communication and language intervention series: Vol. 7. Transitions in prelinguistic communication* (pp. 417–436). Baltimore: Paul H. Brookes Publishing Co.

Reichle, J., York, J., & Sigafoos, J. (Eds.). (1991). *Implementing augmentative and alternative communication: Strategies for learners with severe disabilities.* Baltimore: Paul H. Brookes Publishing Co.

Richard, N.B. (1986). Interaction between mothers and infants with Down syndrome: Infant characteristics. *Topics in Early Childhood Special Education, 6*(3), 54–71.

Siegel-Causey, E., Battle, C., & Ernst, B. (1989). Procedures for enhancing nonsymbolic communication. In E. Siegel-Causey & D. Guess (Eds.), *Enhancing nonsymbolic communication interactions among learners with severe disabilities* (pp. 53–196). Baltimore: Paul H. Brookes Publishing Co.

Siegel-Causey, E., & Ernst, B. (1989). Theoretical orientation and research in nonsymbolic development. In E. Siegel-Causey & D. Guess, *Enhancing nonsymbolic communication interactions among learners with severe disabilities* (pp. 15–51). Baltimore: Paul H. Brookes Publishing Co.

Snow, C. (1977). The development of conversation between mothers and babies. *Journal of Child Language, 4,* 1–22.

Stillman, R., & Battle, C. (1984). Developing prelanguage communication in the severely handicapped: An interpretation of the Van Dijk method. *Seminars in Speech and Language, 5*(3), 159–170.

Stillman, R., & Siegel-Causey, E. (1989). Introduction to nonsymbolic communication. In E. Siegel-Causey & D. Guess (Eds.), *Enhancing nonsymbolic communication interactions among learners with severe disabilities* (pp. 1–13). Baltimore: Paul H. Brookes Publishing Co.

Stone, N.W., & Chesney, B.H. (1978). Attachment behaviors in handicapped infants. *Mental Retardation, 16,* 8–12.

Van Dijk, J. (1966). The first steps of the deaf-blind towards language. *International Journal for the Education of the Blind, 15*(4), 112–114.

Walden, T.A., Blackford, J.U., & Carpenter, K.L. (1997). Differences in social signals produced by children with developmental delays of differing etiologies. *American Journal on Mental Retardation, 102,* 292–305.

Warren, S.F., & Yoder, P.J. (1998). Facilitating the transition from preintentional to intentional communication. In S.F. Warren & J. Reichle (Series Eds.) & A.M. Wetherby, S.F. Warren, & J. Reichle (Vol. Eds.), *Communication and language intervention series: Vol. 7. Transitions in prelinguistic communication* (pp. 365–384). Baltimore: Paul H. Brookes Publishing Co.

Warrick, A. (1988). Socio-communicative considerations with augmentative communication. *Augmentative and Alternative Communication, 4,* 45–51.

Wetherby, A.M., & Prizant, B. (1993). *Communication and Symbolic Behavior Scales (CSBS).* Baltimore: Paul H. Brookes Publishing Co.

Wilcox, M.J., Bacon, C.K., & Shannon, M.S. (1995, December). *Prelinguistic intervention: Procedures for young children with disabilities.* Paper presented at the ASHA Annual Convention, Orlando, FL.

Wilcox, M.J., & Shannon, M.S. (1998). Facilitating the transition from prelinguistic to linguistic communication. In S.F. Warren & J. Reichle (Series Eds.) & A.M. Wetherby, S.F. Warren, & J. Reichle (Vol. Eds.), *Communication and language intervention series: Vol. 7. Transitions in prelinguistic communication* (pp. 385–416). Baltimore: Paul H. Brookes Publishing Co.

Wolfberg, P., Zercher, C., Lieber, J., Capell, K., Matias, S., Hanson, M., & Odom, S. (1999). "Can I play with you?" Peer culture in inclusive preschool programs. *Journal of The Association for Persons with Severe Handicaps, 24*(2), 69–84.

Writer, J. (1987). A movement-based approach to the education of students who are sensory impaired/multihandicapped. In L. Goetz, D. Guess, & K. Stremel-Campbell (Eds.), *Innovative program design for individuals with dual sensory impairments* (pp. 191–223). Baltimore: Paul H. Brookes Publishing Co.

Yoder, P.J., & Warren, S.F. (1998). Maternal responsivity predicts the prelinguistic communication intervention that facilitates generalized intentional communication. *Journal of Speech Language and Hearing Research, 41,* 1207–1219.

Yoder, P.J., Warren, S.F., McCathren, R., & Leew, S.V. (1998). Does adult responsivity to child behavior facilitate communication development? In S.F. Warren & J. Reichle (Series Eds.) & A.M. Wetherby, S.F. Warren, & J. Reichle (Vol. Eds.), *Communication and language intervention series: Vol. 7. Transitions in prelinguistic communication* (pp. 39–58). Baltimore: Paul H. Brookes Publishing Co.

8

Expanding Children's Early Augmented Behaviors to Support Symbolic Development

Cynthia J. Cress

Augmentative and alternative communication (AAC) intervention can concentrate on presymbolic or behavioral strategies, even without incorporating specific aids, boards, or devices. An American-Speech-Language-Hearing Association (ASHA) position paper on AAC included an individual's gestures and behaviors among the other communication modalities that define AAC (ASHA, 1991). A broader working definition of AAC might include anything that helps a person be an effective communicator if traditional means of communication are insufficient. This working definition of AAC includes strategies such as modifying environmental prompts and partner responses, which do not directly modify an individual's communication strategies. Such modifications are considered AAC if those environmental or partner adaptations would not necessarily occur in traditional communication patterns with speaking people. The modalities for early gestural AAC can include any or all of the behaviors listed in Table 8.1.

Even though the field of AAC explicitly recognizes that gestures and other behaviors are critical aspects of AAC systems, there is a common misconception that all AAC systems are necessarily aided or symbolic. When a professional expresses the opinion that a particular child is "not ready for AAC," it usually reflects a perceived limitation at using single-switch voice output or other aided symbolic systems. Yet, there is a continuum of AAC from spontaneous movements to symbolic behaviors, and movements are the earliest forms of AAC expression. Basic AAC intervention includes facilitating

Research for this chapter was supported in part by Grant No. K08 DC00102–01A1 from the National Institute on Deafness and other Communicative Disorders, National Institutes of Health (NIH). The author also appreciates the contributions of the children and families who participated in these research activities, as well as specific reviews of the chapter by Dr. Joe Reichle, Dr. David R. Beukelman, Dr. Janice C. Light, Dr. Christine Marvin, and the Gesture Research Reading Group of Berkeley, California.

Table 8.1. Examples of early gestural expression forms

Forms of early gestural expression	Examples
Spontaneous movements and postural changes	Breathing, looking, squirming
Tactile behaviors and cues	Making postural shifts or functional responses to touch
Vocal behaviors and signals	Sounds, vocalizations, tracheostomy valve noises
Object-oriented behaviors	Banging, exploring, holding, acquiring
Kinesthetic and hand/arm behaviors	Clapping, reaching, participating in routines and games
Contact gestures	Giving, showing, pushing away
Pointing and distal gestures	Reaching palm up, waving, nodding
Conventional and customized signs	Signing MORE or ALL DONE

behaviors, gestures, shared routines, and sounds and does not depend on complex systems or devices. For instance, Light, Roberts, Dimarco, and Greiner (1998) conducted multimodal AAC intervention with a 6-year-old boy with autism that emphasized elaborating his gestural communicative functions and building intentionality, turn taking, joint attention, and communicative initiation. Communicators may demonstrate different skills at comprehending or producing any of these basic communicative components, and initial forms of AAC intervention may primarily involve making changes in partner behaviors and perceptions. AAC, and every other form of communication, starts at birth with social interaction and the earliest behaviors of children. There are no prerequisites to AAC, and no children or adults who are not ready for AAC. Previous research findings that attempted to assign prerequisites to AAC were only considering symbolic forms of communication (Kangas & Lloyd, 1988; Reichle & Karlan, 1985).

AAC strategies to promote specific voluntary communicative acts can begin in infancy and support long-term communication development. Research in the 1990s on typical and atypical language development shows that early communicative behaviors, such as symbolic gestures and joint attention routines, predict the rate and extent of later language development (Harris, Kasari, & Sigman, 1996; Thal, Tobias, & Morrison, 1991; Yoder, Warren, & McCathren, 1998). Early communicators who rely on AAC tend to have limited opportunities and means to express various communicative functions that are associated with advanced language development (Cress, Shapley, et al., 1999). It has been shown that access to AAC is a means to acquire some of the necessary prelinguistic and cognitive skills for language development, but this access is often delayed until assessments that are associated with school entry are conducted (Beukelman & Mirenda, 1998). Even symbolic AAC users will continue to use gestural strategies for some purposes, such as communicating with familiar partners.

This chapter presents 1) an overview of augmented behavior development in AAC, 2) research and other clinical observations about interventions to promote augmented behaviors in early communicators, 3) treatment efficacy research in augmented behaviors, and 4) vignettes that illustrate mixed mode behavioral and symbolic forms of AAC. The sections on augmented behavior intervention include comparisons of behavior development between typically developing and nonspeaking children, as well as focused intervention principles to progress children to a more complex form of communication (i.e., spontaneous behaviors, intentional behaviors, intentional communication, and symbolic communication). The augmented behavior strategies comprise both legitimate communication methods in themselves and supports for further cognitive and communicative development to promote symbolic communication. Augmented behavior strategies can be applied to individuals of all ages who are learning early communicative behaviors; in this chapter, however, early communicators are referred to as *children*, and primary communication partners are called *parents* or *caregivers*. Early AAC strategies also can apply to older individuals with comparable communicative skills, with inevitable adjustment for differences in world experience in older basic communicators.

OVERVIEW OF AUGMENTED BEHAVIOR DEVELOPMENT FOR NONSPEAKING CHILDREN

The general stages of augmented behavioral development parallel those of spoken communication development. Activities that facilitate the transition to more advanced communication strategies are common to both modalities. However, systematic differences are expected because a child's disability may cause limitations in achieving some developmental milestones.

Stages of Augmented Behavior Development

Children's augmented behavior development progresses through three stages of complexity, from 1) partner-perceived communication (perlocutionary stage), to 2) intentional behaviors (illocutionary stage), and 3) symbolic behaviors (locutionary stage) (Bates, Benigni, Bretherton, Camaioni, & Volterra, 1979; Wilcox, Bacon, & Shannon, 1995). Partner-perceived communication can also be divided into substages of spontaneous (reactive) and intentional (proactive) behaviors (McLean & Snyder-McLean, 1987; see also Chapter 2). Children may produce behaviors that represent various stages, and they do not necessarily cease production of simpler gestures when they learn to produce more complex communicative gestures, such as signs or spoken words.

Transition between stages is presumed to occur gradually, and children may produce behaviors that are characteristic of different stages in different contexts.

Partner-Perceived Communication (Perlocutionary Stage)   Communication occurs as a result of a partner's ability to perceive meaning in a child's behavior. Successful communication entirely depends on a partner's ability to attribute meaning to those behaviors. During this stage, the child is not presumed to intend to communicate with the interactive partner but produces one of the following types of perlocutionary behaviors that is interpreted by partners.

Spontaneous Behaviors   Children produce naturally occurring behaviors in response to biological or environmental events. These behaviors tend to be responses to basic preference or dislike for activities, indications of internal state (e.g., hunger, discomfort), or simple attention behaviors to immediate stimuli that prompt partner-attention responses. These behaviors are considered signals, as they are treated as being communicative but are produced by the child without clear intent to influence events or people in the immediate environment. McLean and Snyder-McLean (1987) referred to these behaviors as *reactive perlocutionary* acts that result primarily from responses to internal and external stimuli.

Intentional Behaviors   Children produce behaviors that act on objects or events in the environment that are not specifically directed toward a listener to convey a message. These behaviors include performing direct actions to operate a toy, reaching for or pushing away particular objects, or indicating attention to one or more events in the environment. In some cases, actions toward a listener can be considered noncommunicative intentional behaviors, such as when the child treats the listener as a play object (e.g., chewing on or exploring a parent's hands). Children may show persistence at trying to obtain a desired object but demonstrate limited strategies for directing coordinated attention or requesting behaviors toward the adult nearby. McLean and Snyder-McLean (1987) referred to these behaviors as *proactive perlocutionary* acts, which are goal oriented toward objects or people as reinforcing events but do not signal the child's communicative intentions toward a listener.

Intentional or Purposeful Communication (Illocutionary Stage)   Intentional gestural communication includes behaviors in which the child demonstrates apparent intent to communicate with an interactive partner. Communication occurs as a result of direct action by the child as well as the listener, and communication exchanges are reciprocal and dynamic processes that depend on both child and partner behavior. Some criteria by which intentional communication is inferred include 1) a deliberate attempt to solicit a partner's attention with a gesture, vocalization, or word; 2) evidence of an attempt to convey a specific message; 3) evidence of the child's expecting or waiting for a response from the partner; and 4) evidence of persistence in an attempt to achieve a communication goal (Wetherby & Prizant, 1993). Iacono, Carter, and Hook (1998) proposed that some children with severe and multiple disabilities may use strategies such as persistence or modification of communicative behavior more readily than coordinated visual attention as indicators of intentionality, particularly if children have difficulty producing simultaneous gaze and gesture behaviors. Within intentional communication, McLean and Snyder-McLean (1987) distinguished contact gestures that directly interact with an object (e.g., giving, showing objects) as cognitively simpler behaviors than distal gestures that refer to an object or event without physical contact (e.g., pointing, waving). Rowland and Schweigert (2000) also distinguished unconventional presymbolic acts as an earlier form of intentional communication than conventional acts.

Symbolic Communication (Locutionary Stage)   Children produce clearly intentional communication that can also represent a message in a rule-based and conventionally understood symbol. Symbols can include sign language, spoken or written words, picture symbols, voice output messages, or certain emblematic (symbolic) gestures (e.g., a "come here" gesture).

Transitions Between Stages of Communicative Behaviors

Although communicative experience and practice tend to promote development within any particular stage, particular skills have been proposed as being particularly relevant for prompting transitions between various communicative stages. These transitional behaviors may not occur equivalently in all children, but a combination of factors at a particular developmental stage is presumed to facilitate the expression of more complex communicative behaviors (see Warren & Yoder, 1998, and Wilcox & Shannon, 1998, for more extensive reviews of factors that influence these communicative transitions). For children who rely on gestural AAC, the following factors are particularly important to consider in supporting these developmental transitions.

Spontaneous Behaviors to Intentional Behaviors   Specific AAC intervention is rarely targeted when a child presents only spontaneous (nonintentional) behaviors. Instead, professionals tend to focus on broader cognitive skills that will support communication. For basic communicators, it can be difficult to distinguish elements of cognitive and communicative behaviors; therefore, the specific communicative influences on spontaneous to intentional behavior transitions have not been thoroughly explored. In particular, key influences on development during this phase include cognitive factors such as cause–effect skills and attention to people or objects. Experiential factors such as child imitation and parent responsivity can also have an important facilitative effect on the development of intentional communicative acts (see Chapter 3). Figure 8.1 displays these interactive processes, with sample relationships between child behavior and functional outcome represented in the figure's center column. In all of these processes, the child spontaneously produces an action or gaze behavior that is associated with a verbal, social-interactive, or functional response from a person or toy in the child's environment. The means by which a child learns the association between his or her own behavior and the various responses as well as increases in the production of intentional behaviors are presumed to occur through repeated experience of contingent responses to the behaviors (Dunst & Lowe, 1986).

Intentional Behaviors to Intentional Communication   Additional factors are proposed to support transitions from intentional behaviors to intentional communication, as well as further communicative development (see Figure 8.2). Typical intervention strategies focus on shaping the child's intentional acts toward objects into communicative acts by increasing the child's awareness and solicitation of adult involvement in the intended event. In particular, researchers have proposed that partner responsivity (Yoder & Warren, 1998) and coordinated joint attention (Bakeman & Adamson, 1984) are critical to children's ability to recognize that their intentional behaviors can influence others' behaviors and that these two behaviors can become intentionally communicative acts. For instance, when children consistently shift attention between referents and adult communicators, they are more likely to benefit from the adult responses and initiations about the object or event (Baldwin, 1995).

Intentional Communication to Symbolic Communication   Acredolo and Goodwyn (1990) summarized critical early skills relevant to gesture development that have been viewed as cognitive-social foundations for symbolic gestures. These early skills include 1) understanding communication as an information exchange, 2) demonstrating the intent to communicate, 3) forming context-free concepts that are maintained without visible objects, 4) understanding symbols as representation of ideas (including symbolic play), 5) demonstrating a knowledge of symbols as labels (also known as *naming insight*), and 6) producing speech control for understandable vocalization. The first two of these skills are reported to occur in typical development before 12 months of age and to support early symbolic acquisition. The next three skills are associated with periods of rapid vocabulary acquisition that are typical at about 18 months of age, in which symbolic skills are refined and expanded. The last skill promotes the verbal expression of these intentional and symbolic skills throughout development, but it is clearly impaired in children who may require long-term use of AAC. Although Acredolo and Goodwyn reported that even typically developing children demonstrate some of these skills through naturally occurring symbolic gestures, the most common means for estimating children's acquisition of these early symbolic skills is through their symbolic play and verbal expression. As both vocalization and symbolic play

Construct	Potential processes		Target outcome
	Behavior	Consequence	
Imitation	Child acts →	Parent repeats the child's action	Child repeats his or her own behavior—later also repeats parent's new behaviors.
Attention (later joint attention)	Child looks at parent →	Parent acts while the child looks	Child looks more and longer at parent—later looks at parent's activities and focus.
Parent responsivity	Child acts →	Functional response Interactive response Parent feedback	Child increases activity that receives response—later anticipates the type of response to particular behaviors.
Play and cause–effect behaviors	Child acts →	Toy or activity response	Child increases behavior that activates toy—later engages in planned activation of toys.

Figure 8.1. Interactive processes that support intentional behavior development in typically developing children.

225

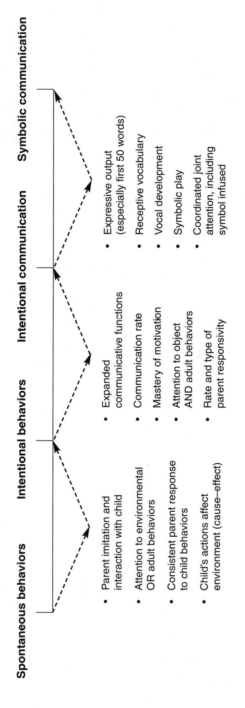

Figure 8.2. Factors that influence transitions between communicative milestones.

skills are related to physical control skills, they may not be reliable estimates of symbolic skills for children who typically rely on AAC systems.

Limitations of Using Gestural and Communicative Milestones from Typical Development

Because few databases of normative information have been established to present specific developmental norms for children with various disabilities, most gestural communication predictions tend to be based on milestones for typically developing children. This practice presents a tacit assumption that critical features of children's gesture development will be similar for children who rely on AAC and children who speak. Dunst and Lowe (1986) proposed a developmental model of communicative competence for nonspeaking children younger than 2 years of age. Their model presents a sequence of behavior development that is similar to typical development: behavior state; recognitory; contingency; instrumental; and triadic interaction among the child, the object, and the partner, including several levels of verbal skills. Yet, several researchers have noted that early gesture production in nonspeaking children may be misinterpreted due to partners' difficulty in judging the intentionality or function of a child's gesture (Iacono et al., 1998). Wilcox, Kouri, and Caswell (1990) suggested that the variations in partner ability to interpret behavior of toddlers with developmental delay are not attributed to children's movement and communication abilities alone. Although nonspeaking children are expected to proceed through gestural milestones that are similar to those of typically developing children (e.g., Iverson & Thal, 1998), these gestures are generally more subtle, variable over time, and different from expected behaviors in nonspeaking children (Iacono et al., 1998; Yoder & Feagans, 1988). Yoder (1987) found that infants with disabilities tended to produce communicative or emotional behaviors that were more difficult for mothers to interpret than gestures that typically developing children provide. This difficulty increased with the severity of disability.

Few tests have been adapted for children who are nonspeaking, so practitioners who conduct early communication and cognitive assessment tend to use standardized tests with mostly surface adaptations for input and output modes (Guerette, Tefft, Furumasu, & Moy, 1999). For instance, published adaptations of the Battelle Developmental Inventory (BDI; Newborg, Stock, Wnek, Guidibaldi, & Svinicki, 1984), the Sequenced Inventory of Communication Development (Hedrick, Prather, & Tobin, 1984), and the adapted Uzgiris and Hunt Scales of Infant Psychological Development (Dunst, 1980) maintain the same behavioral and task expectations for children with physical disabilities but allow for specific differences in the precision or degree of support in target behaviors. Most of the behaviors used to estimate cognitive and communicative skills in such measures are heavily weighted by physical or vocal skills that are difficult for many children who are nonspeaking. For instance, children who have no use of their hands or voice, regardless of their cognitive skills, cannot pass 75% of the Bayley Scales of Infant Development–Second Edition (Bayley, 1993) cognitive scale test items for children 4–22 months of age. If typical assessment measures are based on many skills that are unachievable for young children who are nonspeaking, then it will be difficult to establish alternative milestones or expectations for early AAC by using these measures alone.

Several factors could influence the extent to which practitioners can effectively apply assessment expectations from typical communication development to children who rely on AAC:

- Much of early learning typically involves physically acting on the world, which is difficult for children with physical impairments.
- Many early communicative routines that are familiar to parents involve hand or vocal skills, both of which may be unavailable to some children.
- Some children may not have a clear kinesthetic sense of their own body's movements, which makes it difficult to relate their behaviors to play or interaction effects.
- Parents may not recognize children's unusual or subtle movements as being intentional or communicative behaviors, and they may not respond as often to these actions.
- Motor delays in children's behaviors may limit their early awareness of the relationship between their own behaviors and other events.
- Many of children's early communicative attempts may be unsuccessful (e.g., using breathing as an attention signal), and children may grow passive with repeated communicative failure.
- Some children's early communicative attempts may not be addressed by a listener; in turn, this may lead to using challenging behavior as a repair strategy.
- If children have severely limited expressive skills and cannot easily try out new behaviors to explore their use in interaction, then they may learn communication in a primarily receptive role that limits their linguistic and communicative development.
- Children who rely on AAC may have specific sensory or attention impairments that further limit their ability to process the function of words, concepts, or partner responses.

INTERVENTION STRATEGIES TO
PROMOTE AUGMENTED BEHAVIOR TRANSITIONS

Given the multiple sources of variability in development and assessment of early communication behaviors for children who rely on AAC, intervention strategies must be flexible enough to account for children's skills and learning processes as more complex augmented behaviors develop. Each of the following sections highlights one of the following augmented behavior transitions: spontaneous behaviors to intentional behaviors in early AAC, intentional behaviors to intentionally communicative gestures, and intentional gestures to symbolic gestures. Within each section, evidence of key transitional behavior patterns is compared for typically developing children and nonspeaking children. These comparisons are then applied to principles of intervention for early behavioral AAC.

Spontaneous Behaviors to Intentional Behaviors in Early AAC

Children who produce primarily spontaneous behaviors that result from emotions or behavioral states must rely on partners to interpret the meaning of their behaviors. Because children who are making the transition from spontaneous to intentional behaviors may not recognize that their own behaviors influence the world around them, introducing new communicative behaviors through modeling is unlikely to be the most effective intervention strategy. Instead, most intervention strategies involve partner responses to the spontaneous signals that a child produces, such as a child's arm, body, facial, or attention behaviors. The partner provides reactions that interpret the probable intent of the child's behavior and helps the child associate the communicative or functional response with the child's own behaviors.

Figure 8.3 provides examples of some specific possible associations between a child's spontaneous behaviors and partner responses in early AAC. The child's role is limited to the spontaneous gaze or movement behaviors that he or she may produce in a given circumstance, and possible adult or environmental responses to these behaviors are outlined in the middle column. This figure repeats the constructs that influence transitions from spontaneous to intentional behaviors, which are listed in Figure 8.1. Figure 8.3 adds some possible complications that are associated with physical impairments in the far column. For instance, a child may have limited physical control, which restricts his or her active initiation of behaviors that can cause a result in toys (cause–effect learning), or selective control of his or her visual attention for looking steadily at objects or partners. Physical or visual limitations may also restrict a child's awareness of his or her own actions as well as the parent's ability to recognize and respond to the child's actions. With such a tentative link between child behaviors and parent or environmental responses, it may be more difficult for children with physical impairments to learn the association between their behavior and the resulting consequences in their world. The following sections discuss some strategies by which children with severe disabilities who rely on spontaneous behaviors might develop intentional behaviors. These strategies include gesture imitation, joint attention, partner interaction style and responsivity, and cause–effect play strategies.

Construct	Potential processes		Complications of physical impairment
	Behavior	*Consequence*	
Imitation	Child acts →	Parent repeats the child's action	The child may not have access to this activity, even if he or she has recognizable movements.
Attention (later joint attention)	Child looks at parent →	Parent acts while the child looks	Head control or sensory processing problems may limit initiation of gaze.
Parent responsivity	Child acts Child is aware of own act	Parent is aware of child's act → Functional response → Interactive response → Parent feedback	The child may have a limited kinesthetic sense of his or her own movement. Early behaviors may be difficult for parents to identify.
Play and cause–effect behaviors	Child acts →	Toy or activity response	Limited movement may not allow free exploration of the world.

Figure 8.3. Complications of physical impairment that may affect intentional behavior development.

230

Gesture Imitation   Imitation is an early way to practice behaviors and interaction without understanding why those behaviors are important (Camaioni, 1989). Speaking children practice vocally imitating sounds they hear by cooing and babbling for several months before they recognize the social and communicative significance of those sounds. Imitation is a person-focused behavior that does not necessarily require triadic focus on both interactants as well as an object of interest (Masur & Ritz, 1984). Adults can also scaffold children's early imitation experiences by adapting their own imitation of children's actions and by initiating or maintaining imitation sequences in response to children's spontaneous behaviors (e.g., Masur, 1997; Masur & Rodemaker, 1997). Children who have motor limitations may have less opportunity to experience using vocal or gestural behaviors in imitation to learn that they are meaningful.

Imitation and Nonspeaking Children   Children with physical impairments tend to be less likely to spontaneously imitate behaviors and gestures than other children at similar developmental ages (Cress, Andrews, & Reynolds, 1998). On Piagetian cognitive scales, Cress and colleagues found that children with physical impairments scored consistently lower on gestural and verbal imitation tasks relative to their other cognitive skills. If children are less likely to spontaneously imitate and practice the communicative behaviors addressed to them, then they may be less effective at learning from the modeling and prompting strategies that are common to many intervention plans.

In addition to child factors that might limit spontaneous imitation, some evidence suggests that parents may initiate relatively few behaviors that children with physical impairments can successfully imitate. A detailed analysis of unstructured parent–child interactions for a subset of the families in the study by Cress and colleagues (1998) showed that parents of children with physical disabilities infrequently initiated gesture imitation acts in free play. This analysis categorized the types of behaviors initiated by children and by parents that successfully or unsuccessfully elicited responses in their partners. Adults tended to frequently expand or verbally translate movements of children with physical impairments but rarely directly imitated children's unique movements in ways that the children could easily reproduce. Specifically, when prompting imitation from their children, parents tended to initiate vocal acts that were impossible for their children to imitate more than gestural acts that were within the children's skills. In contrast, parents of typically developing children usually tailor their behavioral and vocal prompting to their perceptions of the children's cognitive skills (Bornstein & Tamis-LeMonda, 1997; Camaioni, 1989). Brand and Ashburn (1999) proposed a type of "motherese" for gestures, as they found that mothers produce more gestural attention-getting features (interactiveness, enthusiasm, proximity to partner) and highlighting features (repetition and reduced complexity) when demonstrating toys for infants than other adults do. For children who are already symbolic, parental expectation of spontaneous imitation may be less critical for learning in social interactions. Yet, if children with physical impairments are less likely to imitate spontaneous movements during early development, then learning strategies by which these children can make the transition from spontaneous behaviors to intentional behaviors to intentional communication may be restricted.

It is possible that limited gestural imitation in children with physical impairments results directly from physical limitations in producing deliberate movements. Children who are nonspeaking would be expected to have poor verbal imitation skills because of limited vocal control, and they might be presumed to have similar limitations in other aspects of motor control that restrict gestural imitation. In the Cress and colleagues (1998) study, however, accommodations were made for children's movement impairments in the sampling procedures and children still showed reduced gesture imitation. For instance, gestures modeled for children were taken from their inventories of the signaling behaviors that they produced spontaneously in play and interaction. Children were credited with imitation if they spontaneously attempted to produce a modeled behavior, even if they were unsuccessful (e.g., posturing). Some children imitated behaviors during toy play that they did not imitate or initiate spontaneously out of the play context (e.g., imitating an adult's pounding his or her hand on a music toy but not imitating the same hand motion on the floor without a toy). The functional responses of toys (e.g., music playing) or the social responses of people may provide support for children to imitate modeled acts that accomplish immediate goals, which they may not imitate spontaneously without adult- or activity-based prompting. Our data suggest that children with physical impairments perform at selectively poorer levels when imitating decontextualized movements than when producing the same movements in play or communicative contexts.

Cress and colleagues (1998) proposed that children with physical impairments may limit decontextualized behaviors that have a low functional cost–benefit ratio, such as spontaneous gesture imitation. If children experience a high motor cost in initiating and controlling movement, then they may be reluctant to produce these difficult behaviors without clear functional or social benefits. This reluctance may be explained by matching theory, in which the likelihood of a behavior's being produced is influenced by the immediacy, rate, and quality of reinforcement as well as the physical effort that is required (see Mace & Roberts, 1993). Initially, typically developing children may imitate gestural behaviors without understanding their purpose because these behaviors are relatively easy to produce in interaction.

Gesture Imitation and Early AAC Intervention   Gesture imitation has been used as an analogue of lexical production for children who have expressive language delays. For instance, Thal and Bates (1988) asked children to imitate adult models of symbolic gestures, such as pushing a car or feeding a baby by using either a food-related object or placeholder object (e.g., a block that represents a spoon). Children who were late talkers successfully imitated symbolic gestures as well as age-matched peers and significantly better than language-matched peers. Thal and Tobias (1994) also found that late talking children produced gestures in sequenced gesture imitation tasks more often than spontaneous gestures. Symbolic gesture imitation or production is a common strategy for estimating the symbolic representation skills of prelinguistic vocal children. Yet, if children who rely on AAC are less likely to imitate gestures out of context, then they may also be less able to demonstrate their language skills by the imitation of symbolic gestures. Decontextualized gestures may not be an accurate estimate of symbolic and expressive language potential for children who have physical as well as expressive language impairments.

Imitation is a frequently used prompting mechanism for many early intervention procedures, such as modeling and play-based stimulation, and children are tacitly expected to already demonstrate spontaneous imitation of adult behaviors for modeling strategies to be effective. For instance, modeling is successful as a nondirective intervention strategy if children spontaneously attempt to incorporate the modeled behaviors into their own communication efforts (e.g., Hwang & Hughes, 1995; Kaiser, Yoder, & Keetz, 1992). Children are able to use imitation to learn to recognize their impact on other people's behaviors because they can experience imitative routines that are scaffolded by parents long before they initiate intentional behaviors or communication (Masur & Ritz, 1984). Typically developing children may incorporate behaviors that they learned in imitation into spontaneous communication because such exploratory behaviors are not difficult to produce. If children find exploratory behaviors physically difficult to produce, then they may be less likely to spontaneously attempt or practice the modeled behaviors in communication events without specific prompting.

Several programs designed to promote communicative gestures in children place a heavy emphasis on learning direct imitation behaviors outside of play or communicative contexts (e.g., Sternberg, McNerney, & Pegnatore, 1985). The risk in teaching imitation as a decontextualized skill is that it may not carry over to effective interactive communication. This is a particular concern for children with autism (Stone, Ousley, & Littleford, 1997). Some children with autism may have a wide range of motor behaviors that they understand but do not use to initiate communication without prompts (e.g., see Attwood, Frith, & Hermelin, 1988), and increasing their repertoire of decontextualized behaviors may not be the most effective communicative intervention strategy.

Early imitation is likely to be most successful if partners imitate the child's behavior exactly and contingently (Wilcox et al., 1995). For children with physical impairments, this may involve imitating unusual or unconventional behaviors that children use communicatively. For instance, rather than prompting a child to wave "bye-bye" with the conventional wave, a parent might prompt imitation of "bye-bye" using the child's idiosyncratic movement, such as a lip smack or head tilt. Parents may also initiate simple turn-taking routines, such as trading head shakes with children, to promote monitoring and matching adult behaviors in a social context. As children's communicative skills increase, these idiosyncratic movements will be replaced or supplemented with more conventional forms to facilitate comprehension by unfamiliar partners.

Joint Attention   Coordinated joint attention—shifting attention back and forth between a targeted object and partner—is critical for children to learn the correct association between words and their referents (Bakeman & Adamson, 1984). Successful language learners acquire very early skills at checking for and directing adult attention (Baldwin, 1995). Children who consistently respond to prompts for joint attention (i.e., turning to follow an adult verbal prompt and pointing cue) tend to show faster language development than children who do not (Mundy & Gomes, 1998). Receptive language development in children with Down syndrome is also associated with the amount of joint attention activity and parent responses to children's attention and interest (Harris et al., 1996).

Joint Attention and Nonspeaking Children   Many children with medical complications or disabilities have difficulty maintaining or effectively initiating joint attention (e.g., Landry, 1995; Landry & Chapieski, 1990). Specific deficits of social and joint attention initiation have provided a basis for differential diagnosis of autism from other types of developmental disabilities (Mars, Mauk, & Dowrick, 1998; Osterling & Dawson, 1994). Reasons for impaired joint attention in autism may relate to underlying perceptual, cognitive, or social difficulties that are associated with autism (Mundy & Sigman, 1989; Wetherby, Prizant, & Hutchinson, 1998). Children with physical impairments demonstrate fewer joint attention acts than expected for their language age, which may be related to the physical cost of producing the act for a relatively low functional or social benefit (Cress et al., 1999). Nonetheless, even children with expressive language delay and no further physical impairments performed at a poorer level than age-matched peers in producing early forms of joint attention behaviors such as showing or pointing (Thal & Tobias, 1994), even though they generally used communicative gestures more frequently than age- and language-matched peers (Thal & Tobias, 1992). These results taken together suggest that the specific link between joint attention initiation and expressive skills for children with severe communication impairments goes beyond a simple association between physical competence and gestural initiation skills.

Because AAC requires children to frequently shift attention among the listener, the activity, and their communication method or system, the ability to control complex attention management is particularly important for effectively using AAC. Adamson, Russell, and McArthur (1997) found that verbal and pictured symbols can add an additional layer of complexity at simple and coordinated levels of joint attention. In particular, children who rely on eye gaze–commenting strategies must learn to clearly emphasize multiple gaze shifts between the partner and the referent or symbol to ensure partner understanding. If the parents and children do not share communicative modes, as typically occurs with AAC users, parents may have difficulty understanding and providing the kinds of joint attention support required. In other cross-modal communication between deaf children and hearing mothers, hearing mothers tend to be less consistent at systematically obtaining children's visual attention before signing than deaf mothers, who specifically move or relate a specific sign within the child's visual space (Spencer, Bodner-Johnson, & Gutfreund, 1992). Parents of children who rely on AAC may need specific coaching in recognizing early eye-pointing behaviors and helping children clearly distinguish simple gaze shifts from deliberate eye-pointing gestures.

If a child and an adult do not share a mutually understandable communicative mode, both partners may spend more interaction time communicating about easily interpretable acts, such as behavior regulation and social interaction, than about joint attention acts. Day (1986) found that 3-year-old deaf children of hearing parents tended to produce significantly more social and imperative communicative acts than informational (i.e., joint attention) acts. Cress and colleagues (1999) found that nonspeaking children with physical impairments demonstrated as many behavior regulation acts as expected for their developmental age, but they produced significantly fewer joint attention acts. Although these patterns may be accepted in basic early communication, continued limitation in joint attention acts and communicative functions will have a long-term impact on children's interactive and linguistic development.

Joint Attention and Early AAC Intervention   If children who rely on AAC are at particular risk for joint attention initiation, then it is critical that early intervention address this communicative function. Promoting early joint attention initiation includes encouraging the child to give or transfer objects of interest to a partner. During activities with a joint focus of attention, adults can provide opportunities for the child to comment and request information by waiting and looking expectantly (Wetherby, 1996). Promoting joint attention with objects that activate independently may both promote simple attention and provide enough novelty to prompt children to comment on the activity (e.g., a wind-up toy, a book with tactile activities, a vibrating ball). In addition, children may indicate an early version of joint attention with a partner during social play before showing joint attention to objects.

Many existing joint attention procedures commonly used in AAC are inconsistent with evidence from typical vocabulary acquisition. For instance, Tomasello and Farrar (1992) demonstrated that 18-month-old children learned new vocabulary more effectively when it was introduced within their current joint attention focus. Yet, adults often introduce new augmented behaviors or symbols without first establishing child attention to the referent—for example, coaching the child to touch the symbol before experiencing the activity. Instead, presenting models for an alternative "more" gesture or symbol that is just beyond the child's fingers as he or she reaches for a desired toy both follows the child's attention and naturally adds the new strategy to the child's existing communicative intent. Interrupting an ongoing activity that occurs in behavior chain interruption (e.g., Goetz, Gee, & Sailor, 1985) creates a similar attention to the referent at the point of a communicative opportunity, but this action is adult initiated rather than child initiated.

Promoting an effective response to joint attention prompts depends on exploring possible reasons for why the child does not already follow the adult's point, head-movement, or voice cue. Children who rely on AAC are less likely to spontaneously shift their gaze between objects and communicative partners, both at intentional communication stages (Cress et al., 1999) and at intentional behavior stages (Bartels, Cress, & Marvin, 2001), but neither physical nor visual processing skills entirely account for this difference. Relatively passive ways to promote a look in children who do not follow a joint attention prompt include using lights or other bright objects to help the child track from the adult's face to the target, then reinforcing this with a verbal and gestural "look" cue. Children with poor head or eye control may particularly benefit from a touch cue to reinforce that the child's gaze is the relevant behavior to which the adult is responding, as gaze is a multipurpose act that does not always convey communicative intent.

Parent Interaction Style and Responsivity   Parent responsivity is one of the more reliable predictors of early communicative transitions (Yoder & Warren, 1998), and numerous research projects have reported that a parent's directive communicative style is associated with poorer communication patterns in their children (see Chapter 3). For instance, Tannock, Girolametto, and Siegel (1992) found that parent directiveness was associated with fewer child initiations. Even with typically developing children, however, adult directiveness may not always have a negative association with child behavior. Researchers have also noted types of appropriate parent directiveness, in which parent directiveness that follows the child's action and attention can actually support communicative development (e.g., Akhtar, Dunham, & Dunham, 1991). In these circumstances, directiveness that redirects the child's attention forces the child to split his or her attention and cognitive processing between activities, but directiveness that follows the child's attention may provide useful cues or reinforcement to accomplish children's functional and communicative goals.

Parent Interaction Style and Responsivity in Nonspeaking Children   Experience with directive parental styles may not necessarily discourage communicative initiation in children with disabilities. Most research about children with disabilities such as Down syndrome (Floyd & Phillippe, 1993; Maurer & Sherrod, 1987) and cerebral palsy (e.g., Hanzlik, 1990) has found that parents of children with disabilities are more directive than parents of typically developing children. Children with physical impairments tended to rely on a responsive role in gestural interactions more than expected for developmental age peers (Cress et al., 1999), and nonspeaking people of all ages are at risk for disproportionately responsive communication patterns (Light, 1988). Nevertheless, Romski, Sevcik, and colleagues found that in interactions with familiar partners, children with mental retardation who were nonsymbolic initiated and repaired communication frequently by using gestural and vocal strategies (Romski, Sevcik, Reumann, & Pate, 1989; Romski, Sevcik, Robinson, & Bakeman, 1994).

Furthermore, parents of children with a disability may not be as directive as commonly reported in the literature. Cress, Moskal, and Benal (2001) found that parents of nonspeaking children with physical impairments were not significantly more directive during free play than parents of typically developing children, and they were significantly less directive than the parents of children with cerebral palsy in the Hanzlik (1990) study. The discrepancy across investigations may relate to the type of play that is sampled. Most studies of directiveness ask parents to engage in object play with their children, a task that is inherently difficult and associated with low success for children with physical impairments. Parent directiveness may be an indirect (and possibly appropriate) compensation for perceived limitations of children on these tasks. The Cress, Moskal, and Benal data included free play in which toys were available, but parents could successfully initiate and control routines or other physical activities without the need for parent directiveness (e.g., beginning a tickling routine that children could initiate with a body lean or vocalization). Thus, parents of nonspeaking children may structure interactions so that children's gestural and vocal behaviors can play a natural role in initiating and responding to parents' communication. Marfo (1992) and Tannock (1988) also suggested that directiveness may be an adaptive parent prompting strategy to support difficult play or interaction activities for children with other developmental disabilities.

Parents may naturally incorporate adult-initiated elements into routines that encourage children's vocal as well as gestural communicative development. For instance, Yoder and Davies (1992) found that preschool children with developmental delays at one to two word stages tended to produce more frequent language and more diverse vocabulary in routines than in nonroutines. Yet, they also found that parents tended to ask more questions during the routines and elicited more child language in routines that are typically judged as being directive (e.g., book routines of "What's this?"). They proposed that, if the parents' questions continue the child's topic, intervention strategies involving "test questions" to which the adult already knows the answer may reflect naturally occurring patterns of routine interaction.

Parent Responsivity in Early AAC Intervention   Several researchers have demonstrated that improving parent recognition and response to children's intentional behaviors significantly improves the development of intentional communication for children with developmental disabilities (e.g., Wilcox et al., 1995; Yoder & Warren, 1998). Researchers have been less successful at demonstrating the effectiveness of parent responsivity intervention for children who do not yet show intentional behaviors (Yoder & Warren, 1999). For spontaneous behavior communicators, failure to respond meaningfully to parent feedback may reflect children's difficulty in identifying the behavior that is being reinforced, as well as associating their own behavior with the response that they received. Better methods are needed for helping children who rely on spontaneous behaviors to recognize this connection.

A key factor for children who rely on AAC at early developmental stages is providing them with concrete feedback about which of their behaviors elicits parental responses. Children who do not yet consistently demonstrate intentional behaviors and do not necessarily anticipate results of their own actions cannot be assumed to routinely associate their own behaviors with the functional or parental responses that they receive. The graphic representation of parent responsivity in Figure 8.3 illustrates this challenge. For children to understand the effect of their behavior on an event, they must both recognize that they have moved and causally link that movement with the response. Children with physical impairments, particularly those with frequent involuntary movements, may have limited kinesthetic awareness of their movements. If parents increase the specificity of their feedback to help their children recognize which movement has elicited a response, they will likely help their children learn to associate the appropriate behavior with the resulting event.

One strategy to help children explicitly associate specific movements with social-interactive responses is to provide concrete touch cues that identify the specific child behavior that the parent is reinforcing. Various studies illustrate this association. Typically developing infants smiled and looked at their parents more when given touch cues even if the parents were instructed to be silent and expressionless (Stack & Arnold, 1998), and parents spontaneously tended to increase active touching when attempting to elicit smiles from infants (Stack, LePage, Hains, & Muir, 1996). Mothers tended to touch infants less when a toy was introduced into the interaction, but touch cues were effective at increasing infant involvement with toys (Colburne, Stack, Bentley,

& Switkin, 1998). Because very early communicators are unlikely to interpret the meaning of the parent's verbal response, a touch response may help them concretely identify the relevant action and associate their own behavior with the functional response that they received. Children are likely to understand a touch that reinforces their own spontaneous behavior before responding to a touch prompt for initiating behaviors.

As with any aspect of individual differences and communication, it is necessary to account for multiple aspects of parent–child play and interaction before interpreting the role of parent interaction style. Directiveness may be an appropriate parental compensation in tasks that are difficult for children who rely on AAC. As many behavior signals by nonspeaking children are difficult to interpret, it is helpful to keep a Communication Signal Inventory (CSI; Blackstone, 1991; see also Chapter 2) to highlight behaviors that parents perceive as meaningful, as well as ways that all partners respond systematically to these behavior signals. Instructional strategies, such as milieu instruction with structured questions and activities (e.g., Kaiser et al., 1992), may be a functional means for promoting children's intentional communication if they already demonstrate intentional behaviors and the parents already recognize and respond to children's communicative signals (Yoder & Warren, 1998; see also Chapter 3). Intervention can guide parents in ways to be directive in response to children's communicative intents, such as helping children communicate about a task in which they are clearly interested (e.g., Wilcox et al., 1995). Even within familiar routines, intervention strategies may also need to include parents' modeling of a waiting response to compensate for the increased latency of a child's action.

Cause–Effect and Play Strategies   Children with physical impairments are usually better at controlling cause–effect skills that affect other people's behavior than those that directly affect toys or events. For instance, children can often initiate social routines with parents by using idiosyncratic or subtle behaviors that may unsuccessfully affect most physical toys. Typically developing children tend to learn cause–effect skills without much adult coaching, through simple interaction with available toys that are physically easy for them to use. Nevertheless, all children who learn to generalize toy-related cause–effect skills to communication must receive environmental prompting of and responses to their interactive initiations (social reinforcement). Some cause–effect and means-end activities can actually foster a passive communication style if they are primarily adult directed rather than child directed. For instance, when children's primary communicative signals are confirmations or protests to offered choices, they tend to have difficulty initiating with those signals, as "yes" or "no" cannot introduce a new topic.

Cause–Effect and Symbolic Play in Nonspeaking Children   Estimates of cognitive skills in play assessments often emphasize toy-based cause–effect skills in early development (e.g., Bayley, 1993). Yet, early play scales from typical development inadequately represent play for children with physical impairments who may rely on social interaction to learn cause–effect skills. Children with disabilities may be able to physically complete only simple motor acts with objects (e.g., gazing, mouthing, banging), which result in lower scores on typical play scales (e.g., Belsky & Most, 1981). Rating children with physical impairments on the Carpenter (1987) play scale ranked some of the most symbolically skilled children as scoring low on play, and it disregarded other complexities in play (Cress & LaMontagne, 2001). For instance, the most complex play scored on the Carpenter scale for eye pointing to desired objects would be *visual regard* (i.e., looking passively toward a play object), which is a much simpler play behavior than gestural requesting. Olswang and Pinder (1995) found that children with cerebral palsy who could use their hands tended to demonstrate a wider variety of object play strategies as their coordinated looking and attention skills increased. For children with severely limited physical skills, however, this association between attention and play skills may not be as easy to establish.

Alternative strategies for measuring play skills in children who rely on AAC are necessary, and they can provide different impressions of children's cognitive and linguistic abilities. For instance, structured symbolic play with dolls has identified limited play schemes for toddlers with expressive language delay (Rescorla & Goossens', 1992). Yet, Thal and Tobias (1994) proposed that these limited structured play schemes do not necessarily show a systematic deficit in symbolic capability but, rather, a specific difficulty in demonstrating this skill in creative situations that require abstract symbolic application. Thal and Tobias found that late talkers with poor symbolic play schemes were equivalent to age-matched peers when measured by spontaneous symbolic gesture imitation or production as a label in confrontation naming (e.g., pretending to fly a plane). Possible reasons why abstract symbolic play skills for children with disabilities are limited include a "stylistic" difference in play, a developmental lag in symbol use, or a deficit in retrieving stored symbolic representation (Rescorla & Goossens', 1992). Many children who rely on AAC may demonstrate additional limitations in symbolic play due to physical limitations in controlling multiple play schemes (e.g., scooping, stirring, feeding dolls) that are used on symbolic play scales.

For reasons beyond physical or sensory limitations, symbolic play may not be equally indicative of language skills for children who rely on AAC. Guerette and colleagues (1999) adapted a play-based cognitive assessment battery that minimizes specific motor responses to help discriminate play characteristics that are associated with physical versus cognitive skills. Symbolic play that is observable in children with disabilities is also influenced by environmental factors such as classroom arrangement, the amount of space for play, the length of play sessions, listener behaviors, task complexity, and the quantity and social nature of the toys used (Rettig, 1998). For instance, as symbolic play tasks increase in complexity, children with autism perform at lower levels than developmental age peers, even when assessors prompt the children in symbolic play tasks (Amato, Barrow, & Domingo, 1999; Rinaldi, Dawson, Meltzoff, & Osterling, 1997). If nonspeaking children have limited access strategies or support in communication by partners, then they are unlikely to be able to demonstrate their symbolic play skills in standard assessment measures.

Cause–Effect and Symbolic Play in Early AAC Intervention Behaviors that demonstrate cause–effect relationship skills need not be separated from social activities. It is extremely important for a child to control, manage, and understand the behavior of others. Parents often create unique interactive routines with nonspeaking children that take advantage of actions and/or sounds that their children can control. It is physically and logistically more difficult for children with physical impairments to control toys than to control a person who can adapt to or scaffold the child's behavior. Intervention strategies need to include person-focused cause–effect activities, as well as object-directed play, for children who are still developing these skills.

Practitioners working with children who rely on AAC need better scales to incorporate the skills presumably developed in object play into observations of social play that children with disabilities can control. For instance, the concept that is learned by placing objects close together involves *association*. Children with limited motor skills may learn association by manipulating their own body's relationship to others in play. Assessments of play and associated cognitive skills that use the physical behaviors of typically developing children (e.g., Guerette et al., 1999) may artificially lower estimates of play skills for nonspeaking children. Thus, alternative cognitive assessments in object and social play for children with physical impairments are being developed (Cress & Anderson, 2001).

Intentional Behaviors to Intentionally Communicative Gestures

Many of the factors discussed regarding the transition from spontaneous behaviors to intentional behaviors also support the development of intentional communication. For instance, parent responsivity continues to support communication long after spontaneous and intentional behaviors develop. The following sections highlight additional factors of communicative functions, communication rate, and mastery motivation that may contribute to the development of intentional communication. Each factor is discussed in relation to both nonspeaking children and early AAC intervention. See Figure 8.2 for a graphic representation of these factors that influence communicative transitions.

Communicative Functions Most children produce behavior regulation (controlling someone else's behavior) earlier and more frequently in development than other communicative functions such as joint attention. For toddlers with typical development, Crais and Day (2000) reported a detailed hierarchical development of specific gestures by age for communicative functions such as requesting objects, requesting actions, protesting, seeking attention, commenting, requesting information, and playing social games. Many of these communicative forms occurred at substantially different ages than reflected in standardized assessment instruments. Wetherby and Rodriguez (1992) found that on average, children who were prelinguistic conveyed behavior regulation in 42% of their communication acts during structured play and in only 25% of communication acts during unstructured play. As children become more able to represent abstract concepts in the late toddler years, more of their communication and conversation revolves around sharing information and commenting rather than strictly expressing wants and needs. In typical conversations of preschool children and their parents at home, only 17% of utterances conveyed specific requests and refusals for environmental control of events (Ball, Marvin, Beukelman, Lasker, & Rupp, 1999).

Communicative Functions in Nonspeaking Children   Research has demonstrated that children with various communicative impairments produce more limited communicative functions than typically developing peers. On the Communication and Symbolic Behavior Scales (CSBS; Wetherby & Prizant, 1993), adults with profound mental retardation compared with typically developing peers 1) produced more behavior regulation acts and fewer joint attention acts, 2) were less responsive, and 3) communicated with primarily untranscribable or vowel-like vocalizations (Ogletree, Wetherby, & Westling, 1992). Similarly, Brady, McLean, McLean, and Johnston (1995) found that adults with severe to profound mental retardation who rely on nonsymbolic gestures initiated more proto-imperative (behavior regulation) than protodeclarative (joint attention) acts when given equal opportunity for both types of acts. Cress and colleagues (1999) found a similar imbalance in behavioral regulation and social interaction over joint attention functions in young children who rely on AAC.

In addition to differences in cognitive development, communicative experience may contribute to children's use of different communicative forms. Nonspoken communication in general tends to be more ambiguous and less intelligible than spoken communication (Kent, 1993). Infants with severe cognitive and physical impairments tend to produce behavior cues that are different from those of typically developing children, and these altered cues are more difficult for even trained observers to interpret (Yoder, 1987). Because parents are more likely to respond to communication that clearly relates to their children's want and needs, such as behavior regulation acts (Flanagan, Coppa, Riggs, & Alario, 1994), these kinds of communicative acts may receive more consistent feedback from parents whose children are at risk for being nonspeaking. If children's communication development reflects the parental feedback that is received, children who rely on AAC might learn to produce more of the behaviors that successfully elicit parent responses and fewer of the complex behaviors, such as joint attention, that may trigger communication breakdowns.

Children who have limited use of communicative forms and functions are also more likely to experience difficulty repairing communication breakdowns. If children who use early AAC provide minimal breakdown repair, then a substantial burden of interpreting the message remains with the listener even after the children become intentional communicators. Persons relying on gestural AAC are more likely to repeat than revise their communicative messages after communication breakdowns (Calculator & Delaney, 1986) and produce few repairs (Brady et al., 1995; McLean, McLean, Brady, & Etter, 1991). Cress and colleagues (1999) also found that children with physical impairments produced fewer repairs than developmental-age peers, although children with physical impairments tended to appropriately apply modification strategies when produced as repairs (see Chapter 10 for an expanded discussion of communication repair).

Children who are skilled at expressing wants and needs through behavioral and gestural strategies may find it difficult to represent joint attention or word labels without more formal symbol or signing strategies. McLean and colleagues (1991) found that nonsymbolic communicators with severe mental retardation tended to initiate relatively few and only proto-imperative communication acts (e.g., requests for objects or help) if they used only contact gestures that directly touch the referent or receiver. The only communicators who produced proto-declarative communication acts (e.g., requests for attention to an object or event) also demonstrated consistent use of distal gestures (e.g., pointing or gesturing towards referents without touching them). Distal gestures are more removed from the communicative referent and, therefore, are more clearly representative or symbolic than contact gestures.

Communicative Functions and Early AAC Intervention   Many of the behaviors that are easy for children without disabilities to produce are not easy for children with disabilities, even if children demonstrate these behaviors under some circumstances, and the behaviors are less likely to be spontaneously transferred across settings without a clear goal or functional result (Cress et al., 1998). Therefore, focused interventions may be necessary to target specific communicative functions, such as joint attention communication acts, that are at risk in children who rely on AAC.

Many AAC interventions focus on wants and needs much longer than is developmentally or functionally appropriate for children. If children who use AAC are already at risk for having restricted communication forms (i.e., limited to wants and needs), interventionists need to increase the emphasis on promoting less frequent forms and functions, such as commenting and requesting information. Coordinated intervention for resolving communication breakdowns and increasing the clarity and interpretability of children's signals to partners may also support the expression of new and more varied communicative functions. Not all children who rely on AAC may take as active a role as expected in independently practicing and applying strategies across different communicative domains or functions, even when children are clearly motivated to learn and influence their environment. Children with various disabilities who require AAC are also at risk for being passive communicators at several points throughout childhood and adulthood (Buzolich & Wiemann, 1988; Sweeney & Engwis, 1996), and they may not always demonstrate strategies that they are capable of producing. Limited experience with the effectiveness of alternative early communication strategies in changing the behavior of others may also limit the extent to which children demonstrate intentional communication.

For young children who have a limited range of motor behaviors, skills such as eye pointing may be particularly important for reference and labeling activities as well as more basic attention monitoring functions (with simple gaze shifts). As eye pointing is considered a distal gesture, it may be more difficult for children to initially control joint attention behaviors with gaze than with proximal gestures such as touching. Also, because eye-pointing behaviors (including simple visual scanning) tend to accomplish multiple purposes for a child, it is necessary to provide additional support in helping children make their eye-pointing behaviors distinct from other behaviors and in helping parents learn to interpret and reinforce children's early indications of joint attention.

Communication Rate   Children's rate of communicative acts has been associated with later expressive vocabulary and symbolic development in typically developing children (Wetherby, Cain, Yonclas, & Walker, 1988) as well as in children with developmental delays (McCathren, Yoder, & Warren, 1999). It is presumed that using gestural labels for symbolic acts reflects a similar reliance on mentally representing objects as spoken-word production (Acredolo & Goodwyn, 1988; Bretherton et al., 1981). These developmental associations provide communication-based predictors for a child's readiness to develop symbols and words, which is preferable to age or developmental age–based estimates, such as the Piagetian Stage V "prerequisite" for symbol acquisition that was previously proposed for AAC users (Shane & Bashir, 1980).

Communication Rate in Nonspeaking Children   In situations that are structured to prompt for communication initiations, people with disabilities have demonstrated frequent initiations in their total communicative interaction (McLean et al., 1991; Wetherby, Yonclas, & Bryan, 1989). Ogletree and colleagues (1992) found that school-age children with profound mental retardation produced communicative acts at an equivalent rate to typically developing children at similar developmental ages in structured play interactions. Individual children with mental retardation who had relatively high rates of expressive communicative acts tended to produce more types of communicative functions and better coordination of gestures and vocalizations, although this effect was not significant for the group data. Intentional communicators with developmental disabilities, including AAC users, also demonstrate an association between a communication rate of one act per minute and the onset of symbolic behaviors in structured play tasks with adults (Wilcox et al., 1995). Relative to developmental peers, children with physical impairments showed a somewhat reduced rate during communication temptations, but multiword communicators consistently produced faster communication rates than prelinguistic or one-word intentional communicators (Cress et al., 1999).

Communication Rate and Early AAC Intervention   Because communicative initiation rate is relatively easy to assess, practitioners can build on this assessment information and target intervention at both improving a child's use of current gestural communication and presenting new symbolic strategies. Although AAC is typically associated with slower communication rates, nonspeaking children who clearly understand the role of their communication in an interaction are likely to initiate communication promptly when opportunities are presented, even if completing the communicative act takes longer due to motor difficulty or limited partner interpretation. Children who rely on AAC need to clearly anticipate that their listener will both understand and respond to their communicative act before they will initiate an elaborate AAC strategy such as eye pointing or partner-assisted scanning.

The physical and sensory restrictions associated with AAC will limit the potential rate of communication through augmented behaviors (as well as other symbolic forms of AAC), and interventionists should be cautioned in their application of communication rate estimates beyond intentional communication stages. Although research indicates that children with physical impairments can achieve gestural communication rates that approach one act per minute for simple requests or comments in structured play tasks, as children gain more complex communication skills, their rate does not increase as quickly as expected for typically developing children (Cress et al., 1999). Cress and colleagues found that nonspeaking children produced a slower rate of communication acts than typically developing children at all communication stages beyond the prelinguistic stage, and the difference from typical development was significantly larger for children with multiword and better communication. Therefore, children who rely on AAC may be able to learn new signs or symbols quickly from limited exposure (i.e., *fast mapping,* or learning words from as little as 1–2 modeled or incidental presentations) earlier than might be predicted from communicative rate estimates that are derived from typically developing children. The clinical implication is that each communicative act will take longer for the children to compose as they integrate multiple modes to produce complex messages, and that communication rate may not be correlated with message complexity or interactive skill beyond early communication.

Mastery Motivation   Mastery motivation, the drive to attempt to master tasks for the intrinsic feeling of self-efficacy, can be measured in children as young as 4 months of age and is demonstrated in children's earliest gestures and play strategies (Morgan, MacTurk, & Hrncir, 1995). Acredolo and Goodwyn (1990) proposed that children are likely to attempt mastery of gestures to fulfill their need for self-produced interaction with the environment. Mastery motivation is a measure of how well a child's interest and goal-directed focus leads to active exploration and problem solving regarding a task. Qualities such as persistence and the range of attempted strategies in resolving problems and play tasks are typical ways of measuring mastery motivation in young children (McCall, 1995). Children tend to demonstrate optimum mastery motivation on tasks that are neither too easy nor too hard, as they can solve easy problems without trying new strategies and will give up quickly if problems are too hard.

Mastery Motivation and Self-Efficacy in Nonspeaking Children   Some researchers have proposed that children with various disabilities have more limited mastery motivation than typically developing children. For instance, several researchers have found some differences in mastery motivation measures from developmental peers for children with mental retardation (MacTurk, Vietze, McCarthy, McQuiston, & Yarrow, 1985; Ruskin, Mundy, Kasari, & Signam, 1994), spina bifida (Landry, Copeland, Lee, & Robinson, 1990), and cerebral palsy (Blasco, Hrncir, & Blasco, 1990). This research may be confounded by task difficulty and the theoretical construct of mastery motivation (Hupp & Abbeduto, 1991), which are difficult to assess in a standard way, particularly for children with physical impairments. Hauser-Cram (1996) found no differences between mastery motivation for children with developmental disabilities and developmental peers when it was measured as persistence or goal-oriented motivation in successfully completing puzzles or cause–effect tasks. Nonetheless, parents of children with physical disabilities have rated their children as being less motivated and more likely to seek out easier or familiar activities during free play than children without disabilities (Jennings, Connors, Stegman, Sankaranaryan, & Mendelsohn, 1985).

Learned helplessness is a related concept that is frequently associated with many people with disabilities, including adults who rely on AAC. It occurs when communicative or activity attempts are repeatedly met with failure and the AAC user has no perceived strategies for resolving the failure (Sweeney & Engwis, 1996). Jennings, Connor, and Stegman (1988) observed that, at 3 years of age, children with physical impairments showed equivalent curiosity but less persistence than their peers, but by 4 years of age, they began to consistently choose easier and less novel tasks. Children who were relatively less motivated at 3 years of age also tended to show low motivation at 4 years of age, which suggests that mastery motivation patterns even among children with significant disabilities are individually stable patterns.

The severity of physical disability has not been significantly associated with the degree of mastery motivation (Jennings et al., 1988). In research with children ages 1–2 years, Hauser-Cram (1996) found that children with motor impairments did not differ in persistence, goal orientation, positive affect, or competence in play from other children without disabilities at similar developmental levels. The critical element for the development of mastery motivation in the children with physical impairments was the extent to which parents created environments in which children could learn and be encouraged to self-initiate problem-solving ability. Creating meaningful interaction and play tasks that can be independently managed by children with severe motor or sensory limitations is, however, one of the ongoing challenges that confronts the fields of AAC and assistive technology.

Mastery Motivation and Early AAC Intervention   To successfully select and manage multiple AAC modalities, children must demonstrate creativity in attempting alternative strategies to solve a problem. Persistence in conveying an exact message that a child wants to convey is necessary to overcome the frequent communication breakdowns or compromises in messages that are common in AAC applications. Because mastery motivation is a distinct characteristic from other aspects of cognition or communication, reliable assessments of mastery motivation might help to predict successful acquisition of augmented communication beyond the prediction from children's motor or cognitive skills.

If mastery motivation were solely an intrinsic characteristic, then it would not be easily susceptible to intervention. Yet, many researchers have proposed that parent-provided opportunities and reinforcement for successful task exploration directly influence mastery motivation development (e.g., Hauser-Cram & Shonkoff, 1995). Helping parents develop skills in gauging task difficulty and prompting child independent exploration and persistence may foster improved mastery motivation. Mastery can be learned by persistence in social tasks as well as in physical tasks (Linke & Cress, 2001). Tools such as the CSI (see Chapter 2) can help in providing structure for partners to recognize subtle signals and in planning consistent social responses by all interactants.

Intentional Gestures to Symbolic Gestures

All of the previous factors that affect development continue to affect transitions from intentional gestures to symbolic gestures (see Figure 8.2). Additional factors that are particularly relevant for this stage include expressive and receptive vocabulary development, as well as the special case of vocal gesture development as part of a multimodal communication system in early AAC.

Expressive Vocabulary   Symbolic gesture production has been associated with expressive language development. Relative to language-age peers, late-talking children who have equivalent comprehension skills and increased communicative gesture production eventually reach expressive language scores that are appropriate for their chronological age (Thal & Tobias, 1992). Late talkers who are delayed in comprehension produce significantly fewer gestures of all types than typically developing children (Thal et al., 1991). During periods of rapid vocabulary acquisition, children also tend to produce multischeme play schemes (McCune-Nicolich, 1981) that demonstrate skill at combining symbolic representations. Other skills that tend to co-occur with rapid expressive language development in children include simple categorization (e.g., sorting objects into two groups) and fast mapping (Mervis & Bertrand, 1994).

Expressive Vocabulary in Nonspeaking Children   Children with limited verbal expression may not be able to demonstrate the extent of their expressive vocabulary potential, as they depend on the vocabulary that is available in their AAC system and/or linguistic and spelling capacity. Even children who use AAC with maximum access to expressive vocabularies are at risk for reduced expressive vocabulary in communication samples because the rate restrictions on communicative output tends to reduce the length and complexity of output (Venkatagiri, 1995). Skilled adult AAC communicators still tend to produce fewer expressive utterances than speaking peers, and they experience more receptive than expressive communication with speaking partners (Buzolich & Wiemann, 1988). If this pattern is also true for young children who rely on AAC, then their expressive communication experience is likely to be similarly restricted, which may affect vocabulary development in ways that have not yet been determined.

Nonspeaking children with limited access to vocabulary are also less likely to demonstrate an expressive vocabulary of 50 words as early as they are actually capable of having a "burst" of rapid expressive vocabulary development. Yet, the so-called vocabulary burst that is associated with verbal output in speaking children may not mark the first point at which children separate concepts from objects and events or understand the purpose of naming as a generative language activity (Acredolo & Goodwyn, 1990). Once the cognitive foundations are in place, there is considerable difference among typically developing children in their rate of gesture versus speech acquisition. For instance, one of the typically developing children in the Acredolo and Goodwyn (1989) study had 40 symbolic gestures before showing a spoken vocabulary burst from 7 to 68 words at 19 months of age. This child seemed to have the cognitive skills for representing close to 50 words gesturally before that skill was demonstrated through the verbal modality. Similar research is likely to show even more variability in the coordination of gesture and spoken communication modes in children who rely on AAC.

Expressive Vocabulary and Early AAC Intervention   Symbolic gesture production has been associated with expressive language skills of late-talking children, who may rely on gestural communication longer than typically developing children (Thal & Tobias, 1992). Typically developing children who produced more symbolic gestures as infants tended to have better expressive language scores than infants with fewer gestures (Acredolo & Goodwyn, 1988). Brown (1998) taught children (ages 19–23 months) who had expressive language delays to produce a symbolic gesture (e.g., opening hands to indicate *book*) by using a combination of child modeling and parent training. Children who were trained in symbolic gesture production produced an equivalent number of spoken words and rate of change in expressive vocabulary to age-matched peers at an 8-month follow-up. In contrast, children who received only verbal or no instruction remained below age expectations in language expression. This suggests that symbolic gesture training can be a strategy for improving vocal expression as well as other forms of language and symbolic development. Yet, if children who rely on AAC are less likely to imitate communicative gestures out of context (as discussed in this chapter's section on imitation development), then this symbolic gesture training needs to be embedded in meaningful communicative contexts for children.

In addition, for children who rely on AAC and are expected to communicate with gestural and other nonvocal strategies long-term, additional intervention may be necessary to facilitate expression. For instance, children with gestural strategies such as eye pointing may need extra intervention to learn to refer to concepts that are removed in time and space, as these items do not have a visual referent. Children who eye point may develop strategies of looking in the direction of absent objects or marking the referent spatially within visual space (e.g., looking up for things that happened in the past versus looking down for future events). Nonetheless, these strategies are not likely to be easily interpretable unless codeveloped or coached with communication partners.

Receptive Vocabulary   Parent reports on inventories such as the MacArthur Communication Development Inventory (CDI; Fenson et al., 1993) have consistently reflected children's receptive vocabulary size as well as other standardized measures. Receptive vocabulary does not seem to be a good predictor of expressive vocabulary acquisition rate, however, as children may have receptive vocabularies from 50 to 200 or more words before demonstrating a language burst (Bates, Bretherton, & Snyder, 1988). Nevertheless, poorer receptive vocabulary (as well as symbolic gesture production) does help

distinguish late talkers who fail to catch up with developmental expectations (i.e., those who have true delays) from children that meet developmental norms by late toddlerhood (i.e., those who are "late bloomers") (Thal
et al., 1991).

Receptive Vocabulary and Gesture Comprehension in Nonspeaking Children
Parents who complete receptive vocabulary measures for children with disabilities are likely to underestimate children's repertoires as the children's vocabulary increases beyond common nouns and routines, particularly if parents and children do not share a communicative modality (Prezbindowski,
Spencer, & Lederberg, 1999; Yoder, Warren, & Biggar, 1997). If the primary
way that parents recognize nonspeaking children's knowledge of terms is by
introducing them and gauging the child's response, then this estimate depends
on whether the vocabulary has been presented in context and whether parents
recognize children's meaningful responses. It is also possible that older nonspeaking children who do not yet use words in a broadly symbolic way (i.e.,
intentional communicators) may build a larger repertoire of situation-de-
pendent vocabulary than typically developing children.

    Little research has addressed the extent to which children who rely
on AAC comprehend gestures beyond the gestures included in the CDI (Fenson et al., 1993) and reviews (e.g., Iverson & Thal, 1998) of gesture comprehension in typically developing children. Mundy and Gomes (1997, 1998) reported that children's skills at responding to joint attention cues from parents
(e.g., pointing at an interesting event and saying, "Look") correlated with expressive language in typically developing children 14–18 months old. In older
children who rely on symbolic AAC, Hunt-Berg (1996) found adult pointing
cues between the symbol and the referent object facilitated children's learning
of novel graphic symbol labels better than pointing to the symbol alone. Because children shifted gaze between the symbol and the object in both conditions, Hunt-Berg attributed the observed difference to the role of the dual
point in disambiguating the adult's intended referent for the child. Heller, Alberto, and Romski (1995) found similar results for preschool intentional communicators with mental retardation who learned to recognize the partner's
referent more effectively if the partner provided cues of partial objects or de-
pictive movements with the spoken label.

    Preliminary indications suggest that children with physical disabilities
may begin to play labeling games (e.g., "Show me the [object name]") later than
speaking children with similar language comprehension skills (Cress, 1999).
Therefore, traditional receptive vocabulary assessments are likely to underestimate these children's vocabulary comprehension. Traditional receptive vocabulary assessments that emphasize pointing to items on command also may
be mismatched with the communicative experience and needs of children who
may have had restricted world experience because of medical limitations as-

sociated with their disability (e.g., children who are tube fed may not know many food-related words). It is particularly difficult to recognize comprehension of function words such as *of* or *the* in repertoires of nonspeaking children, as these words are not associated with observable characteristics and are usually judged by expressive vocabulary in verbal children. Caution should be taken in interpreting vocabulary checklists for nonspeaking children who may have artificially high floors or low ceilings in their scores.

Receptive Vocabulary and Early AAC Intervention   Various concepts in children's early AAC systems can be initiated at gestural levels of communication to promote particular content vocabulary for receptive communication. For instance, "What's that?" is a key phrase to include in AAC behavioral or symbolic systems for encouraging active initiation of joint attention as well as for giving children the means to solicit information that builds receptive vocabulary skills. Children who do not yet successfully integrate picture- or device-based symbols into their AAC system can still learn to ask or answer questions such as "What's that?" with simple sign or gestural strategies. Other activities in which children use their available AAC strategies for multiple purposes (e.g., eye pointing to both label and request objects) are also likely to help broaden children's semantic skills in ways that are comparable to those of typically developing children.

Teaching children to "point to the (object name)" may have limited generalization to other aspects of language use. For instance, in isolated activities, adults with profound mental retardation could comprehend functional gestures (e.g., spinning a top) that were already in their expressive repertoire as effectively as unknown gestures in a "give me the (object name)" task (Duker, van Deursen, de Wit, & Palmen, 1997). Yet, adults in this study did not consistently associate the "give me" cue with gestures in their behavioral repertoire, which suggests that establishing a receptive repertoire of gestures does not automatically promote association with the expressive or communicative use of those gestures. Even learning to recognize symbols or representative gestures is best conducted in the context of realistic and effective communicative activities.

Vocal Behavior Development: A Special Case of Gestures   Although children who are nonspeaking are at risk for not developing spoken words, most children can use some kinds of vocalizations in combination with or for many of the same purposes as physical gestures. Some of the predictive factors for spoken language in children with developmental disability or who are late talkers may also apply to children who are at risk for being nonspeaking. The timing of canonical babbling (consonant-vowel syllables that have a crisp transition, e.g., /dada/, /ti/, /ne/) is a good predictor of many aspects of language development in typically developing children (Oller, Eilers, Neal, &

Cobo-Lewis, 1998). Late talkers tend to have consistently late and/or reduced canonical babbling (Paul, 1998; Paul & Fountain, 1999; Thal, Oroz, & McCaw, 1995). For children with developmental disabilities who are late talkers, canonical babbling also predicts speech development (Yoder et al., 1998). Other factors that predicted who would be "functional speakers" in the Yoder and colleagues study at a 1-year follow-up include the children's ratio of expressive to receptive vocabulary inventory and their rate of behavior regulation initiation.

Vocal Behaviors in Nonspeaking Children   Some of these typical predictive factors for vocal gesture development may not apply to nonspeaking children with physical impairments. For instance, children with poor motor initiation and control may not play freely with syllables in the same fashion as children with intact motor systems. Children with Down syndrome produced sequences of vocal development from quasivowels through canonical syllables (e.g., /ba/, /da/) that were similar to those of typically developing children (Steffens, Oller, Lynch, & Urbano, 1992). Yet, Oller and colleagues (1998) also found that children with Down syndrome and other disabilities were at risk for not producing reduplicated canonical babbling, and this was negatively correlated with expressive language development. Some children with severe physical impairment seem to move directly from single syllable sounds to meaningful word use without ever passing through a stage of reduplicated syllables (Cress, 1999). Children who do not produce clearly distinguished syllables until late in their communicative development may already use even simple sounds and syllables meaningfully when they are produced. For children who rely on AAC, there may be a conflict between what is easy and commonly seen in children without physical impairments and what is consistently and effectively produced by nonspeaking children.

Vocal Behaviors and Early AAC Intervention   Better assessment and intervention strategies are needed for spoken language development in children with severely restricted syllable sets, as well as other skills that may compensate for limited canonical babbling and expressive production. Some tools for adapted play allow children to actively select sounds to combine in babbling-like activities, which may fulfill some of the developmental functions of independent babbling for typically developing children (Ferrier, Fell, Mooraj, Delta, & Moscoe, 1996). Children's motor systems are still developing in ways that cannot be predicted, and the early intervention period is too early in the development process to give up on further improvement in speech skills. Almost all children who can produce a voice will use sounds in some ways that are interpretable to listeners. It is generally considered a positive sign for continued vocal development when children continue to learn new sounds or new variations on the sounds that they are producing (Romski & Sevcik, 1996).

Specific strategies for supporting vocal development in children who produce only a few sounds may depend to some extent on whether the child can produce sounds or vocalizations consistently when desired, as well as the range of sounds that the child produces under different circumstances. Table 8.2 presents more specific examples of the relationship between vocal intervention strategies and the stages of typical vocal development (Stoel-Gammon, 1998). If children are producing primarily vowel sounds, then partners can provide functional and verbal responses to the children's spontaneous vocalizations, as well as focus on tactile feedback on the mouth or throat to alert children to the parts of the body that produce sounds. Children who can produce reactive sounds or turn taking within social environments may respond to partners who echo children's sounds and gradually introduce new sounds that are potentially within the children's repertoires. Associating different sounds with different activities in the environment, such as pairing simple physical activities with different vocalizations (varying in phoneme, pitch, or duration of vocalization) can help to increase children's variety and awareness of different sounds from vowels through simple babbling (Cress & Ball, 1998). Children who can produce more complex sounds without hesitation may be able to insert sounds into familiar routines or respond to prompts for vocalizations within activities (e.g., "vroom" sounds when driving a car, "ga" to get out of a chair). As children's vocalizations approximate words or are used in one-to-one correspondence with specific meanings, partners can expand on and imitate children's utterances in patterns that are similar to those of typically developing children. If children with physical impairments are less likely to initiate gestural imitation than typically developing children (Cress et al., 1998), partners may need to consider alternative strategies in addition to vocal imitation for promoting vocal gesture development.

Table 8.2.   Typical vocal development and vocal intervention suggestions

Age*	Form* (speech)	Function* (communication)	Intervention ideas
Birth–2 months	Sounds (phonation)	Reflexive sound making	Give tactile response to spontaneous vocalizations.
2–3 months	Cooing	Reactive sounds, turn taking	Echo child's sounds; gradually try new sounds.
4–6 months	Simple babbling	Activity-based interaction	Pair sounds with physical activities and routines.
6–11 months	Canonical babbling	Communicative interaction	Pause in routines and prompt for vocalization.
12 months +	Jargon	Communication, first words	Imitate and expand child's word approximations.

* *Source:* Stoel-Gammon (1998).

EDUCATIONAL IMPLICATIONS: AUGMENTED
BEHAVIOR INTERVENTION FOR NONSPEAKING CHILDREN

Some research has clearly demonstrated the efficacy of early AAC intervention for improving augmented and other forms of AAC behaviors. More efficacy research is needed to reflect the full range of early intervention strategies already in practice, particularly for children at the earliest stages of augmented behavior development.

Treatment Efficacy of Gestural
Intervention with Nonspeaking Children

Systematic investigations have demonstrated success in applying various types of AAC interventions with children beginning at 3–8 years chronological age (e.g., Culp, 1989; Goossens', 1989; Kobacker & Todaro, 1992). Some research has shown successful AAC use with individual older children and adults at cognitive ages of 18–36 months (Gobbi, Cipani, Hudson, & Lapenta-Neudeck, 1986; Keogh & Reichle, 1985; Romski, Sevcik, & Adamson 1999). Wilcox and colleagues (1995) and Yoder and Warren (1998, 1999) demonstrated that improving parent recognition and responsivity for child intentional behaviors can support intentional communication development in young children with developmental delays, including some children who are nonspeaking or have physical impairments.

   Some researchers have investigated the transition from behavioral to symbolic forms of AAC in young children. Pinder and Olswang (1995) and Pinder, Olswang, and Coggins (1993) conducted small-group and single-case intervention research that demonstrated success in improving intentional communication for children with physical impairments who were as young as 11–14 months old. Romski and Sevcik (see Chapter 14) have conducted research on the success of the System for Augmenting Language (SAL), an intervention in symbolic forms of AAC demonstrated for children ages 3 years and older. Preliminary results suggest that most of the children learned symbolic forms of AAC using this strategy, and specific factors that distinguish the few children who did not successfully acquire symbolic AAC have not yet been determined. Similarly, Rowland and Schweigert (2000) reported that most of the 41 children with developmental disabilities (who had an average age of 6 years) learned to use tangible symbols through longitudinal intervention to some extent, except for five children who initially demonstrated only intentional behaviors and one child who demonstrated preintentional behaviors. No intervention research to date has addressed the success of AAC intervention that helps nonspeaking children younger than 3 years of age make the transition from spontaneous behaviors to intentional and symbolic forms of communication.

Potential strategies for gestural intervention in early AAC users are derived from research with children who are typically developing, have language delays or disorders, or have hearing impairments. For instance, young infants can successfully change aspects of their environment using switches (e.g., Behrmann & Lahm, 1983; Brinker & Lewis, 1982; Rosenberg & Robinson, 1987), although the use of these skills for communication occurs later in development and has not been systematically examined in young children. Intervention programs for children with language delays, such as the Hanen Program, address behavioral communication improvement through 1) interaction-promoting strategies to encourage child initiation and balanced turn taking; 2) language-modeling strategies, including responsive labels and comments; and 3) child-oriented strategies, such as responding to the child's attention and interpreting the child's cues (Tannock et al., 1992). Tannock and colleagues found that increasing the responsivity of parents of preschool children with developmental delays increased the children's use of vocal turns but did not improve communicative and linguistic development more than it did in the control group.

Although nonspeaking children with physical impairments may have limited ability to produce exact signed models from conventional systems, considerable research suggests that sign language can be an effective, natural way to extend early behaviors and communicative gestures into symbolic communication for young nonspeaking children. Acredolo and Goodwyn found that even typically developing children can use spontaneous symbolic gestures "to augment fledgling attempts at symbolic verbal words" for ideas that children did not have the words to express, and even parents who were unfamiliar with American Sign Language could successfully promote these gestures (1990, p. 36). Spontaneous symbolic gesturing does not delay but, instead, supports verbal language development in typically developing children, as gesture production accounted for variance in children's verbal vocabulary more than factors related to gender, birth order, or parent education (Acredolo & Goodwyn 1988).

Several authors have proposed that sign language intervention may provide a developmental advantage for some children, particularly those who benefit from the following: physical shaping of signs, gestural-motor experience, visual direct feedback of success, or reduced emphasis on fine motor neurological control associated with verbal speech (Orlansky & Bonvillian, 1988). Caselli and colleagues (1998) proposed a similar gestural advantage for young children with Down syndrome. In intervention, children with Down syndrome 8–20 months old showed fewer delays in learning "augmented signs" as verbal labels than in learning verbal words, and they learned signs as proficiently as children of similar developmental ages who did not have disabilities (Abrahamsen, Cavallo, & McCluer, 1985). In contrast, when speech is proportionately advantaged relative to gestures, children may produce simple early gestures such as pointing much later than expected. Bertrand, Mervis, and Neu-stat (1998) found that children with Williams syndrome first produced point-ing gestures at a median age of 36 months compared with 12 months for chil-dren with Down syndrome, although the children with Williams syndrome demonstrated better verbal skills.

Incorporating Traditional AAC Strategies into Gestural Assessment and Intervention

Specific intervention strategies may be provided to introduce voice output de-vices and picture symbols into children's earliest communicative interactions. It is important to consider the ways in which augmented behaviors interact with other formal AAC strategies at all levels of communication development.

Communication "Tools" Model to Estimate Relative Difficulty of Gestural AAC   When planning AAC intervention, it is necessary to con-sider the complexity of the various behavioral and symbolic strategies that a child needs to control to accomplish a communicative goal. Thal and col-leagues (1991) showed a parallel relationship between language and gesture at four periods of typical development that can influence the gradual incorpo-ration of complexity into gestural intervention for nonspeaking children (see Table 8.3). For instance, children tend to develop decontextualized gestural labels during the approximate time periods in which they develop verbal labels and names. As children develop beyond multiword and multigesture combi-nations, they are likely to demonstrate coordinated sequences of actions and/or utterances that represent familiar routine events as whole "cultural scripts" (e.g., buying food at a store, playing house).

The full array of communicative behaviors and aids that are available to children can be considered communicative "tools" that children gradually learn to control to be successful augmented communicators. The first tool that children must learn to control is their own body (a one-tool system), and

Table 8.3.   Parallel relationships between language and gesture at four periods of typi-cal development

Age (months)	Language	Gesture
9–10	Intentional communication Vocal routines	Intentional communication Gestural routines
12–13	Vocal labels or names Decontextualization	Gestural labels or names Decontextualization
20	Multiword speech	Multischeme gesture combinations
24–30	Grammaticization	Sequences Cultural scripts

From Thal, D., Tobias, S., & Morrison, D. (1991). Language and gesture in late talkers: A 1-year follow-up. *Journal of Speech and Hearing Research, 34,* 604; reprinted by permission.

operation of any other types of tools relies on controlling some type of behavior, including eye gaze, sound, or movement. Most of the early tools are not necessarily physical objects but separate aspects of interaction that children use to accomplish communicative goals (e.g., a message is a type of tool). Even spontaneous communicators are likely to have a repertoire of signals that they produce consistently that familiar partners recognize, regardless of whether those signals are produced with the intent to communicate to a partner.

Table 8.4 presents a communication tools model, which has been proposed for estimating the numbers and types of communicative demands that a given interactive task places on the child (Cress, 2001). External communicative tools can be added to the child's own behavior to form communicative signals of two or more tools. For instance, "affecting other person's behavior" tends to be one of the early second tools a child uses. A child might smile (controlling his or her own behavior) to directly elicit a social response from an adult (influencing the adult's behavior) as a two-tool system of the child's behavior initiation plus affecting another person. Similar two-tool systems may combine the child's behavior with a toy (e.g., shaking a rattle) or with a communicative intent (e.g., vocalizing a distinct protest sound). Other communicative tools that speaking children may add to more complex messages include anticipation of a specific response, language, and spoken-word output.

Specific communicative tools that are common to early AAC users include a symbolic representation (e.g., a representative picture symbol or sign), an external device (e.g., a switch that plays a prerecorded message), and the spoken voice output of such a device. The external device and its voice output message are considered separate tools, as children can interact with the physical device without attending to the voice output that is produced. Also, the task of deciding to communicate by using an external device that is not

Table 8.4. Application of communicative tools model to a child's request for "more tickle" by choosing a voice output switch with a particular picture symbol

Type of communicative tool	Example
Child initiates a behavior	Reaches own arm out and controls its movement . . .
+ Toy or other direct object	and pushes switch with arm movement
+ Message content	and child enjoys and wants to continue tickle game
+ Symbolic representation	and chooses picture symbol representing "tickle"
+ External device	and controls a nonbehavioral means of communication
+ Language	and conveys specific semantic content: More tickle
+ Voice output	and hears "more tickle" from device
+ Affects other person's behavior	and partner attends to and interacts with child
+ Communicative outcome	and child anticipates/reacts to specific tickle activity

Note: Copyright © 2001 Cynthia J. Cress.

part of one's body is presumed to add cognitive load to the previous communication task, which is presented by the voice output of the message alone.

Conventionalizing Gestures into Mixed Modality Symbolic AAC Systems

Both behavioral and symbolic strategies can co-occur at all stages of development, and a child is not expected to fully complete gestural development before he or she is introduced to symbolic communication. Ideally, children who rely on AAC would be exposed to symbolic AAC in natural communicative interactions starting in early infancy, in a similar fashion to the ways that typically developing children are exposed to spoken language. This chapter concludes with vignettes that are designed to provide examples of conventionalizing gestures into mixed modality AAC systems. Children and adults may continue to use multiple simultaneous strategies—including gesture, vocal, partner, and other AAC means—to help disambiguate potentially confusing communication throughout the life span. Conventional linguistic signs or formal symbolic systems are effectively introduced as natural extensions of children's successful behavioral and gestural communication.

Using Voice Output to Facilitate Developing Intentional Behaviors

Linda is a 17-month-old girl who was developing typically until she experienced brain damage from encephalitis at 12 months of age. She sits upright with support, and she has frequent writhing hand and arm behaviors that appear to be involuntary. Linda makes occasional faint vocalizations, but her parents have not been able to associate these with any meaning, and she does not give consistent signals of pain or discomfort. Cortical visual impairment interferes with Linda's responses to people and objects, although her parents perceive that some lighted or noisy events capture her attention briefly. Her parents have difficulty judging what activities she enjoys, as Linda's responses do not vary much across situations. She most consistently calms or orients to musical toys and hearing familiar voices. Other spontaneous signals that her parents recognize include slight push-away gestures, eyebrow wrinkling when overstimulated, or tongue smacking when thirsty. Although Linda activates music toys with hand-over-hand guidance and sometimes activates toys with her spontaneous movements, she has not yet consistently shown intentional behavior skills to control these toys. Linda's parents perceive that she has activity preferences but find her communication signals difficult to interpret.

Linda's parents would like to develop a repertoire of play activities that elicit clear responses so that they can provide feedback for these signals, which will help Linda develop awareness of controlling interaction in the world around her. Because she responds most consistently to music and familiar voices, one intervention goal involves providing a consistent means for Linda to control a device that plays her mother's voice. A simple voice output switch plays a recording of her mother speaking a familiar interactive phrase. The switch is held near Linda's right arm, which she favors, so that some of her writhing movements will activate the switch incidentally, thereby making use of her spontaneous gesture production. Her mother provides additional vocal response when Linda hits the switch. Initially, the delay between switch activations is several minutes, and Linda does not seem to associate her movements with the voice output response. After several successful activations, Linda's arm movements change pattern from their cyclic motion. She begins to pause before continuing movement, and she stretches her arm toward the switch location. At times, Linda looks briefly toward the switch before reaching her arm, apparently targeting the switch deliberately by using hand–eye coordination. As she demonstrates these associated behaviors, her parents touch her arm or face to provide feedback that these are the relevant behaviors for achieving the response in this interaction. As Linda learns that these specific movements consistently affect her environment, she can also expand similar movements to control other interactive activities, such as touching her parent's arm in the same placement to initiate a vocal or social response.

Formalizing Existing Behavioral Strategies into Symbolic Gestures

Neil is an 18-month-old boy who has spina bifida with Arnold Chiari malformation. He has good fine motor control in his hands but paralysis below his waist. He uses a ventilator and heart monitor, and he has independently developed effective strategies for making vocal sounds around his tracheostomy valve to express emotions and get attention from adults. Neil enjoys music toys, books, blocks, and cars, and he will frequently explore a toy intently to try out its different functions. His parents and support staff play many different kinds of routine games with him, and they have recognized at least 12 intentional communication behaviors that Neil produces for different messages. For instance, he will reach and flap his hands toward people for things that he wants and turn his head and hide his face from activities that he does not want. His parents have created a CSI and a picture notebook that show Neil making these gestures so that all of his communicative partners can respond consistently.

Neil produces a face-hiding gesture frequently as his primary way of refusing activities, and his parents would like to see him using more conventional strategies. Currently, they simply take the activity away when Neil shows refusal and give him brief verbal responses (e.g., "Oh, I guess you don't want it"). With AAC intervention, they add two elements to their response to this gesture: 1) touching Neil's hands to emphasize what he did to communicate and 2) immediately modeling a more conventional strategy that accomplishes the same purpose. The new, modeled gesture is a push away with one hand, which Neil occasionally uses to refuse items at the dinner table. This is being gradually shaped into a one-handed "all done" sign. Thus, when Neil hides his face, his parents touch his hands to acknowledge Neil's existing signal. Neil's parents also help him produce the push-away gesture and look toward them in response to his signal initiation as they take away the refused activity. As Neil realizes that specific gestures symbolize ideas and convey an exact message more effectively than broad gestures, he will use more of these formalized gestures across a variety of communicative contexts.

Incorporating Symbols, Strategies, and Devices into Routines to Supplement Gestures   Tina is a 22-month-old girl with physical impairments and other developmental disabilities of unknown origin. She can sit independently on the floor and can scoot a short distance by hitching her feet and her bottom. She demonstrates marked effort to make vowel-like vocalizations but has difficulty using her voice when she first attempts to make sounds. She likes to control switch toys, particularly ones that play music or loud sounds, and she tends to prefer short periods of play and shifting activities frequently. Tina will pay attention to adult activities but tends to play with toys by herself (e.g., banging, mouthing) rather than giving them to an adult for help. Her longest and most focused interaction tends to be in social play, especially in familiar routines with her parents. For instance, her father will begin a familiar tickle routine and Tina will watch him and giggle in anticipation of the tickle. The clearest signal that her parents interpret as requesting "more tickle" is Tina's occasionally looking and vocalizing at her parents during pauses.

Tina's parents would like her to play a more active role in interactions and communicating with them in play. As she already likes to operate switches and play tickle with her father, one intervention goal involves combining these skills for communication. She is given a voice output switch that is programmed with the message "more tickle." Her father starts a few turns of the tickle routine until Tina begins looking at him expectantly. Then the voice output switch is placed within her reach and visual field, directly between Tina and her father, to add a new strategy to her existing behavioral strategy of looking. Tina may look away from her father to activate the switch and listen to the sounds. Each time she pushes the "more tickle" switch, her father repeats the message and starts another tickle turn, touching Tina's face to reinforce her as she looks again to anticipate the tickle. At first, Tina hits the switch and seems to be puzzled by the separate activity of the tickling. After a few turns of experiencing these two familiar events together, Tina pauses after hitting the switch to look expectantly at her father for the tickle routine without additional touch cues. In this way, her parents perceive that she is beginning to understand the relationship between the voice output device and the communicative message conveyed and to add a new strategy for requesting "more tickle" that directly builds on her current gestural repertoire.

Systematizing Existing Gestural AAC Strategies   Tyler is a 24-month-old boy with spastic cerebral palsy. He sits in adapted seating and has difficulty opening and controlling his hands well enough to grasp and release objects. He can make vowel sounds and a few consonants when he is appropriately positioned, but he tends to use a variety of eye-pointing and partner-assisted communication strategies as his primary expressive modes. Tyler's parents report that he has a receptive vocabulary of more than 300 words and can eye point promptly and accurately to most common objects, locations, or activities. He initiates communication frequently and persistently, and he combines ideas in his symbolic play and eye-pointing messages. Tyler anticipates complex events, such as watching for the red bag that holds the best toys and getting excited when it appears several minutes later. He selects choices from verbal options offered by parents by vocalizing, eye pointing, or calming and smiling, and he can respond to multiple rapidly offered choices from adults.

Tyler's parents are exploring various electronic AAC devices with him, but they would also like more symbolic versions of Tyler's existing strategies to take advantage of his language skills and provide more independence in informally structured communication interactions. Two extensions of his existing gestural strategies are incorporated into his intervention: 1) an eye-gaze board with picture symbols and 2) partner-assisted scanning with topic boards for play and other choice-making activities. For instance, Tyler's existing strategy for requesting more bubbles with eye pointing was to look or vocalize toward the adult during this activity. With single picture symbols mounted on a clear board, Tyler is prompted to add onto his existing gaze strategy a look toward the symbol and back to the adult to express specific linguistic information to the adult. Because multiple symbols, objects, and interactants are available for eye pointing as well, Tyler quickly learns to build multiword utterances with eye pointing by using this simple strategy.

Topic boards of symbols and words associated with specific play activities are added to his choice-making activities to provide similar access to specific vocabulary in different interactive contexts. For instance, for playing with a doctor kit, a topic board was created with objects, activities, verbs, descriptive words, and comments that would be typical for this play script (e.g., "Ouch!"). Tyler's partners were coached not only to offer choices as they typically would but also to point to the picture symbols that represent those concepts to help Tyler focus and anticipate choices. As Tyler learns the choices that are available on the board, he can more rapidly choose rows and columns that represent his ideas. He can also reject the board in favor of more open-ended eye pointing or topical-choice strategies for items that are not reflected on any board. In addition to expressing specific linguistic messages, partner-assisted scanning provides interactive practice with formal scanning strategies that will be useful for controlling row-column scanning on an electronic AAC device. As Tyler's literacy skills improve, both eye pointing and partner strategies can be refined for more exact low-tech communication to supplement electronic strategies.

Augmented Input of Both Gestural and Symbolic Strategies   Erica is a 28-month-old girl with oral-motor control difficulties. She runs and plays with toys in a fashion similar to her older brothers who have no identified disabilities, although all of her siblings also have been slow to develop coordinated or planned movements such as going down stairs and throwing a ball. She enjoys complex play activities such as books and puzzles, and she often initiates elaborate gestural or play routines with familiar and unfamiliar partners. Erica produces some vowel sounds and /m/ sounds with effort, but she tends to posture and show particular difficulty in initiating speech sounds when she tries to do so deliberately. At times, Erica's parents will notice her babbling to her toys, but she rarely can repeat those same sounds again after her parents imitate what she is saying. When Erica gets frustrated or excited, she produces a loud high-pitched squeal that can communicate a variety of messages.

Her parents suspect that speech-motor control issues, such as developmental apraxia of speech, are limiting Erica's vocal development, and they would like her to use gestural and symbolic strategies while she is building her speech skills. Her family members have begun learning sign language and consistently model their sentences to Erica by using signs. For instance, when Erica points to the cows in her farm book, her mother prompts Erica to look and signs YES, BIG BROWN COW. Erica pays close attention to these signs and successfully initiates at least 50 signs for a variety of communicative functions. She is rapidly learning new signs and reducing many indications of communicative frustration, and her family considers this an effective method for her current communication. Nevertheless, when Erica is either frustrated or does not know the sign for something that she cannot point to or get, she still uses squealing or other agitated behaviors.

Picture symbols and spontaneous hand-drawn images are used to represent ideas for which either Erica or her family members do not know the sign. For instance, during doll play, Erica pointed to the doll's bottom and flapped her hands at her mother in a recognized "I don't know" signal. Her mother signed options for DIRTY and STINKY and quickly drew images to represent the concepts *wet* and *change,* for which she did not know the signs. When her mother read and pointed to the *wet* image, Erica smiled and pointed to *wet* and signed BABY DIAPER. Similar multimodal sign, gesture, symbol, and drawing strategies are used to offer choices that clarify Erica's message when she is frustrated. Once her parents determine Erica's intended message, it is added to her "mad" topic board so that she can anticipate a strategy for conveying these important messages when she is angry and cannot express this through signs or gestural signals.

CONCLUSION

Augmented behaviors are integral to AAC at all levels of communicative development and should be included in AAC intervention for all children. Augmented behaviors and partner responses to these behaviors may constitute a major intervention focus for spontaneous communicators, although incorporation of aided AAC is possible even at these earliest stages. As children continue to develop communication skills, a greater intervention focus will be placed on transitions to more formal and conventional AAC strategies, although even skilled AAC users will still rely on behaviors for some purposes. It is important that the introduction of new conventional communicative strategies is contingent on children's production of familiar behavior strategies to build on familiar contexts and communicative functions and to only introduce "one hard thing at a time." In early AAC intervention, the "one hard thing" that is introduced will vary in different interactions, including new communicative forms, functions, or partners.

REFERENCES

Abrahamsen, A.A., Cavallo, M.M., & McCluer, J.A. (1985). Is the sign advantage a robust phenomenon? From gesture to language in two modalities. *Merrill-Palmer Quarterly, 31,* 177–209.

Acredolo, L., & Goodwyn, S. (1988). Symbolic gesturing in normal infants. *Child Development, 59,* 450–466.

Acredolo, L.P., & Goodwyn, S.W. (1989, April). *Symbolic gesturing in normal infants: A training study.* Paper presented at the Society for Research in Child Development Conference, St. Louis, MO.

Acredolo, L.P., & Goodwyn, S.W. (1990). Sign language in babies: The significance of symbolic gesturing for understanding language development. *Annals of Child Development, 7,* 1–42.

Adamson, L.B., Russell, C.L., & McArthur, D. (1997, April). *Joint attention and symbols at the end of infancy.* Poster presented at the Society for Research in Child Development Conference, Washington, DC.

Akhtar, N., Dunham, F., & Dunham, P.J. (1991). Directive interactions and early vocabulary development: The role of joint attentional focus. *Journal of Child Language, 18,* 41–49.

Amato, J., Barrow, M., & Domingo, R. (1999). Symbolic play behavior in very young verbal and nonverbal children with autism. *Infant-Toddler Intervention, 9*(2), 185–194.

American Speech-Language-Hearing Association (ASHA). (1991). Report: Augmentative and alternative communication. *Asha, 33*(Suppl. 5), 9–12.

Attwood, A., Frith, U., & Hermelin, B. (1988). The understanding and use of interpersonal gestures by autistic and Down's syndrome children. *Journal of Autism and Developmental Disabilities, 18*(2), 241–257.

Bakeman, R., & Adamson, L.B. (1984). Coordinating attention to people and objects in mother–infant and peer–infant interaction. *Child Development, 55,* 1278–1289.

Baldwin, D.A. (1995). Understanding the link between joint attention and language. In C. Moore & P.J. Dunham (Eds.), *Joint attention: Its origins and role in development* (pp. 131–158). Mahwah, NJ: Lawrence Erlbaum Associates.

Ball, L.J., Marvin, C.A., Beukelman, B.R., Lasker, J., & Rupp, D. (1999). Generic talk use by preschool children. *Augmentative and Alternative Communication, 15*(3), 145–155.

Bartels, K., Cress, C.J., & Marvin, C.A. (2001). *Gaze-shift patterns of pre-intentional children with physical impairments and children with typical development.* Manuscript submitted for publication.

Bates, E., Benigni, L., Bretherton, I., Camaioni, L., & Volterra, V. (1979). *The emergence of symbols: Cognition and communication in infancy.* San Diego: Academic Press.

Bates, E., Bretherton, I., & Snyder, L. (1988). *From first words to grammar: Individual differences and dissociable mechanisms.* New York: Cambridge University Press.

Bayley, N. (1993). *Manual for the Bayley Scales of Infant Development–Second Edition.* San Antonio, TX: The Psychological Corp.

Behrmann, M., & Lahm, L. (1983). Critical learning: Multiply handicapped babies get on-line. In M. Behrmann & L. Lahm (Eds.), *Proceedings of the National Conference on the Use of Microcomputers in Special Education* (pp. 181–193). Hartford, CT: Educational Resources Information Center.

Belsky, J., & Most, R.K. (1981). From exploration to play: A cross-sectional study of infant free play and behavior. *Developmental Psychology, 17,* 630–639.

Bertrand, J., Mervis, C.B., & Neustat, I. (1998, April). *Communicative gesture use by preschoolers with Williams syndrome: A longitudinal study.* Presentation at the International Conference on Infant Studies, Atlanta, GA.

Beukelman, D.R., & Mirenda, P. (1998). *Augmentative and alternative communication: Management of severe communication disorders in children and adults* (2nd ed.). Baltimore: Paul H. Brookes Publishing Co.

Blackstone, S. (1991). Intervention framework. In S. Blackstone (Ed.), *Technology in the classroom: Communication module.* Rockville, MD: American Speech-Language-Hearing Association Publications.

Blasco, P.M., Hrncir, E.J., & Blasco, P.A. (1990). The contribution of maternal involvement to mastery performance in infants with cerebral palsy. *Journal of Early Intervention, 14*(2), 161–174.

Bornstein, M.H., & Tamis-LeMonda, C.S. (1997). Maternal responsiveness and infant mental abilities: Specific predictive relations. *Infant Behavior and Development, 20*(3), 283–296.

Brady, N., McLean, J.E., McLean, L.K., & Johnston, S. (1995). Initiation and repair of intentional communication acts by adults with severe to profound cognitive disabilities. *Journal of Speech and Hearing Research, 38,* 1334–1348.

Brand, R.J., & Ashburn, L. (1999, April). *"Motionese": Extending "motherese" beyond language to motion.* Poster presented at the Society for Research in Child Development conference, Albuquerque, NM.

Bretherton, I., Bates, E., McNew, S., Shore, C., Williamson, C., & Beeghly-Smith, M. (1981). Comprehension and production of symbols in infancy–An experimental study. *Developmental Psychology, 17,* 728–736.

Brinker, R.P., & Lewis, M. (1982). Making the world work with microcomputers: A learning prosthesis for handicapped infants. *Exceptional Children, 49*(2), 163–170.

Brown, C. (1998, June). *Symbolic gesture training in children with early signs of expressive language delay.* Paper presented at the Symposium in Child Language Disorders, Madison, WI.

Buzolich, M.J., & Wiemann, J.M. (1988). Turn taking in atypical conversations: The case of the speaker/augmented-communicator dyad. *Journal of Speech and Hearing Research, 31,* 3–18.

Calculator, S.N., & Delaney, D. (1986). Comparison of non-speaking and speaking mentally retarded adults' clarification strategies. *Journal of Speech and Hearing Disorders, 51*(3), 252–258.

Camaioni, L. (1989). The role of social interaction in the transition from communication to language. In A. de Ribaupierre (Ed.), *Transition mechanisms in child development: The longitudinal perspective* (pp. 109–125). New York: Cambridge University Press.

Carpenter, R.L. (1987). Play scale. In L.B. Olswang, C. Stoel-Gammon, T.E. Coggins, & R.L. Carpenter (Eds.), *Assessing prelinguistic and early linguistic behaviors in developmentally young children* (pp. 44–77). Seattle: University of Washington Press.

Caselli, M.C., Vicari, S., Longobardi, E., Lami, L., Pizzoli, C., & Stella, G. (1998). Gestures and words in early development of children with Down syndrome. *Journal of Speech, Language, and Hearing Research, 41,* 1125–1135.

Colburne, K.A., Stack, D.M., Bentley, V.M., & Switkin, M.C. (1998, April). *Mothers' and infants' use of touch during face-to-face play with and without objects.* Poster presented at the 11th Biennial International Conference on Infant Studies, Atlanta, GA.

Crais, E., & Day, D. (2000, November). *Gesture development from six to twenty-four months.* Presentation at the American Speech-Language-Hearing Association convention, Washington DC.

Cress, C.J. (1999, November). *Augmenting play and communication for young children with physical impairments.* Presentation at the American Speech-Language-Hearing convention, San Francisco.

Cress, C.J. (2001). *The "tools" of early communication: A conceptual model for children relying on technology for communication.* Manuscript submitted for publication.

Cress, C.J., & Anderson, V. (2001). *An adapted play analysis scheme for describing complexity of play in children with physical impairments.* Manuscript in preparation.

Cress, C.J., Andrews, T.A., & Reynolds, C.D. (1998, April). *Gestural imitation and contingent parent responses in non-speaking children with physical impairments.* Paper presented at the International Conference on Infant Studies, Atlanta, GA.

Cress, C.J., & Ball, L. (1998, June). *Strategies for promoting vocal development in young children relying on AAC: Three case illustrations.* Paper presented at the Rehabilitation Engineering and Assistive Technology Association of America (RESNA) Annual Conference, Minneapolis, MN.

Cress, C.J., & LaMontagne, J.L. (2001). *Play patterns of infants with physical impairment across interactants and play characteristics.* Manuscript in preparation.

Cress, C.J., Moskal, L., & Benal, A. (2001). *Parent directiveness in social and object play with their children with physical impairments.* Manuscript submitted for publication.

Cress, C.J., Shapley, K., Linke, M., Havelka, S., Dietrich, C., Elliott, J., & Clark, J. (1999, November). *Intentional communication patterns in young children with physical impairments.* Presentation at the American Speech-Language-Hearing Association convention, San Francisco.

Culp, D. (1989). Developmental apraxia and augmentative or alternative communication—A case example. *Augmentative and Alternative Communication, 5,* 27–34.

Day, P.S. (1986). Deaf children's expression of communicative intentions. *Journal of Communication Disorders, 19,* 367–385.

Duker, P.C., van Deursen, W., de Wit, M., & Palmen, A. (1997). Establishing a receptive repertoire of communicative gestures with individuals who are profoundly mentally retarded. *Education and Training in Mental Retardation and Developmental Disabilities, 32*(4), 357–361.

Dunst, C.J. (1980). *A clinical and educational manual for use with the Uzgiris and Hunt Scales of Infant Psychological Development.* Baltimore: University Park Press.

Dunst, C.J., & Lowe, L.W. (1986). From reflex to symbol: Describing, explaining, and fostering communicative competence. *Augmentative and Alternative Communication, 2*(1), 11–18.

Fenson, L., Dale, P.S., Reznick, J.S., Bates, E., Thal, D., Hartung, J., Pethick, S., & Reilly, J. (1993). *MacArthur Communicative Development Inventory (CDI): User's guide and technical manual.* San Diego: Singular Publishing Group.

Ferrier, L.J., Fell, H.J., Mooraj, A., Delta, H., & Moscoe, D. (1996). Baby-babble-blanket: Infant interface with automatic data collection. *Augmentative and Alternative Communication, 12*(2), 110–121.

Flanagan, P.J., Coppa, D.F., Riggs, S.G., & Alario, A.J. (1994). Communication behaviors of infants of teen mothers: An exploratory study. *Journal of Adolescent Health, 15,* 169–175.

Floyd, F.J., & Phillippe, K.A. (1993). Parental interactions with children with and without mental retardation: Behavior management, coerciveness, and positive exchange. *American Journal on Mental Retardation, 97*(6), 673–684.

Gobbi, L., Cipani, E., Hudson, C., & Lapenta-Neudeck, R. (1986). Developing spontaneous requesting among children with severe retardation. *Mental Retardation, 24,* 357–363.

Goetz, L., Gee, K., & Sailor, W. (1985). Using a behavior chain interruption strategy to teach communication skills to students with severe disabilities. *Journal of the Association for Persons with Severe Handicaps, 10,* 21–30.

Goossens', C. (1989). Aided communication intervention before assessment: A case study of a child with cerebral palsy. *Augmentative and Alternative Communication, 5,* 14–26.

Guerette, P., Tefft, D., Furumasu, J., & Moy, F. (1999). Development of a cognitive assessment battery for young children with physical impairments. *Infant-Toddler Intervention, 9*(2), 169–184.

Hanzlik, J.R. (1990). Nonverbal interaction patterns of mothers and their infants with cerebral palsy. *Education and Training in Mental Retardation, 25*(4), 333–343.

Harris, S., Kasari, C., & Sigman, M.D. (1996). Joint attention and language gains in children with Down syndrome. *American Journal on Mental Retardation, 100*(6), 608–619.

Hauser-Cram, P. (1996). Mastery motivation in toddlers with developmental disabilities. *Child Development, 67,* 236–248.

Hauser-Cram, P., & Shonkoff, J.P. (1995). Mastery motivation: Implications for intervention. In R.H. MacTurk & G.A. Morgan (Eds.), *Mastery motivation: Origins, conceptualizations, and applications* (pp. 257–272). Stamford, CT: Ablex Publishing Corp.

Hedrick, D., Prather, R., & Tobin, A. (1984). *Sequenced Inventory of Communication Development* (2nd ed.). Los Angeles: Western Psychological Service.

Heller, K.W., Alberto, P.A., & Romski, M.A. (1995). Effect of object and movement cues on receptive communication by preschool children with mental retardation. *American Journal on Mental Retardation, 99*(5), 510–521.

Hunt-Berg, M. (1996). *Learning graphic symbols: The role of visual cues in interaction.* Unpublished doctoral dissertation. Lincoln: University of Nebraska–Lincoln.

Hupp, S.C., & Abbeduto, L. (1991). Persistence as an indicator of mastery motivation in young children with cognitive delays. *Journal of Early Intervention, 15*(3), 219–225.

Hwang, B., & Hughes, C. (1995). Effects of social interactive strategies on early social-communicative skills of a preschool child with developmental disabilities. *Education and Training in Mental Retardation and Developmental Disabilities, 30*(4), 336–349.

Iacono, T., Carter, M., & Hook, J. (1998). Identification of intentional communication in students with severe and multiple disabilities. *Augmentative and Alternative Communication, 14*(2), 102–114.

Iverson, J.M., & Thal, D.J. (1998). Communicative transitions: There's more to the hand than meets the eye. In S.F. Warren & J. Reichle (Series Eds.) & A.M. Wetherby, S.F. Warren, & J. Reichle (Vol. Eds.), *Communication and language intervention series: Vol. 7. Transitions in prelinguistic communication* (pp. 59–86). Baltimore: Paul H. Brookes Publishing Co.

Jennings, K.D., Connors, R.E., & Stegman, C.E. (1988). Does a physical handicap alter the development of mastery motivation during the preschool years? *Journal of the American Academy of Child and Adolescent Psychiatry, 27,* 312–317.

Jennings, K.D., Connors, R.E., Stegman, C.E., Sankaranaryan, P., & Mendelsohn, S. (1985). Mastery motivation in young preschoolers: Effect of a physical handicap and implications for educational programming. *Journal of the Division for Early Childhood, 9,* 162–169.

Kaiser, A.P., Yoder, P.J., & Keetz, A. (1992). Evaluating milieu teaching. In S.F. Warren & J. Reichle (Series Eds. & Vol. Eds.), *Communication and language intervention series: Vol. 1. Causes and effects in communication and language intervention* (pp. 9–47). Baltimore: Paul H. Brookes Publishing Co.

Kangas, K.A., & Lloyd, L.L. (1988). Early cognitive skills as prerequisites to augmentative and alternative communication use: What are we waiting for? *Augmentative and Alternative Communication, 4*(4), 211–221.

Kent, R.D. (1993). Speech intelligibility and communicative competence in children. In S.F. Warren & J. Reichle (Series Eds.) & A.P. Kaiser & D.B. Gray (Vol. Eds.), *Communication and language intervention series: Vol. 2. Enhancing children's communication: Research foundations for intervention* (pp. 223–239). Baltimore: Paul H. Brookes Publishing Co.

Keogh, W., & Reichle, J. (1985). Communication intervention for the "difficult-to-teach" severely handicapped. In S. Warren & A.K. Rogers-Warren (Eds.), *Teaching functional language* (pp. 157–194). Austin, TX: PRO-ED.

Kobacker, N., & Todaro, M.P. (1992, August). *Use of assistive devices by a preschooler with autism.* Presentation at the International Society for Augmentative and Alternative Communication (ISAAC) International Conference, Philadelphia.

Landry, S.H. (1995). The development of joint attention in premature low birth weight infants: Effects of early medical complications and maternal attention-directing behaviors. In C. Moore & P.J. Dunham (Eds.), *Joint attention: Its origins and role in development* (pp. 223–250). Mahwah, NJ: Lawrence Erlbaum Associates.

Landry, S.H., & Chapieski, M.L. (1990). Joint attention of six-month-old Down syndrome and preterm infants: I. Attention to toys and mother. *American Journal on Mental Retardation, 94,* 488–498.

Landry, S.H., Copeland, D., Lee, A., & Robinson, S. (1990). Goal-directed behavior in children with spina bifida. *Journal of Developmental and Behavioral Pediatrics, 11,* 306–311.

Light, J. (1988). Interaction involving individuals using augmentative and alternative communication systems: State of the art and future directions. *Augmentative and Alternative Communication, 4*(2), 66–82.

Light, J., Roberts, B., Dimarco, R., & Greiner, N. (1998). Augmentative and alternative communication to support receptive and expressive communication for people with autism. *Journal of Communication Disorders, 31,* 153–180.

Linke, M., & Cress, C.J. (2001). *Mastery motivation in object and social play for children with physical impairments.* Manuscript submitted for publication.

Mace, F.C., & Roberts, M. (1993). Factors affecting selection of behavioral interventions. In S.F. Warren & J. Reichle (Series Eds.) & J. Reichle & D.P. Wacker (Vol. Eds.), *Communication and language intervention series: Vol. 3. Communicative alternatives to challenging behaviors: Integrating functional assessment and intervention strategies* (pp. 113–133). Baltimore: Paul H. Brookes Publishing Co.

MacTurk, R., Vietze, P.J., McCarthy, M.E., McQuiston, S., & Yarrow, L.J. (1985). The organization of exploratory behavior in Down syndrome and nondelayed infants. *Child Development, 56,* 573–581.

Marfo, K. (1992). Correlates of maternal directiveness with children who are developmentally delayed. *American Journal of Orthopsychiatry, 62*(2), 219–233.

Mars, A.E., Mauk, J.E., & Dowrick, P.W. (1998). Symptoms of pervasive developmental disorders as observed in prediagnostic home videos of infants and toddlers. *Journal of Pediatrics, 132,* 500–504.

Masur, E.F. (1997, April). *Quality of play during mothers' and infants' object-related imitation.* Presentation at the Biennial Meeting of the Society for Research in Child Development, Washington, DC.

Masur, E.F., & Ritz, E.G. (1984). Patterns of gestural, vocal, and verbal imitation performance in infancy. *Merrill-Palmer Quarterly, 30*(4), 369–392.

Masur, E.F., & Rodemaker, J.E. (1997, April). *Mothers' and infants' spontaneous vocal and action imitation in two contexts.* Presentation at the Biennial Meeting of the Society for Research in Child Development, Washington, DC.

Maurer, H., & Sherrod, K.B. (1987). Context of directives given to young children with Down syndrome and nonretarded children: Development over two years. *American Journal of Mental Deficiency, 91*(6), 579–590.

McCall, R.B. (1995). On definitions and measures of mastery motivation. In R.H. MacTurk & G.A. Morgan (Eds.), *Mastery motivation: Origins, conceptualizations, and applications* (pp. 273–292). Stamford, CT: Ablex Publishing Corp.

McCathren, R.B., Yoder, P.J., & Warren, S.F. (1999). Prelinguistic pragmatic functions as predictors of later expressive vocabulary. *Journal of Early Intervention, 22*(3), 205–216.

McCune-Nicolich, L. (1981). Toward symbolic functioning: Structure of early pretend games and potential parallels with language. *Child Development, 52,* 785–797.

McLean, J., & Snyder-McLean, L. (1987). Form and function of communicative behavior among persons with severe developmental disabilities. *Australia and New Zealand Journal of Developmental Disabilities, 13*(2), 83–98.

McLean, J.E., McLean, L.K.S., Brady, N.C., & Etter, R. (1991). Communication profiles of two types of gesture using nonverbal persons with severe to profound mental retardation. *Journal of Speech and Hearing Research, 34,* 294–308.

Mervis, C.B., & Bertrand, J. (1994). Acquisition of the novel name–nameless category (N3C) principle. *Child Development, 65,* 1646–1662.

Morgan, G.A., MacTurk, R.H., & Hrncir, E.J. (1995). Mastery motivation: Overview, definitions, and conceptual issues. In R.H. MacTurk & G.A. Morgan (Eds.), *Mastery motivation: Origins, conceptualizations, and applications* (pp. 1–18). Stamford, CT: Ablex Publishing Corp.

Mundy, P., & Gomes, A. (1997). A skills approach to early language development: Lessons from research on developmental disabilities. In L.B. Adamson & M.A. Romski (Eds.), *Communication and language acquisition: Discoveries from atypical development* (pp. 107–133). Baltimore: Paul H. Brookes Publishing Co.

Mundy, P., & Gomes, A. (1998). Individual differences in joint attention skill development in the second year. *Infant Behavior and Development, 21*(3), 469–482.

Mundy, P., & Sigman, M. (1989). The theoretical implications of joint-attention deficits in autism. *Development and Psychopathology, 1,* 173–183.

Newborg, J., Stock, J.R., Wnek, L., Guidibaldi, J., & Svinicki, J. (1984). *Battelle Developmental Inventory (BDI).* Allen, TX: DLM Teaching Resources.

Ogletree, B.T., Wetherby, A.M., & Westling, D.L. (1992). Profile of the prelinguistic intentional communicative behaviors of children with profound mental retardation. *American Journal on Mental Retardation, 97*(2), 186–196.

Oller, D.K., Eilers, R.E., Neal, A.R., & Cobo-Lewis, A.B. (1998). Late onset canonical babbling: A possible early marker of abnormal development. *American Journal on Mental Retardation, 103*(3), 249–263.

Olswang, L.B., & Pinder, G.L. (1995). Preverbal functional communication and the role of object play in children with cerebral palsy. *Infant-Toddler Intervention, 5*(3), 277–300.

Orlansky, M.D., & Bonvillian, J.D. (1988). Early sign language acquisition. In M.D. Smith & J.L. Locke (Eds.), *The emergent lexicon* (pp. 263–292). San Diego: Academic Press.

Osterling, J., & Dawson, G. (1994). Early recognition of children with autism: A study of first birthday home videotapes. *Journal of Autism and Developmental Disorders, 24*(3), 247–257.

Paul, R. (1998, November). *Predicting outcomes of early expressive language delay.* Presentation at the American Speech-Language-Hearing Association conference, San Antonio, TX.

Paul, R., & Fountain, R. (1999). Predicting outcomes of early expressive language delay. *Infant-Toddler Intervention, 9*(2), 123–135.

Pinder, G.L., & Olswang, L.B. (1995). Development of communicative intent in young children with cerebral palsy: A treatment efficacy study. *Infant-Toddler Intervention, 5*(1), 51–70.

Pinder, G.L., Olswang, L., & Coggins, K. (1993). The development of communicative intent in a physically disabled child. *Infant-Toddler Intervention, 3*(1), 1–17.

Prezbindowski, A.K., Spencer, P.E., & Lederberg, A.R. (1999, April). *The MacArthur Communication Development Inventory as an assessment tool of vocabulary development for deaf children.* Poster presentation at the Biennial Meeting of the Society for Research in Child Development, Albuquerque, NM.

Reichle, J., & Karlan, G. (1985). The selection of an augmentative system in communication intervention: A critique of decision rules. *Journal of The Association for Persons with Severe Handicaps, 10,* 146–156.

Rescorla, L., & Goossens', M. (1992). Symbolic play development in toddlers with expressive specific language impairment (SLI-E). *Journal of Speech and Hearing Research, 35,* 1290–1302.

Rettig, M. (1998). Environmental influences on the play of young children with disabilities. *Education and Training in Mental Retardation and Developmental Disabilities, 33*(2), 189–194.

Rinaldi, J.A., Dawson, G., Meltzoff, A.N., & Osterling, J. (1997, April). *Autistic children exhibit symbolic and functional play impairments even in prompted conditions.* Presentation at the Biennial Meeting of the Society for Research in Child Development, Washington, DC.

Romski, M.A., & Sevcik, R.A. (1996). *Breaking the speech barrier: Language development through augmented means.* Baltimore: Paul H. Brookes Publishing Co.

Romski, M.A., Sevcik, R.A., & Adamson, L.B. (1999). Communication patterns of youth with mental retardation with and without their speech-output communication devices. *American Journal on Mental Retardation, 104*(3), 249–259.

Romski, M.A., Sevcik, R.A., Reumann R., & Pate, J. (1989). Youngsters with moderate or severe mental retardation and severe spoken language impairments: I. Extant communication patterns. *Journal of Speech and Hearing Disorders, 54,* 366–373.

Romski, M.A., Sevcik, R.A., Robinson, B.F., & Bakeman, R. (1994). Adult-directed everyday communications of youth with mental retardation using the System for Augmenting Language. *Journal of Speech and Hearing Research, 37*(3), 617–628.

Rosenberg, S.A., & Robinson, C.C. (1987). *Sensorimotor correlates of performance on a switch task by pupils with multiple handicaps.* Unpublished manuscript, University of Nebraska–Omaha.

Rowland, C., & Schweigert, P. (2000). Tangible symbols, tangible outcomes. *Augmentative and Alternative Communication, 16*(2), 61–78.

Ruskin, E., Mundy, P., Kasari, C., & Sigman, M. (1994). Object mastery motivation of children with Down syndrome. *American Journal on Mental Retardation, 98,* 499–509.

Shane, H.C., & Bashir, A.S. (1980). Election criteria for the adoption of an augmentative communication system: Preliminary considerations. *Journal of Speech and Hearing Disorders, 45,* 408–414.

Spencer, P.E., Bodner-Johnson, B.A., & Gutfreund, M.K. (1992). Interacting with infants with a hearing loss: What can we learn from mothers who are deaf? *Journal of Early Intervention, 16*(1), 64–78.

Stack, D.M., & Arnold, S.L. (1998). Changes in mothers' touch and hand gestures influence infant behavior during face-to-face interchanges. *Infant Behavior and Development, 21*(3), 451–468.

Stack, D.M., LePage, D.E., Hains, S., & Muir, D.W. (1996, April). *Qualitative changes in maternal touch as a function of instructional condition during face-to-face social interactions.* Poster at the International Conference on Infant Studies, Providence, RI.

Steffens, M.L., Oller, D.K., Lynch, M., & Urbano, R.C. (1992). Vocal development in infants with Down syndrome and infants who are developing normally. *American Journal on Mental Retardation, 97*(2), 235–246.

Sternberg, L., McNerney, C.D., & Pegnatore, L. (1985). Developing co-active imitative behaviors with profoundly mentally handicapped students. *Education and Training of the Mentally Retarded, 20*(4), 260–267.

Stoel-Gammon, C. (1998). Role of babbling and phonology in early linguistic development. In S.F. Warren & J. Reichle (Series Eds.) & A.M. Wetherby, S.F. Warren, & J. Reichle (Vol. Eds.), *Communication and language intervention series: Vol. 7. Transitions in prelinguistic communication* (pp. 87–110). Baltimore: Paul H. Brookes Publishing Co.

Stone, W.L., Ousley, O.Y., & Littleford, C.D. (1997). Motor imitation in young children with autism: What's the object? *Journal of Abnormal Child Psychology, 25*(6), 475–485.

Sweeney, L.A., & Engwis, P. (1996, August). *Perceived levels of initiation among individuals experiencing significant communication challenges.* Presentation at the ISAAC International Conference, Vancouver, Canada.

Tannock, R. (1988). Mothers' directiveness in their interactions with their children with and without Down syndrome. *American Journal on Mental Retardation, 93*(2), 154–165.

Tannock, R., Girolametto, L., & Siegel, L.S. (1992). Language intervention with children who have developmental delays: Effects of an interactive approach. *American Journal on Mental Retardation, 97*(2), 145–160.

Thal, D., & Bates, E. (1988). Language and gesture in late talkers. *Journal of Speech and Hearing Research, 31,* 115–123.

Thal, D.J., Oroz, M., & McCaw, V. (1995). Phonological and lexical development in normal and late-talking toddlers. *Applied Psycholinguistics, 16,* 407–424.

Thal, D.J., & Tobias, S. (1992). Communicative gestures in children with delayed onset of oral expressive vocabulary. *Journal of Speech and Hearing Research, 35,* 2181–1289.

Thal, D., & Tobias, S. (1994). Relationships between language and gesture in normally developing and late-talking toddlers. *Journal of Speech and Hearing Research, 37,* 157–170.

Thal, D., Tobias, S., & Morrison, D. (1991). Language and gesture in late talkers: A 1-year follow-up. *Journal of Speech and Hearing Research, 34,* 604–612.

Tomasello, M., & Farrar, M.J. (1992). Joint attention and early language. *Child Development, 57,* 1454–1463.

Venkatagiri, H.S. (1995). Techniques for enhancing communication productivity in AAC: A review of research. *American Journal of Speech-Language Pathology, 4*(4), 36–45.

Warren, S.F., & Yoder, P.J. (1998). Facilitating the transition from preintentional to intentional communication. In S.F. Warren & J. Reichle (Series Eds.) & A.M. Wetherby, S.F. Warren, & J. Reichle (Vol. Eds.), *Communication and language intervention series: Vol. 7. Transitions in prelinguistic communication* (pp. 365–384). Baltimore: Paul H. Brookes Publishing Co.

Wetherby, A.M. (1996, June). *Communication assessment with infants and toddlers for early identification and intervention planning.* Paper presented at the American Association of Home-Based Early Interventionists Regional Conference, Omaha, Nebraska.

Wetherby, A.M., Cain, D.H., Yonclas, D.G, & Walker, V.G. (1988). Analysis of intentional communication of normal children from the prelinguistic to the multiword stage. *Journal of Speech and Hearing Research, 31,* 240–252.

Wetherby, A.M., & Prizant, B. (1993). *Communication and Symbolic Behavior Scales (CSBS).* Baltimore: Paul H. Brookes Publishing Co.

Wetherby, A.M., Prizant, B.M., & Hutchinson, T.A. (1998). Communicative, social/affective, and symbolic profiles of young children with autism and pervasive developmental disorders. *American Journal of Speech-Language Pathology, 7*(2), 79–91.

Wetherby, A.M., & Rodriguez, G.P. (1992). Measurement of communicative intentions in normally developing children during structured and unstructured contexts. *Journal of Speech and Hearing Research, 35,* 130–138.

Wetherby, A.M., Yonclas, D.G., & Bryan, A.A. (1989). Communicative profiles of preschool children with handicaps: Implications for early identification. *Journal of Speech and Hearing Disorders, 54*(2), 148–158.

Wilcox, M.J., Bacon, C.K., & Shannon, M.S. (1995, November). *Prelinguistic intervention: Procedures for young children with disabilities.* Paper presented at the ASHA Annual Convention, Orlando, FL.

Wilcox, M.J., Kouri, T.A., & Caswell, S. (1990). Partner sensitivity to communication behavior of young children with developmental disabilities. *Journal of Speech and Hearing Research, 55*(4), 679–693.

Wilcox, M.J., & Shannon, M.S. (1998). Facilitating the transition from prelinguistic to linguistic communication. In S.F. Warren & J. Reichle (Series Eds.) & A.M. Wetherby, S.F. Warren, & J. Reichle (Vol. Eds.), *Communication and language intervention series: Vol. 7. Transitions in prelinguistic communication* (pp. 385–416). Baltimore: Paul H. Brookes Publishing Co.

Yoder, P.J. (1987). Relationship between degree of infant handicap and clarity of infant cues. *American Journal of Mental Deficiency, 91*(6), 639–641.

Yoder, P.J., & Davies, B. (1992). Do children with developmental delays use more frequent and diverse language in verbal routines? *American Association on Mental Retardation, 97*(2), 197–208.

Yoder, P.J., & Feagans, L. (1988). Mothers' attributions of communication to prelinguistic behavior of developmentally delayed and mentally retarded infants. *American Journal on Mental Retardation, 93*(1), 36–43.

Yoder, P.J., & Warren, S.F. (1998). Maternal responsivity predicts the prelinguistic communication intervention that facilitates generalized intentional communication. *Journal of Speech, Language, and Hearing Research, 41,* 1207–1219.

Yoder, P.J., & Warren, S.F. (1999). Maternal responsivity mediates the relationship between prelinguistic intentional communication and later language. *Journal of Early Intervention, 22*(2), 126–136.

Yoder, P.J., Warren, S.F., & Biggar, H.A. (1997). Stability of maternal reports of lexical comprehension in very young children with developmental delays. *American Journal of Speech-Language Pathology, 6*(1), 59–64.

Yoder, P.J., Warren, S.F., & McCathren, R.B. (1998). Determining spoken language prognosis in children with developmental disabilities. *American Journal of Speech-Language Pathology, 7*(4), 77–87.

9

Considerations in Teaching Graphic Symbols to Beginning Communicators

Krista M. Wilkinson and William J. McIlvane

Professionals in the field of language and communication intervention have long argued that the success of any effort depends on the integration of diverse perspectives and theoretically grounded research (Bowler, 1991; Kaiser, 1993; Light & Lindsay, 1991; Schiefelbusch & Lloyd, 1974; Warren & Reichle, 1992). Yet, the diversity of potential augmentative and alternative communication (AAC) users as well as the AAC system itself often preclude simple wholesale adaptation of theories or models generated in other disciplines (Blockberger, 1995; Bowler, 1991; Gerber & Kraat, 1992). Therefore, it may be most useful to consider specific aspects of AAC when evaluating the contributions of other disciplines. In this chapter, we integrate perspectives from several disciplines as they relate to the unique demands of teaching graphic symbols. We begin by surveying some relatively well-known issues about graphic modes used with beginning communicators. We then describe how state-of-the-art methodology in various disciplines might well be adapted to meet specific intervention goals. Finally, we consider how to evaluate the appropriateness of graphic symbol intervention for individuals.

CONSIDERATIONS OF THE GRAPHIC MODE ITSELF

To begin a consideration of any communication mode, one must ask the following: What do symbols offer in general? Many beginning communicators effectively use nonverbal modes of communication that include vocalization or

Funding for the manuscript preparation was supported by the National Institute of Child Health and Human Development (NICHD) Grant No. HD 25995 and an NICHD FIRST grant to K.M. Wilkinson (Grant No. R29-11 R29 HD35107–01A1). We thank our colleagues at the Shriver Center for their insights during the conceptualization of this paper, as well as Laura Becker for her review.

nonsign gestures (e.g., points, reaches, head nods; cf. Romski & Sevcik, 1996; Romski, Sevcik, & Adamson, 1997). Why is it of interest to introduce a more abstract or conventionalized communication mode? Consider the challenge of referencing a friend who is not present or planning activities for the upcoming weekend. With access only to gestural signals, discussions of such topics are virtually impossible, as such signals are limited to the immediate "here and now" context (Rowland & Schweigert, 1989). Thus, introduction of a symbolic mode—be it speech, sign, or graphic symbols—may be an important first step to foster further learning.

Advantages and Disadvantages of the Graphic Symbol Mode

For many individuals, a conventional symbol vocabulary takes the form of unaided speech or sign. For others, however, graphic symbols may be the mode of choice, either transitionally or as a long-term component of the communication system. In this section, we consider the benefits and drawbacks of using graphic symbols and raise some issues to consider when choosing among available sets.

Memory Load   One significant advantage of graphic symbols is that they decrease the memory demands of lexical access. Words and signs are dynamic; once produced, they "disappear" unless repeated. Furthermore, to produce a word or sign, the speaker or signer must retrieve the symbol from his or her own memory. Graphic symbols, in contrast, are static in time and space; they remain visible on the display page at all times. Therefore, users need only scan the already visible symbols on a display to access or retrieve vocabulary.

The different lexical access routes of spoken versus graphic symbols parallel the distinction in cognitive psychology between recall and recognition memory. To recall something, an individual must retrieve an item from memory, with few or no cues provided. In recognition memory, the item is presented to the individual and used as a cue for memory (e.g., the individual might be asked if he or she had seen this item previously). Recognition memory tasks are substantially less difficult than recall tasks, even for young children and individuals with disabilities (Hamilton & Ghatala, 1994). Because graphic symbol displays require the user only to scan the display until the desired symbol is found, they take advantage of recognition rather than recall. Reduction in the lexical access demands could be useful for individuals who have memory or lexical retrieval problems (cf. Light & Lindsay, 1991). Some clinical evidence supports this proposal. Kravitz, Littman, and Cassidy (1996) reported that an individual who used both signs and pictures for output reliably produced longer utterances when using pictures than when using signs, perhaps because retrieval was facilitated by the presence of the pictures on the board.

Alternate Access   Graphic symbols can be placed on a fixed display (i.e., an unmoving board) and programmed to allow either direct selection or scanning responses. Consequently, individuals who have difficulty with articulation or hand control (e.g., the problems with planning and executing motor sequences that are associated with apraxia) may benefit from the alternate access provided by aided symbols. The alternative access modes may also be valuable for individuals with general cognitive delay. Released from the mechanics of speech or sign production, such individuals might better be able to focus their attention on the content of communication. Nevertheless, aided communication makes operational demands that are inherent to neither speech nor sign (Light, 1997b). For users who gain access to their symbols through direct selection, a relatively precise point-based response is required. Users who are not able to select directly from among a display must learn to select symbols via a scanning technique, anticipating the arrival of the cursor on the visual symbol of choice and responding in time to select that item. High-technology electronic communication devices require the additional skills in turning them on, maintaining their function by charging batteries, moving between different display pages, and so forth. Thus, although aided symbols remove some of the motor and cognitive constraints of speech and sign, they themselves place certain unique demands on users.

Rate of Message Preparation   Perhaps the most frustrating property of graphic modes is the often prolonged time that is required for message preparation. Beukelman and Mirenda pointed out that the rates of word production in AAC modes are often "only a fraction of those achieved by natural speakers" (1998, p. 74). In part, this rate reduction is due to the very same factors that can be advantages; that is, 1) an external visual array is available to be scanned for each message and 2) the implementation of an alternate but usually slower access strategy. Thus, benefits of recognition memory and alternate access must be weighed with the toll that is taken on communication outcomes such as message preparation.

A reduction in production rate can have several consequences. Speaking partners may dominate the communication exchange (Calculator & Dollaghan, 1982; Farrier, Yorkston, Marriner, & Beukelman, 1985; Light, Collier, & Parnes, 1985a, 1985b), ultimately inhibiting independent communication (McNaughton & Light, 1989). Furthermore, many conversational patterns—such as narratives, small talk, or jokes—have reduced efficacy if they are produced too slowly. King, Spoeneman, Stuart, and Beukelman (1995) suggested that fast-moving, conventionalized exchanges (e.g., "Hi, how are you?" "Fine, and you?") may constitute one third of typical conversations. Individuals who are limited in their capability to participate are therefore likely at a disadvantage.

Rate enhancement strategies have been offered to address this problem. Whole words, full sentences, or letter or word prediction strategies can be programmed into aided AAC devices. Letter or word prediction has been reported to accelerate message preparation (Higginbotham, 1992; Newell et al., 1992; Venkatigiri, 1993). One study, however, showed that word prediction increased text generation rate only for new users (i.e., speaking adults without disabilities who are using a mouth pointer; Koester & Levine, 1996). The rate was substantially reduced for a group of individuals with spinal cord injury who had previous experience with mouth-pointer typing. For experienced users, the cognitive or perceptual demands may have interfered with potential enhancement benefits. Even when rate enhancement is successful, message preparation time may remain dramatically reduced relative to that of speech or sign modes (e.g., Koester & Levine, 1996). The somewhat conflicting results emphasize the point made by Newell and colleagues (1992): The potential impact of rate enhancement may vary depending on the individual user, the level of his or her experience, the outcome being measured, and the short- or long-term goals.

The use of rate enhancement strategies by beginning communicators has yet to receive much attention. Logically, it would seem most effective to introduce rate enhancement strategies from the outset of AAC interventions. This suggestion is supported by the previously described findings by Koester and Levine (1996). Yet, there is the question of how rate enhancement strategies might influence the development of language in beginning communicators. It is still unknown whether tactics such as adding preprogrammed sentences to an AAC device alter the learning landscape and, perhaps, negatively affect the language-learning process (Bedrosian, 1997; Romski et al., 1997). This issue clearly has significant implications for choosing symbol vocabulary for AAC users. Therefore, questions of how preprogrammed messages interact with early linguistic development are considered further in the section "Vocabulary Content and Linguistic Development."

Symbol and Display Size   Another potential disadvantage of graphic symbol modes concerns the number of symbols that can be displayed at any given time. A visual communication display is by necessity limited in its physical size and the number of symbols it can display. A tiny display might be highly portable, but its symbols would be virtually impossible to see and select; a very large display might contain many readable symbols, but it would be cumbersome to carry.

The number of available symbols has important consequences. As the number of symbols displayed decreases, so does the diversity of topics that are readily accessible to the AAC user. Yet, the addition of numerous symbols is not simple. A user's visual acuity and motor coordination must be considered in terms of the density of a stimulus array (see Chapter 12). Furthermore, Mizuko, Reichle, Ratcliff, and Esser (1994) reported that typically developing preschoolers showed increasing difficulty in a basic memory task as the size of the stimulus array increased. This difficulty was particularly apparent when a scanning response, rather than direct selection, was required. Although this finding was obtained from typically developing children who used speech rather than AAC modes, it suggests that array sizes and scanning-based responses place specific demands on memory and attentional resources. By implication, it seems logical that any beginning AAC user with memory or attention limitations might benefit from smaller array sizes.

Range of Meaning for Nonspelling Users   For many graphic mode users who are not literate, the range of meanings that can be expressed may be limited. Individuals with literacy skills can generate any word by combining individual letters and, thus, are unconstrained in this regard. Users without access to writing, however, are restricted to the vocabulary that intervention teams select for or with them. Vocabulary selection and updating is therefore one of the most fundamental activities for intervention. Because of the wide-ranging implications, we consider the issues of vocabulary selection in greater detail in the sections of this chapter that address selecting symbols to foster linguistic development.

Summary   Graphic symbols offer both advantages and disadvantages for users. Reduced communication rate or lack of symbol diversity may be the most conspicuous limitations for individuals with high-level or intact lexical competence, for whom issues of conversational competence are most pressing. Yet, any AAC candidate, including beginning communicators, may be hampered by these factors. Interventions must therefore address these potential issues from the outset to provide the most effective long-term treatment possible.

Considerations for Choosing the Symbol Set: Physical Characteristics

Selecting the type of symbols to include on aided communication displays requires the interventionist to consider the physical features of the symbols. In this section, we discuss graphic symbols in terms of their visual features and internal organization, and we consider how these features might affect symbol learning or use. An evaluation of how such features of symbols may relate to specific assessment and teaching strategies is addressed in the ensuing "Considerations in Instruction of Graphic Symbols" section of this chapter.

Iconicity   The term *iconicity* has been used to describe the visual similarities, or the relationship, between a symbol and its referent. Some symbols are more iconic than others. For instance, a photograph of a dog is more iconic than a sketched line drawing of a dog because the photograph shares a greater degree of physical similarity with the actual referent. Symbol iconicity is an issue that is unique to graphic and gestural modes because, with a few exceptions (e.g., onomatopoeia, animal noises), similarity of medium and referent is not common in speech.

Highly iconic pictures may facilitate symbol learning or use, as well as interpretation by communication partners, particularly if no voice output communication aid (VOCA) is used. Often, the level of a symbol's iconicity is measured by the ease with which a viewer can guess a symbol's meaning or understand the rationale for linking the symbol with its referent. Many studies of symbol "guessability" have compared the overall iconicity of different symbol sets (e.g., Blissymbols versus Mayer-Johnson's Picture Communication Symbols [PCS] or other media) or different symbols within sets (Bloomburg, Karlan, & Lloyd, 1990; Goossens', 1984; Hurlbut, Iwata, & Green, 1982; Mirenda & Locke, 1989; Mizuko & Reichle, 1989; Sevcik & Romski, 1986). These studies tended to support that more realistic (i.e., iconic) representations are more easily guessed and learned than less iconic representations (e.g., Fuller, 1997; also see Sevcik, Romski, & Wilkinson, 1991, for a review).

There has been growing recognition that the iconicity of any individual symbol likely differs from individual to individual, and it may differ for individuals with and without cognitive impairments (Light & Lindsay, 1991; Sevcik et al., 1991; Stephenson & Linfoot, 1996). What is clearly iconic for a typically developing preschooler may be completely opaque (i.e., unguessable) for an individual with cognitive impairments (Franklin, Mirenda, & Phillips, 1996). As Stephenson and Linfoot noted, the iconicity of any stimulus is "a characteristic determined by the observer, rather than intrinsic to the picture" (1996, p. 246).

In addition, Stephenson and Linfoot (1996; see also Blockberger, 1995) pointed out that even recognition of similarity between a symbol and its referent may not be sufficient to ensure that an individual will put that symbol to communicative use. In a comprehensive cross-cultural and interdisciplinary analysis, Stephenson and Linfoot identified several factors that might influence an individual's ability to use pictures as symbols. These factors include a familiarity with pictures in general (i.e., an understanding of the medium itself), the ability to understand pictures as more than simple patterns on a two-dimensional surface (i.e., understanding of the pattern as a representation of something other than itself), and the ability to use those representations to provide information and/or to guide behavior (i.e., symbolic picture use).

Each of these levels of understanding is necessary to meet the goal of symbol use, and demonstration of only one level of understanding may not ensure demonstration of others. For instance, some individuals with severe disabilities or individuals who have limited experience with pictures can match photographs in an identity matching task, in which the task is to select a photograph that is identical to one displayed among several available choices. This suggests that they are capable of discriminating the pattern within the photograph. Nevertheless, these same individuals may not match the photograph to the real-world object it depicts, which is termed *feature matching to sample* or *arbitrary matching to sample* and is described further in the section "Assessing Relationships Among Nonidentical Visual Stimuli" (Dixon, 1981). Thus, the individuals apparently fail to recognize the picture as a representation of something other than itself. Stephenson and Linfoot (1996) also described evidence from a study that involved people whose cultures provided little experience of photographs as a medium of expression. The participants were adults who learned to name objects depicted within pictures, thereby showing an understanding of pictures being representational. Yet, when they were asked to sort either the objects themselves or the photographs of the objects into categories, these individuals had more difficulty sorting the photographs than the objects. The problems arose in *using* the pictoral representations as symbolic aids during categorization tasks. Thus, "perception of similarity between the picture and the object . . . is not a sufficient basis for use of pictures as symbols" (Stephenson & Linfoot, 1996, p. 248).

For some children, miniature three-dimensional objects may be considered rather than two-dimensional objects, which are more common. These three-dimensional symbols are most often scale models of larger objects, but they may also include parts of larger objects (e.g., a tab from a soda can) or associated objects. Several observers have suggested that such tangible, three-dimensional symbols may be particularly useful for individuals who function at the lowest developmental levels (Kravitz, Littman, & Cassidy, 1996; Rowland & Schweigert, 1989). The use of miniature objects for representations, however, has been critiqued (e.g., DeLoache, 1995; Stephenson & Linfoot, 1996). DeLoache conducted research on miniature objects as representational in young children. She found that children at age 2.5 years had difficulty viewing the miniature object as an object (in and of itself) and, simultaneously, as a representation of some other object. The dual nature of miniature objects (object and symbol) appeared to confuse these children; by age 3, however, the children had no such difficulty. This research, which was conducted independent of research in AAC, nevertheless seems consistent with some findings in the AAC field that miniature objects may be more difficult for users than some two-dimensional symbols (Mirenda & Locke, 1989). In fact, it may be that miniature objects are better for individuals who are developmentally more advanced and can understand the dual roles of such objects.

Issues of Stimulus Organization   In addition to general issues of iconicity, a second factor may influence discriminability, learnability, or recall of visual symbols. *Stimulus organization* refers to the physical features of the symbol itself. To provide a familiar example, consider the uppercase letters X and R. When an uppercase letter X is divided either horizontally (into left and right sides) or vertically (into top and bottom halves), the resulting halves mirror one another. In contrast, an uppercase letter R does not divide into even halves, horizontally, vertically, or otherwise. Research in perception and learning suggests that stimuli that are constructed with regular, matching features are easier to recognize than irregular stimuli (Carlin & Soraci, 1993; Soraci, Carlin, Deckner, & Baumeister, 1990).

Several research studies have suggested that this effect also exists in AAC. Romski, Sevcik, Pate, and Rumbaugh (1985) evaluated the relative discriminability of printed words versus lexigrams in nonspeaking individuals with severe mental retardation. Lexigrams are arbitrary symbols that are constructed from graphic elements (e.g., circles, lines, squiggles). Like written words, they are completely noniconic, yet their elements are superimposed rather than transcribed linearly. Thus, lexigrams have horizontal and/or vertical regularity, whereas written words do not. Participants showed higher accuracy in an identity matching task with the lexigrams than with written words. Brady and McLean (1996) extended this inquiry to determine whether differences occurred in learnability and recall for individuals with severe mental retardation who used speech for communication. Again, lexigrams showed an advantage over written words. These two studies suggest that the organization of the stimulus itself is salient for most individuals, regardless of cognitive level.

Considerations for Arranging the Symbols

A unique feature of graphic modes is that they require the symbols to be arranged on some external display device. It is therefore the responsibility of the intervention team to organize the symbols in a manner that is meaningful to users and to allow smooth transitions between different displays containing those symbols.

Organization of the Lexicon Itself   Different approaches vary in the extent to which they recommend organizational structures for symbols. *Symbol sets* offer symbols as stand-alone items, with no specific recommendations for organization. Nonetheless, organization strategies are available for such sets. For instance, the Fitzgerald key system recommends arranging symbols by form/class (grammatical) category, oftentimes through color coding (cf. Beukelman & Mirenda, 1998). Another method of organization is to divide symbols by activity, such as having a snack page or a basketball page in an individual's binder of AAC symbols (see Mirenda, 1985; see also Beukelman & Mirenda, 1998, for a detailed discussion). In contrast, *symbol systems* constrain symbol use/arrangement, so that different symbols can take on different meanings depending on the context. An example of this is the iconic encoding of the Minspeak (Baker, 1982) and the Blissymbolics (McNaughton & Kates, 1980) systems. Both systems use relationships among symbols and symbol modifiers to allow for communication generativity (see Beukelman &

Mirenda, 1998, for a description). Clinically, each type of approach has certain advantages and drawbacks that have been articulated in the literature (Blockberger, 1995; Bruno, 1989; Light, Lindsay, Siegel, & Parnes, 1990). The key issue reflected in each of these approaches is the need to arrange the aided AAC user's lexicon meaningfully. From a developmental standpoint, it might seem most desirable to organize the symbols along the same system that governs the spoken lexicon. The logic is that beginning AAC users might benefit from a structure that is consistent with the typical language user's experience. Yet, this logic has two fundamental problems. First, despite years of research, there is still little consensus on exactly how the spoken lexicon is organized. Some questions remain unresolved. Are categories structured around sets of features or more general prototypes (e.g., Lakoff, 1987; Rosch & Mervis, 1975)? Are networks of categories structured hierarchically (along the lines of the original [Collins & Quillian, 1969] or later variations [Collins, Gathercole, Conway, & Morris, 1993]) or along parallel distributed paths (Rumelhart & McLelland, 1986)?

The second problem is that, even if the organization of a spoken lexicon were known, there is no assurance that such an organization would be most efficient for use with people with the disabilities that lead to use of graphic modes (e.g., Bedrosian, 1997). The extent to which the path of language development in augmented communicators resembles that of typical speakers is still unknown, although research efforts have been initiated (Romski et al., 1997; Wilkinson, Romski, & Sevcik, 1994). Nor is it clear how different symbol types affect the course of development (Bedrosian, 1997; Blockberger, 1995; Light, 1997b). Development of a meaningful symbolic organization is essential, particularly for beginning communicators who have no preexisting linguistic/symbolic structure upon which to map aided systems. Because virtually no research exists on this problem, organization of the lexicon is clearly an area where further research will be essential to guiding best practice efforts.

Relationship of Displays within the Lexicon to One Another   As noted, the graphic symbol lexicon must be arranged externally on a visual display. Previously, we emphasized that only a certain number of symbols can appear on any single display page. Taken together, these two points beg a final decision in aided AAC: how to arrange individual display pages in relation to one another.

There are two primary methods for relating display pages, a fixed display versus a dynamic display. In fixed displays, each page display is a physical entity that is distinct from the other pages. The symbols on each page stand alone and remain in fixed position. To shift from one fixed display page to another, the entire overlay is physically removed and replaced. Variants on this are low-technology paper notebooks in which each page displays a set of symbols and the user flips through to find each symbol. Conversely, in dynamic displays, computer-based pages are linked to one another electronically. A symbol on one page of a dynamic display may be a link that does not itself have communicative meaning but, rather, sends the user to a different page. For instance, a symbol in the lower right corner of a dynamic display may say- FOOD PAGE; by pressing it, the user is presented with a new screen that lists different types of food. Pages are changed automatically by the computer instead of manually, as is done in a fixed display.

Dynamic displays offer a rapid and independent means of gaining access to vocabulary, thereby eliminating the essential but time-consuming tasks of retaining all overlay pages in one place, locating the appropriate new overlays when a switch is needed, and removing and replacing the current overlay page. Nonetheless, dynamic displays may be difficult for some users because of the relatively complex skills needed to understand the hierarchical relationships of symbols on different pages and the virtual replacement of one visual display with another. For a user who does not understand that a symbol can be used to represent an individual concept (*food*) as well as a relational one (*go to food page*), dynamic displays may not be the most appropriate display type.

Both dynamic and multipage displays require certain memory skills on the part of the user. Fixed displays require memory for the page location on which specific symbols appear. For instance, the learner must recall whether the symbol for *milk* appears on the snack page, the dinner page, or both. Dynamic displays present additional memory demands. The user must recall not only the page location but also the path that he or she must travel to reach the target page. For instance, to reach the *milk* symbol, the user might have to travel from the main page to the food page and, finally, to the drinks page. To do this the individual must maintain memory/attention for the original target (*milk*) while responding to other potentially distracting targets within the path (i.e., the access symbols on the food/snack pages). This task thus involves both memory and attention, because recall must be maintained not only across delay but across the intervening symbol selections. Dynamic displays in particular might therefore not be the option of choice for individuals with short-term memory problems or difficulties maintaining attention. Clearly, decisions about the relation of the pages to one another must be made on an individual basis, depending on the type of understanding that the communicator brings to the learning situation.

Vocabulary Content and Linguistic Development

One of the most pressing issues confronting AAC interventionists is the selection and use of a functional vocabulary that can change with the needs of the user (Beukelman, McGinnis, & Morrow, 1991; Carlson, 1981; Light 1997b; Paul, 1997). When the vocabulary is to be represented on external aided symbol displays, it is essential to consider how those symbols will interact with the beginning communicator's intrinsic skills and knowledge. Again, little is known about the language development of individuals who are candidates for using aided AAC modes (Bedrosian, 1997; Paul, 1997; Romski et al., 1997). Furthermore, it is not known how the different available symbol sets or systems influence the course of development or whether certain systems are more or less likely to maximize linguistic potential. In this section, we consider some of the most critical issues surrounding graphic symbol vocabulary selection and its potential effect on linguistic development.

Prestored Language Units and the Development of Language   As noted previously, prestored language units such as full sentences programmed into a single symbol have the potential to enhance communication rate, particularly for small talk or other important language functions. When considering beginning communicators, however, several authors have questioned whether the use of prestored language units could be detrimental because the units involve fully formed, unanalyzed linguistic units. What if the programmed unit is syntactically more sophisticated than the learner is currently capable of constructing independently (Light, 1997b)? If users are provided with preprogrammed sentences, how will they learn to construct sentences of their own (Bedrosian, 1997)?

Analysis of typical development may provide some clues. The most prevalent pattern of morphosyntactic development is evolution from producing single words (oftentimes nouns) to two-word phrases, followed by sophisticated sentences constructed by adding words or grammatical morphemes (Brown, 1973; Nelson, 1973). This pattern suggests that children build their sentences from single "holophrase" units, which are combined in systematic ways. Under this analysis, unanalyzed blocks such as preprogrammed sentences would be an unusual, even atypical, event. Yet, although this model describes a large proportion of early syntactic development, Nelson (1973, 1981) and others (e.g., Peters, 1983) reported a second "language-learning style" that a substantial minority of typically developing children demonstrate. These children, whom Nelson (1981) called "expressive" learners, produce a large number of formulas or preset sentences, such as "I want it" or "Stop it," often for purposes of maintaining social interactions. Nelson noted that these children are characterized by their use of vocabulary and syntax that are "embedded in what appeared to be unanalyzed formulas or routines rather than novel constructions" (1981, p. 172). Nelson made the point that no child ever adopts one style to the exclusion of the other; single units and unanalyzed formulas appear in the speech of all typically developing children. Differences among children are a matter of degree rather than of kind.

These data on the inclusion of formulaic or unanalyzed sentences in the speech of typically developing children are invaluable to a discussion of using preprogrammed sentences in aided AAC. The data strongly suggest that the spoken equivalent of preprogrammed messages (i.e., formulas) are not unusual in typical development and often serve social functions. Two implications result for aided vocabulary programming. First, prestored messages may not, by themselves, hinder language development. Furthermore, the current AAC practice of including preprogrammed messages to make small talk or tell jokes appears to coincide directly with the functions that are served by formulaic speech in typical development. Clearly, research is necessary to determine the actual effect of different types of prestored messages on aided language development. Until that time, however, there is evidence to suggest that prestored messages can function as one component in a larger symbol system, even in typical development.

Selecting Symbols to Foster Linguistic Development: Object Words

Many interventions for beginning communicators have targeted symbols for objects as the initial vocabulary, on the premise that concrete and highly preferred referents (e.g., food, favorite toys) would foster the best initial learning (Yovetich & Young, 1988). The inclusion of tangible, easily pictured referents is clearly essential for beginning communicators. Yet, it is equally important to ensure that aided vocabulary is able to keep pace with the changing needs of the communicator (see Chapter 7). We describe several types of studies that support the critical role of object-label as well as nonobject vocabulary in fostering the language development of beginning augmented communicators (Adamson, Romski, Deffebach, & Sevcik, 1992; Wilkinson & Murphy, 1998; Wilkinson et al., 1994).

The "Iconicity" section of this chapter makes reference to questions about the level of specificity that should be represented in the vocabulary items. Fundamentally, the question concerns whether symbol meanings should be explicit ("Oreo," "Spot"), general ("cookie," "dog"), or broad ("snack," "pet"). Each different level of specificity has certain practical advantages and drawbacks in terms of its picturability as well as its potential range of referents. To some extent, the user's practical needs will dictate the level of specificity for individual symbols, and a mix of symbols will likely be necessary. Valuable information is also available from studies of spoken language development (cf. Blockberger, 1995; Schlosser, 1997). The levels of specificity that we have thus far called *explicit, general,* or *broad* parallel different levels of categories that have been defined in the cognitive and developmental language literatures since the 1970s. The most general level ("snack," "pet") encompasses many different types of items and is referred to as a *superordinate category level.* The most explicit level ("Oreo," "Spot"), which refers to specific types of items or even individual items, is called the *subordinate category level.* The level in between ("cookie," "dog") is called the *basic category level.* As described by Schlosser, "Basic-level categories share the greatest amount of features, including overall appearance, function, and terms" (1997, p. 5). All dogs share certain features (they bark, are furry, and pant to keep cool) that are not necessarily shared by members of the superordinate category (mammal) and tend to be refined in the subordinate level (a fox terrier has short fur, a Lhasa Apso has long fur). Substantial research suggests that the basic category level is the most salient and the earliest-developing basis for categorization in typically developing children as well as in individuals with developmental disabilities (e.g., Daehler, Lonardo, & Bukatko, 1979; Hayes & Taplin, 1993; Horton & Markman, 1980; Hupp & Mervis, 1982; Mervis & Crisafi, 1982; Rosch, Mervis, Gray, Johnson, & Boyes-Braem, 1976; Sperber & McCauley, 1984; Tager-Flusberg, 1985; Waxman & Gelman, 1986). Word learning in the earliest years also is most likely to involve basic-level meanings (Golinkoff, Shuff-Bailey, Olguin, & Ruan, 1995). What does this mean for AAC intervention with beginning communicators? Although little research has been conducted, the consistency of the findings with speakers who are developing both typically and atypically allows relative confidence in assuming the likely salience of the basic level for most language learners, including those who use aided symbols. If this is true, it suggests that the inclusion of basic-level object labels might best serve early learners, at least at the outset of vocabulary growth.

Selecting Symbols to Foster Linguistic Development: Social-Regulatory Words   In considering vocabulary other than object labels, many studies since Nelson (1973) have revealed that the vocabulary of preschoolers through older adults includes a large number of nonobject words (Barrett & Diniz, 1989; Beukelman, Jones, & Rowan, 1989; Gopnik, 1988; Marvin, Beukelman, & Bilyeu, 1994; Stuart, Vanderhoof, & Beukelman, 1993). Language provides us with a tool for sharing information and organizing other people's behavior (Bruner, 1981). Thus, one significant function that is expressed in early vocabulary is the regulation of social interactions. In the AAC field, Adamson and colleagues (1992) studied the effects of providing access to social-regulative terms to 13 individuals with severe cognitive impairments who were learning to use visual-graphic symbols. The terms included greetings, politeness terms, and affirmation and negation terms. Despite the fact that the vocabulary content was not concrete or easily picturable, students showed little difficulty in learning the meanings. Furthermore, after the social words were added, the students showed increased production of social-communication functions, indicating that they appreciated the functions that were served by those words. A second study also reported the facilitative effect of nonobject vocabulary, this time on the AAC users' linguistic development (Wilkinson et al., 1994). Wilkinson and colleagues (1994) examined the symbol combinations that 7 of the 13 individuals produced (the other 6 produced no combinations). The symbols on the communication boards were all "single-unit" meanings—that is, symbols referred either to individual items (e.g., "hot dog") or, in the case of nonobject meanings, to individual concepts (e.g., "more," "please," "finished"). Virtually no combinations were produced prior to the inclusion of social-regulatory words. Furthermore, the vast majority (86%) of symbol combinations contained at least one nonnominal symbol, and the meanings expressed in these combinations were consistent with those of early word combinations. These reports have demonstrated the importance of social-regulatory functions for language in individuals who are learning to use aided symbols.

Selecting Symbols to Foster Linguistic Development: Person-Reference Words Another vocabulary category is words that reference people. Family and social networks are an integral topic of conversations for individuals without disabilities (Beukelman et al., 1989; Marvin et al., 1994; Stuart et al., 1993). Research has also explored person-centered conversation in individuals with developmental disabilities (Wilkinson & Murphy, 1998; see also Wilkinson, Murphy, & Bakeman, 1999). A preliminary analysis of conversational topics obtained during the dyadic leisure activities of students with mental retardation and of an adult without disabilities revealed that more than one third of the students' utterances (36%) contained references to people. Striking differences in the amount of person reference were found for the eight individuals who used speech as their primary mode of communication, compared with eight similar individuals who were nonspeaking (some of whom had access to aided symbols). Among those who used speech, a mean of 42% of utterances referenced people. Among those who used nonverbal means, only half that number of utterances (22%) contained person references. The reason for this difference has not yet been explored. It does suggest, however, that discussions about people might be limited in the communications of individuals who use AAC modes, and it argues for the inclusion of such vocabulary in the displays and interventions that are designed for nonspeaking individuals.

Summary

In this section, we have considered some relatively well-known issues in augmentative communication regarding the use of graphic symbol modes. Our intent has been to enrich the current understanding of these issues through a thorough analysis of how knowledge from other disciplines could inform decision making concerning graphic symbol selection/organization. In the next section, we turn directly to an analysis of the specific constraints that are involved in teaching graphic, rather than spoken or signed, symbols.

CONSIDERATIONS IN ASSESSING
CANDIDATES FOR GRAPHIC SYMBOL USE

Fundamental to many of the decisions about intervention involving graphic symbol use is an understanding of the learner's strengths and limitations. A systematic assessment is necessary to determine not only the types of symbols, displays, and vocabulary content that are best suited to the learner but also the most facilitative intervention approach. In this section, we describe a general approach to such assessment for beginning communicators.

Stimulus Control Approaches as a Structure for Augmenting Current Practice

Collaboration between developmental and behavioral scientists has examined ways in which language studies could be enriched through adaptation of stimulus control methodologies (e.g., Wilkinson, Dube, & McIlvane, 1996; Wilkinson & McIlvane, 1997b). *Stimulus control* refers to the relationship between an individual and the environmental conditions that influence that individual's behavior. For instance, consider the behavior of a person who is expecting an incoming telephone call. Most people do not simply pick up the receiver randomly. Rather, they wait for the ring, and only upon hearing the ring do they lift the receiver. Thus, the ring signals the listener as to the appropriate time for "telephone-answering" behavior, and the absence of the ring signals to the listener that answering the telephone would likely be fruitless. Thus, the person's answering the telephone is under the stimulus control of the telephone ringing. Analysis of this type of relationship of the individual's behavior to available environmental signals is the subject of stimulus control research.

Stimulus control analysis can be adapted to explore factors that influence learning and behavior in diverse areas, including lexical development (Wilkinson et el., 1996; Wilkinson & McIlvane, 1997b) and category formation (Wilkinson & McIlvane, in press). One strength of stimulus control approaches is their detailed analyses of the diverse influences on behavior and analysis of the principles that underlie learning. In this section, we illustrate how these principles might guide assessment and intervention for beginning augmented communicators.

Techniques for Assessing Existing Skills

As a general rule, it is easier to elaborate and/or transform existing behavior than to create behavior anew. Therefore, one typically begins by conducting a behavioral assessment to determine which skills the candidate already has and which must be taught. The nature of the assessment depends to some degree on the nature of the symbol system that is to be mastered, but a few general principles can be articulated that apply to all systems. Then, principles for guiding intervention can be identified. Figure 9.1 presents a flowchart of the four areas of assessment that are discussed in this section, including assessment of 1) sensitivity to the consequences of behavior, 2) simple discrimination of identical visual stimuli, 3) relationships among nonidentical visual stimuli

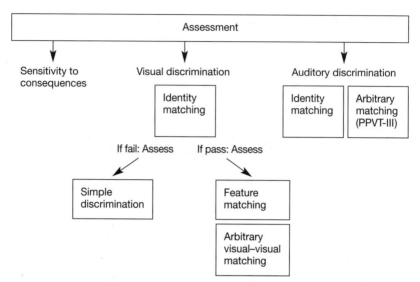

Figure 9.1.   Flowchart for assessing the skills of potential AAC users. (Key: PPVT-III = Peabody Picture Vocabulary Test–III [Dunn & Dunn, 1997].)

(through feature matching and arbitrary visual–visual matching), and 4) discrimination among auditory stimuli.

Sensitivity to Consequences of Behavior   Communication serves a variety of functions (e.g., requesting, expressing affection, providing information). From the user's perspective, any symbolic communication system will be effective only if the consequences of an individual communication act are consistent with its intended function (i.e., a communication request results in satisfaction of the stated need). During initial assessment, it is necessary to determine what types of feedback (i.e., consequences) best motivate each individual learner. For instance, if social feedback is to be integrated into a teaching procedure, it is necessary to determine whether the learner responds appropriately to feedback such as "Yes, good job" or "No, that's not right." With beginning communicators, one cannot simply assume that such consequences will motivate the user—either because he or she is not motivated by social praise or because he or she has extremely limited comprehension.

To make such a determination empirically, assessment must explore whether provision of the positive feedback ("Yes, good job") indeed leads to the user's reproducing the target behavior and, furthermore, whether provision of the negative feedback ("No, that's not right") leads to a reduction in the rate of the target behavior. Experimental verification of the utility of this type of assessment has been reported (McIlvane, Dube, & Callahan, 1996; see also Neef, Shade, & Miller, 1994). It is important to note that the teacher must also ascertain whether those consequences continue to be effective over time. In addition, it is important that target behaviors that are evaluated during an assessment of sensitivity to feedback should be well within the learner's current capabilities. Otherwise, it would be impossible to know whether an apparent lack of sensitivity to feedback is truly due to unresponsiveness to consequences. Rather, it might be due to a lack of understanding of the presented task (see Chapter 4 for further discussion of examining the consequences for behavioral acts).

Assessing Discrimination Among Identical Visual Stimuli   The next assessment step is to determine whether the learner can distinguish among the stimuli that are to serve as symbols. For visual stimuli, a common and useful procedure is *identity matching to sample*. In this task, the learner is presented with an array of two or more comparison stimuli. The learner is then presented with another stimulus (the sample), which is physically identical to one of the comparison stimuli. This procedure is illustrated in Figure 9.2. The task is to identify the comparison stimulus that is identical to the sample. When a student can match *any* set of novel stimuli without explicit training, generalized identity matching is in place. Generalized identity matching reveals that the learner can distinguish among the presented stimuli. Existing generalized identity matching skills therefore permit efficient, easy-to-survey discrimination skills.

Some individuals will demonstrate identity matching to sample skills; others will not. There are two possible reasons for failure. One is that the person cannot discriminate between the two stimuli that are being presented; in other words, he or she cannot tell the stimuli apart. If this is the case, attempts to implement instruction procedures will likely fail. Another possible reason is that the person does not understand the task; that is, although he or she can tell the stimuli apart, the individual does not understand that the choice among comparisons depends on the sample displayed. If this is the case, the interventionist must implement procedures to teach the learner this skill.

How might one determine which of the two problems underlies failure in identity matching? It is possible to determine whether the problem lies in discrimination among stimuli by implementing what is called a *simple discrimination procedure* (Serna, Dube, & McIlvane, 1997), which is illustrated in Figure 9.3. Two choices may be presented. One of the two choices is arbitrarily designated as the correct stimulus. Every time the individual responds to that stimulus, he or she receives positive consequences (whatever has been identified to motivate that learner). Each time he or she chooses the other stimulus, no consequence or error feedback is delivered. Ample evidence suggests that if the learner can discriminate among the stimuli and is sensitive to the consequences, he or she will quickly begin to select the correct stimulus preferen-

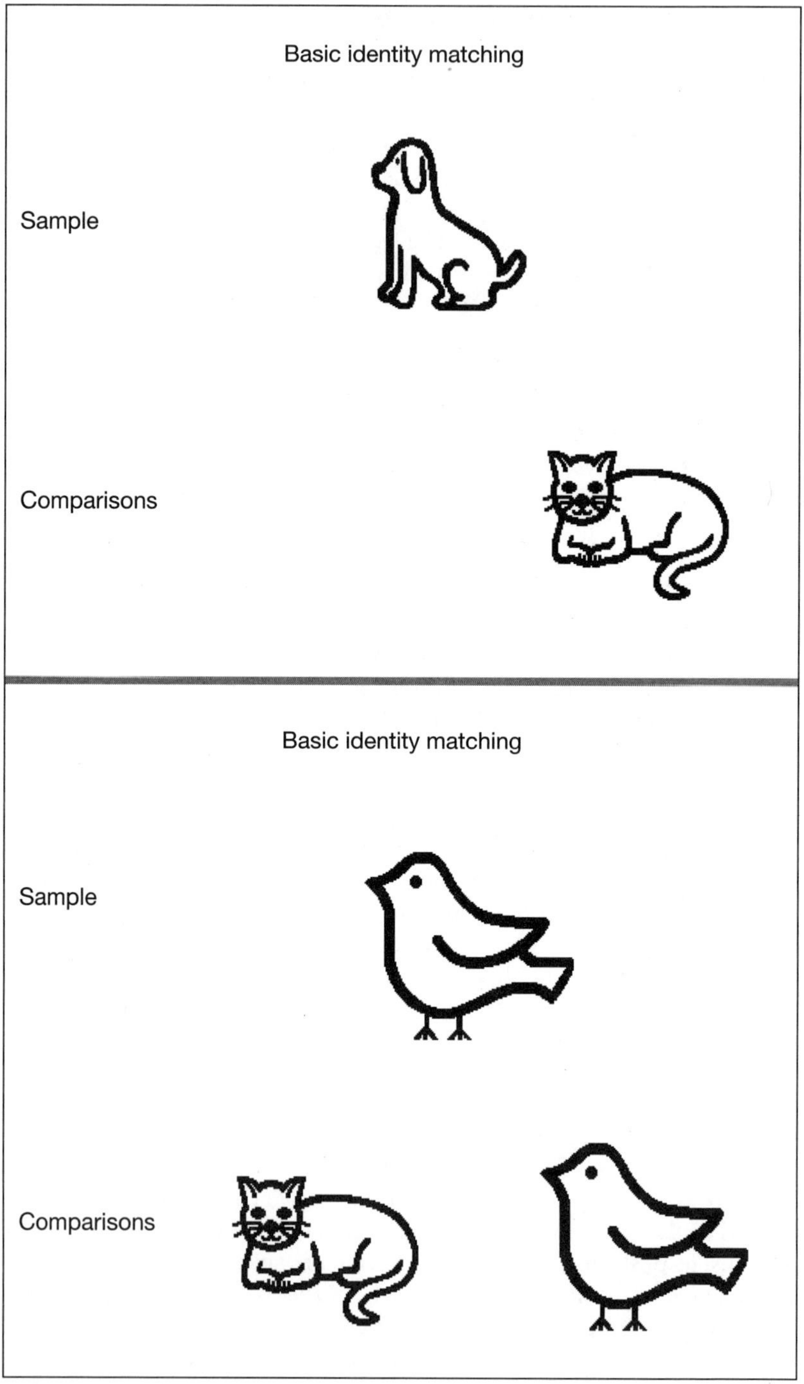

Figure 9.2. Example of an identity matching to sample procedure. (Picture Communication Symbols, Copyright 1981–2001, Mayer-Johnson, Incorporated, all rights reserved. The PCS used in this chapter were taken from the Boardmaker™ software program and were used with permission [1-800-588-4548; www.mayer-johnson.com]).

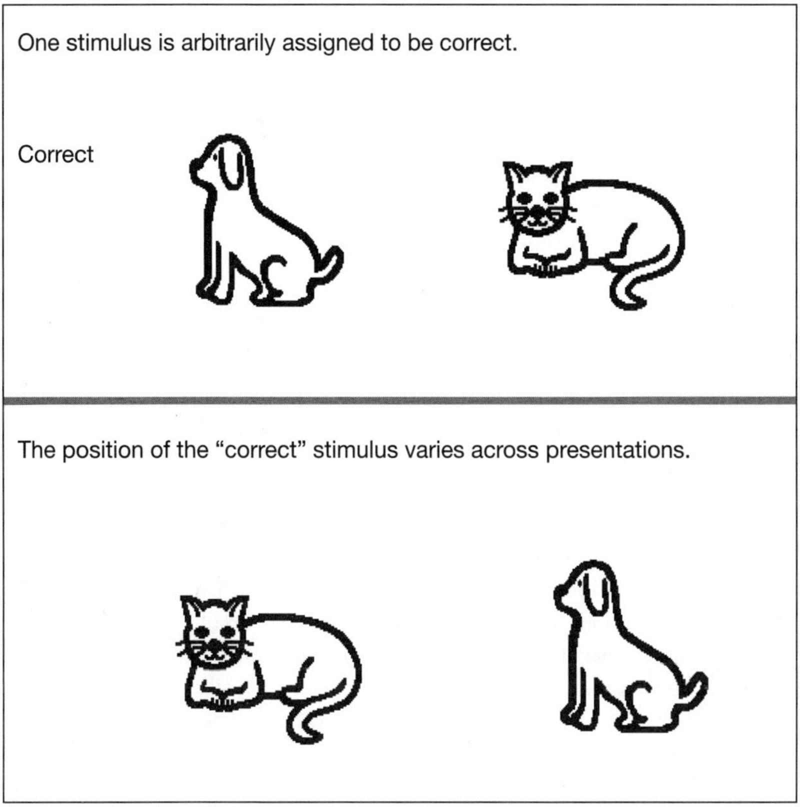

One stimulus is arbitrarily assigned to be correct.

Correct

The position of the "correct" stimulus varies across presentations.

Figure 9.3. Example of a simple discrimination procedure. (Picture Communication Symbols, Copyright 1981–2001, Mayer-Johnson, Incorporated, all rights reserved. The PCS used in this chapter were taken from the Boardmaker™ software program and were used with permission [1-800-588-4548; www.mayer-johnson.com]).

tially. Failure on simple discrimination would suggest a problem in telling the stimuli apart, implying that these stimuli would be inappropriate for use with this learner. Success on this task, alternately, would suggest that implementing teaching procedures would be fully justified (see the section "Step 1: Establishing the Basic Response for Visual Symbol Use" for details on such procedures).

Assessing Relationships Among Nonidentical Visual Stimuli   Identity matching tasks can serve as an initial screen for an individual's ability to discriminate among and conditionally match stimuli that are identical to one another. Yet, the majority of stimuli that an AAC user will encounter, and which ones will form the basis for vocabulary, will involve symbols and referents that are not identical. Even the miniature objects that are sometimes used as symbols on visual communication boards differ from their referents in scale.

Thus, two other matching procedures that are of particular interest in many AAC applications are *feature matching to sample* and *arbitrary matching to sample*.[1] In feature matching, the individual is asked to match stimuli with similar but not identical physical features. One example is matching a photograph and a line drawing of an object, as illustrated in Figure 9.4. As the figure shows, the Mayer-Johnson PCS bear a certain physical resemblance to the photographs to which they refer; thus, they have a certain amount of iconicity. Feature-based matching can be generalized in a manner similar to identity matching; the learner can match novel objects and pictures without explicit training. Yet, as discussed in the previous "Iconicity" section, the ability to match physically identical stimuli does not mean that a learner can also display feature matching. Some learners who can match symbol to symbol and independently match object to object still seem to have difficulty relating the symbols with their corresponding objects, even when the symbols share some features (cf. Dixon, 1981). For such individuals, the relationships are not transparent but, rather, arbitrary; consequently, this skill must be taught.

Arbitrary matching is procedurally similar to identity and feature matching, except that the comparison stimulus to be selected shares no features with the sample; this is illustrated in Figure 9.5. Written words or other clearly noniconic representations (e.g., lexigrams, many Blissymbols) are examples of symbols that involve arbitrary relations with referents. Yet, arbitrary relations can also exist even among symbols that might be considered iconic. For instance, some individuals might be able to guess the meanings of specific Blissymbols or at least understand the relationship once it is explained to them. Other individuals, however, might never perceive the physical basis for these very same relationships. Because these individuals do not perceive the physical basis for the symbol–referent relationship, those symbols are arbitrary to them and, consequently, must be taught. The "Establish an Initial Vocabulary" section in this chapter gives suggestions for facilitating relationships between visual stimuli such as these, for either feature or arbitrary relations.

Assessing Discrimination Among Auditory Stimuli   The ability to discriminate among auditory stimuli is essential for comprehending speech. It is therefore important to determine whether a child can distinguish between

---

[1] Both of these procedures involve matching stimuli that are not identical to one another. The difference between feature and arbitrary matching reflects the extent to which symbol and referent share features; this concept is very similar to *iconicity*, which was described previously in this chapter. Because both involve matching of nonidentical stimuli, they might be classified as being *nonidentity* matching procedures. We choose not to use this umbrella term, however, because it can have multiple meanings. For some, the term *nonidentity matching* refers to what has also been called *nonmatching to sample* or *oddity response*. That is, rather than requiring participants to select the choice that does match the sample, the task is to identify the comparison that does not match (recall the Sesame Street segment that instructs viewers to find the thing that does not match). To avoid the multiple potential meanings, we will work on the level of the terms *feature matching* and *arbitrary matching*.

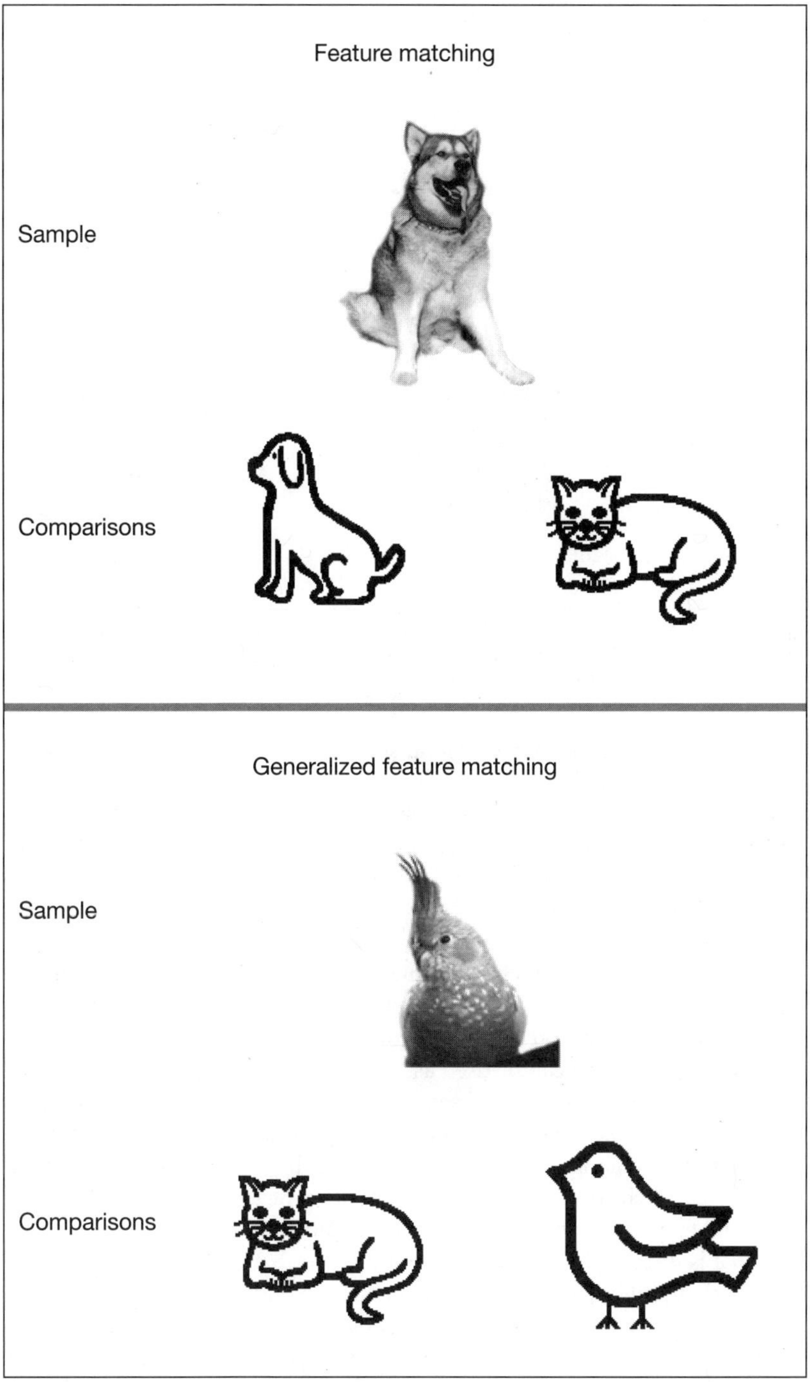

Figure 9.4. Example of a feature matching to sample procedure. (Picture Communication Symbols, Copyright 1981–2001, Mayer-Johnson, Incorporated, all rights reserved. The PCS used in this chapter were taken from the Boardmaker™ software program and were used with permission [1-800-588-4548; www.mayer-johnson.com]).

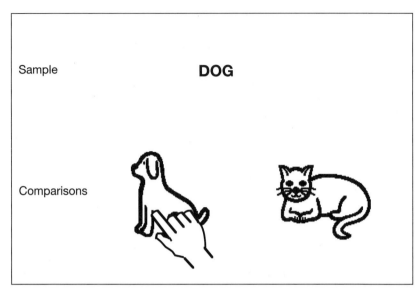

Figure 9.5. Example of an arbitrary visual–visual matching to sample procedure. (Picture Communication Symbols, Copyright 1981–2001, Mayer-Johnson, Incorporated, all rights reserved. The PCS used in this chapter were taken from the Boardmaker™ software program and were used with permission [1-800-588-4548; www.mayer-johnson.com]).

words that sound minimally different, such as "bat" and "pat." Assessing auditory discrimination is of particular interest in augmentative communication because of the apparent role of speech comprehension in language-learning outcomes. As Romski and colleagues noted, individuals who enter AAC intervention with some existing speech comprehension skills show an accelerated profile of AAC learning and use, whereas those with little speech comprehension show slower, more deliberate, and perhaps more limited learning outcomes (see Chapter 14). Having some existing relationships among spoken words and visual referents seems to provide a stepping stone for learners.

An additional reason to assess auditory discrimination in AAC users is that an auditory signal can be used as an access method in scanning. In scanning, each symbol is highlighted sequentially. Most often, the scanning selection technique is executed by using a visual cursor, such as a light signal moving across the symbols. Once the light reaches the targeted symbol, the user activates a switch to select the desired message. Scanning is appropriate for users who may not be able to directly select symbols. Nevertheless, visual scanning that is directed by a light may not be appropriate for all users, including those with visual impairments. In such cases, an auditory signal may be substituted. The word or phrase represented by each symbol is spoken aloud sequentially until the user hears the targeted word and activates the switch. If this method is to be implemented, it is essential to be confident in the user's ability to discriminate among the auditory stimuli that comprise the symbol array.

Logically, one might use the same approach for assessing discrimination and matching of auditory stimuli as for visual stimuli. For instance, we previously proposed that identity matching of visual stimuli can help determine whether the individual can discriminate among the symbols of interest. Implementation of such a procedure for auditory signals is not as simple as it is for visual stimuli. There is no easy procedure for assessing discrimination by using an identity matching format, because auditory stimuli lose their intelligibility when presented at the same time. One possibility is a procedure in which two auditory stimuli are presented one at a time and the learner is required, for example, to raise his or hand if the stimuli are the same and to keep his or her hand still if the stimuli are different. Many learners with severe cognitive disabilities, however, have difficulty learning *not* to respond. Although habituation or preferential looking paradigms have been used with younger children (e.g., Werker, Cohen, Lloyd, Casasola, & Stager, 1998) and are common in audiometric testing, they are difficult to adapt for older individuals. Researchers are trying to develop useful alternatives (e.g., Serna, Jeffery, & Stoddard, 1996; Soraci, Stoddard, Serna, McIlvane, & Carlin, 1994), yet none has thus far proven entirely satisfactory and appropriate for all learners. This remains an area in which further research is clearly mandated.

Assessing arbitrary relations among auditory and visual stimuli is a less challenging prospect. In fact, most familiar language comprehension tests, such as the Peabody Picture Vocabulary Test–III (PPVT-III; Dunn & Dunn, 1997), exemplify procedures that are designed to assess arbitrary relationships between auditory (spoken words) and visual (picture) stimuli. As illustrated in Figure 9.6, two or more pictures are displayed in this procedure. The learner is to select the picture that corresponds to the name dictated (i.e., spoken) by the examiner. Obviously, there is no physical similarity between a dictated name and a picture; the relationship is arbitrarily established by convention among English speakers. Assessment of auditory–visual arbitrary matching, as done in the PPVT-III, is a relatively standard yet essential component of many assessments. The potential impact of comprehension on outcomes in AAC intervention attests to this assessment's value.

CONSIDERATIONS IN INSTRUCTION OF GRAPHIC SYMBOLS

Language intervention for individuals with severe communication limitations has undergone several transitions. Many early efforts implemented pull-out intervention, in which therapy focused on structural forms of language. As the role of semantics (meaning) and pragmatics (use) in early communication development became broadly recognized (Bruner, 1983), programs shifted to functional interventions that were conducted within daily communication en-

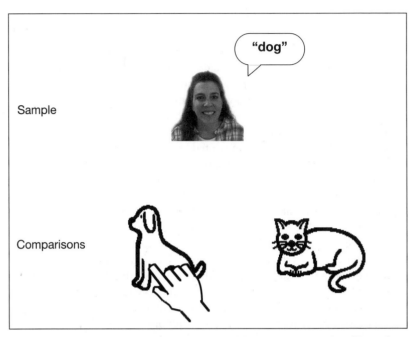

Figure 9.6. Example of an arbitrary auditory–visual matching to sample procedure. (Picture Communication Symbols, Copyright 1981–2001, Mayer-Johnson, Incorporated, all rights reserved. The PCS used in this chapter were taken from the Boardmaker™ software program and were used with permission [1-800-588-4548; www.mayer-johnson.com]).

vironments (Romski & Sevcik, 1993). Yet, an integrated program of structured and functional intervention may best suit some children's needs and preferences (Beukelman & Mirenda, 1998; Yoder, Kaiser, & Alpert, 1991). State-of-the-art functional intervention strategies exist (see Chapters 1 and 14 for a summary). This section focuses on how structured procedures might complement functional interventions.

Particularly in the early stages of teaching, it is desirable to establish structured routines as a context for teaching (Linfoot, 1994; McLean, 1993; see Saunders & Spradlin, 1991, for a discussion of teaching routines). The nature of such routines will vary according to the learner's entry skills and the teaching objectives (Yoder et al., 1991). Establishing certain types of skills (e.g., discrimination of one symbol from another) may require a series of highly structured discrete teaching trials, as in the previously described matching to sample procedures. Some familiar standardized assessment instruments offer such routines. For instance, if the individual can be tested via standard instruments such as the PPVT-III, then the use of items from a test is a convenient way to establish an initial teaching routine. If such assessment is not possible, the next step should be an assiduous search for skills such as those described in the previous section. The next step is to define the targeted teaching objectives and methods. The following discussion gives a four-step process of structured routines that may be used in AAC interventions.

Two figures chart the progress of this section. Figure 9.7 illustrates the relationship between assessment and teaching techniques when the symbols and referents all involve visual stimuli. Figure 9.8 illustrates how the inclusion of spoken words might also be integrated within the assessment and teaching procedures. To assist matching the text and figure illustrations, each section heading includes the step number that is illustrated graphically in the figures. Thus, whereas the text details each of the four procedures, the figures allow a quick overview of the relationship among the procedures either for visual or auditory stimuli.

Step 1: Establish the Basic Response for Visual Symbol Use

For the beginning communicator who does not speak or sign, touching visual symbols to indicate wants or needs is often an explicit teaching goal. Such point-based responses serve as the basis for many access strategies in aided AAC. Yet, this selection-based response is not always part of the individual's repertoire. The first step, therefore, is to identify a relatively simple task within which the response could be mastered.

On the surface, identity matching to sample (pointing to a picture that is identical to a sample picture) seems to be a logical starting point. As noted previously, however, certain individuals may show clear ability to discriminate visual stimuli (perhaps through successful performance on simple discrimination tasks) yet still face difficulties when asked to perform identity-based matching. In Figure 9.7, these individuals would "pass" simple discrimination assessments yet "fail" at identity matching. The difficulty, therefore, lies in conditionally pointing to a comparison upon the presentation of a sample. Thus, teaching this fundamental behavior is of great interest.

A number of methods have been proposed to assist with this performance. Since the 1970s, a variety of methods have been studied for teaching identity matching. Trial-and-error methods have a notoriously poor track record (e.g., Richmond & Bell, 1986; Sidman & Stoddard, 1967). Some children can be taught via procedures such as delayed prompting or stimulus fading, in which prompts are provided and then gradually withdrawn (Dube, McIlvane, Mackay, & Stoddard, 1987; Halle 1987; Sidman, 1977). Yet, Serna and colleagues (1997) noted that these procedures may show mixed success rates (Dube et al., 1993) unless extensive training is conducted (Saunders, Johnston, Tompkins, Dutcher, & Williams, 1997).

Another option that makes use of "attentional capture" may also be effective in teaching matching to sample with some individuals. This task takes advantage of a phenomenon called *popout* or *oddity*, which involves stimuli that differ on some dimension (e.g., shape). As illustrated in the top of Figure 9.9,

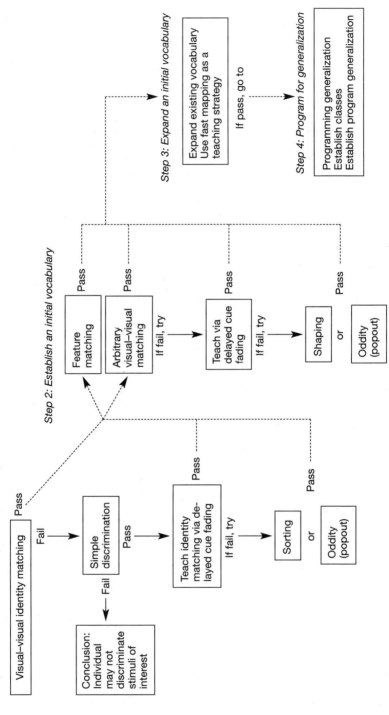

Figure 9.7. Flowchart for teaching visual matching. Steps to take in teaching visual discriminations.

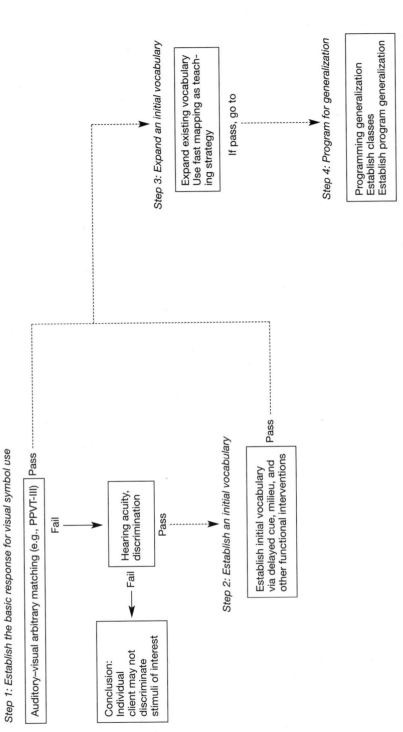

Figure 9.8. Flowchart for teaching auditory matching. Steps to take in teaching auditory–visual discriminations. (Key: PPVT-III = Peabody Picture Vocabulary Test–III [Dunn & Dunn, 1997].)

299

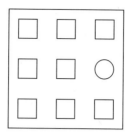

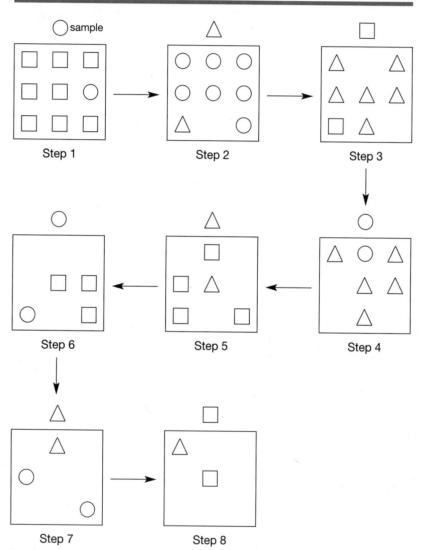

Figure 9.9. Example of oddity task as a means of teaching identity matching. (Figure from "Guiding visual attention in individuals with mental retardation" by R.W. Serna & M.T. Carlin in INTERNATIONAL REVIEW OF RESEARCH IN MENTAL RETARDATION, Volume 24, edited by L.M. Glidden, copyright © 2001 by Academic Press, reproduced by permission of the publisher.)

a single stimulus (e.g., a circle) is presented, surrounded by multiple exemplars of the second stimulus (e.g., squares). The presentation of the single stimulus amidst multiple other stimuli serves to guide the viewer's attention to that one odd stimulus, thereby making that stimulus appear to "pop out." This phenomenon, which is well-documented in cognitive psychology (Wolfe, Cave, & Franzel, 1989), has been integrated with training measures to teach identity matching (Mackay, Soraci, Carlin, Chechile, & Dennis, 1999; Soraci et al., 2001). As illustrated in Figure 9.9, this procedure initially presents a sample (e.g., a circle in Step 1) and a comparison array that guides the viewer's attention to the correct comparison by using the oddity/popout arrangement. As the participant selects correctly, the number of comparisons drops (from nine in Step 1, to eight in Step 2, and so forth). Ultimately, by the final step (Step 8), the participant can only select correctly based on the sample, thereby making this a true matching to sample task. This procedure has been proved effective with typically developing children (Soraci et al., 2001) as well as with some individuals who have developmental disabilities (Serna & Carlin, 2001).

Another method for teaching individuals who have trouble with direct selection-based matching to sample is to begin by asking them to sort stimuli into groups (see Figure 9.10). Sorting of stimuli into groups or kinds is a task that is within the grasp of typically developing children at early developmental levels (Clark & Clark, 1977; Gopnik & Meltzoff, 1992). Serna and colleagues (1997) studied the effects of introducing sorting tasks to five individuals with severe mental retardation. These individuals had failed to learn selection-based identity matching through other teaching procedures. When asked to sort the stimuli into groups, the participants had little trouble. Furthermore, the experience of sorting identical objects appeared to then enhance the participants' subsequent selection-based identity matching performance. Perhaps the physical matching (placing two items directly next to each other) provided the participants with greater information about the task, thus facilitating the slightly more abstract performance of simply pointing to one item when presented with another.[2]

Step 2: Establish an Initial Vocabulary

Once communication and matching skills are established, it is necessary to design an individualized program to integrate those skills into the teaching routine. Establishing the first instances of symbol–referent relationships can be a time-consuming and painstaking process. Although some individuals can rapidly build sizable symbol vocabularies, others show slower and more limited

---

[2] Note the apparent similarities with the strategies that underlies the Picture Exchange Communication System (PECS; Bondy & Frost, 1994), which also has reportedly provided scaffolding for communication to individuals who otherwise may have difficulty with selection-based access methods.

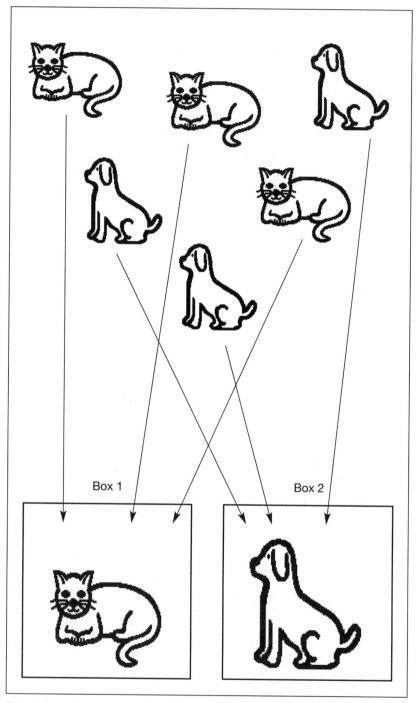

Box 1

Box 2

Figure 9.10. Example of a sorting procedure. Top of figure: Individual is presented with a set of items. Bottom of figure: Individual physically places each item into the box that contains its match. (Picture Communication Symbols, Copyright 1981–2001, Mayer-Johnson, Incorporated, all rights reserved. The PCS used in this chapter were taken from the Boardmaker™ software program and were used with permission [1-800-588-4548; www.mayer-johnson.com]).

acquisition outcomes (Romski & Sevcik, 1993, 1996). Furthermore, candidates for AAC intervention are not a homogeneous group but, rather, display a broad range of behavioral abilities and disabilities. For this reason, it is not possible in this chapter to describe prescriptive solutions to the myriad of individual learning problems that will be encountered. It may be helpful, however, to describe a multistep strategy that will be useful in most teaching situations.

Teaching Visual–Visual Matching   As noted, routines that are based on matching to sample can be one route to learning the relationship between the symbols and their referents. The previously discussed assessment of generalized identity and generalized feature-based matching would be a useful point of entry. For our purposes, consider an individual who has mastered some generalized feature-based matching, whose educational goals include the acquisition of additional symbols. Yet, assessment has indicated that the individual does not immediately match targeted new symbols to their real-world referents. The task of the education team is to facilitate the acquisition of relations that are, to the learner, arbitrary in nature.

As with identity matching, easily implemented delayed cue or fading procedures may be used to teach nonidentity matching; however, their effectiveness remains unclear (Oppenheimer, Saunders, & Spradlin, 1993). Halle (1987) provided a summary of how such teaching procedures can be integrated directly within communication environments, illustrating the potential gains of using both structured and natural communication intervention techniques. Yet, when these procedures do not succeed in teaching arbitrary relations, more elaborate techniques are required. One approach, for example, uses computer-based morphing procedures to transform pictures gradually and systematically into symbols. This is illustrated in Figure 9.11. This shaping technique begins directly with the learner's existing identity- or feature-based matching skills and then builds from the existing capability. Over the course of the shaping procedure, a new performance is generated. Shaping is somewhat time and labor intensive, and there are cases in which it fails to generate the performance of interest (Serna & Carlin, 2001). Yet, it can be effective (as reported by Carr, Wilkinson, Blackman, & McIlvane, 2000) and, thus, provides an additional avenue for teaching children who have an especially hard time learning symbolic relations. (Although comprehensive review of shaping technology is beyond the scope of this chapter, see McIlvane, 1992, for a summary.)

Step 3: Expand an Initial Symbol Vocabulary

Once the individual learns an initial symbol repertoire, what methods are most effective for teaching additional vocabulary? Partner modeling can be extremely effective (Romski & Sevcik, 1996). This method is best implemented in functional environments (see Chapter 14). Also available are methods for

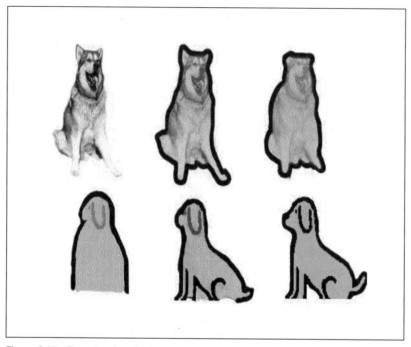

Figure 9.11. Example of a shaping procedure. (Picture Communication Symbols, Copyright 1981–2001, Mayer-Johnson, Incorporated, all rights reserved. The PCS used in this chapter were taken from the Boardmaker™ software program and were used with permission [1-800-588-4548; www.mayer-johnson.com]).

augmenting this learning environment. We describe one such method that has been adapted from both developmental language and stimulus control research.

Studies of normative language development have suggested that word learning involves two phases of acquisition. Children's very first words are acquired through a slow, one-at-a-time learning pattern. After a certain period, there is an apparent explosion in children's vocabulary (Bloom, Lifter, & Broughton, 1985). Children learn perhaps nine new words each day during their preschool years (Carey, 1982; based on Templin, 1957). A phenomenon called *fast mapping* has been proposed to account for this rapid vocabulary explosion. In fast mapping, children obtain a "quick, initial, partial understanding of a word's meaning" (Rice, 1989, p. 152) after even brief exposure to the new word. At least in part, fast mapping seems to make use of children's ability to perceive a distinction between 1) novel words and items and 2) already known words and items. When children hear a novel word, they appear to search for a novel item as its referent and reject items that already have labels (Wilkinson & McIlvane, 1997a). Thus, a contrast of known/unknown allows children to ascertain word meaning when they are confronted with a new label.

Fast mapping of spoken words has been reported not only for typically developing children but also for individuals with language impairments (Dollaghan, 1987; Rice, Buhr, & Nemeth, 1990) and mental retardation (Chapman, Kay-Raining Bird, & Schwartz, 1990; Mervis & Bertrand, 1995). Romski, Sevcik, Robinson, Mervis, and Bertrand (1995) also conducted a study regarding fast mapping of aided symbols (new lexigrams). A novel graphic symbol was added to a display that included several already known symbols. Would the participants select a novel item when the experimenter pointed to the new visual graphic symbol? Fast mapping was demonstrated by students with the most advanced learning patterns in that sample. Therefore, most individuals, even those who are candidates for aided communication modes, demonstrate fast mapping.

Wilkinson and colleagues (1996) noted *learning by exclusion,* which is a convergence among the methods, questions, and findings of the fast mapping literature and a parallel line of inquiry in stimulus control. In this analysis, the authors argued that the two disciplines were in fact studying the same phenomenon. Wilkinson and Green (1998) tested this proposal in an empirical study that integrated the two methodologies for purposes of vocabulary expansion. They found that, if the teaching was structured in a specific way, 8 of the 10 individuals with severe cognitive and communication limitations were able to learn two nonsense word-referent relationships through adapted fast mapping/exclusion procedures (see Wilkinson & Green, 1998, for details). Since then, the research has successfully adapted the procedure for teaching Mayer-Johnson PCS as well as sight-word vocabulary for inclusion in aided communication systems (Wilkinson & Albert, in press). Although in its early stages, adaptations from fast mapping and exclusion research offer promising methods for augmenting symbol vocabularies for graphic symbol users.

Other Considerations: How Many Symbols?   A fundamental debate in clinical intervention concerns adding symbols to a communication board. How many symbols should be placed on the display? One might make multiple symbols available as soon as possible, allowing the user to learn whichever symbols are most salient to him or her. This approach suffers from the possibility that a completely new user might be confused by a profusion of symbols and have difficulty learning any individual symbol. Another commonly used option is to begin with a very small set, adding new symbols as earlier ones become understood (Beukelman & Mirenda, 1998). Romski and Sevcik (1996) reported research support for the efficacy of this method in a comprehensive 2-year assessment of symbol learning in school and home environments by youth with mental retardation.

How many symbols constitute a "very small set"? One logical approach is to start with a single symbol and build from there. This method can often be successful (Romski & Sevcik, 1993). Nonetheless, it can also be problematic for some students. For instance, an early study (Romski, Sevcik, & Pate, 1988) used didactic teaching methods to teach lexigram meanings. The first symbol meaning was introduced in a three-part sequence. First, the symbol appeared on a display with other symbols that were only faintly visible. Once the learner understood the relationship between touching the symbol and receiving a reward that was associated with the symbol, the same symbol was placed in three different locations on the display. The respondent could touch any one of the locations to receive the reward. Finally, other symbols on the display were made as visible as the first one, although only a response to the first symbol was associated with a reward. Romski and colleagues (1988) reported that acquisition of the single lexigram meaning through this procedure took, on average, 1,002 trials. Acquisition of a second lexigram took even longer (1,278 trials); however, learning then appeared to proceed with relative ease (with means of 152 and 278 for the third and fourth lexigrams, respectively).

What might account for the learning difficulties, particularly with the second symbol? In part, problems may have reflected use of didactic instruction alone. Another possible reason is also suggested in stimulus control research by McIlvane, Dube, Kledaras, Iennaco, and Stoddard (1990). They noted that because the symbol and/or its referent is presented in isolation, the learner does not have to attend to any specific features of either the symbol or the referent to respond correctly. Only when the symbol or the referent is directly contrasted with another is it necessary for the learner to actively distinguish the unique features of each. If so, beginning instruction by teaching just a single symbol runs the risk of "actually encourag[ing] subjects to ignore the [symbol]" (McIlvane et al., 1990, p. 285). To avoid this problem, inclusion of at least two symbols may constitute the best "small set" on which to build a further vocabulary.

Class Membership (Categories)   An essential component or consequence of lexical development is the formation and stabilization of categories. Categorization is central to many of one's abilities to integrate, understand, and subsequently predict one's experiences (Bruner, Goodnow, & Austin, 1956). Learners acquire not only the relationship between a particular word and its referent but also the relationship of the word between other words and referents within the lexicon. Yet, the processes by which categories are formed and expanded, and the rules governing relations among concepts, are still poorly understood (Lakoff, 1987). It is not surprising, then, that the categorization skills of clinical groups also remain a research challenge.

We have proposed that methodology stemming from stimulus control analysis may offer promise for evaluating category membership and expansion (Wilkinson & McIlvane, 1997b, in press). We have detailed the overlaps between accepted criteria for determining symbolic functioning in psycholinguistics (i.e., Bates, 1979) and a stimulus control model of arbitrary class formation, called *stimulus equivalence* (Sidman, 1994). The proposed methodology offers an operationalized approach that may allow investigators to trace directly how a relationship between two distinctly different stimuli (e.g., a Lhasa apso and the cartoon character Snoopy) may emerge simply by virtue of their shared experience with a third stimulus (i.e., the word *dog*). We are currently conducting ongoing research that seeks to verify the utility of this approach for studying language categories (Wilkinson, Becker, & McIlvane, 2000). Through this effort, we hope to identify areas that might best adapt equivalence methods for questions that are of interest to researchers and professionals who are interested in category formation.

Step 4: Program for Generalization

A concern for any intervention, particularly one that involves structured teaching, is the generalization of skills or knowledge to functional use (e.g., Halle, 1987; Hart & Rogers-Warren, 1978). Many people believe that cross-task or cross-environment generalization is a mysterious, poorly understood phenomenon. Yet, a case may also be made that most or all of the basic scientific principles for influencing generalization outcomes have been discovered and articulated. By way of background, Kirby and Bickel (1988) made an early effort to articulate stimulus control principles that undergird the various techniques for programming for generalization (cf. Stokes & Baer, 1977). Their paper has had little impact on the field, however. Also underappreciated in relationship to the problem of generalization is the extensive research on stimulus classes and stimulus equivalence (Sidman, 1994). What follows is an effort to provide an overview of a stimulus class account of generalization.

The Roles of Feature and Arbitrary Classes in Teaching   Figure 9.12 illustrates how a goal of teaching may be described as establishing appropriate, highly reliable relationships between target stimulus classes and target behavior. One example is when a Mayer-Johnson symbol is reliably matched with photographs of the object, the object itself, and also with the dictated name. Here, the learner behaves in the same way toward all members of the target stimulus class, matching all of the stimuli to one another. Furthermore, the learner also reliably excludes other nontarget stimuli from that class, thus not matching the target Mayer-Johnson symbol to photographs or names of different objects.

Figure 9.13 presents a diagrammatic overview of the teacher's task in establishing behavior in initial teaching environments. At the outset, the individual's behavior may be described as showing little reliable relationship to the target stimulus classes. The individual may select the incorrect photograph from a group of comparisons when presented with the Mayer-Johnson symbol

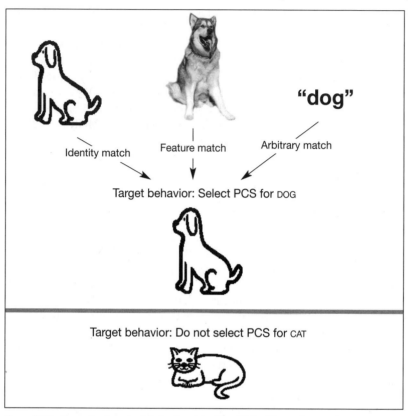

Figure 9.12. Example of a potential stimulus class. (Key: PCS = Picture Communication Symbols.) (Picture Communication Symbols, Copyright 1981–2001, Mayer-Johnson, Incorporated, all rights reserved. The PCS used in this chapter were taken from the Boardmaker™ software program and were used with permission [1-800-588-4548; www.mayer-johnson.com]).

(i.e., the target stimulus class occasions "other" behavior) or, conversely, the person may select the Mayer-Johnson symbol when presented with a photograph of some other item (i.e., other stimulus classes occasion the target behavior). In addition, the consequences in the environment may contribute to a lack of reliable performance. If the student elicits giggles from his or her peers upon selecting incorrectly, and if those giggles are motivating for the student, then unreliable responding will likely continue to occur (see Chapter 4 for a discussion of social functions that are associated with child behavior).

Intervention procedures should reduce the competition from unwanted sources and, therefore, increase the reliability of the relationship between the stimulus class and the learner's behavior. The teacher's goal is that at the end of intervention the target behavior (i.e., selecting the correct symbol) occurs only in the presence of the target stimulus class (i.e., the spoken word, the

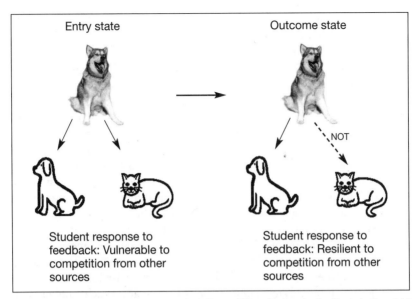

Figure 9.13. Example of the interventionist's challenge. (Picture Communication Symbols, Copyright 1981–2001, Mayer-Johnson, Incorporated, all rights reserved. The PCS used in this chapter were taken from the Boardmaker™ software program and were used with permission [1-800-588-4548; www.mayer-johnson.com]).

photo, or the object) and never in the presence of other stimulus classes (i.e., stimuli concerning other objects). Under other conditions (i.e., when symbols concerning other objects are present), other behavior occurs.

The Roles of Feature and Arbitrary Classes in Generalization   *Generalization* refers to a learner's ability to maintain his or her behavior in new environments. Generalization can only occur if three conditions are met. First, it must be possible for the learner to produce the target behavior in the generalization context (e.g., the AAC symbol must be available and accessible within the new environment). Second, the consequences that helped establish and maintain the communication during teaching must exist in the generalization environment. A corollary of this second condition is that other sources of feedback in the generalization environment must not compete with the consequences that were constructed within teaching. It is here that problems such as peer behavior (e.g., the giggling described previously) may often interfere. The learner may respond reliably to the teacher's feedback when peers are not present; however, in a generalization environment that includes peers, there will be competition from these naturally occurring sources of feedback. If the response is not resilient to such competition, then there is effectively a return to conditions similar to those prior to intervention, and generalization will be weak or absent. Note, however, that this is not a problem of capability for generalization per se; rather, it is a problem of structuring the feedback to with-stand competition from other sources.

Third, at least some member(s) of the target stimulus class must be present in the generalization environment, as there must be some continuity between the teaching and the generalization environments. Analysis of the difference between feature classes and arbitrary classes, however, allows a novel extension of traditional approaches to behavioral analyses of generalization (e.g., Horner, Dunlap, & Koegel, 1988). Specifically, this distinction allows the notion that two types of stimulus classes—feature and arbitrary classes—can be involved in generalization (e.g., Mackay, Stromer, & Serna, 1998). Making use of feature classes for generalization, a teacher could arrange for physically similar stimuli to be present in both the teaching and generalization environments. Yet, consider how the environments could be arranged to allow arbitrary classes to facilitate generalization. As noted previously, the arbitrary class does not entail common physical features. Rather, stimuli become class members when they are mutually substitutable within a given context. For purposes of communication, a photograph and a symbol can be used in lieu of the actual object. To promote generalization, one can arrange for such mutually substitutable stimuli to be present in both the teaching and generalization environments. For example, a student who is taught to sit quietly when his or her teacher says "Quiet" in the classroom and also has learned to read the printed word *quiet* aloud in some other environment may sit quietly in the presence of the word *quiet* on a printed sign (e.g., in a hospital hallway), although he or she has not been taught explicitly to do so. Thus, factors that promote generalization need not be restricted to physically similar stimuli but, rather, can function as members of a larger category.

Summary

It has been our intent in this section to illustrate general principles that might guide assessments that are relevant to graphic symbol instruction and to highlight specific strategies for including structured teaching within intervention. A distinction between feature and arbitrary classes allows analysis of how both feature-based and more abstract category-based classes can contribute to generalization. For beginning communicators, identification of all the potential environmental supports is a valuable exercise to ensure success.

WHO MIGHT BENEFIT FROM GRAPHIC SYMBOL INTERVENTION?

AAC intervention can benefit many individuals, even perhaps young children who are still only at risk for speech-language delays (Romski & Sevcik, 1996).

Recognition of this fact may be considered a shift from earlier approaches, in which certain fundamental skills were argued to be prerequisites for AAC intervention. Yet, accepting AAC as an appropriate clinical response to language risk or impairment is not a simple proposition. As we have discussed, many factors will be involved. In this section, we turn from considerations of the aided symbol mode itself and evaluate some user characteristics that might influence one's ability to use graphic symbols. Is the user capable of manipulating a graphic symbol mode at all? If so, will the graphic symbols add anything to the individual's communicative repertoire? What teaching methods are best suited to the individual's skill levels?

A phenomenon noted by several authors is a profile in which a learner produces between one and four signs or picture symbols but seems to have substantial difficulty learning any more than that (Kravitz et al., 1996; McLean, 1993; Rowland & Schweigert, 1989). Communicators with these profiles appear to prefer nonsymbolic modes to the limited symbols that appear within their repertoires (Cirrin & Rowland, 1985; McLean, McLean, Brady, & Etter, 1991; Ogletree, Wetherby, & Westling, 1992). Are these individuals using their small number of pictures or signs symbolically? Will ongoing symbol instruction lead to greater symbol acquisition or use? Or is there some cognitive or linguistic "cusp" that is fundamentally difficult for these individuals (McLean, 1993)? What factors contribute to the advancement from physical gesture use to active pointing and conventionalized gesture to the use of symbols?

Some authors have speculated that the emergence of symbolic behavior may follow the sequence in typical development (Ogletree et al., 1992; Rowland & Schweigert, 1989) and may even be loosely tied to developmental functioning level (Kravitz et al., 1996). Kravitz, however, cautioned that noting associations between developmental skills level and symbolic functioning is a separate issue from that of "cognitive prerequisites" (personal communication, 1999). At the outset of the formalization of AAC as a discipline, many scholars believed that cognitive development preceded language learning. Consequently, AAC interventionists considered the idea that certain cognitive skills were necessary prior to intervening with picture symbols (e.g., Shane & Bashir, 1980). Subsequent research made it clear that no individual cognitive skill is itself prerequisite for starting intervention (Reichle & Karlan, 1985; Romski & Sevcik, 1988; Zangari, Kangas, & Lloyd, 1988). Nonetheless, as many have pointed out (Beukelman & Mirenda, 1998; Kravitz et al., 1996; Rowland & Schweigert, 1989), the level of developmental functioning can be useful for guiding both assessment and intervention goals.

In what ways can developmental skills level help estimate and guide language goals? It appears that receptive language level may be associated with facility in learning aided symbols (see Chapter 14). In addition to comprehension, Kravitz and colleagues (1996) suggested other potential cognitive markers. Using a scale to estimate developmental level (the Callier-Azusa scale; Stillman & Battle, 1985), their clinical research suggested that a critical point of transition from presymbolic intentional communication to truly symbolic picture use occurs at the developmental level from 12 to 18 months. Prior to 12 months developmental age, symbol instruction of any sort is oftentimes difficult and, for the learner, frustrating. From 12 to 18 months developmental age, symbols can be learned but they are acquired slowly. Finally, after 18 months developmental age, learning begins to occur more rapidly, and individuals are likely to use the symbols in flexible ways for multiple functions. These clinical observations are virtually identical to the pattern of word learning that has been observed in typical development (e.g., Bates, 1979). Evaluation of developmental level, either cognitive or language based, may therefore be a productive avenue for identifying assessment or outcome goals. Clearly, research attention is needed to verify the clinical observations that have thus far formed the basis for these suggestions.

CONCLUSION

We began this chapter with a discussion of fundamental psychological and linguistic processes that must be considered when initiating a graphic symbol system with a beginning AAC user. We then outlined in more detail how stimulus control principles might be useful when actually implementing the symbol system clinically. An integration of stimulus control principles in assessment and intervention permits the evaluation of discrimination and matching skills that are fundamental to graphic symbol use. We have argued that stimulus control principles can be applied to complement naturally based protocols, yet they can also provide guidelines for troubleshooting problems that arise in graphic symbol instruction.

The stimulus control principles that we discussed apply to skills in discriminating and learning either visual or auditory symbol discriminations. In either modality, it is necessary to begin by establishing some response skill that allows the evaluator to be confident that the learner discriminates between the target symbols. If the user does not discriminate, those symbols are unlikely to be useful as a communication mode. Although in the visual modality standard identity matching to sample is often used as an index of a learner's ability to discriminate stimuli, failure on identity matching tasks may not in fact reflect failure to discriminate. Rather, it may reflect a lack of understanding of the task at hand. The use of a simple discrimination task can help determine whether failure at identity matching is task related or truly a reflection of inability to discriminate. If the learner demonstrates the ability to identify symbols on simple discrimination, then strategies such as delayed cue or fading procedures, sorting tasks, or even oddity tasks may induce the identity matching to sample performance. With an auditory task, fewer procedures are available short of standard hearing acuity and discrimination tasks; however, these tasks will provide some information about the user's auditory discrimination skills.

Once discrimination has been assessed and a basic response identified, it is possible to begin establishing the initial vocabulary. Assessment of a client's ability to perform visual feature matching to sample tasks as well as arbitrary matching to sample tasks will provide information about that client's existing visual symbol skills. Individuals who demonstrate no feature-based or arbitrary matching may learn initial visual–visual relationships through delayed cue procedures, fading procedures, oddity tasks, or perhaps stimulus shaping procedures. Individuals who do show some feature-based or arbitrary matching, or who learn it through the specified procedures, are ready to begin expanding the vocabulary. Expansion of an existing vocabulary is often accomplished not only through naturalistic interventions but also through methods based on fast mapping methodologies. Finally, it is essential to program principles that support generalization of learning in order for learning to be useful across multiple and diverse environments.

The stimulus control principles can be implemented at each stage in order to foster maximum performance. If at any point learning begins to break down, the procedures allow a systematic means of evaluating what behaviors may be involved. Such structured analysis is a valuable addition to the naturalistic intervention strategies that are best suited to promoting functional use.

In sum, issues that are related to graphic symbol instruction range from considerations of the symbols themselves to teaching issues to considering which individuals graphic symbols might best benefit. These three issues are interwoven and mutually influence one another. For instance, the physical similarities of some symbols and their referents is a unique issue in initially selecting the symbol, but it will also be a consideration during assessment and intervention. Furthermore, the ability to use symbols that physically resemble their referents may depend on the symbol and the individual's developmental level. We have attempted to highlight how such diverse issues interrelate. In addition, we have identified principles that might help guide attempts to integrate structured assessment and instruction into existing interventions for beginning communicators.

REFERENCES

Adamson, L.B., Romski, M.A., Deffebach, K., & Sevcik, R.A. (1992). Symbol vocabulary and the focus of conversations: Augmenting language development for youth with mental retardation. *Journal of Speech and Hearing Research, 35,* 1333–1343.

Baker, B. (1982). Minspeak: A semantic compaction system that makes self-expression easier for communicatively disabled individuals. *Byte, 7*(9), 186–202.

Barrett, M.D., & Diniz, F.A. (1989). Lexical development in mentally-handicapped children. In M. Beveridge, G. Conti-Ramsden, & I. Leuder (Eds.), *Language and communication in mentally handicapped people* (pp. 3–32). London: Chapman & Hall/CRC.

Bates, E. (1979). *The emergence of symbols: Cognition and communication in infancy.* San Diego: Academic Press.

Bedrosian, J.L. (1997). Language acquisition in young AAC system users: Issues and directions in future research. *Augmentative and Alternative Communication, 13,* 179–185.

Beukelman, D.R., Jones, R.S., & Rowan, M. (1989). Frequency of word usage by nondisabled peers in integrated preschool classrooms. *Augmentative and Alternative Communication, 5,* 243–248.

Beukelman, D.R., McGinnis, J., & Morrow, D. (1991). Vocabulary selection in AAC. *Augmentative and Alternative Communication, 7,* 171–185.

Beukelman, D.R., & Mirenda, P. (1998). *Augmentative and alternative communication: Management of severe communication disorders in children and adults* (2nd ed.). Baltimore: Paul H. Brookes Publishing Co.

Blockberger, S. (1995). AAC intervention and early conceptual and lexical development. *Journal of Speech-Language Pathology and Audiology, 19,* 221–232.

Bloom, L., Lifter, K., & Broughton, J. (1985). The convergence of early cognition and language in the second year of life: Problems in conceptualization and measurement. In M. Barrett (Ed.), *Children's single-word speech* (pp. 149–180). New York: John Wiley & Sons.

Bloomburg, K., Karlan, G., & Lloyd, L. (1990). The comparative translucency of initial lexical items represented by five graphic symbols and sets. *Journal of Speech and Hearing Research, 33,* 717–725.

Bondy, A., & Frost, L. (1994). The Picture Exchange Communication System (PECS). *Focus on Autistic Behavior, 9,* 1–19.

Bowler, D.M. (1991). Need for theory in studies of augmentative and alternative communication. *Augmentative and Alternative Communication, 7,* 127–132.

Brady, N.C., & McLean, L.K. (1996). Arbitrary symbol learning by adults with severe mental retardation: A comparison of lexigrams and printed words. *American Journal on Mental Retardation, 100,* 423–427.

Brown, R. (1973). *A first language.* Cambridge, MA: Harvard University Press.

Bruner, J. (1981). The social context of language acquisition. *Language and Communication, 1,* 155–178.

Bruner, J. (1983). *Child's talk: Learning to use language.* New York: Norton.

Bruner, J.S., Goodnow, J.J., & Austin, G.A. (1956). *A study of thinking.* New York: John Wiley & Sons.

Bruno, J. (1989). Customizing a Minspeak system for a preliterate child: A case example. *Augmentative and Alternative Communication, 5,* 89–100.

Calculator, S., & Dollaghan, C. (1982). The use of communication boards in a residential setting: An evaluation. *Journal of Speech and Hearing Disorders, 47,* 281–287.

Carey, S. (1982). Semantic development: The state of the art. In E. Wanner & L.R. Gleitman (Eds.), *Language acquisition: The state of the art* (pp. 265–293). Cambridge, MA: The MIT Press.

Carlin, M.T., & Soraci, S.A. (1993). Similarities in the detection of stimulus symmetry by persons with and without mental retardation. *American Journal on Mental Retardation, 98,* 336–348.

Carr, D., Wilkinson, K.M., Blackman, D., & McIlvane, W.J. (2000). Equivalence classes in individuals with minimal verbal repertoires. *Journal of the Experimental Analysis of Behavior, 74,* 101–114.

Carlson, F. (1981). A format for selecting vocabulary for the nonspeaking child. *Language, Speech, and Hearing Services in the Schools, 12,* 240–245.

Chapman, R.S., Kay-Raining Bird, E., & Schwartz, S.E. (1990). Fast mapping of words in event contexts by children with Down syndrome. *Journal of Speech and Hearing Disorders, 55,* 761–770.

Cirrin, F.M., & Rowland, C.M. (1985). Communicative assessment of nonverbal youths with severe and profound mental retardation. *Mental Retardation, 23,* 52–62.

Clark, H.H., & Clark, E.V. (1977). *Psychology and language: An introduction to psycholinguistics.* Orlando, FL: Harcourt.

Collins, A.M., & Quillian, M.R. (1969). Retrieval time from semantic memory. *Journal of Verbal Learning and Verbal Behavior, 8,* 240–247.

Collins, A.M., Gathercole, S.E., Conway, M., & Morris, P.E. (1993). *Theories of memory.* Mahwah, NJ: Lawrence Erlbaum Associates.

Daehler, M., Lonardo, R., & Bukatko, D. (1979). Matching and equivalence judgments in very young children. *Child Development, 50,* 170–179.

DeLoache, J.S. (1995). Early understanding and use of symbols: The model model. *Current Directions in Psychological Science, 4,* 109–113.

Dixon, L.S. (1981). A functional analysis of photo-object matching skills of severely retarded adolescents. *Journal of Applied Behavior Analysis, 14,* 465–478.

Dollaghan, C.A. (1987). Fast mapping in normal and language-impaired children. *Journal of Speech and Hearing Disorders, 52,* 218–222.

Dube, W.V., Iennaco, F.M., & McIlvane, W.J. (1993). Generalized identity matching to sample of two-dimensional forms in individuals with intellectual disabilities. *Research in Developmental Disabilities, 14,* 457–477.

Dube, W.V., McIlvane, W.J., Mackay H.A., & Stoddard, L.T. (1987). Stimulus class membership established via stimulus-reinforcer relations. *Journal of the Experimental Analysis of Behavior, 47,* 159–175.

Dunn, L.M., & Dunn, L.M. (1997). *Peabody Picture Vocabulary Test–Third Edition.* Circle Pines, MN: American Guidance Service.

Farrier, L.D., Yorkston, K.M., Marriner, N.A., & Beukelman, D.R. (1985). Conversational control in nonimpaired speakers using an augmentative communication system. *Augmentative and Alternative Communication, 1,* 65–73.

Franklin, K., Mirenda, P., & Phillips, G. (1996). Comparisons of five symbol assessment protocols with nondisabled preschoolers and learners with severe intellectual disabilities. *Augmentative and Alternative Communication, 12,* 63–77.

Fuller, D.R. (1997). Initial study into the effects of translucency and complexity on the learning of Blissymbols by children and adults with normal cognitive abilities. *Augmentative and Alternative Communication, 13,* 30–39.

Gerber, S., & Kraat, A. (1992). Use of a developmental model of language acquisition: Applications to children using AAC systems. *Augmentative and Alternative Communication, 8,* 19–32.

Golinkoff, R.M., Shuff-Bailey, M., Olguin, R., & Ruan, W. (1995). Young children extend novel words at the basic level: evidence for the principle of categorical scope. *Developmental Psychology, 31,* 494–507.

Goossens', C.A. (1984). The relative iconicity and learnability of verb referents differentially represented by manual signs, Blissymbols, and Rebus symbols: An investigation with moderately retarded individuals. *Dissertation Abstracts International, 45,* 809A.

Gopnik, A. (1988). Three types of early word: The emergence of social words, names and cognitive-relational words in the one-word stage and their relation to cognitive development. *First Language, 8,* 49–70.

Gopnik, A., & Meltzoff, A. (1992). Categorization and naming: Basic level sorting in eighteen-month-olds and its relation to language. *Child Development, 63,* 1091–1103.

Halle, J. (1987). Teaching language in the natural environment: An analysis of spontaneity. *Journal of the Association for Persons with Severe Handicaps, 12,* 28–37.

Hamilton, R., & Ghatala, E. (1994). *Learning and instruction.* New York: McGraw-Hill.

Hart, B., & Rogers-Warren, A. (1978). Milieu language training. In R.L. Schiefelbusch (Ed.), *Language intervention strategies : Vol. 2* (pp. 193–235). Baltimore: University Park Press.

Hayes, B.K., & Taplin, J.E. (1993). Development of conceptual knowledge in children with mental retardation. *American Journal on Mental Retardation, 98,* 293–303.

Higginbotham, D.J. (1992). Evaluation of keystroke savings across five assistive communication technologies. *Augmentative and Alternative Communication, 8,* 258–272.

Horner, R.H., Dunlap, G., & Koegel, R.L. (1988). *Generalization and maintenance: Life-style changes in applied settings.* Baltimore: Paul H. Brookes Publishing Co.

Horton, M.S., & Markman, E. (1980). Developmental differences in the acquisition of basic and superordinate categories. *Child Development, 51,* 708–719.

Hupp, S., & Mervis, C.B. (1982). Acquisition of basic object categories by severely handicapped children. *Child Development, 53,* 760–767.

Hurlbut, B.I., Iwata, B.A., & Green, J.D. (1982). Nonvocal language acquisition in adolescents with severe physical disabilities: Blissymbol versus iconic stimulus formats. *Journal of Applied Behavior Analysis, 15,* 241–248.

Kaiser, A.P. (1993). Introduction: Enhancing children's social communication. In S.F. Warren & J. Reichle (Series Eds.) & A.P. Kaiser & D.B. Gray (Vol. Eds.), *Communication and language intervention series: Vol. 2. Enhancing children's communication: Research foundations for intervention* (pp. 3–9). Baltimore: Paul H. Brookes Publishing Co.

King, J., Spoencman, T., Stuart, S., & Beukelman, D.R. (1995). Small talk in adult conversations: Implications for AAC vocabulary selection. *Augmentative and Alternative Communication, 11,* 260–264.

Kirby, K.C., & Bickel, W.K. (1988). Toward an explicit analysis of generalization: A stimulus control interpretation. *The Behavior Analyst, 11,* 115–129.

Koester, H., & Levine, S. (1996). Effects of a word prediction feature on user performance. *Augmentative and Alternative Communication, 12,* 155–168.

Kravitz, E., Littman, S., & Cassidy, K. (1996, August). *Meeting the communication needs of adults with severe developmental disabilities.* Symposium presented at the Seventh Biennial Conference of the International Society for Augmentative and Alternative Communication, Vancouver, Canada.

Lakoff, G. (1987). *Women, fire, and dangerous things: What categories reveal about the mind.* Chicago: University of Chicago Press.

Light, J. (1997a). "Communication is the essence of human life": Reflections on communicative competence. *Augmentative and Alternative Communication, 13,* 61–70.

Light, J. (1997b). Let's go star fishing: Reflections on the contexts of language learning for children who use aided AAC. *Augmentative and Alternative Communication, 13,* 158–171.

Light, J., Collier, B., & Parnes, P. (1985a). Communicative interaction between young nonspeaking physically disabled children and their primary caregivers: Part I–Discourse patterns. *Augmentative and Alternative Communication, 1,* 74–83.

Light, J., Collier, B., & Parnes, P. (1985b). Communicative interaction between young nonspeaking physically disabled children and their primary caregivers: Part II–Communicative functions. *Augmentative and Alternative Communication, 1,* 98–107.

Light, J., & Lindsay, P. (1991). Cognitive science and augmentative and alternative communication. *Augmentative and Alternative Communication, 7,* 186–203.

Light, J., Lindsay, P., Siegel, L., & Parnes, P. (1990). The effects of message and coding techniques on recall by literate adults using AAC systems. *Augmentative and Alternative Communication, 6,* 184–201.

Linfoot, K. (1994). Functional communication and the role of context. In K. Linfoot (Ed.), *Communication strategies for people with developmental disabilities: Issues from theory and practice* (pp. 124–155). Baltimore: Paul H. Brookes Publishing Co.

Mackay, H., Soraci, S.A., Carlin, M.T., Chechile, M.A., & Dennis, N.A. (1999, March). Guiding visual attention in young children. In *Proceedings of the 32nd Annual Gatlinburg Conference on Research and Theory in Mental Retardation and Developmental Disabilities* (p. 106).

Mackay, H.A., Stromer, R., & Serna, R. (1998). Emergent behavior and intellectual functioning: Stimulus classes, generalization, and transfer. In S. Soraci & W.J. McIlvane (Eds.), *Perspectives in intellectual functioning: A survey of research approaches* (pp. 287–310). Stamford, CT: Ablex Publishing Corp.

Marvin, C.A., Beukelman, D.R., & Bilyeu, D. (1994). Vocabulary use patterns in preschool children: Effects of context and time sampling. *Augmentative and Alternative Communication, 10,* 224–236.

McIlvane, W.J. (1992). Stimulus control analysis and nonverbal instructional methods for people with intellectual disabilities. In N.W. Bray (Ed.), *International review of research in mental retardation* (Vol. 18, pp. 55–109). San Diego: Academic Press.

McIlvane, W.J., Dube, W.V., & Callahan, T.D. (1996). Attention: A behavior analytical perspective. In G.R. Lyon & N.A. Krasnegor (Eds.), *Attention, memory, and executive function* (pp. 97–117). Baltimore: Paul H. Brookes Publishing Co.

McIlvane, W.J., Dube, W.V., Kledaras, J.B., Iennaco, F.M., & Stoddard, L.T. (1990). Teaching relational discrimination to individuals with mental retardation: Some problems and possible solutions. *American Journal on Mental Retardation, 95,* 283–296.

McLean, J.E., McLean, L.K.S., Brady, N.C., & Etter, R. (1991). Communication profiles of two types of gesture using nonverbal persons with severe to profound mental retardation. *Journal of Speech and Hearing Research, 34,* 294–308.

McLean, L.K. (1993). Communication intervention for adults with severe mental retardation. *Topics in Language Disorders, 13,* 47–60.

McNaughton, D., & Light, J. (1989). Teaching facilitators to support the communication skills of an adult with severe cognitive disabilities: A case study. *Augmentative and Alternative Communication, 5,* 35–41.

McNaughton, S., & Kates, B. (1980). The application of Blissymbolics. In R.L. Schiefelbusch (Ed.), *Nonspeech language and communication* (pp. 303–321). Baltimore: University Park Press.

Mervis, C.B., & Bertrand, J. (1995). Acquisition of the novel-name nameless–category (N3C) principle by young children who have Down syndrome. *American Journal on Mental Retardation, 100,* 231–243.

Mervis, C.B. & Crisafi M.A. (1982). Order of acquisition of subordinate-, basic-, and superordinate-level categories. *Child Development, 53,* 258–266.

Mirenda, P. (1985). Designing pictorial communication systems for physically able-bodied students with severe handicaps. *Augmentative and Alternative Communication, 1,* 58–64.

Mirenda, P., & Locke, P. (1989). A comparison of symbol transparency in nonspeaking persons with intellectual disabilities. *Journal of Speech and Hearing Disorders, 54,* 131–140.

Mizuko, M., & Reichle, J. (1989). Transparency and recall of symbols among intellectually handicapped adults. *Journal of Speech and Hearing Disorders, 54,* 627–633.

Mizuko, M., Reichle, J., Ratcliff, A., & Esser, J. (1994). Effects of selection techniques and array sizes on short-term visual memory. *Augmentative and Alternative Communication, 10,* 237–244.

Neef, N.A., Shade, D., & Miller, M. S. (1994). Assessing influential dimensions of reinforcers on choice in students with serious emotional disturbance. *Journal of Applied Behavior Analysis, 27,* 575–583.

Nelson, K. (1973). Structure and strategy in learning to talk. *Monographs of the Society for Research in Child Development, 38,*(1–2).

Nelson, K. (1981). Individual differences in language development: Implications for development and language. *Developmental Psychology, 17*, 170–187

Newell, A.F., Arnott, J.L., Booth, L. Beattie, W., Brophy, B., & Ricketts, I.W. (1992). Effect of the "PAL" word prediction system on the quality and quantity of text generation. *Augmentative and Alternative Communication, 8*, 304–311.

Ogletree, B.T., Wetherby, A.M., & Westling, D.L. (1992). Profile of the prelinguistic intentional communicative behaviors of children with profound mental retardation. *American Journal on Mental Retardation, 97*, 186–196.

Oppenheimer, M., Saunders, R.R., & Spradlin, J.E. (1993). Investigating the generality of the delayed-prompt effect. *Research in Developmental Disabilities, 14*, 425–444

Paul, R. (1997). Facilitating transitions in language development for children using AAC. *Augmentative and Alternative Communication, 13*, 141–148.

Peters, A. (1983). *The units of language acquisition.* New York: Cambridge University Press.

Reichle, J., & Karlan, G. (1985). The selection of an AAC system in communication intervention: A critique of decision rules. *Journal of The Association for People with Severe Handicaps, 10*, 146–156.

Rice, M. (1989). Children's language acquisition. *American Psychologist, 44*, 149–156.

Rice, M.L., Buhr, J.C., & Nemeth, M. (1990). Fast mapping word-learning abilities of language-delayed preschoolers. *Journal of Speech and Hearing Disorders, 55*, 33–42.

Richmond, G., & Bell, J. (1986). Comparison of trial-and-error and graduated stimulus change procedures across tasks. *Analysis and Intervention in Developmental Disabilities, 6*, 127–136.

Romski, M.A., & Sevcik, R.A. (1988). Augmentative and Alternative Communication systems: Considerations for individuals with severe intellectual disabilities. *Augmentative and Alternative Communication, 4*, 83–93.

Romski, M.A., & Sevcik, R.A. (1993). Language learning through augmented means: The process and its products. In S.F. Warren & J. Reichle (Series Eds.) & A.P. Kaiser & D.B. Gray (Vol. Eds.), *Communication and language intervention series: Vol. 2. Enhancing children's communication: Research foundations for intervention* (pp. 85–104). Baltimore: Paul H. Brookes Publishing Co.

Romski, M.A., & Sevcik, R.A. (1996). *Breaking the speech barrier: Language development through augmented means.* Baltimore: Paul H. Brookes Publishing Co.

Romski, M.A., Sevcik, R.A., & Adamson, L.B. (1997). A framework for studying how children with developmental disabilities develop language through augmented means. *Augmentative and Alternative Communication, 13*, 172–178.

Romski, M.A., Sevcik, R.A., & Pate, J. (1988). Establishment of symbolic communication in persons with severe retardation. *Journal of Speech and Hearing Disorders, 53*, 94–107.

Romski, M.A., Sevcik, R.A., Pate, J.L., & Rumbaugh, D.M. (1985). Discrimination of lexigrams and traditional orthography by nonspeaking severely retarded persons. *American Journal of Mental Deficiency, 90*, 185–189.

Romski, M.A., Sevcik, R.A., Robinson, B.F., Mervis, C.B., & Bertrand, J. (1995). Mapping the meanings of novel visual symbols by youth with moderate or severe mental retardation. *American Journal on Mental Retardation, 100*, 391–402.

Rosch, E., & Mervis, C.B. (1975). Family resemblances: Studies in the internal structure of categories. *Cognitive Psychology, 7*, 573–605.

Rosch, E., Mervis, C.B., Gray, W.D., Johnson, D.M., & Boyes-Braem, P. (1976). Basic objects in natural categories. *Cognitive Psychology, 8*, 382–439.

Rowland, C., & Schweigert, P. (1989). Tangible symbols: Symbolic communication for individuals with multisensory impairments. *Augmentative and Alternative Communication, 5*, 226–234.

Rumelhart, D.E., & McLelland, J.L. (1986). *Parallel distributed processing: Explorations in the microstructure of cognition (2 volumes)*. Cambridge MA: The MIT Press.

Saunders, K.J., Johnston, M.D., Tompkins, B.F., Dutcher, D.L., & Williams, D.C. (1997). Generalized identity matching of two-dimensional forms by individuals with moderate to profound mental retardation. *American Journal on Mental Retardation, 102,* 285–291.

Saunders, R.R., & Spradlin, J.E. (1991). A supported routines approach to active treatment for enhancing independence, competence, and self-worth. *Behavioral Residential Treatment, 6,* 11–37.

Schiefelbusch, R.L., & Lloyd, L.L. (1974). Introduction. In R.L. Schiefelbusch & L.L. Lloyd (Eds.), *Language perspectives: Acquisition, retardation, and intervention* (pp. 1–16). Baltimore: University Park Press.

Schlosser, R.W. (1997). Nomenclature of category levels in graphic symbols, Part I: Is a flower a flower a flower? *Augmentative and Alternative Communication, 13,* 4–13.

Serna, R.W., & Carlin, M.T. (2001). Guiding visual attention in individuals with mental retardation. In L.M. Glidden (Ed.), *International review of research in mental retardation* (Vol. 24, pp. 321–357). San Diego: Academic Press.

Serna, R.W., Dube, W.V., & McIlvane, W.J. (1997). Assessing same/different judgments in individuals with severe intellectual disabilities: A status report. *Research in Developmental Disabilities, 18,* 343–368.

Serna, R.W., Jeffery, J.A., & Stoddard, L.T. (1996). Establishing go-left/go-right auditory discrimination baselines in an individual with severe mental retardation. *The Experimental Analysis of Human Behavior Bulletin, 14,* 18–23.

Sevcik, R.A., & Romski, M.A. (1986). Representational matching skills of persons with severe retardation. *Augmentative and Alternative Communication, 2,* 160–164.

Sevcik, R.A., Romski, M.A., & Wilkinson, K.M. (1991). Roles of graphic symbols in the language acquisition process for persons with severe cognitive disabilities. *Augmentative and Alternative Communication, 7,* 161–170.

Shane, H., & Bashir, A. (1980). Election criteria for the adoption of an augmentative communication system: Preliminary considerations. *Journal of Speech and Hearing Disorders, 45,* 408–414.

Sidman, M. (1977). Teaching some basic prerequisites for reading. In P. Mittler (Ed.), *Research to practice in mental retardation, Vol. II* (pp. 353–360). Baltimore: University Park Press.

Sidman, M. (1994). *Equivalence relations: A research story*. Boston: Authors Cooperative.

Sidman, M., & Stoddard, L.T. (1967). The effectiveness of fading in programming a simultaneous form discrimination for retarded children. *Journal of the Experimental Analysis of Behavior, 10,* 3–15.

Soraci, S.A., Carlin, M.T., Deckner, C.W., & Baumeister, A.A. (1990). Detection of stimulus organization: Evidence of intelligence-related differences. *Intelligence, 14,* 435–447.

Soraci, S.A., Mackay, H., Carlin, M.T., Dennis, N.A., Chechile, N.A., & Lee, M. (2001). *Guiding visual attention in children*. Manuscript in preparation.

Soraci, S.A., Stoddard, L.T., Serna, R.W., McIlvane, W.J., & Carlin, M.T. (1994). Auditory spatial location in auditory-visual matching to sample: A preliminary investigation. *The Experimental Analysis of Human Behavior Bulletin, 12,* 14–16.

Sperber, R., & McCauley, C. (1984). Semantic processing efficiency in the mentally retarded. In P.H. Brooks, R. Sperber, & C. McCauley (Eds.), *Learning and cognition in the mentally retarded* (pp. 141–163). Mahwah, NJ: Lawrence Erlbaum Associates.

Stephenson, J., & Linfoot, K. (1996). Pictures as communication symbols for students with severe intellectual disability. *Augmentative and Alternative Communication, 12,* 244–255.

Stillman, R., & Battle, C. (1985). *The Callier-Azusa Scales for the Assessment of Communicative Abilities*. Dallas: University of Texas, Callier Center.

Stokes, T.F., & Baer, D.M. (1977). An implicit technology of generalization. *Journal of Applied Behavior Analysis, 10,* 349–367.

Stuart, S., Vanderhoof, D., & Beukelman, D.R. (1993). Topic and vocabulary use patterns of elderly women. *Augmentative and Alternative Communication, 9,* 95–110.

Tager-Flusberg, H. (1985). Basic level and superordinate level categorization by autistic, mentally retarded, and normal children. *Journal of Experimental Child Psychology, 40,* 450–469.

Templin, M. (1957). *Certain language skills in children: Their development and interrelationship*. Minneapolis: University of Minnesota Press.

Venkatigiri, H.S. (1993). Efficiency of lexical prediction as a communication acceleration technique. *Augmentative and Alternative Communication, 9,* 161–167.

Warren, S.F., & Reichle, J. (1992). The emerging field of communication and language intervention. In S.F. Warren & J. Reichle (Series Eds. & Vol. Eds.), *Communication and language intervention series: Vol. 1. Causes and effects in communication and language intervention* (pp. 1–8). Baltimore: Paul H. Brookes Publishing Co.

Waxman, S., & Gelman, R. (1986). Preschoolers' use of superordinate level relations in classification. *Cognitive Development, 1,* 139–156.

Werker, J.F., Cohen, L.B., Lloyd, V.L., Casasola, M., & Stager, C.L. (1998). Acquisition of word-object associations by 14-month old infants. *Developmental Psychology, 34,* 1289–1309.

Wilkinson, K.M., & Albert, A. (in press). Adaptations of fast mapping for vocabulary intervention with augmented language users. *Augmentative and Alternative Communication.*

Wilkinson, K.M., Albert, A., & Green, G. (1999, November). *Fast mapping of sight-word vocabulary: A case study*. Poster presented at the American Speech-Language-Hearing Association Annual Convention, San Francisco.

Wilkinson, K.M., Becker, L.B., & McIlvane, W.J. (2000, August). *Stimulus equivalence as a model for category learning and expansion*. Symposium conducted at the Annual Meeting of the American Psychological Association, Washington, DC.

Wilkinson, K.M., Dube, W.V., & McIlvane, W.S. (1996). A cross-disciplinary perspective on studies of rapid word mapping in psycholinguistics and behavior analysis. *Developmental Review, 16,* 125–148.

Wilkinson, K.M., & Green, G. (1998). Implications of "fast mapping" for vocabulary expansion in individuals with mental retardation. *Augmentative and Alternative Communication, 14,* 162–170.

Wilkinson, K.M., & McIlvane, W.J. (1997a). Blank comparison analysis of emergent symbolic mapping in young children. *Journal of Experimental Child Psychology, 67,* 115–130.

Wilkinson, K.M., & McIlvane, W.J. (1997b). Contributions of stimulus control perspectives to psycholinguistic theories of vocabulary development and delay. In L.B. Adamson & M.A. Romski (Eds.), *Communication and language acquisition: Discoveries from atypical development* (pp. 25–48). Baltimore: Paul H. Brookes Publishing Co.

Wilkinson, K.M., & McIlvane, W.J. (in press). Methods for studying symbolic behavior and category formation: Contributions of stimulus equivalence research. *Developmental Review.*

Wilkinson, K.M., & Murphy, N. (1998). References to people in the communications of female and male youths with mental retardation. *Research in Developmental Disabilities, 19,* 201–224.

Wilkinson, K.M., Murphy, N.A., & Bakeman, R. (1999). Consideration of alternative accounts of gender-linked speech patterns in individuals with mental retardation. *Research in Developmental Disabilities, 20,* 255–268

Wilkinson, K.M., Romski, M.A., & Sevcik, R.A. (1994). Emergence of visual-graphic symbol combinations in children with mental retardation using an augmented communication system. *Journal of Speech and Hearing Research, 37,* 883–896.

Wolfe, J.M., Cave, K.R., & Franzel, S.L. (1989). Guided search: An alternative to the feature integration model for visual search. *Journal of Experimental Psychology: Human Perception and Performance, 15,* 419–433.

Yoder, P.J., Kaiser, A.P., & Alpert, C.L. (1991). An exploratory study of the interaction between language teaching methods and child characteristics. *Journal of Speech and Hearing Research, 34,* 155–167.

Yovetich, W., & Young, T. (1988). The effects of representativeness and concreteness on the "guessability" of Blissymbols. *Augmentative and Alternative Communication, 4,* 35–39.

Zangari, C., Kangas, K., & Lloyd, L.L. (1988). Augmentative and alternative communication: A field in transition. *Augmentative and Alternative Communication, 4,* 60–65.

10

Breakdowns and Repairs in Conversations Between Beginning AAC Users and Their Partners

Nancy C. Brady and James W. Halle

The long-term goals for most individuals who participate in a communication intervention program include being able to initiate, maintain, and appropriately end conversations. Each phase of conversation can be described in terms of a complex set of rules, discriminations, and behaviors. One of the most important yet difficult challenges facing the augmentative and alternative communication (AAC) field is trying to teach the necessary skills for successfully negotiating a conversation. Studying aspects of conversational exchanges between dyads at various levels of communication proficiency is one strategy that may advance the field's knowledge about what and how to teach individuals who are learning to use AAC.

One does not have to delve very far into the literature or venture beyond casual observations to learn that individuals at all levels of communication proficiency frequently encounter communication breakdowns (Alexander, Wetherby, & Prizant, 1997; Brady, McLean, McLean, & Johnston, 1995; Brinton & Fujiki, 1989; Golinkoff, 1986; Tomasello, Conti-Ramsden, & Ewert, 1990). For example, breakdowns may occur when one member of a dyad does not understand her or his partner's communication attempt. This lack of understanding could be due to a multitude of factors, such as the manner in which the communication attempt was produced or competing environmental factors (e.g., noise).

Although breakdowns frequently interrupt the flow of conversation, competent communicators learn to negotiate these breakdowns seamlessly

---

Support for writing this chapter was provided from the following sources: National Institute of Child Heatlth and Human Development (NICHD) Grant No. PO1 HD18955 and U.S. Department of Education Grant #H029D960035.

to maintain conversation (Brinton, Fujiki, Winkler, & Loeb, 1986). Focusing on how competent communicators repair communication breakdowns may provide some potentially teachable strategies for AAC users to maintain conversations. Strategies to negotiate breakdowns are the primary focus of this chapter.

In this chapter, we examine the role of communication breakdowns and repairs in conversations between beginning AAC users and their communicative partners. First, we describe a communication breakdown, then examine why communication breakdowns appear to be particularly prevalent in conversations between AAC users and their partners. We review literature regarding prevalence of communication breakdowns as well as describe some of their causes. Also reviewed are the types of communication repair strategies that have been observed in conversations between AAC users and their communication partners. In addition, we examine the correlation between the causes of communication breakdowns and the repair strategies that AAC users employ in their conversations with speaking individuals. The focus of this comparison is to identify possible interventions that are valid across communication modes and to define directions for further research.

EXAMPLES OF BREAKDOWNS AND REPAIRS

A communicative exchange begins when one individual initiates an interaction with another individual. Typically, following this initiation, the communication partner responds and the exchange may continue until one of the partners discontinues the interaction. Even between eloquent and sophisticated communicators, however, it is common to encounter minor disruptions in the continuous flow of turn taking that constitutes a conversation. These interruptions constitute a communication breakdown. Communication breakdowns may be caused by many different factors. For example, a listener may not hear or may misunderstand a speaker's utterance, as illustrated in the following sample dialogue.

Example 1:
Speaker 1: "I would like the club sandwich, please."
Speaker 2: "White bread or wheat?"
Speaker 1: "What?"
Speaker 2: "Would you like white bread or wheat bread on your sandwich?"
Speaker 1: "Oh, wheat, please."

The second turn for Speaker 1 marks the start of a communication breakdown between these two conversational partners. Speaker 1 indicates a communication breakdown by uttering a nonspecific request for clarification,

"What?" (Brinton & Fujiki, 1989). Speaker 2's response to this request for clarification is called a repair attempt. In this example, the repair attempt was successful because Speaker 1 indicated an understanding of Speaker 2's repair attempt.

Conversations by less linguistically skilled speakers also are marked by instances of communication breakdowns and subsequent repairs. The following dialogue from Wetherby, Alexander, and Prizant (1998, p. 135) represents a 20-month-old child's attempt to comment on a flag hanging in the street.

Example 2:
Child: "/fag, fag/"
Mother: What?
Child: "/fag, fag/" while pointing to a flag
Mother: What?
Child: "/tag, tag/" while pointing to the flag
Mother: "Oh, pretty flag!"
Child: Smiles and stops pointing

Similar to Example 1, the communication breakdown in Example 2 also is signaled by a nonspecific request for clarification (i.e., "What?"). The child first attempts to repair by adding a gesture (a point) to her utterance. This attempt is unsuccessful, as indicated by the mother's second request for clarification. The child's second attempt to repair involves changing the phonology of the word approximation. Although the word approximation /tag/ seems less like *flag* than her original utterance, the mother correctly interprets /tag/ and this repair attempt is successful.

Communication repair attempts have also been observed by individuals who communicate with nonsymbolic gestures and vocalizations (Brady et al., 1995; Golinkoff, 1986). The occurrences of nonverbal communicative repairs are often cited as one of the earliest signs that an infant is communicating intentionally (Bates, Benigni, Bretherton, Camaioni, & Volterra, 1979). Examples of nonverbal repairs include repeating or modifying communicative gestures or vocalizations.

The next two examples represent breakdowns and repair attempts in dyads composed of a speaking and a nonspeaking individual. In Example 3, the participant was an individual who communicated with nonsymbolic gestures and his partner was a speaking individual.

Example 3:
Participant: Attempts to blow up a balloon, then gives the balloon to his partner
Partner: "No, I don't want it." (Partner gives balloon back to Participant.)

Participant: Places balloon up to the partner's lips and vocalizes
Partner: "Oh, you want me to do it, huh?" (Partner blows up bal-
loon.)
Participant: Smiles and watches the balloon

The partner's first response does not match the intended effect of the participant. That is, based on the resolution of this episode, it appears that the
participant was requesting that the partner blow up the balloon. The partner,
however, responded as if the participant were giving the balloon to the partner.
This type of breakdown is referred to as a *topic shift*, which is discussed in the
"Differences in Types of Breakdowns" section of this chapter.

Example 4 illustrates a communication breakdown and repair sequence
that is similar to those described in Golinkoff's (1986) study, wherein she reported the communicative repairs of three children who were observed at 14
months of age and then again at approximately 16 and 18 months of age.

Example 4:
Child: Vocalizes and points to request a toy that is out of reach
Mother: Offers him the wrong toy
Child: Shakes his head "no" and continues pointing
Mother: Offers him another toy
Child: Fusses, shakes his head "no," and points again
Mother: Offers him another toy
Child: Accepts the toy, smiles, and discontinues pointing

The child's persistence in pointing serves to repair this communication
breakdown. Thus, communicative repairs are critical even at these early stages
of communication development.

Individuals who have developmental disabilities often communicate with
behaviors similar to those illustrated in Examples 3 and 4. In addition to these
conventional gestures, some individuals with developmental disabilities also
use idiosyncratic and challenging behaviors to communicate (Carr & Durand,
1985; Reichle & Wacker, 1993). Although a growing literature is devoted to analyzing the communicative functions of challenging behaviors, it may prove
fruitful to consider the role that challenging behaviors play in communication
breakdown sequences.

Challenging Behaviors as Communicative Repairs

Behaviors that are described as challenging or socially unacceptable may also
be described as communicative repair attempts. Since the mid-1980s, researchers
have considered challenging behavior as being communicative (Carr & Durand, 1985; Horner & Carr, 1997; O'Neill et al., 1997). The challenging behavior of children who have developmental disabilities and no formal language

system may enable them to influence people in their environment in intended and desired ways. We hypothesize that, in some contexts, problem behavior may be a form of repair, and it is in these contexts that we wish to extend the topographies that are typically considered repairs.

From an operant conceptual perspective, communicative acts such as requests and protests are labeled *mands* (i.e., a response that is "reinforced by a characteristic consequence and is therefore under the functional control of relevant conditions of deprivation or averse stimulation"; Skinner, 1957, p. 35). When previously reinforced behavior is no longer reinforced, extinction occurs (Catania, 1984). Thus, when a request form is not understood or is misunderstood by the listener, a breakdown ensues and reinforcement is not immediately forthcoming. It is well known that behavior that is undergoing extinction may be repeated, that its frequency and intensity may increase, and that often its topography becomes more varied. Consider the following example, in which a young child, who has no language and a small repertoire of communicative forms, approaches her teacher, who is busily preparing materials for the next large-group activity.

Example 5:
>Child: Vocalizes softly while shifting her gaze between the teacher and the door
>Teacher: No response
>Child: Gently touches the teacher and vocalizes
>Teacher: Still does not attend to child
>Child: Begins to scream loudly
>Teacher: Immediately takes the child by the hand and says, "Be quiet! Show me what you want!"
>Child: Stops screaming and leads the teacher to the drinking fountain in the hallway

In this example, the child attempted two initial forms of request (first a vocalization, then a touch combined with a vocalization), neither of which was successful. Only the third form, the loud scream, produced the student's intended outcome (i.e., to get a drink in the hallway). The child was differentially reinforced for a coercive topography, whereas two socially acceptable attempts were extinguished. The child may learn that when the teacher is busy, screaming is an effective request form. Likewise, the teacher may learn that when screaming occurs, immediate attention will terminate the unpleasant response. The insidious feature of this interaction is that neither the child nor the teacher intended to strengthen screaming as a repair strategy, but the coercive and salient nature of the response evoked attention in a situation in which the more subtle forms did not.

Whether these challenging behaviors are called *communicative repairs* or *behaviors undergoing extinction,* the implication is the same—children will attempt to obtain a desired outcome by engaging in additional behavior. The additional behavior may be a repetition, an intensified version, or a variation of the original response. It also might be a distinctly different behavior that shares the same function of gaining access to an item or an event. All of these alternatives can be viewed as means that the child uses to "get the message across" to the listener. Unfortunately, some of these topographies are coercive and unpleasant to others and, therefore, are labeled as problems. An especially insidious feature of this dynamic is that the very topographies that are labeled problems may become the most effective communicative acts in terms of producing intended outcomes.

Thus far, we have provided examples of many different communication breakdowns and repair strategies from a variety of communicators, including speakers and individuals who use gestures. The following section focuses on communication breakdown and repair sequences in dyads that include AAC users.

COMMUNICATION BREAKDOWNS OF AAC USERS

Communication breakdowns occur with some frequency in all interactions. At high frequencies, however, they may disrupt the fluidity of conversations. Limited repair strategies may also compromise conversational flow. We begin this section with a discussion of the prevalence and significance of communication breakdowns in dyads that include AAC users.[1] The following sections describe different types of breakdowns that occur in dyads that include AAC users, as well as strategies used to repair these breakdowns.

Prevalence of Breakdowns

Communication breakdowns appear to occur with high frequency when one or both members of a dyad use AAC. O'Keefe and Dattilo (1992) observed that conversational breakdowns occur frequently in AAC dyads, even when AAC users have extensive symbolic repertoires and can produce multiword utterances.

One of the problems in reporting the prevalence of communication breakdowns and repairs stems from the methodology that is employed to study them. Frequently, communication repairs are studied in contrived contexts.

---

[1] Throughout this chapter, we refer to *AAC dyads* as being composed of one AAC user and one speaker or one nonsymbolic communicator and his or her speaking partner. We discuss graphic and gestural modes of AAC, including sign systems and natural gestures. Yet, we do not focus on children who are learning sign language and have parents who are deaf and members of the Deaf community because, in this instance, sign language is the primary form of communication rather than an AAC system.

That is, researchers will often ensure a consistent number of repair opportu-nities by telling communication partners to purposely create communication breakdowns. For example, communication partners are told to respond to par-ticipants' communication attempts by asking "What?" or a similar request for clarification (Anselmi, Tomasello, & Acunzo, 1986; Brinton & Fujiki, 1991). Con-versation partners may be told to emit a certain number of requests for clari-fication during a conversation (Ansel, McNeil, Hunker, & Bless, 1983; Calcu-lator & Delaney, 1986), or they may follow a more specific script that indicates precisely when to request clarification (Brady et al., 1995; Light, Collier, & Parnes, 1985). Two obvious advantages to this methodology are that all partic-ipants receive an equal number of opportunities to repair communication break-downs and a great deal of behavior can be sampled in a relatively short period of time. If the aim of the research is to compare repair strategies across children, then equal numbers of opportunities are advantageous. Such methodology will not, however, provide information on how frequently communication break-downs occur in more natural situations. To address this disadvantage, some studies have included free play or other unscripted conversation contexts (Golinkoff, 1986; Light et al., 1985; Tomasello et al., 1990).

To learn how frequently communication breakdowns occur in natural conversations, the conversations should be recorded and the frequency of break-downs documented. Several studies have recorded the frequencies of com-munication breakdowns between two speaking individuals (Coggins & Stoel-Gammon, 1982; Golinkoff, 1986; Tomasello et al., 1990). In one of the few studies that reported communication breakdowns between AAC users and their partners, Light and colleagues (1985) observed young AAC users in both structured interactions with a clinician and in free play interactions with their primary caregivers. In the free play context, caregivers and children were given a set of toys and told to "play, converse, and interact as you normally would at home" (p. 100). Experimenters recorded several different communicative functions, including requests for clarification by the child or the parent and provision of clarification by the child or the parent. The authors reported that the parents requested clarification following 11.4% of their children's turns in conversation. The authors did not record other types of communication breakdown, however, such as topic shifts. One of the major findings of the Light and colleagues study was that parents frequently chained together sev-eral questions that required short responses rather than ask more open-ended questions that could require lengthy responses. The authors felt that this par-ticular interaction style increased AAC users' communication success and de-creased communication breakdowns.

Calculator and Dollaghan (1982) recorded and analyzed the communi-cation functions of seven individuals who communicated by selecting Blis-symbols on a communication board. Most of the participants also communicated with gestures or spoke a few single word utterances. The participants were between 8 and 25 years of age and had moderate to profound mental retardation. Participants were observed during the opening 30 minutes of their classroom day. Calculator and Dollaghan (1982) found that teachers requested clarification following 28% of the AAC users' communication attempts. In addition, teachers changed topics following 8% of student initiations, and many of these topic changes could have resulted in communication breakdowns (see the ensuing discussion regarding the types of communication breakdowns). Therefore, the AAC users in the Calculator and Dollaghan study encountered communication breakdowns following approximately a third of all communication attempts. This proportion is notably higher than that reported by Light and colleagues (1985). Differences in sampling contexts, familiarity of communication partners, and definitions of breakdowns may have contributed to differences in proportions of breakdowns reported in these two studies.

Is the prevalence of communication breakdowns in AAC dyads higher than in dyads with speaking children? Tomasello and colleagues (1990) observed speaking children at ages 1 year, 3 months and 1 year, 9 months during two free-play contexts—once with their mothers and once with their fathers. Breakdowns were recorded when parents asked for clarification, shifted topics, or failed to acknowledge their child's utterance. Results revealed that breakdowns occurred with mothers during 7% of interactions at age 1 year, 3 months and during 21% of interactions at age 1 year, 9 months. Breakdowns occurred with fathers during 13% of interactions at age 1 year, 3 months and during 31% of interactions at age 1 year, 9 months. Golinkoff (1986), however, reported higher proportions of breakdowns in her study of typically developing preverbal infants. Nearly half of the parent–child communication episodes that she observed contained a communication breakdown. This high proportion of communication breakdowns may be due, in part, to different communicative proficiency among children in the studies. For the most part, the infants in Golinkoff's study used deictic gestures and were just beginning to attempt a few spoken words. Thus, their gestures, unlike words or symbols, could have referred to any number of objects or events. This ambiguity could have lead to the frequent breakdowns that Golinkoff reported. In addition, Golinkoff observed mothers and their children during mealtimes rather than in a free play context. (The motivational aspects of different contexts are discussed in the "Motivational Variables" section of this chapter.)

It is difficult to compare the results from the studies of typically developing speaking children with the studies of AAC users because of differences in observational contexts, communication partners, developmental levels, and definitions of breakdown. The available data on the prevalence of communication breakdowns in AAC users do not, however, suggest that breakdowns are substantially more prevalent with this group than with speaking children.

It may be that communication breakdowns seem particularly frequent in AAC dyads because negotiating breakdowns in AAC dyads requires more time and energy than in speaking dyads (Buzolich & Wiemann, 1988). Thus, partners may react more to the quality of repair strategies by AAC users than to the number of breakdowns. Before we review AAC users' repair strategies, however, let us consider some of the factors that contribute to communication breakdowns in AAC dyads.

Causes of Breakdowns in Speakers and AAC Users

As discussed previously, all communicators experience breakdowns in communication. Nevertheless, a discussion of some of the causes of these breakdowns, as well as the unique features of AAC that contribute to communication breakdowns, may illuminate areas in which to concentrate future interventions to enhance AAC conversations.

Intelligibility   An area that is relevant to breakdowns in AAC dyads is the intelligibility of the AAC system. Communication partners more easily understand some AAC systems than others (Beukelman & Mirenda, 1998; Rotholz, Berkowitz, & Burberry, 1989). Intelligibility of graphic AAC may be influenced by whether there is voice output and, if so, the quality of the voice output. For example, newer generations of synthesized speech are much more intelligible than earlier versions (Beukelman & Mirenda, 1998).

The intelligibility of graphic AAC without voice output depends on how well graphic symbols represent objects, events, or ideas. For example, a picture of a cow may represent milk to some but not all communication partners. In addition, the intelligibility of graphics depends on a listener's willingness to make inferences about a symbol's meaning and to establish close physical proximity with the AAC user. That is, the listener must be close enough to view the symbol.

Typically, beginning AAC users have a small vocabulary array from which to choose. This may lead to general requests or comments that lead to a breakdown. For example, if a beginning communicator selects a symbol that represents *want,* then a likely response would be a request for clarification (e.g., "*What* do you want?"). Similar problems may ensue when an AAC user would like some chips but selects a symbol for *cookie* because it is the only snack symbol available.

The aforementioned problems are not limited to graphic forms of AAC. Communication breakdowns also follow gestural AAC, and the intelligibility of the gesture affects communicative success. Some natural gestures, such as pointing, are readily understood by unfamiliar communication partners. Yet, specific referents may be vague because these gestures do not refer to specific objects or events (i.e., a child may be referring to countless objects by pointing out the window). Signs from sign systems or sign languages are less ambiguous, but they are only comprehensible to those who are familiar with the sign system (Iverson & Thal, 1998).

Conversational Timing   In addition to these system characteristics, differences in the nature and flow of conversations between AAC users and speaking partners may contribute to breakdowns. Conversation is a complex series of events that has been described in terms of the synchrony of timing between speakers' turns (Garvey, 1977; Newman & Smit, 1989). For example, speaking children have been found to moderate their pause rates to match those of their conversational partners (Newman & Smit, 1989). Pause times between turns with an AAC user are likely to be much longer than between two speakers because of the increased production time associated with AAC (Beukelman & Mirenda, 1998). That is, the time from the end of the speaker's utterance until the end of the AAC user's subsequent utterance is much longer than in a conversation with two speakers. These increased pause times may lead to confusion regarding when one speaking turn ends and another begins (Buzolich & Wiemann, 1988). This is compounded by the fact that many individuals combine different forms of AAC. They may select symbols sometimes, nod their head, or simply smile at other times. This variability in response modes makes it difficult for communication partners to predict turn transfers and participate in a fluid exchange.

Partner Unfamiliarity with AAC   Finally, many communication partners may be unfamiliar with AAC and nonsymbolic communication. This unfamiliarity may lead to breakdowns (Farrier, Yorkston, Marriner, & Beukelman, 1985). Conversations between AAC users and speaking partners may require some period of calibration to adjust sensitivity to greater pause times between turns. For example, a speaking partner may be unsure how or when to respond to AAC. The partner may respond before the AAC user is finished forming an utterance, or the partner may fail to recognize the end of an AAC user's turn and wait for more communication. Speaking partners of AAC users frequently repeat the AAC utterance before they respond to it, thus creating even a more atypical interaction pattern (Buzolich & Wiemann, 1988; Calculator & Delaney, 1986).

REPAIR STRATEGIES USED IN AAC DYADS

Not only do AAC users frequently encounter communication breakdowns, but there also is some evidence that individuals who communicate with AAC may not have adequate strategies to repair these breakdowns when they occur. Light and colleagues (1985) analyzed the interactions of eight graphic AAC users and their primary caregivers. These eight children were younger than 6 years of age and communicated by selecting Blissymbols on a nonelectronic board. As stated previously, the children encountered communication breakdowns following roughly 11% of their utterances during a free play context. The mean percentage of children's utterances that repaired communication breakdowns was only 5%, however, indicating that the AAC users did not repair many breakdowns. The authors commented that the caregivers primarily assumed responsibility for repairing the conversations in this study. When the children did attempt to provide clarification, they usually repeated their message in its original form. As discussed in the "Differences in Types of Repair Strategies" section of this chapter, depending on the source of the breakdown, repetition may not be an efficient way to repair specific types of communication breakdowns.

In addition to the free play context, Light and colleagues (1985) included a structured context. The structured context was intended to elucidate whether anticipated restrictions in the participants' range of communication functions were attributable to child limitations or to characteristics of the caregiver–child interaction. In the structured context, each of the eight children was provided with an opportunity to request clarification and an opportunity to repair a scripted communication breakdown. The opportunity for the child to request clarification was established when the clinician purposely mumbled a statement. An opportunity for the child to repair was established when the clinician responded to a child's utterance by saying, "I don't understand." All eight children responded to both of these opportunities, even though one child had never provided clarification and six children had never requested clarification during interactions with their caregivers. Apparently, the children recognized the breakdowns more readily in the structured contexts. It would be interesting to compare the breakdowns across conditions to identify the salient cues that facilitated the children's requests for clarifications and repair attempts in the structured context.

Calculator and Delaney (1986) used a semistructured context to examine repair behaviors used by five AAC users and five speakers, all of whom had developmental disabilities. All of the participants were able to combine spoken words (if they were speakers) or symbols (if they were AAC users). The AAC users had between 191 and 229 symbols available on their nonelectronic communication boards. The participants engaged in unstructured conversation with the experimenter, but this individual purposely provided a request for clarification when cued by a second experimenter. Each participant interacted with an examiner during a conversation of approximately 75 minutes. During this conversation, the experimenter produced 40 clarification requests. Calculator and Delaney found that all of the participants responded to the requests for clarification and there was little difference between the speakers and the nonspeakers. Yet, the authors commented that the types of repair strategies used by all of the participants (speakers and nonspeakers) differed from strategies used by typically developing children at similar stages of language development (Brown Stages II or III; Brown, 1973). The participants in the Calculator and Delaney study usually attempted to repair by repeating their original utterances, whereas typically developing children in other studies more frequently revised their original utterance (Gallagher, 1977; Tomasello et al., 1990).

Ciocci and Baran (1998) used a similar elicitation strategy to examine communication repairs produced by young children who were learning to use a total communication system (signs combined with speech).[2] Sixteen children participated: eight children with profound hearing impairments and eight typically developing children. All of the children were between 4 and 7 years old, and those with hearing impairments had been learning total communication for at least 2 years. The authors, however, did not provide information about the language level of the participants. Ciocci and Baran implemented two different elicitation tasks—free play and structured elicitation. The free play tasks involved the experimenter and the participant's playing together with a variety of toys and games. The structured elicitation task consisted of the experimenter and the child's looking at picture books together. During conversations in each of these tasks, the experimenter presented 10 "stacked sequences" of three communication breakdowns. A *stacked sequence* is when several breakdowns (e.g., "Huh?" "What?" "I don't understand") follow successive repair attempts (Brinton & Fujiki, 1989). Both groups of children in the Ciocci and Baran study responded to nearly all of the communication breakdowns presented to them. Yet, there were some differences in the ways in which the two groups responded. The children in both groups most often attempted to repair by revising their original utterances. Compared with the speaking children, however, the children who used total communication added information to their original utterances more often. The authors noted that children from the total communication group often repaired with gestures and pantomimes. In addition, they made larger signs and signed more slowly during repair attempts. It may be that the children who used total communication added information more often because they had more means by which to do so. That is, they could use multiple topographies in their repair attempts.

Thus far, we have discussed the importance of studying communication breakdowns and repairs as well as some of the logistical concerns that surround conducting this research with AAC users. We have described some of the conditions under which breakdowns and repairs are observed and which variables may account for differences in these observations. The following sections describe more thoroughly the differences between types of communication breakdowns and types of repair attempts. We propose that by distin

---

[2] Although the participants in this study had profound hearing impairments and such individuals typically are not considered to be AAC users, this study is discussed because the methods are applicable to multimode AAC users.

guishing the differences between these types of breakdowns and the repairs that AAC users employ, we may learn more about the specific conditions that lead to breakdowns and how best to negotiate a successful repair.

TYPES OF COMMUNICATION BREAKDOWNS AND REPAIRS

Several different types of communication breakdowns and repairs were mentioned in the preceding discussion, but we have not yet adequately described these different types of breakdowns and repairs or the potential relationships between breakdown and repair types. The types of repair strategies often appear to depend on the specific nature of the breakdown. For example, if a specific part of an utterance is unintelligible, then it is likely that a more specific request for clarification—one that asks for the specific missing piece of information—will be issued. This analysis of different types of breakdowns and repairs lays the foundation for some possible interventions presented in the "Educational Implications" section of this chapter.

Figure 10.1 presents a flowchart of a conversational exchange in which an AAC user encounters a communication breakdown. The figure is intended to show many of the possible sequences of events in an exchange that is initiated by an AAC user. Breakdowns may also occur following an initiation by the speaking member of the dyad, but there are few empirical studies of these types of breakdowns. Hence, we focus on interactions initiated by an AAC user. Steps that appear in boxes represent communications by the AAC user. Steps that appear in circles represent communications by the partner. For example, suppose an AAC user gestures toward the refrigerator (an initiated communication act, represented in the top box). A communication partner might respond by looking at the refrigerator, then at the AAC user and asking, "What?" (represented in the left-hand side of the top-most circle). The AAC user may attempt to repair the exchange by handing her partner a symbol representing *drink* (a modification, represented by the middle box). The partner might respond by opening the refrigerator and offering a favorite beverage (represented by the left of the smaller circles, beneath the "Repair Attempts by AAC User" box). Finally, the AAC user might drink the beverage, smile, and otherwise depict satisfaction (represented by the bottom box). As indicated by the flowchart, any of several different communication breakdown types may be followed by any of several repair attempts. The next section describes the three types of communication breakdowns that are listed in Figure 10.1.

Differences in Types of Breakdowns

Assume that one member in a communication dyad initiates a communication act. Following that initiation, some type of communication breakdown may occur. The occurrences of communication breakdowns may be detected in the

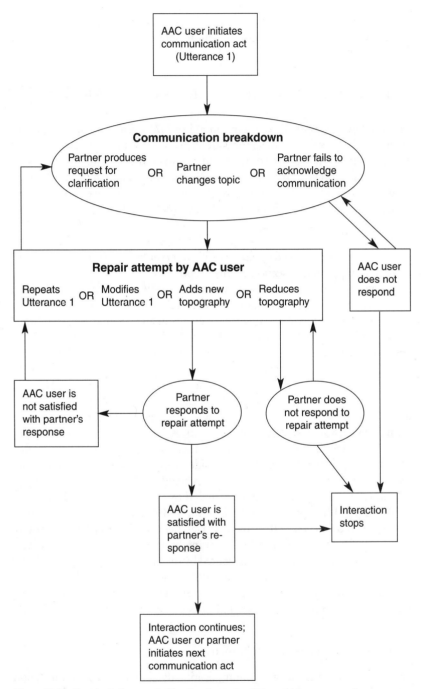

Figure 10.1. Flowchart of a conversational exchange in which an AAC user encounters a communication breakdown.

course of unscripted conversations (Golinkoff, 1986; Tomasello et al., 1990), or different types of breakdowns may be scripted into an interaction (Brady et al., 1995; Brinton, Fujiki, Loeb, & Winkler, 1986). We use the terms *requests for clarification, ignore,* and *topic shift* to describe three frequently encountered types of breakdowns. In this chapter's section on interactions between types of breakdowns and repairs, we discuss how interactions between these types of communication breakdowns and subsequent repair attempts may determine relative success in negotiating communication breakdowns.

Requests for Clarification   Requests for clarification (e.g., "What?" "Pardon?") are obvious indications that a breakdown in communication has occurred. Requests for clarification may be further broken down into specific and nonspecific requests. Saying "What?" would be an example of a nonspecific request, whereas asking, "Did you say ____?" (in which the blank indicates a particular word) would be considered a specific request (Paul & Cohen, 1984).

Ignore   In addition to requests for clarification, there are other types of communication breakdowns. For example, one member may basically ignore the communicative attempts of the partner. Conti-Ramsden, Hutcheson, and Grove (1995) and Tomasello and colleagues (1990) included the category of breakdown non-acknowledgments to describe these types of breakdowns. *Breakdown non-acknowledgment* is defined as the adult's failing to provide verbal or nonverbal acknowledgment of the child's utterance when one is seemingly needed. Similarly, Brady and colleagues (1995) included the category *ignore* to describe when the experimenter purposely ignored the participants' communicative attempts.

In actual conversations, it is likely that the breakdowns that we have placed in the ignore category are comprised of many subtypes. For example, a listener may ignore a speaker if he or she is preoccupied and does not realize that a communication act is directed toward him or her. Alternatively, a listener may ignore a speaker if he or she hears the speaker but would rather not comply with the speaker's utterance. A listener may also ignore a misunderstood utterance instead of requesting clarification. This last scenario seems most probable if the listener is not very motivated to understand the speaker or if the negotiation episode has proceeded for many turns without resolution.

Topic Shift   Another possible response to a communication attempt is to shift the topic. Although changing a topic is a vital part of conversation, some topic changes constitute communication breakdowns. A communication breakdown occurs if a child asks for help obtaining an object and his or her parent tries to redirect the child to a different object. This is considered a breakdown because the child's communication intent is not honored or acknowledged. Tomasello and colleagues (1990) used the term *breakdown topic shift* to refer to such occurrences. In their study, a breakdown topic shift was recorded when a parent replied to a child's utterance by changing the topic in a way that seemed to indicate a lack of comprehension. In some studies, researchers have found it difficult to determine whether topic shifts were due to a lack of comprehension or parents' trying to change topics even if they do understand their child's intent, so they have described both types of breakdowns as topic shifts (Bruegger, 2000; Pasek, 1999). Often in these studies, breakdowns that are categorized as a *breakdown topic shift* involved a partially unintelligible child utterance (Tomasello et al., 1990).

Similar to the breakdown topic shift category, Brady and colleagues (1995) used the category of *wrong response*. In the wrong response condition, the experimenter purposely violated the participant's apparent communicative intent. For example, if the participant seemed to request help in opening a container—first by trying to open the container and then by giving it to the experimenter—the experimenter might comment, "Yes, doesn't that look good?" Wilcox and Webster (1980) used a similar approach and referred to this condition as a *misunderstanding*. During the misunderstanding condition, the experimenter responded to requests as if the child was issuing a declarative (Wilcox & Webster, 1980).

Differences in Responsiveness to Types of Breakdowns   Some research suggests that individuals are likely to respond to certain breakdown types more often than they respond to others. For example, requests for clarification are particularly compelling (Gallagher & Darnton, 1978). Pragmatically speaking, requests for clarification demand a response, whereas the other types of breakdown do not necessarily demand a response (Garvey, 1977; Tomasello et al., 1990). That is, when a listener asks, "What?" or says, "I beg your pardon," the rules of conversation compel one to reply.

These rules of conversation may not necessarily apply with very young children or individuals who have developmental disabilities, however, because they may not comprehend the semantics or pragmatics of these rules. For example, Wilcox and Webster (1980) found significantly more responses to their misunderstanding condition than to nonspecific requests for clarification (i.e., "What?"). Participants in Wilcox and Webster's (1980) study were between 17 and 24 months of age and had expressive language equivalent to Brown's Stage I (Brown, 1973). Brady and colleagues (1995) found that more participants (all of whom had severe developmental disabilities and communicated with gestures) responded to the ignore condition than to the request for clarification condition, although this difference was not statistically significant.

Differences in Types of Repair Strategies

As shown in Figure 10.1, following any of the previously described types of communication breakdown, the speaker or AAC user may respond in a number of ways. The AAC user may not respond to the communication breakdown, or he or she may attempt to repair the failed communication. Based on data regarding speaking and gesturing dyads, we expect that most individuals will attempt to repair communication breakdowns (Wetherby et al., 1998).

Repetitions   Probably the most basic type of repair strategy is to repeat one's original utterance. Calculator and Delaney (1986) noted that exact repetitions were the most frequent type of communication repair strategy for both speakers and AAC users. Ansel and colleagues (1983) also found that speakers with dysarthria most often attempted to repair by repeating all or part of their original utterance. Bruegger (2000) found that at 13 and 24 months of age, speaking children used repetitions more often than attempting other repair strategies. Repetitions have not, however, been the most frequently observed strategies in most other studies of speaking dyads.

Modifications   Although many different terms and definitions have been used (e.g., *recasts, revisions, recodings, modifications*), a number of studies have found that repairs that somehow modified original utterances occurred more often than other repair types (Coggins & Stoel-Gammon, 1982; Furrow & Lewis, 1987; Gallagher, 1977; Golinkoff, 1986; Tomasello et al., 1990; Wetherby et al., 1998). For example, Coggins and Stoel-Gammon reported that the four children in their study, each of whose expressive language was at Brown Stage 1 (Brown, 1973), used revision most often during repair attempts. Revised utterances differed from their original utterances in phonology, syntax, or lexicon.

In Brady and colleagues' (1995) study of repairs by adults who used gestures and had severe developmental disabilities, recasts occurred more often than repetitions, or additions. In addition, recasts occurred more often than other repair types in Joyner's (1999) study of communication repairs by children with developmental disabilities between the ages of 4 and 6 years. The range of expressive communication observed in these children was from beginning gesture use to single word utterances. The preverbal participants in Golinkoff's (1986) study also modified original utterances more often than they repeated utterances. The differences between proportions of repetitions and modifications were not very great in Golinkoff's study, however. In their studies, Brady and colleagues (1995), Golinkoff (1986), and Joyner (1999) considered even slight modifications to be revisions. For example, a frequently occurring recast in the Brady and colleagues study was that a participant showed an object in his or her original communication act, then gave the object to the experimenter in his or her repair attempt. Thus, *recast* or *revision* may describe a change in the content of the message or a change in the form used to convey that message.

Additions and Reductions   In addition to the previously discussed types of repair strategies, some authors have described repairs in terms of the addition or reduction of a word, gesture, or symbol. Additions and/or reductions typically differ from modifications in that modifications substitute one form of responses for another. Additions add something new to the form of the original utterance, and reductions include a subset of the forms that were presented in the original utterance. For example, Brady and colleagues (1995) described repairs as *additions* when repair attempts added a gesture or vocalization that was not part of the original utterance to the original gesture or vocalization. Golinkoff (1986) used the term *augmentation* to describe repairs that were similar to Brady's *additions*.

In contrast to adding information, individuals may repair by subtracting aspects of their original utterance. Tomasello, Farrar, and Dines (1983) used the term *reduction* to describe repairs that were shorter than the participant's original utterances. The participants in Tomasello and colleagues' (1990) study were speaking children, but reductions can also be a category for nonverbal repairs. Bruegger (2000) identified repairs as *simplifications* if the child repaired by reducing the speech or gestures that were used in the original utterance. For example, a child may convey the original communication with a point plus vocalization but use only a point during the repair attempt.

Differences in Types of Repair Across Ages and Stages of Development   Most of the literature on communicative repairs in young children presumes that the mechanisms or processes that determine repairs emerge as children develop. Often, the dependent variables in these descriptive studies include the percentage of repairs in response to breakdowns. Furthermore, general categories of repair (e.g., repetitions, modifications) are assessed, and their developmental trajectories are monitored. There are at least two possible interpretations of observed differences in repairs at different ages. First, the changes may be due to some maturational or developmental trend. Second, motivational variables may account for the differences. Each possibility is explored in the following sections.

Developmental Trends   Alexander and colleagues (1997) examined repairs in four groups of typically developing children. Each group represented a different language stage (prelinguistic, early one-word, late one-word, and multiword), and there was a difference in mean age of 2–3 months between groups. One of their primary findings was that only 2 of the 120 participating children failed to repair—and these two children were 8-month-old infants. Alexander and colleagues also reported on developmental trends in the use of repetitions (increased from prelinguistic to early one-word, then decreased) and modifications for which the trends were the inverse of repetitions, generally increasing with age. Wetherby and colleagues (1998) concluded that the changes in repair types reported by Alexander and colleagues might reflect a developmental trend.

Similarly, Golinkoff (1986) reported that infants changed their repair types across three mealtime observations, completed at 12, 14, and 16 months of age. Significantly fewer substitutions were observed in the first observation, as compared with the second and third observations. By the third observation, the children were more likely to substitute a different communicative signal for the original signal. For example, a child may point in his or her initial communication attempt, then repair by naming the object. This type of repair would become possible because the child has developed a larger communicative repertoire, which includes words. Thus, a child who has a number of different strategies to ask for a cookie has more options for repairing a failed request for a cookie than a child who has only acquired two different means of requesting. The size of a participant's communication repertoire appears to be an important variable that affects communication repairs by beginning communicators. Other changes in linguistic abilities also seem to affect repairs. Gallagher (1977) observed that children who were more linguistically advanced revised by elaborating utterances more often than children who were less linguistically advanced. As children were able to use more advanced language and phonology, their repairs reflected these skills.

Concomitant with these changes in linguistic abilities are changes in children's social development (Adamson & Bakeman, 1985; Bates, Bretherton, Beeghly-Smith, & McNew, 1982; Franco & Butterworth, 1996; Snow, 1991). Children become increasingly adept at taking another person's perspective during an interaction (Bretherton, McNew, & Beeghly-Smith, 1981). These social developments seem germane to the development of repair skills. It is reasonable to assume that children will better identify and repair the cause of a communication breakdown when they are able to consider their partner's perspective in the interaction. Golinkoff's (1986) finding that substitutions increase with age may reflect not only an increase in verbal repertoire but also an increase in perspective taking. Developments of perspective taking are difficult to measure, however, particularly in beginning communicators. An additional problem in identifying social developmental bases for repairs is that other powerful variables interact with developments in linguistic and social behaviors, such as the child's motivation level.

Motivational Variables   Motivational logic is an alternative to the developmental logic that was presumed in the previously described studies. That is, children may be more likely to repair communication breakdowns when their motivation regarding the intended outcome is high. According to this explanation, a child would not repair unless he or she is sufficiently motivated to produce another response or the intended outcome is worth the effort that is required to respond.

Support for the motivational logic can be found in the Alexander and colleagues (1997) study. There were no differences between the percentages of breakdowns responded to by the prelinguistic and the late one-word groups—both failed to repair on 12% of the occasions presented. In addition, the group that had the least number of nonresponses was the one-word group, whose members' mean age was younger than 15 months—not the oldest group at the multiword stage. These findings do not represent a smooth developmental trajectory and might be better explained by focusing on the specific occasions presented and by determining the reinforcing value of these occasions for each participant.

Similarly, findings by Brinton, Fujiki, Winkler, and Loeb (1986) could be explained by motivational variables instead of development of persistence. Brinton and colleagues (1986) presented stacked requests for clarification to children who were 5–9 years old and had language learning disabilities. The authors studied the results of the children's repairs and found that the children produced more inappropriate responses or failed attempts to the second and third clarification requests than their typically developing peers. The authors interpreted the findings as evidence that children with less developed language may lack the persistence that is needed to respond repeatedly to the stacked clarification requests. Another possibility is that the study participants lacked motivation to persist.

If we stop to consider situations in which speaking adults persist, clearly motivation plays a role. If a woman suspects that she has just won the lottery and is calling to confirm the winning number, she is likely to persist in asking the official to repeat the number until she is sure that she heard correctly. In other circumstances, however, the likelihood that one will persist in negotiating communication breakdowns depends on specific conditions. For example, if a person asks his or her boss for a raise and the request is rejected, the person's decision about whether to persist depends on many factors (e.g., his or her belief that the raise is deserved, his or her relationship with the boss, a history of the boss's decisions—are they final, or are they characterized by "waffling"?). In addition, the person's need for the raise will likely affect his or her motivation to persist.

This concern about motivation is crucial to the entire literature on communicative repairs and persistence. It implies that a critical control procedure is necessary to examine repairs: The motivational value of the communicative exchange (i.e., what the speaker intends or anticipates as an outcome) needs to be equated. When motivation or reinforcing value is not controlled, then a failure to repair may be due to one's inability (lack of readiness) to repair or it may be due to low motivation. It may not be worth another response to produce the intended effect. Such an interpretation becomes even more probable in stacked breakdown sequences because greater effort and additional responses are required of the child. Rather than invoking failure to persist as a developmental explanation, a more parsimonious alternative might be that it is not worth the time and effort to maintain the exchange. This analysis of response effort is similar to that described in research on the matching law discussed in Chapter 4.

Some evidence that supports the importance of motivation emanates from findings of differences in responsiveness across different communicative functions. Cirrin and Rowland (1985); McLean, McLean, Brady, and Etter (1991); and others have found that individuals with severe mental retardation are more likely to respond to opportunities to request than to respond to opportunities to comment. The motivation for a request is gaining access to a desired item or event, whereas the motivation for a comment is to maintain social interaction. Social interaction may not be reinforcing for many individuals with developmental disabilities. Even typically developing children have been observed to repair more breakdowns following requests than following comments (Shatz & O'Reilly, 1990). Another possible explanation for decreased repairs in commenting situations is that the repair is not necessary to obtain reinforcement. Given that the reinforcer for commenting is social interaction, it may not be as important to repair because the communicator maintains social interaction, even if the listener does not attend to the precise comment (J. Light, 2000, personal communication).

INTERACTIONS BETWEEN TYPES OF BREAKDOWNS AND REPAIR

In addition to changes across developmental periods, different response types have been linked to different types of breakdown conditions (Anselmi et al., 1986; Brady et al., 1995; Furrow & Lewis, 1987; Garvey, 1977; Wilcox & Webster, 1980). That is, participants have been found to attempt different types of repairs following different types of breakdowns. This has been noted as an important indication that participants in these studies not only attempted to repair communication breakdowns, but they also tried to tailor their repairs according to the source of a communication breakdown. Fey, Warr-Leeper, Webber, and Disher (1988) summarized research from young speaking children and concluded that different request types determine the forms of clarification attempted. For example, Anselmi and colleagues (1986) found that children at Brown Stage II of language development (Brown, 1973; mean length of utterance = 2.0 to 2.5) repeated more following a nonspecific request for clarification (e.g., "What?") and provided specific missing information more often following a specific request for clarification (e.g., "What color did you say?").

Differences have also been reported in beginning communicators. Brady and colleagues (1995) compared different repair types in response to five different breakdowns conditions:

1. The experimenter ignored the communication attempt while pretending to be occupied with another activity.

2. The experimenter ignored the communication attempt but attended to the participant.
3. The experimenter requested clarification.
4. The experimenter shrugged.
5. The experimenter responded inappropriately according to the apparent intent of the participant.

The authors categorized repairs as repetitions, recasts, or additions. They found that significantly fewer additions occurred in response to the ignore condition than in the other breakdown conditions. This finding suggests that even participants with very limited communication repertoires may adapt their repair strategy to suit the perceived source of breakdown.

What would it mean if someone did not tailor his or her repair strategy according to the perceived source of breakdown? This lack of fine tuning could be interpreted as a *pragmatic disability*—that is, a disability in the way an individual socially uses language. Geller (1998) noted that children with autism tended to attempt to repair communication breakdowns but failed to add specific linguistic information to clarify their original message. Paul and Cohen (1984) found that participants with autism were significantly less likely to give a specific response to a request for clarification than participants with mental retardation. Similarly, Calculator and Delaney (1986) found that their participants with developmental disabilities most frequently repaired by repeating their original utterances rather than trying a different way to communicate.

Thus, it appears that, in these studies, many communicators with developmental disabilities responded to communication breakdowns, but they did not respond differentially to different types of communication breakdowns. This nondifferential responding may hinder success in negotiating communication breakdowns. In reference to Figure 10.1, it may be that following specific signals for repair (presented in the circles) with specific types of repairs (presented in the boxes) results in more efficient, successful communication. For example, it may be most efficacious to repeat one's utterance following a nonspecific contingent query, whereas it may be best to add a vocalization following an ignored utterance. Research is needed to determine whether individuals who are learning to use AAC respond differntially to different types of breakdowns. This type of research has the potential to discover appropriate intervention targets for facilitating negotiations of communication breakdowns.

Response Classes and Conversational Repairs

How does a beginning communicator learn to use a specific repair strategy in response to particular breakdowns? Once again, an operant learning paradigm may be useful in addressing this question. When differing responses such as vocalizing, reaching, gesturing, or handing a picture all produce the same functional outcome (e.g., obtaining a drink of water), then the responses are said to constitute a response class. The notion of *response class* provokes an important question: If differing responses share the same function, then why is one particular member of the class selected relative to the others? In a sense, the different members compete with one another. In situations similar to the current one, the response that has proven to be most efficient is the one that is most likely to be selected. Mace and Horner and their colleagues have elaborated some of the criteria that determine response efficiency (Horner & Day, 1991; Lalli, Mace, Wohn, & Livezey, 1995). These include 1) immediacy, quality, and schedule of reinforcement and 2) the physical and cognitive effort that is required to make the response. Horner and Day (1991) demonstrated that when any variable that determines efficiency is manipulated, the members of the class change in probability of occurrence. For example, a newly taught response became the most probable member when it 1) required less effort than the other members, 2) produced reinforcement on a richer schedule than the other members, or 3) produced more immediate reinforcement than the other members.

The implications of the response class notion for repairs are direct and pervasive. Conceptually, the notion that varying responses exist in a child's repertoire and compete with one another, depending on the exigencies of any particular situation, is novel and potentially explanatory. Clinically, this notion provides a strategy for intervention such that particular members of the class might be selected intentionally to receive an immediate response from listeners, thus strengthening the response, whereas others might intentionally be ignored or extinguished, thus weakening the response.

In the case of challenging behaviors, a new response (e.g., pointing to a picture in a communication book) might be taught as a replacement for disruptive behavior. This may circumvent the need for a disruptive repair attempt such as screaming. Baer (1981) discussed the imposition of a model for the structure of behavior by including a description of response classes. He described positively and negatively co-occurring classes in which the probability of occurrence of all the members varied either directly or inversely. That is, when the rate of one member in the class is changed, other members' rates will change in either the same or the opposite direction. Repair is a case of a negatively co-occurring response class because when one member is strengthened, other members are weakened (under the same conditions or in the same context). Lalli and colleagues (1995) provided an empirical demonstration of a response class hierarchy that was composed of problem behavior. The authors found that the members were organized in a sequence such that a therapist's response to an early member in the sequence meant that later members rarely occurred. A response to a later member, however, meant that earlier members were consistently produced. There may be a number of situations in which an individual uses different members of the same class of repair behaviors because of their past history of success.

SUCCESS OF REPAIR STRATEGIES

Some repair strategies appear to be more successful in negotiating particular breakdown episodes. That is, when individuals use particular repair strategies, they may be more likely to obtain their desired result. For example, children may be more likely to obtain the food item they are requesting if they repair by adding a pointing gesture to their vocalization. The pointing gesture serves to specify the referent. Similarly, beginning communicators may be more likely to obtain something (e.g., a drink of water) when their repair attempts include screaming (see Example 5, presented at the beginning of this chapter). In these scenarios, success is equivalent to efficiency in obtaining what one wants. Thus, a more efficient negotiation episode would be judged as more successful. Measures such as the number of repairs preceding the successful outcome or the time required to negotiate the communication breakdown would be helpful in comparing the efficiency of different repair strategies. Variables that seem likely to influence the efficiency of a repair include the previously discussed variables of an individual's motivation to obtain the end result and the response effort that is required to repair.

An additional variable that contributes to the relative success of different repair strategies is the history of interactions between members of the dyad. Two listeners may be equally familiar to a child, yet depending on the child's history of listener responsiveness to repairs, the child may produce one type of repair in the presence of Listener 1 and a second type in the presence of Listener 2. This can be explained easily by listeners' differential responses to particular repair topographies (see the previous discussion about response class). An example may be instructive. Imagine a mother who is quite responsive to Paul, her 5-year-old son with autism. When she does not understand his first signal, she extends her hand to allow Paul to lead her to the item he wants. Now imagine a teacher who has 20 students, including Paul. When Paul first signals, his teacher is busy, and although she hears his vocalization, she cannot attend to it immediately. He soon begins to scream. At this point, the teacher stops what she is doing and accompanies Paul to the object of his request. If this pattern of differential responding by Paul's mother and teacher is repeated over and over, Paul may learn to repair differently with his mother and his preschool teacher. Paul's "success" will depend on his ability to discriminate the appropriate repair strategy to use with each listener.

Successful conversations are not always reflected in efficiency in obtaining wants, however. Light (1988) pointed out that if one views the goal of conversation as maintaining social interactions through extended conversations, then lengthy negotiation episodes would be considered a strength. AAC users have been observed to have shorter interactions than speaking communicators. Calculator and Dollaghan (1982) observed shorter exchanges between dyads composed of AAC users than between dyads composed of two speakers. One reason for shorter interactions may be that dyads with AAC users do not participate in lengthy episodes to negotiate communication breakdowns. For example, an AAC user may attempt once or twice to repair a failed communication attempt, but he or she is not as likely to enter into an extensive exchange in which both members of the dyad actively attempt to determine the specific nature of the communication breakdown. Such exchanges are limited to situations in which one or both members of the dyad are extremely motivated to negotiate the communication breakdown.

To lengthen interactions, it may be beneficial to teach children who use AAC to ask for clarification by providing clear signals that a communication breakdown has occurred. O'Keefe and Dattilo (1992) taught three adults, who had mental retardation and communicated by selecting graphic symbols on communication boards, to follow their responses to questions with another question. For example, when asked, "What's your name?", participants were taught to answer with a response such as, "Nancy. What's yours?" The goal of this intervention was to increase the length of interactions between AAC users and their speaking partners. All three participants increased their use of this strategy during intervention. Strategies similar to this could be used that teach AAC users to recruit requests for clarification. For example, AAC users could periodically end their utterance with the question, "Do you understand?"

EDUCATIONAL IMPLICATIONS

Research is still needed to explore how communication breakdowns and repairs influence AAC users' communication success. Nevertheless, education planners may benefit from considering some of the points discussed in this chapter. For example, it seems beneficial not only to evaluate an AAC user's skills in initiating communication and responding to others but also to evaluate the communicator's skills in repairing communication breakdowns. Both the unscripted observations and scripted interaction methods discussed in this chapter should prove useful as part of such assessment.

If an AAC user seldom attempts to repair communication breakdowns, then it seems appropriate to target repair strategies in intervention. Furthermore, an educator's evaluation might indicate that an AAC user always employs one repair strategy, such as repeating his or her original communication, regardless of differences in types of communication breakdown. In this case, it might be beneficial to teach the learner to try different repair strategies under different conditions.

In addition, educators may wish to review this chapter's discussions about working with children and older individuals who have challenging behaviors. An analysis of the conditions that surround challenging behavior could indicate that the behavior occurs when other communication attempts fail. In such a case, interventions should focus not only on teaching more appropriate alternative behavior but also on increasing partner responsiveness to earlier communication attempts.

CONCLUSION

The literature reviewed in this chapter provides evidence that individuals at all levels of communicative proficiency will attempt to repair communication breakdowns. These repair attempts appear to reflect persistence in communicating. This persistence is critical to communicative success and development.

We have also described differences in the repair strategies that beginning communicators use when faced with different types of communication breakdowns. Although these strategies differ in form from the types of repairs that speaking individuals issue, we have shown that beginning communicators, including beginning AAC users, will often attempt to repair in much the same way as speakers. That is, sometimes they repeat their utterances, and other times they modify the form of their utterances or add additional forms to their original communication attempt.

We have gone one step further and attempted to explain how an individual learns to use these different repair strategies in different breakdown conditions. Theoretically, individuals may learn to use different responses in different breakdown contexts in the same way that individuals learn to select responses from a response class: through processes of differential reinforcement. Research is needed to investigate this theory. The results of such research may demonstrate how individuals can learn to use different repair strategies in the face of different types of communication breakdowns or with different communication partners. Because some repair strategies are deemed unsatisfactory, such as challenging behavior repairs, efforts to teach replacement strategies are worthwhile.

Research that demonstrates how to teach effective repair strategies should advance efforts toward improving AAC users' conversational interactions. Although negotiating conversation breakdowns is but one aspect of maintaining conversation, it is a necessary aspect in light of the frequency with which AAC dyads encounter communication breakdowns.

REFERENCES

Adamson, L.B., & Bakeman, R. (1985). Affect and attention: Infants observed with mothers and peers. *Child Development, 56,* 582–593.

Alexander, D., Wetherby, A., & Prizant, B. (1997). The emergence of repair strategies in infants and toddlers. *Seminars in Speech and Language, 18*(3), 197–212.

Ansel, B.M., McNeil, M.R., Hunker, C.J., & Bless, D.M. (1983). The frequency of verbal and acoustic adjustments used by cerebral palsied dysarthric adults when faced with communicative failure. In W.R. Berry (Ed.), *Clinical dysarthria* (pp. 85–106). San Diego: College-Hill Press.

Anselmi, D., Tomasello, M., & Acunzo, M. (1986). Young children's responses to neutral and specific contingent queries. *Journal of Child Language, 13,* 135–144.

Baer, D. (1981). The imposition of structure on behavior and the demolition of behavioral structures. In R. Dienstbier (Ed.), *Nebraska symposium on motivation* (Vol. 29, pp. 217–254). Lincoln: University of Nebraska Press.

Bates, E., Benigni, L., Bretherton, I., Camaioni, L., & Volterra, V. (1979). *The emergence of symbols: Cognition and communication in infancy.* San Diego: Academic Press.

Bates, E., Bretherton, I., Beeghly-Smith, M., & McNew, S. (1982). Social bases of language development: A reassessment. In H.W. Reese & L.P. Lipseitt (Eds.), *Advances in child development and behavior* (pp. 7–75). San Diego: Academic Press.

Beukelman, D.R., & Mirenda, P. (1998). *Augmentative and alternative communication: Management of severe communication disorders in children and adults* (2nd ed.). Baltimore: Paul H. Brookes Publishing Co.

Brady, N.C., McLean, J.E., McLean, L.K., & Johnston, S. (1995). Initiation and repair of intentional communication acts by adults with severe to profound cognitive disabilities. *Journal of Speech and Hearing Research, 38,* 1334–1348.

Bretherton, I., McNew, S., & Beeghly-Smith, M. (1981). Early person knowledge as expressed in gestural and verbal communication: When do infants acquire a "theory of mind"? In M.E. Lamb & L.R. Sherrod (Eds.), *Infant social cognition: Empirical and theoretical considerations.* Mahwah, NJ: Lawrence Erlbaum Associates.

Brinton, B., & Fujiki, M. (1989). *Conversational management with language-impaired children.* Gaithersburg, MD: Aspen Publishers.

Brinton, B., & Fujiki, M. (1991). Responses to requests for conversational repair by adults with mental retardation. *Journal of Speech and Hearing Research, 34,* 1087–1095.

Brinton, B., Fujiki, M., Loeb, D.F., & Winkler, E. (1986). Development of conversational repair strategies in response to requests for clarification. *Journal of Speech and Hearing Research, 29,* 75–81.

Brinton, B., Fujiki, M., Winkler, E., & Loeb, D. (1986). Responses to requests for clarification in linguistically normal and language-impaired children. *Journal of Speech and Hearing Disorders, 51,* 370–378.

Brown, R. (1973). *A first language: The early stages.* Cambridge, MA: Harvard University Press.

Bruegger, A. (2000). *Communication breakdowns and repairs by children at 13 and 24 months of age.* Unpublished manuscript, University of Minnesota, Minneapolis.

Buzolich, M.J., & Wiemann, J.M. (1988). Turn taking in atypical conversations: The case of the speaker/augmented-communicator dyad. *Journal of Speech and Hearing Research, 31,* 3–18.

Calculator, S., & Dollaghan, C. (1982). The use of communication boards in a residential setting: An evaluation. *Journal of Speech and Hearing Disorders, 47,* 281–287.

Calculator, S.N., & Delaney, D. (1986). Comparison of nonspeaking and speaking mentally retarded adults' clarification strategies. *Journal of Speech and Hearing Disorders, 51,* 252–259.

Carr, E.G., & Durand, V.M. (1985). Reducing behavior problems through functional communication training. *Journal of Applied Behavior Analysis, 18,* 111–126.

Catania, A.C. (1984). *Learning.* Upper Saddle River, NJ: Prentice Hall.

Ciocci, S.R., & Baran, J.A. (1998). The use of conversational repair strategies by children who are deaf. *American Annals of the Deaf, 143*(3), 235–245.

Cirrin, F.M., & Rowland, C.M. (1985). Communicative assessment of nonverbal youths with severe/profound mental retardation. *Mental Retardation, 23,* 52–62.

Coggins, T.E., & Stoel-Gammon, C. (1982). Clarification strategies used by four Down's syndrome children for maintaining normal conversational interaction. *Education and Training of the Mentally Retarded, 17,* 65–67.

Conti-Ramsden, G., Hutcheson, G.D., & Grove, J. (1995). Contingency and breakdown: Children with SLI and their conversations with mothers and fathers. *Journal of Speech and Hearing Research, 38,* 1290–1302.

Farrier, L.D., Yorkston, K.M., Marriner, N.A., & Beukelman, D.R. (1985). Conversational control in nonimpaired speakers using an augmentative communication system. *Augmentative and Alternative Communication, 1,* 65–73.

Fey, M.E., Warr-Leeper, G., Webber, S.A., & Disher, L.M. (1988). Repairing children's repairs: Evaluation and facilitation of children's clarification requests and responses. *Topics in Language Disorders, 8*(2), 63–84.

Franco, F., & Butterworth, G. (1996). Pointing and social awareness: Declaring and requesting in the second year. *Journal of Child Language, 23,* 307–336.

Furrow, D., & Lewis, S. (1987). The role of the initial utterance in contingent query sequences: Its influence on responses to requests for clarification. *Journal of Child Language, 14,* 467–479.

Gallagher, T. (1977). Revision behaviors in the speech of normal children developing language. *Journal of Speech and Hearing Research, 20,* 303–318.

Gallagher, T.M., & Darnton, B.A. (1978). Conversational aspects of the speech of language-disordered children: Revision behaviors. *Journal of Speech and Hearing Research, 21,* 118–135.

Garvey, C. (1977). The contingent query: A dependent act in conversation. In M. Lewis & L.A. Rosenblum (Eds.), *Interaction, conversation, and the development of language* (pp. 63–93). New York: John Wiley & Sons.

Geller, E. (1998). An investigation of communication breakdowns and repairs in verbal autistic children. *The British Journal of Developmental Disabilities, 44*(87), 71–85.

Golinkoff, R.M. (1986). 'I beg your pardon?' The preverbal negotiation of failed messages. *Journal of Child Language, 13,* 455–476.

Horner, R.H., & Carr, E.G. (1997). Behavioral support for students with severe disabilities: Functional assessment and comprehensive intervention. *Journal of Special Education, 31,* 84–104.

Horner, R.H., & Day, H.M. (1991). The effects of response efficiency on functionally equivalent competing behaviors. *Journal of Applied Behavior Analysis, 24*(4), 719–732.

Iverson, J.M., & Thal, D.J. (1998). Communicative transitions: There's more to the hand than meets the eye. In S.F. Warren & J. Reichle (Series Eds.) & A.M. Wetherby, S.F. Warren, & J. Reichle (Vol. Eds.), *Communication and language intervention series: Vol. 7. Transitions in prelinguistic communication* (pp. 59–86). Baltimore: Paul H. Brooks Publishing Co.

Joyner, J. (1999). *Communication repairs of children with severe language impairments during play.* Unpublished manuscript, University of Minnesota, Minneapolis.

Lalli, J., Mace, F.C., Wohn, T., & Livezey, K. (1995). Identification and modification of a response-class hierarchy. *Journal of Applied Behavior Analysis, 28,* 551–559.

Light, J. (1988). Interaction involving individuals using augmentative and alternative communication systems: State of the art and future directions. *Augmentative and Alternative Communication, 4,* 66–82.

Light, J., Collier, B., & Parnes, P. (1985). Communicative interaction between young nonspeaking physically disabled children and their primary caregivers: Part II– Communicative functions. *AAC Augmentative and Alternative Communication, 1,* 98–107.

McLean, J.E., McLean, L.K.S., Brady, N.C., & Etter, R. (1991). Communication profiles of two types of gesture using nonverbal persons with severe to profound mental retardation. *Journal of Speech and Hearing Research, 34,* 294–308.

Newman, L.L., & Smit, A.B. (1989). Some effects of variations in response time latency on speech rate, interruptions, and fluency in children's speech. *Journal of Speech and Hearing Research, 32,* 635–644.

O'Keefe, M., & Dattilo, J. (1992). Teaching the response-recode form to adults with mental retardation using AAC systems. *Augmentative and Alternative Communication, 8,* 224–233.

O'Neill, R.E., Horner, R.H., Albin, R., Sprague, J., Storey, K., & Newton, J.S. (1997). *Functional assessment and program development of problem behavior: A practical handbook.* Pacific Grove, CA: Brooks/Cole Thomson Learning.

Pasek, M. (1999). *Communication repair strategies of typically developing children.* Unpublished manuscript, University of Minnesota, Minneapolis.

Paul, R., & Cohen, D. J. (1984). Responses to contingent queries in adults with mental retardation and pervasive developmental disorders. *Applied Psycholinguistics, 5,* 349–357.

Reichle, J., & Wacker, D.P. (Vol. Eds.). (1993). *Communication and language intervention series: Vol. 3. Communicative alternatives to challenging behavior: Integrating functional assessment and intervention strategies.* Baltimore: Paul H. Brookes Publishing Co.

Rotholz, D.A., Berkowitz, S.F., & Burberry, J. (1989). Functionality of two modes of communication in the community by students with developmental disabilities: A comparison of signing and communication books. *The Journal of The Association for Persons with Severe Handicaps, 14,* 227–233.

Shatz, M., & O'Reilly, A.W. (1990). Conversational or communicative skill? A reassessment of two-year-olds' behaviour in miscommunication episodes. *Journal of Child Language, 17,* 131–146.

Skinner, B.F. (1957). *Verbal behavior.* New York: Appleton-Century-Crofts.

Snow, C.E. (1991). The language of the mother–child relationship. In M. Woodhead, R. Carr, & P. Light (Eds.), *Becoming a person* (pp. 195–210). New York: Routledge.

Tomasello, M., Conti-Ramsden, G., & Ewert, B. (1990). Young children's conversations with their mothers and fathers: Differences in breakdown and repair. *Journal of Child Language, 17,* 115–130.

Tomasello, M., Farrar, J., & Dines, J. (1983). Young children's speech revisions for a familiar and an unfamiliar adult. *Journal of Speech and Hearing Research, 27,* 359–363.

Wetherby, A.M., Alexander, D.G., & Prizant, B.M. (1998). The ontogeny and role of repair strategies. In S.F. Warren & J. Reichle (Series Eds.) & A.M. Wetherby, S.F. Warren, & J. Reichle (Vol. Eds.), *Communication and language intervention series: Vol. 7. Transitions in prelinguistic communication* (pp. 135–159). Baltimore: Paul H. Brookes Publishing Co.

Wilcox, M.J., & Webster, E.J. (1980). Early discourse behavior: An analysis of children's responses to listener feedback. *Child Development, 51,* 1120–1125.

11

Visual Assessment
Considerations for the Design of AAC Systems

Bonnie L. Utley

Successful design of augmentative and alternative communication (AAC) systems for beginning communicators must accommodate the full range of physical and sensory characteristics presented by each learner. This chapter has three purposes: 1) to review multiple dimensions of sensory functioning that apply to beginning communicators who may be undergoing consideration for an AAC system, 2) to provide an overview of essential information regarding common physical and sensory characteristics that affect the design of AAC for some of the most challenging beginning communicators—those with combined physical and sensory disabilities, and 3) to share a sequence of critical questions and corresponding assessment methods that relate to the design of AAC for beginning communicators with severe or multiple disabilities. The critical questions and sample assessment procedures are intended to illustrate a systematic and scientific approach to the design of personalized AAC systems. The process of conducting multiple assessments on a series of observable visual responses, followed by collective interpretation of results within the framework of a collaborative team, serves as an example of inquiry in action. In the case of AAC design, the process of posing and answering a personalized set of questions regarding a beginning communicator's sensory and physical functioning may be a useful framework for team members as they strive to support each learner's entry into successful communication.

This chapter is based on a series of assumptions that must underlie the deliberations of team members as they proceed through assessment and decision making. These assumptions fall into three distinct areas: 1) assumptions regarding the existence of a positive, working relationship among two or more

---

This chapter is meant to supplement, not supplant, the expertise of an ophthalmologist, optometrist, neurologist, and/or other medical professional.

team members and medical professionals who specialize in visual impairments; 2) assumptions regarding the composition of the team of school professionals who serve the learner and his or her family; and 3) assumptions regarding the background knowledge of the beginning communicator that each team member brings to the decision-making process regarding the personalized design of an AAC system. These three overaching assumptions are detailed next.

Assumptions regarding the existence of a positive working relationship among two or more team members and medical professionals who specialize in visual impairments:

• Team members have productive working relationships with medical professionals, as the assessment data and hypotheses generated by these procedures are *not* diagnostic but informational in nature.

• Assessment results obtained from these procedures permit team members to make informed judgments about important AAC decisions such as eye preference, preferred distance of visual regard, and the arrangement of symbols on a display surface. These judgments, however, must always be considered as working hypotheses that are subject to ongoing data collection and analysis, as well as the input of medical professionals.

• The knowledge and skills that may be acquired as a function of this chapter permit team members to be better informed regarding the complexity of the visual system and its interaction with posture and movement in some of the most challenging beginning communicators. It is hoped that this information will lead team members to advocate for ongoing, rigorous treatment of visual disorders as appropriate.

Assumptions regarding the composition of the team of school professionals who serve the learner and his or her family:

• Team members share a common set of values that underlie their work. These values include a commitment to be learner centered and family friendly, as well as a willingness to adopt multiple processes of inquiry (including both quantitative and qualitative elements) in the evaluation of their efforts to design, implement, and modify AAC systems.

• The team is comprised of professionals who possess in-depth knowledge and skills within their own disciplines, as well as a disposition toward sharing their respective discipline-referenced frameworks with their fellow team members (Utley & Rapport, 2000).

• The team operates through consensus decision making rather than democratic or autocratic processes, and members cultivate the use of strong interpersonal skills to resolve conflict as it arises.

• Team members defer to one anothers' discipline-referenced frameworks as suggested by the results of data collection and interpretation and/or as suggested by regulatory and legal guidelines (Rapport, 1995).

Assumptions regarding the background knowledge of the beginning communicator that each team member brings to the decision-making process:

- All team members conduct their own discipline-referenced assessments that contribute to a thorough understanding of the beginning communicator *prior* to entering the decision-making process regarding the design of a personalized ACC system.
- The team commits to having two or more members concurrently conduct the assessment procedures described in this chapter. This collaborative process permits multiple frames of reference (and the resulting alternative interpretations of various learner behaviors) to be identified and resolved (Campbell, 2000; Dunn, 1996).

Many beginning communicators have complex learning characteristics. It is only through the collective expertise of a well-functioning team that the best hope for a successful AAC system can be realized. To that end, this chapter content is organized into three sections. The first section provides an overview of some of the sensory skills that team members who design AAC should assess. These skills include fixation; tracking, scanning, and gaze shift; and considerations regarding the interpretation of atypical posture and patterns of visual regard that are common to many beginning communicators. The first section addresses these postural and sensory responses in the absence of neuromuscular involvement (i.e., the abnormal muscle tone and reflex activity often associated with a label "cerebral palsy"). Assessment for these students is conducted for the purpose of verifying the presence or absence of these selected visual and visual-motor skills, with follow-up intervention to support development of necessary skills. If intervention on visual and visual-motor skills is indicated as a result of careful assessment, then it should occur within the context of functional routines. In this way, visual and visual-motor skills are developed as embedded skills, which are necessary to ensure partial or full participation in meaningful tasks, as opposed to isolated sensory responses (Guess & Helmstetter, 1986; Silberman, Sacks, & Wolfe, 1998; Utley & Nelson, 1992; Utley, Roman, & Nelson, 1998).

The second section of the chapter addresses common physical characteristics that complicate sensory functioning for beginning communicators and challenge team members as they plan personalized AAC systems. The second section includes an overview of environmental considerations that may affect the success of a system. These include overall positioning, including seating and head support, as well as lighting.

The third and final section describes a model of assessment and decision making that is based on a series of critical questions. These critical questions are accompanied by a number of sample assessment procedures that may serve as a guide for team members as they address specific design features of an AAC system. Also included are suggested data sheets and guidelines for interpreting the data that are generated through implementation of this model.

GENERAL SENSORY
CHARACTERISTICS OF BEGINNING COMMUNICATORS

Learners who need an AAC system may have been assigned a number of diagnostic labels that pertain to cognitive limitations (e.g., mental retardation, autism and other pervasive developmental disorders), as well as labels that are specific to physical disabilities (e.g., cerebral palsy) and visual impairments (e.g., strabismus). Many learners have been given multiple diagnostic labels. For beginning communicators without severe limitations in posture and movement, a number of sensory skills that contribute to effective AAC use are easily documented by using a variety of informal and formal measures. Team members can determine whether a particular beginning communicator has typical sensory functioning through direct observation and careful review of medical records. The visual behaviors to be documented are listed as a series of questions in Table 11.1.

Table 11.1.   Categories of observation and sample questions to determine whether a learner has typical sensory skills

Category 1: Overall appearance of eyes

Do the learner's eyes appear clear with pupils of equal size?

Do the learner's eyes appear to be free of discharge?

Category 2: Orientation and mobility

Does the learner visually regard novel and familiar objects that are located within an area that is bound by the width of the shoulders and the length of the arms?

Does the learner move toward or away from objects, events, or people in his or her environment?

Doe the learner avoid obstacles in his or her path?

Category 3: Coordinated movement of both eyes

Do the learner's eyes move freely within the bony orbits of the skull?

Do the eyes move together to view objects, events, or people in the environment at mid-line? (Note: If the eyes are coordinated, viewing a stimulus at mid-line closer than a few feet distant will produce convergence of the two eyes [i.e., both eyes roll nasally].)

Do the eyes move together to view objects, events, or people to either side of mid-line? (Note: If the eyes are coordinated, viewing an object to the left or right of mid-line without head movement in the same direction will produce eye movements that are parallel [i.e., to view an object to the right side of mid-line, the right eye moves temporally and the left eye moves nasally].)

Category 4: Visual-motor behaviors

Does the learner engage in tracking, scanning, and gaze shift?

Does the learner reach and touch objects accurately?

Does the learner transport objects through space and release those objects accurately?

Table 11.2 provides definitions and examples of visual and visual-motor skills that are essential to AAC access. Of particular relevance to AAC decision making is the visual-motor skill *scanning*, which is essential to a beginning communicator's ability to engage in choice making.

A second essential skill for successful access to AAC is visual tracking. Beginning communicators must be able to watch the actions of peers and adults in the communication environment. Askvig's (1990) work is a fine supplementary source for guidance in these two areas; it provides detailed instructions regarding the assessment of scanning on a series of "mock" communication displays. The display surfaces include samples ranging from 3 to 8 visual stimuli so that a beginning communicator's ability to scan a range of different arrays can be assessed. The procedures described can be modified to document an early communicator's ability to respond visually to switch location, object cues, or the position in space of a potential communication partner (either a peer or an adult). Johnson, Baumgart, Helmstetter, and Curry (1996) extended Askvig's efforts to include a data sheet designed to document tracking skills, as well as a summary of a learner's ability to scan. Many of the general assessment tools for young children—such as the Bayley (1969), Dunst's (1980) work on the Uzgiris and Hunt Scales of Infant Psychological Development, and the HELP: Hawaii Early Learning Profile (VORT Corporation, 1995)—also address a series of additional, more general assessment

Table 11.2.   Definitions and examples of selected visual and visual-motor skills

Term	Definition
Fixation	Actively aligns the line of sight (i.e., the visual axis) of one or both eyes on a stationary object or person
	Example:
	Looks at an object cue that represents *art class*
Scanning	Visually searches for an object or person among a display of visual stimuli
	Example:
	Looks sequentially at the row of numerals on a number line affixed to the desk to locate the numeral 5
Tracking	Visually follows a moving stimulus
	Example:
	Watches continuously as the lunchroom employee ladles chili into the bowl
Gaze Shift	Shifts visual fixation in space from one visual stimulus to another
	Example:
	Looks first at one photograph and then another on the bulletin board display of class members

From Utley, B.L. (1994). Providing support for sensory, postural, and movement needs. In L. Sternberg (Ed.), *Individuals with profound disabilities* (3rd ed., pp. 132). Austin, TX: PRO-ED; adapted by permission.

procedures for many of the visual and visual-motor skills that are listed in Tables 11.1 and 11.2. These assessment resources are extremely helpful in guiding decision making for beginning communicators whose visual skills are typical (i.e., not interfered by delayed or absent head control, abnormal muscle tone, or reflex activity).

In addition to assessment of the visual and visual-motor skills described in Tables 11.1 and 11.2, a related area that may influence AAC decision making for teams of school professionals is the posture and form of visual regard that is adopted by some beginning communicators. Examples include beginning communicators who prefer to view an object or communication partner by adjusting the trunk (i.e., the learner leans forward or backward) or to either side (i.e., the beginning communicator turns to the left or right side). The child's adapted trunk posture may match or differ from the orientation of his or her head in space. The child may turn his or her head to view an object, communication display, or communication partner out of the corner of one eye, or the learner may turn his or her head to regard the field of view with only one eye. In the former observation, the learner may be using *eccentric viewing*—an adaptive response to a limited visual field in which a person views a preferred object, action, or person by deliberately averting the line of sight (i.e., the imaginary line that extends outward from the center of a person's eyes) to one side of the visual stimulus. This behavior permits the learner to use peripheral vision, rather than the more precise central vision, to regard an object or person. In the latter observation, a beginning communicator may be attempting to isolate the use of one eye by using the bridge of the nose as an occluder (i.e., any stimulus present in the visual field that blocks light rays from entering one or both eyes). This atypical head posture is a helpful adaptation if a learner has 1) vision that is asymmetrical (i.e., differs between the two eyes) in clarity or refractive (i.e., bending) power or 2) an unequal visual field due to eye muscle irregularities or scotomata (i.e., blind spots). Some of these conditions may be difficult to assess in learners who present challenging behaviors in assessment situations or whose current levels of receptive and expressive communication skills preclude their comprehension of complex directions. Measuring the learner's motor accuracy when he or she is able to adopt the position freely provides a framework that may be helpful in determining whether the learner is using eccentric fixation or other atypical head or trunk positions adaptively. Informal observations of the learner's preferred head and trunk position are conducted as he or she engages in highly preferred activities. The observers note whether the learner's ability to retrieve a preferred object or engage in rewarding social interaction occurs readily under conditions of independent posture and/or patterns of visual regard. If observations consistently reveal that a learner is able to reach and touch objects with ease and accuracy without concomitant viewing of those same objects, then the head and/or trunk position may be considered adaptive and should be permitted. If motor accuracy is poor under conditions of self-selected head and/or trunk position, then the team's decision making becomes more complicated, and a number of questions must be posed. These questions include the following:

1. Is the head and/or trunk position that this learner readily adopts a habit that may need to be replaced?
2. Is the head or trunk position a function of the learner's poor motivation to actively engage the world around him or her?
3. Is the learner's atypical head or trunk position an expression of avoidance of the objects, actions, and people in the environment?

All of these questions may need to be answered by the team's collecting additional data as outlined in the final section of this chapter, combined with the team's thorough understanding of the beginning communicator's learning characteristics.

PHYSICAL CHARACTERISTICS THAT COMPLICATE SENSORY FUNCTIONING FOR BEGINNING COMMUNICATORS

This section's content is designed to illuminate AAC assessment and decision making as it pertains to learners with one of the most significant challenges to teams of school professionals—that is, learners who have suspected visual impairments combined with disorders in posture and movement. The most common diagnostic label that is assigned to students with atypical posture and movement is *cerebral palsy*. Among the wide range of physical disabilities found in beginning communicators, cerebral palsy occurs most often—in approximately 2.4 per 1,000 live births (Pellegrino, 1997). For learners with cerebral palsy, the occurrence of concomitant visual impairments ranges from 23%–64%, depending on the type and distribution of motor impairment that is associated with the condition (Pellegrino, 1997). Rosen (1998) has provided a detailed description of the most common sensory impairments that occur in learners with cerebral palsy, specifically impaired motility (i.e., voluntary eye movements)—including difficulties in tracking, strabismus (i.e., the visual axes of the two eyes are not parallel), and nystagmus (i.e., involuntary oscillating eye movements). Sacks (1998) stated that most teachers of students who are visually impaired report that more than 50% of the children and youth assigned to their caseloads have vision loss with additional disabilities. According to Batshaw and Shapiro, "More than half of children with mental retardation requiring extensive supports and one quarter of children requiring intermittent supports have sensory impairment, of which visual impairments, especially strabismus and refractive errors, are the most common" (1997, p. 349). Given the prevalence of sensory disabilities in learners with cerebral palsy, it is highly likely that many beginning communicators will require the collective expertise of multiple team members to assess and address multiple needs in the design of AAC.

Implications of Physical Disabilities
for the Design and Implementation of AAC Systems

All children and youth with cerebral palsy have disorders in posture and movement. These disorders manifest in various ways including abnormalities in muscle tone, reflex activity, and automatic movements, as well as delayed or arrested motor development. Comprehensive resources for the team as to the nature and expression of these manifestations are found in Campbell (2000), Rosen (1998), and Utley (1994). A more concise summary of each characteristic follows.

Abnormalities in Muscle Tone   *Muscle tone* may be defined as the degree of tension or stiffness in a muscle group. *Normal muscle tone* may be described as muscle tension (in individual muscles as well as muscle groups) that is sufficient to permit upright posture and resistance to the force of gravity as well as to support coordinated movements into and away from gravity (Campbell, 2000). *Abnormal muscle tone may* be described as above normal (i.e., hypertonia), below normal (i.e., hypotonia), or fluctuating (i.e., muscle tone that ranges from low tone to higher than normal tone on a momentary basis). Abnormal muscle tone may be distributed symmetrically or asymmetrically throughout a person's body. For example, if only one lateral side of the person's body is affected (i.e., hemiplegia), an increase in muscle tone may be observed that appears as internal rotation of the extremities (i.e., the arm and leg of the involved side turn inward toward the body mid-line) as well as increased flexion (i.e., bending at the joints).

Abnormalities in Reflex Activity   A second characteristic of many learners with cerebral palsy is the presence of primitive or abnormal reflexes. Reflexes change the amount and distribution of muscle tone throughout the body and may have an impact on a beginning communicator's ability to engage in voluntary visual behavior. Although a number of abnormal or primitive reflexes are observed in beginning communicators, the three most common reflexes, and their implications for coordinated visual and visual-motor behaviors, are described next.

The Asymmetrical Tonic Neck Reflex   The asymmetrical tonic neck reflex (ATNR) is described as a primitive reflex because it is controlled by a primitive region of the nervous system; it is typically suppressed and integrated into voluntary movement patterns by 12 months of age. The ATNR is elicited by passive or active lateral rotation of the head (i.e., a head turn to the right or left side) that results in a predictable pattern of muscle tone abnormality. For example, the posture of a learner who manifests an ATNR to the right lateral side reveals extended (i.e., straight) extremities on the face side of the skull, whereas those extremities on the opposite side of the head and body are characterized by flexion. This reflex is sometimes described as the "fencing posture."

The degree to which an ATNR is manifested is variable across learners. For some, the extremely persistent emergence of this reflex (sometimes referred to as *obligatory*) can complicate multiple decision-making elements regarding AAC design and implementation. The communication partner's position in space may need to be planned and monitored carefully to avoid encouraging the beginning communicator to turn his or her head to the side of the reflex. Positioning the communication partner at the learner's mid-line is often recommended to avoid eliciting a lateral movement of the head, which may result in emergence of the reflex.

A second possible outcome of a persistent ATNR is the long-term impact of asymmetrical muscle tone on the muscles that control the orientation of the eyes in the bony orbits of the skull. A set of six muscles (termed the *extraocular muscles*) control eye movements in all directions. The impact of abnormal muscle tone may not be limited to the head, trunk, and extremities; it can extend to the extraocular muscles as well. In some learners with a persistent ATNR, the eyes are pulled to the "face side" of the reflex, resulting in less freedom of the eyes to move in all directions. This, in turn, may limit a learner's ability to view his or her environment through a full 180-degree arc.

The Symmetrical Tonic Neck Reflex   The symmetrical tonic neck reflex (STNR) is considered abnormal because it never appears during normal maturation of the nervous system. Just as with the ATNR, the STNR is elicited by movement of the head. In the STNR, the direction of passive or active head movement that elicits the reflex is movement of the head forward (i.e., the chin flexes to the chest) or backward (i.e., the head and neck extend so the chin is elevated). If the head and neck of a learner with a STNR are flexed so the person's chin moves toward his or her chest, the muscle tone in the upper extremities is characterized by flexion, whereas those of the lower extremities are characterized by extension. Extension of the head and neck produces an opposite increase in abnormal tone (extension of the upper extremities and flexion of the lower extremities). Although much less common than an ATNR in learners with cerebral palsy, the presence of a STNR can have a negative impact on a learner's ability to assume upright posture. It can also affect a learner's ability to alternate head position freely in space between a desktop (the horizontal plane) and his or her peers and teacher (the vertical plane). Of particular significance is the manifestation of the STNR that occurs when a learner looks down at a desktop, tabletop, or wheelchair tray. The presence of the STNR results in withdrawing the arms into a flexion pattern, thereby prohibiting the learner from reaching, touching, and exploring the object of visual regard. It is essential that a learner with any degree of a STNR does not have an AAC display that is presented horizontally on a desktop or wheelchair tray. Experimentation with a variety of other presentation positions—from an angle of approximately 45 degrees to the learner's upper body to a fully upright vertical position—should be evaluated. An assessment procedure to assist team members in selecting the most appropriate plane of presentation is found in the section "Determining the Plane of Presentation and Arrangement of Stimuli on the Display."

The Tonic Labyrinthine Reflex   The labyrinth in the inner ear stimulates the tonic labyrinthine reflex (TLR). The presence of a TLR may be observed when a learner is lying on his or her back with an extended head and neck. In this position, the legs extend and the shoulders retract or pull down into the force of gravity. When the same learner is in a stomach lying (i.e., prone) position with his or her head and neck flexed forward, the hips and knees are flexed and the shoulders protract or roll inward. Although the TLR is most readily observed when a learner is lying on the floor, the presence of a strong TLR may be a factor in AAC decision making. This reflex delays or stops the development of independent sitting and may produce patterns of extension and flexion throughout the body that complicate the maintenance of equilibrium and balance. This manifestation of the reflex leaves some learners without a stable base of support from which they can use their arms and hands readily. Thus, the presence of the TLR may have implications for the development and use of adaptive seating equipment. It is essential that a learner with a TLR be provided with a stable base of support, and support for the head as indicated, to permit the maximum degree of upper extremity function. The relationship between the TLR and AAC is obvious: Exerting energy to maintain upright posture and equilibrium, rather than being able to move freely in search of a particular symbol on an AAC array, can affect a learner's ability to gain access to a control device (e.g., a switch) or to engage in the direct selection of symbols on a display.

Abnormalities in Automatic Movements   One of the foundations for the ability to sit and move comfortably is the development of a number of automatic movement reactions, including righting, equilibrium, and protective reactions. In some learners with physical disabilities, the persistence of primitive reflex activity delays or even prevents the development of the automatic movement reactions. In learners with one or more dominant reflex patterns, the ability to develop complex, voluntary movement and control of posture may be limited. An example of an automatic movement is the righting reaction, during which the eyes and head adjust to remain in alignment with the horizontal plane when the body is tilted in space. A range of equilibrium and protective reactions that compensate for a shift in one's center of gravity may also be absent or delayed in some beginning communicators. These reactions, including the ability to protect oneself when falling from a sitting position, again underscore the necessity for team members to address the need for a stable, secure sitting position (Campbell, 2000; York & Weimann, 1991). A stable base in sitting may enable a beginning communicator to attend more fully to the demands of AAC rather than struggling to maintain posture and control against the force of gravity.

Delayed or Arrested Motor Development   The presence of abnormal muscle tone, either alone or in combination with one or more of the primitive reflexes, interferes with the development of more mature expressions of central nervous system function. In typical learners the integration of primitive reflexes permits the emergence of higher level voluntary movement skills such as head control, sitting, standing, and walking. In some learners with physical disabilities, major motor milestones are affected by the severity, type, and distribution of abnormal posture/muscle tone throughout the body. Some learners have severe neuromuscular problems throughout the trunk, head, and neck. For these individuals, the ability to control breathing, as well as precise mouth and tongue movements, precipitate the need for AAC. Again, as described previously regarding the ATNR, the abnormalities that are associated with severely abnormal muscle tone also affect some students' vision. A direct result of absent or severely delayed head control is a delay in development of the "centering mechanisms" of the eyes. This may be particularly true for learners with "wobbly" heads due to rapidly fluctuating muscle tone. The ability to move the eyes independently from the position of the head may complicate all facets of AAC, including the ability to

- Initiate and sustain eye contact with a communication partner
- Look at a graphic display for a sustained period of time
- Search systematically across an array of graphic symbols to allow an informed "choice"
- "Hold" the location in space of a desired symbol or control mechanism long enough to indicate a clearly identifiable communication "response" (Baumgart, Johnson, & Helmstetter, 1990; Musselwhite & St. Louis, 1988; Orelove & Sobsey, 1996)

For these reasons it is essential that team members select an optimum overall position for each learner to engage in communication interactions.

Team members must also commit to a priority-setting process so that learners who are engaging in communication interactions are free from the expectation that they will simultaneously work on other therapeutic objectives, particularly goals or objectives related to major motor milestones. It may be especially difficult for some learners to maintain upright sitting and head erect behavior while also using their eyes and upper extremities (Campbell, 1987; Rosen, 1998; Utley, 1994). For example, a learner with significantly impaired head control may benefit from a variety of procedures to promote increased use of the neck muscles. Yet, this demand should occur at a time of the day other than when the learner is expected to use his or her vision in a controlled fashion (e.g., to scan and select from an array of communication symbols). For some learners with arrested motor development, attempts to engage in voluntary control of the head *and* eyes concurrently compromise a learner's ability to perform either skill well.

Environmental Assessment

Communication occurs across a range of environments, in which lighting and contrast factors vary broadly. Nonetheless, team members and potential communication partners must be aware of the impact that environmental factors may have on a student's ability to use an AAC system successfully. Physical disabilities complicate decisions regarding adaptations that are necessary to meet combined sensory and physical needs. A simple checklist follows that can be used to evaluate what adaptations are needed in home, school, and community environments (see the Environmental Checklist in the appendix at the end of this chapter). The checklist, when completed by team members simultaneously, represents a beginning strategy to create a personalized set of environmental adaptations. (A more thorough assessment of a particular student's ability to benefit from specific low-vision aids and/or specialized positioning equipment must be made in concert with professionals who are most familiar with the student. See Utley and colleagues [1998] for a more detailed description of environmental factors and the teacher of visually impaired's role in the process of developing personalized supports.)

Organization of the Environmental Checklist   The Environmental Checklist is broken into two dimensions: 1) therapeutic positioning and 2) lighting. To improve the functional utility of the decisions made regarding these checklist items, team members should complete the environmental checklist from the student's perspective (i.e., from the same orientation in space that the student typically occupies). A more detailed description of each checklist dimension follows.

Therapeutic Positioning   Certain checklist items are designed to assist team members in determining whether key aspects of therapeutic positioning are present that may enhance the learner's sensory functioning. These items also explore the learner's physical ability and normalization of muscle tone. The first two checklist items address overall body positioning in sitting and side lying. The items reflect general, desirable attributes of these positions. Nonetheless, team members must collaborate to determine whether all the features of a particular position as described are appropriate for an individual learner. An additional item in this section of the checklist relates to the position of peers and adults during communication interaction. To the extent possible, team members and peers should assume a position for interaction that is on the same plane as the student's face (i.e., all parties should be positioned so that face-to-face regard is facilitated). This adjustment in the communication partner's position may facilitate a more neutral head position in the beginning communicator (i.e., the head is aligned with the body mid-line, neither turned to one lateral side, nor flexed or extended), thereby reducing the likelihood that a learner will adopt a head position that may inadvertently result in abnormal posture, muscle tone, or reflex activity.

The final item in the therapeutic positioning portion of the checklist relates to plane (a horizontal plane, a vertical plane, or an angle in between those points). Plane is essential in determining the presentation of a communication device or display. Selecting the most appropriate presentation plane is particularly difficult for learners who do not have head control. A neutral head position is ideal for many beginning communicators who have both sensory and physical difficulties. For some other learners, however, a position in which the head is turned slightly to one side, flexed, or hyperextended may be more visually functional for the learner. (See the section "Determining the Plane of Presentation and Arrangement of Stimuli on the Display" for more precise guidelines to assess the most functional head position for a learner's participation in communication interaction.)

Learners who benefit from a neutral head position should be enabled to assume and maintain this position throughout the duration of communication interaction. This is true even for learners who are not yet able to maintain the head in a neutral position independently for the length of time that is needed to complete a communication interaction. A range of external supports may be provided to serve this purpose, including the various mechanisms that may be part of a seating device (e.g., support straps, or "wings," that are attached to a wheelchair at head and/or neck level). In addition, an adult or a peer can provide gentle physical support to help the learner maintain an upright head position.

Although the team should consider multiple factors as they select the optimal position for a learner's engaging in communication interaction, using a fully upright position is strongly encouraged. Upright posture in sitting or standing is the most normalized position for conversation in home, school, or work environments; it provides the most enriched view of the environment. Too often, learners spend the day sitting in equipment that is characterized by a reclining "seat-in-space angle." This position may leave the learner with a view of the intersection of the wall and ceiling instead of the view that others see in the same environment. To prevent this undesirable positioning, team members have two options. The first is to make sure that the learner's seating equipment is adjusted to promote a fully upright posture for periods of the school day when communication interaction is a priority. The second option is to maintain the semireclined seat-in-space angle but to support the learner's head and neck for fully erect positioning. This head position permits full face-to-face regard with peers and adults and a more typical view of the classroom, home, or community environment. A more upright head position may also improve the learner's view of his or her hands within the visual field—an essential condition for the development of eye–hand coordination. Interventionists should explore using such full-upright positioning for a learner's communication interactions, even if the seat-in-space angle is reclined for therapeutic reasons. An upright head position also promotes joint attention to people, places, and things in the near and distant environments, which are essential contents of communication interactions.

Again, intervention that is designed to promote head erect behavior should occur at times *other* than those during which the learner has additional demands on his or her energy. For many learners with complex sensory and physical needs, the physical effort that is required to hold the head erect, use visual skills, and participate in communication interaction may produce undesirable changes in muscle tone, thereby lessening motor accuracy (Campbell, 1987; Rosen, 1998; Utley, 1994).

Lighting   The Environmental Checklist is designed to guide team members as they examine two aspects of lighting to enhance communication intervention. These include 1) amount and type of light and 2) the position of light sources. The team's challenge is to create a communication environment that has a sufficient amount of lighting.

Generally, it is desirable to have a combination of light sources available in the communication environment, including natural light from windows and open doors, in addition to typical fluorescent and incandescent sources. The surface of the communication display, or the background surface of a switch or an object cue, should be illuminated evenly. In some situations, a learner may benefit from supplemental incandescent lighting on the communication display to enhance visual discrimination among the various symbols or to make a switch or other three-dimensional communication device stand out. In the latter situation a table lamp or "clip-on" study lamp can be used for supplementary illumination.

Team members must consider two primary factors when providing a supplemental incandescent light source directly on a communication display or device. If a table lamp is used, it should have a weighted base or be attached to the supporting surface with a "C" clamp to prevent tipping. In addition, the shade should be double layered, which permits the outer surface of the shade to remain cool to the touch. This is an important factor when the light source may be positioned close to a learner and his or her peers for prolonged periods of time. The lamp should be fitted with a standard 60- or 75-watt indoor bulb. "Soft white" bulbs should not be used; they diffuse the light too much, substantially lowering light output.

The design of optimal lighting also accounts for the position, or direction, of the light sources. Generally, a learner should be positioned with his or her back to natural light sources (e.g., windows or doors that flood the environment with natural light). This is particularly important for learners who rely on gestural mode input, as facing natural light sources may limit their view of a signing partner to a silhouette. Most primary light sources are in the ceiling. Yet, any supplemental light source should be placed directly over a communication device or display, if necessary, to promote higher contrast between the device and the background surface.

An alternate accommodation is to position a supplemental light source so that the light emanates over the shoulder that is opposite the learner's dominant hand (which is used to activate a communication device or select from an array of symbols). For learners who are essentially monocular (i.e., use one eye only), it is equally important that the illumination from a supplemental light source originates from the same lateral side as the learner's functional eye. For some learners, however, the most functional upper extremity may not be on the same side of the body as the functional eye. In this latter situation, the best approach may be to position the supplemental light source so that it provides even surface illumination on the communication device without shadows.

Team members should consider the "Lighting" section of the checklist for each of several environments (e.g., school cafeteria, classroom, home). Identifying poor lighting conditions that may exist allows team members to implement simple accommodations. Examples of simple accommodations include reversing the student's position during a typical classroom activity (e.g., storytime, opening activities) to reduce glare and improve contrast, giving the student an age-appropriate visor or pair of sunglasses to wear during recess, or adding a clip-on study lamp to a table or wheelchair tray during library time. A teacher of people with visual impairment can often generate extremely creative, practical, and age-appropriate environmental accommodations.

Aggressively designing environmental accommodations is a more appropriate strategy than recommending that learners spend time in more restrictive environments where lighting and glare may be controlled more easily. Communication is an embedded, or cross-environmental, skill. *Embedded skills* are most appropriately identified as learning outcomes that occur throughout the day in all home, school, community, and vocational contexts. Functional vision's importance as part of communication intervention suggests that students must learn to function visually in multiple environments. In this way, beginning communicators may participate to the maximum degree across the full range of environments to which their typical peers have access.

Summary   Two or more team members should work together to complete the Environmental Checklist. Jointly, these team members may guide the productive implementation of environmental assessment by attending to two features. The first is recognizing the need to balance the various environmental modifications that the completed checklist suggests. Simple adjustments to seating posture and head position, the position of materials, and lighting can enhance a beginning communicator's success. Interventionists must also appreciate enhanced functional vision's essential role in the learner's ability to communicate successfully. All learning relies on receiving sensory stimuli. Although time consuming, assessing and modifying factors that enhance sensory functioning constitute priority tasks for the intervention team. Ultimately, every attempt should be made to use communication materials that are typically found in classroom and community environments. For example, students should not be moved to a darkened room or be supported with adjustments that are "overly special" (Giangreco, Edelman, & Dennis, 1991). Again, a balance between carefully planned modifications and normalcy is the desired outcome of this process. More in-depth information regarding environmental adaptation in terms of lighting, contrast, and glare can also be found in Utley and colleagues (1998).

CRITICAL QUESTIONS AND
ASSESSMENT PROCEDURES TO GUIDE AAC DESIGN

The third and final section of this chapter is organized into three parts: 1) determining binocularity or monocularity, 2) determining presentation distance, and 3) assessing visually directed reach and touch. The format of this section consists of a series of questions to be answered by the team. The answers to these questions contribute much needed information that may be useful during the initial AAC design process.

Determining Binocularity or Monocularity

The human visual system is designed to produce single vision by using both eyes (i.e., *binocularity*). This outcome results only when the slightly different images that are transmitted by the eyes are fused into a single image in the cortical region of the brain. Several preconditions must be met for binocular single vision to be present. These preconditions include 1) approximately equal refractive (i.e., bending) power in both eyes; 2) coordinated, conjugate eye movements that result from anatomically correct alignment of the extraocular eye muscles; and 3) an intact visual pathway that transmits the information received by the eyes through a complex electrochemical process to the brain for processing. Of these three preconditions, the second—presence or absence of coordinated, conjugate eye movements—is most easily observed and documented by a team of school professionals. Systematic observation of this precondition's elements assists team members in determining the presence or absence of binocularity in a beginning communicator. Yet, the complexity of the visual system, as well as the reality that not all visual behaviors can be readily observed by school professionals, is further support for collaboration between team members and medical professionals. Although team members may observe poorly coordinated conjugate eye movements, these symptoms may be secondary to a defect in one or both of the other two preconditions for binocularity, evidence of an underlying disease process, or associated with another form of visual impairment that is unknown to the team. A medical professional's confirmation or refutation of a team's impression of weakened or absent binocularity, however, permits the AAC design process to address the condition's impact. The functional outcomes of weakened or absent binocularity (i.e., a potential reduction in the visual field, poor depth perception, or the need for adaptation in head and trunk support and position) constitute an essential element of promoting AAC access. This is particularly true for learners who do not have head control (i.e., who may lack the ability to turn the head to view a display more completely) or upper trunk strength (i.e., who are unable to freely assume an optimal viewing distance).

Conjugate eye movements can occur only when the extraocular eye muscles permit the eyes to move freely in multiple directions (upward, downward, temporally, and nasally) and in a coordinated fashion. The coordinated movements of the two eyes may also be described as *ocular motility*, which is defined as the two eyes' ability to assume a range of positions within the bony orbits of the skull. These positions include

- One eye moving outward (i.e., temporally) and the other rolling nasally when the learner views a person or thing in the periphery without moving his or her head to one lateral side
- Both eyes rolling inward to view a person or object at mid-line (i.e., both eyes roll nasally)
- The eyes remaining in a neutral position when the learner views a distant object

The presence or absence of conjugate eye movements can be documented through observation of the overall appearance of the eyes, the orientation of the eyes in the skull, movement of the eyes in response to the presentation of a visual stimulus, and the alignment or misalignment of the visual axes of both eyes (Campbell, Baumgarner, & Wilcox, 1989; Cress, 1988; Erhardt, 1986; Sobsey & Wolf-Schein, 1996; Utley, 1994). The visual axes may be described as invisible lines that emanate from the centers of both eyes; they are also termed the *lines of sight*. In a person who has typical eyes, the visual axes are parallel when a person views an object at a distance of 6 meters or more, and they converge when a person regards an object at a distance of arm's length and at mid-line. In the latter case, the visual axes converge and both eyes roll nasally to view the near object (Erhardt, 1986). A learner's coordinated, conjugate eye movements can be observed in response to a broad range of sensory stimuli as well as in shifts in a learner's attention to various people and things.

Relevance of Binocularity or Monocularity for Beginning Communicators   Binocularity permits true depth perception and a full visual field. These aspects of binocularity have powerful implications for AAC design, particularly with regard to the location in space of the AAC system and the arrangement of stimuli on a display. For these reasons, determining whether a learner is binocular or monocular is an essential element in system selection. Team members must be able to answer the question, "Is the individual able to visually gain access to the full field of vision that is available to typical learners, or will he or she need to have a system designed for a more narrow field of vision?"

For a number of reasons, some beginning communicators lack binocularity. For some learners, the absence of binocularity may be linked to imbalance in one or more sets of the extraocular eye muscles that control orientation of the eyeballs in the bony orbits of the skull. Sometimes, the muscle imbalance occurs as the result of asymmetrical, abnormal muscle tone or reflex activity that "pulls" one or both eyes into deviation. Conditions that may suggest a lack of binocularity to a team may be determined through careful review of a child's medical records. Table 11.3 displays a list of terms that may appear in a vision report. The presence of any of these terms can alert team members to the possibility of reduced or absent binocularity. Sacks (1998) provided an excellent description of the general range of implication of visual disorders that may influence the acquisition of initial communication skills.

Learners who lack binocular vision but have no additional disabilities may compensate for their loss in a variety of ways. Some learners may turn their heads to view objects or people predominantly with one eye. Others learn to compensate for poor depth perception by using other sources of visual information to cue the relative position of an object or person in the environment. Yet, the successful use of these alternative input forms depends on the learner's background knowledge and experience. For example, a learner who functions in a monocular fashion may use his or her knowledge of the dimensions or size of familiar objects to understand the relative location of those objects in space. Regrettably, many learners with complex combinations of sensory and physical disabilities have had limited opportunities to explore the places and objects that are common to most people in everyday life, thereby limiting the learners' ability to relate to such objects and environments.

For a learner who has both limited experience with objects and severely delayed acquisition of major motor milestones (particularly head control), the

Table 11.3. Medical terms and definitions that may suggest an absence of binocularity

Term	Definition
Strabismus	A visual disorder in which one eye cannot focus on the same object of regard simultaneously with the other eye
Convergent strabismus	Strabismus in which one deviates nasally
	Also called "cross-eye," internal strabismus
	Two levels of the condition: *esophoria* is a tendency of an eye to roll nasally; *esotropia* is the manifest presence of the deviation
Divergent strabismus	Strabismus in which one eye deviates temporally
	Also called "wall-eye," external strabismus
	Two levels: *exophoria* is the tendency of an eye to roll temporally; *exotropia* is the manifest presence of the deviation
Amblyopia ex anopsia	A reduction in visual functioning (often in the absence of an observable malformation or disease process in the eye) that results when the brain fails to process the visual information that is transmitted by one eye
	The condition often results from uncorrected strabismus, as the information transmitted by the deviating eye is too different from that transmitted by the correctly aligned eye to fuse the two views into a single image. Over time, the brain increasingly disregards the input from the deviating eye, and the vision in that eye becomes dim. It may also be caused by unequal refractive errors (i.e., the bending power of the two eyes differs) or a lack of clarity in the lens or cornea.

possibility of monocularity and its impact on AAC design becomes even more complicated. The compensatory head and upper torso positioning that may be readily adopted by a person who is monocular and has no additional disabilities may not be available to a person with multiple disabilities. A learner with multiple disabilities may be incapable of assuming or maintaining a postural adjustment that may facilitate a better view of the immediate environment. Alternatively, team members may prevent the learner from assuming that position because it may complicate support for other therapeutic needs. For example, a learner who is essentially monocular due to a right exotropia (i.e., the right eye rolls manifestly to the temporal side) may turn his or her head to the right side to permit viewing of the immediate environment with the left eye. This behavior may be interpreted as undesirable because it violates the importance that some team members may associate with mid-line posture. Another learner may attempt to lean far forward on a wheelchair tray or desktop to view an object more clearly, a behavior that may be interpreted by some team members as insufficient use of the muscles of the trunk. In reality, most people lean slightly forward to engage in joint attention on an object of interest or to demonstrate interest in a communication partner. It is also typical to support part of the weight of the upper torso on the arm of a chair or to lean on a hand to rest the weight of the head. An analysis of typical posture may give the team guidance in positioning learners for communication intervention so that beginning communicators may adopt compensatory postures more readily. If possible, the ideal situation may be to provide support so that a learner's upper trunk leans forward slightly (a chest restraint may be helpful) during times of high priority communication intervention. In addition, seating equipment should be adjusted so the learner can rest his or her forearms easily on the supporting surface with an angle at the elbows of between 90 and 120 degrees. This position may facilitate initiation of compensatory head and upper body positions that give the learner a better view of an object or a peer and also provide stability for the proximal joints of the shoulder and elbow.

Stability in the proximal joints may also permit increased controlled mobility of the hands and fingers to engage in sign language production, switch activation, or selection within an array of graphic symbols (Campbell, 2000). Again, the suggestion that visual efficiency is a primary factor in decision making regarding positioning does not minimize the need to address other needs as well. An increase in trunk strength is an important goal for many beginning communicators. It is essential that team members design interventions for that purpose and select appropriate opportunities in the context of school, home, and community routines to practice this important motor milestone as well.

Systematic Assessment for Determination of Binocularity or Monocularity   As stated previously, Pellegrino (1997) estimated that 23%–64 % of learners who may need a beginning communication system have visual impairments, many of which are associated with reduced or absent binocularity. Monocularity, combined with poor or absent head control, may limit the learner's ability to visually gain access to the full field of his or her immediate environment; it may also result in poor depth perception. Consequently, it is essential that interventionists determine whether a learner has functional or absent binocularity so that adults, peers, and AAC devices or displays can be presented appropriately in space. The question to be answered is, "Does the learner have binocular vision, and if not, which eye is most functional for the learner to receive visual information?" The team may proceed to answer this question by first reviewing the learner's medical records for evidence of difficulty in this area. In the absence of clear, comprehensive medical records, the team may also conduct simple observations to assess a learner's degree of binocularity.

Observations that may alert the team to potential binocularity problems include rolling one or both eyes in any direction, alternating eye use, and/or persistent deviation of one or both eyes to one lateral side of the body. Systematic observation of binocularity is achieved by conducting a series of four assessment procedures, the results of which are shared with a medical professional. The four procedures are 1) assessing the pupillary consensual response,

2) assessing the corneal light reflection, 3) conducting the cover test, and 4) assessing convergence. Each of these procedures is described more thoroughly in the ensuing sections and tables and figures. Some of these assessment procedures are conducted outside of typical home, school, and community routines. This is necessary because precise observations of the functional visual system may require the use of instructional materials (e.g., a penlight) that are atypical in a learner's daily life.

None of the following four assessment procedures, conducted in isolation, should be interpreted as suggesting reduced or absent binocularity. If the data generated by all four assessment procedures yield consistent results, however, the team may want to share these data with a medical professional who can confirm or refute the findings or give team members an alternative explanation for the results.

Assessing the Pupillary Consensual Response   In people with binocularity, stimulating one eye with a penlight results in immediate constriction of the pupil in the *unstimulated* eye. This response may demonstrate a connection between the two eyes in the visual pathway, thereby indicating that some degree of binocularity may be present. After first observing the unstimulated eye, some medical professionals suggest that the penlight be presented immediately to that same eye to assess whether additional constriction occurs. Additional constriction may show a reduced degree of connection between the two eyes and may support the hypothesis that the learner has reduced or absent binocularity. See Table 11.4 for the specific steps to follow for assessing the pupillary consensual response. Figure 11.1 provides a form to record the data.

Assessing the Corneal Light Reflection   Assessing corneal light reflection is used frequently to help determine the symmetry of both eyes, which is a precondition for binocularity. The procedure consists of presenting a lighted object to a person at mid-line, within arm's reach, and at nose-tip level. If the eyes are aligned, then symmetrical pinpoints of light are reflected on the corneas, just slightly to the nasal side of center in the pupils of both eyes. Although the information obtained from this assessment can be very valuable to a medical professional, some beginning communicators may fail to cooperate when this procedure is conducted in a physician's office. This may occur if the learner fails to understand that it is necessary to keep his or her eyes open and to regard the light actively as it is presented. For this reason, school professionals who are familiar with the procedure may use it to collect data in more familiar environments, thereby assisting medical professionals in determining the presence of binocularity.

Data from assessment of the corneal light reflection are recorded on a diagram of the learner's eyes. The exact location of the pinpoints of light are drawn on the diagram, so asymmetrical pinpoints of light suggest that one eye is rolled nasally or temporally. Poorly aligned eyes may transmit images that

Table 11.4.   Steps for assessing the pupillary consensual response

1. Position the learner so he or she is comfortable in a therapeutic supine (i.e., back-lying) position.

2. Kneel or sit at the learner's head so that you may observe his or her eyes readily.

3. Position an occluder, such as a soft piece of foam or your hand, along the bridge of the learner's nose so that you extend the bridge to effectively block a light stimulus (provided by a small penlight) from reaching both eyes at the same time. Be sure to align the occluder tightly along the bridge so that no light can escape from one side of the face to the other under the occluder. The occluder must be made of a sub-stance that will not harm the learner's eye if he or she moves suddenly

4. Tell the learner that you will be shining a light into one of his or her eyes for a few sec-onds.

5. On the data sheet, note which eye is to be stimulated with the light on the first as-sessment trial.

6. Position yourself to observe the eye opposite of the one to be stimulated and then position the penlight (in an "off" setting) about 4 inches from the eye to be stimulated just above the tip of the learner's nose.

7. Turn on the penlight and watch for instantaneous pupillary constriction (i.e., shrink-ing) of the pupil in the unstimulated eye. (Note: You may also then quickly present the penlight to the previously unstimulated eye to see if additional constriction oc-curs. Remember that if additional constriction does occur, that this may indicate a weakened connection between the two eyes.)

8. Continue this assessment procedure a few trials at a time over several days, until five assessment trials for each eye have been completed. Remember to follow the data sheet in order so that you observe and stimulate each eye randomly.

are too different for the brain to fuse them into a single image. For some learn-ers, one eye and then the other is centered and active during visual regard of an object or person. This alternating condition may produce inconsistent re-sults on this assessment as well as on other measures of binocularity. An in-consistency that may be revealed during the assessment is a pinpoint of light being reflected near the center of one pupil on the first assessment trial and the opposite pattern being observed on one or more subsequent trials. The de-sirable response during this measure is symmetrical reflection of the pinpoints of light in both eyes simultaneously. (As with all of the assessment measures described in this section, it is important that interventionists practice the pro-cedures to gain proficiency and fluency with them and experience in judging a typical response.)

Assessment of the corneal light reflection may be somewhat unpleasant for the learner, as the procedure calls for the light source to be presented di-rectly in front of the face. Team members must conduct each assessment trial quickly to minimize the learner's distress. The learner must actively view the light during this assessment, which may be facilitated by conducting the pro-cedure in a darkened room or, if age appropriate, by inserting the penlight inside of a lightly colored finger puppet to increase interest in the lighted ob-

Eye to be stimulated	Eye to be observed	Constriction observed	Additional constriction observed (optional)
Right	Left	Yes/No	Yes/No
Right	Left	Yes/No	Yes/No
Left	Right	Yes/No	Yes/No
Right	Left	Yes/No	Yes/No
Left	Right	Yes/No	Yes/No
Right	Left	Yes/No	Yes/No
Left	Right	Yes/No	Yes/No
Left	Right	Yes/No	Yes/No
Right	Left	Yes/No	Yes/No
Left	Right	Yes/No	Yes/No

Total number of assessment trials during which constriction occurred in the **left** eye: _____
Did additional constriction occur in response to direct stimulation?   Yes   No

Total number of assessment trials during which constriction occurred in the **right** eye: _____
Did additional constriction occur in response to direct stimulation?   Yes   No

Figure 11.1. Data sheet for recording the results of the assessment of pupillary consensual response.

ject. Table 11.5 lists the specific steps for assessing the corneal light reflection; the recording form is found in Figure 11.2.

Team members can familiarize themselves with the correct position of the corneal light reflection (i.e., where the pinpoints of light are reflected on the cornea if the eyes are typically aligned) by viewing full-face regard photographs of people with typical corneal light reflection. In fact, a full-face photograph of the learner, on which the pinpoints of light are clearly reflected on the corneas, may replace the need for conducting this assessment.

Conducting the Cover Test   The cover test involves using a set of systematic observations to reveal whether one or both eyes are used during the learner's active regard of a high-preference object. During this test, the learner's view of the high-preference object is interrupted by randomly occluding one eye at a time. The learner's reaction or lack of reaction to occlusion is recorded. If the learner reveals a consistent pattern of overt responses to the occlusion

Table 11.5.   Steps for assessing the corneal light reflection

1. Position the learner in a therapeutic sitting or supine (i.e., back-lying) position.
2. Select an age-appropriate finger puppet or other action figure into which the penlight may be inserted. This may increase the interest level of the visual stimulus thereby increasing the probability that the learner will regard the lighted object actively during each assessment trial.

OR

3. Select a dark room for conducting this assessment to increase the learner's interest in the penlight.
4. Position the lighted object (in an "off" setting) about 13 inches away from the learner's face, at mid-line and at the level of the tip of the learner's nose.
5. Activate the lighted object or penlight and ask the learner to look at the object. (Note: Tap or wave the lighted object or penlight to increase the learner's interest level if necessary.)
6. Quickly observe the position of the lighted object's reflection in the learner's eyes, making sure to maintain the correct position of the lighted object as you complete your observation.
7. Turn off the lighted object and record the relative location of the corneal reflections on the data sheet in the spaces provided.
8. Continue the procedure until you have observed the pinpoints of light a total of five times.

Trial 1	
Trial 2	
Trial 3	
Trial 4	
Trial 5	

Total number of assessment trials
during which the corneal light reflection was typical: _____

Figure 11.2.   Data sheet for recording the results of the assessment of the corneal light reflection. Instructions: Determine the typical corneal light reflection that is observed when a learner regards an object at mid-line, approximately 13 inches distant and at the level of the tip of the nose. Then conduct five trials of this assessment procedure. In the blank box next to each trial number, draw the approximate site of the observed reflection.

of one eye (e.g., eye closing, eye rolling, avoidance of the occluder), the observer may infer that the occluded eye transmitted useful visual information. The rationale for the cover test is that a learner will protest the introduction of an occluder in front of a dominant or functional eye but will not protest this action if the occluded eye does not transmit valuable information to the brain.

To conduct the cover test, the observer first establishes the learner's active eye fixation on a preferred object and then introduces an occluder into the visual field from one lateral side of the learner's face. The procedure requires careful observation to determine whether the learner responds to the introduction of the occluder and, if so, the nature of that response. For an individual who understands that he or she must not move his or her head during this assessment, one eye rolling (in either a nasal or temporal direction) upon introduction of the occluder indicates weak or absent binocularity. For many early communicators, who may not understand the interventionist's directions, a broader range of responses may indicate weakened or absent binocularity. For example, learners with upper extremity function and some head control may simply move their heads in response to introduction of the occluder to continue viewing the preferred object. Alternatively, they may attempt to push the occluder out of the visual field.

This assessment should be conducted over several sessions, a few opportunities at a time. The data sheet in Figure 11.3 identifies the specific order in which the eye is to be occluded and which eye is to be observed for each assessment trial. Table 11.6 provides the specific steps for conducting the cover test.

Assessing Convergence   The assessment of convergence is designed to determine the probability of absent or weak binocularity. In convergence, both eyes roll to the nasal side of the nose as an object of regard approaches at midline and nose-tip level. The primary outcomes of the convergence assessment are the determination of whether the learner views an approaching object with predominantly one eye, turns his or her head to facilitate viewing of the object with one eye, and/or turns one or both eye(s) in any direction as the object approaching is viewed. Convergence requires the eye muscles that control the orientation of the eyeballs to work in a coordinated fashion. Observation of smooth, coordinated convergence in both eyes suggests that binocularity may be present. The purpose of conducting the assessment of convergence is to add a fourth set of data that may strengthen a judgment of monocularity or binocularity. The implications for a beginning communicator pertain to monocularity's impact on the visual field within which an AAC display and potential communication partners are located. For beginning communicators with monocularity, the field of view is restricted. This knowledge is essential for team members who plan (and modify, as appropriate) the environments in which the beginning communicator functions. Table 11.7 lists the specific procedures for observing convergence; the accompanying data sheet is found in Figure 11.4.

Learner's Response

Learner's name: _____   Date: _____

	Occlude	Observe	Rolls unoccluded eye	Moves head to avoid introduction of the occluder	Pushes occluder out of the line of sight	Closes one or both eyes		Other	No response
Trial 1	R	L				R	L		
Trial 2	L	R				R	L		
Trial 3	R	L				R	L		
Trial 4	R	L				R	L		
Trial 5	L	R				R	L		
Trial 6	R	L				R	L		
Trial 7	L	R				R	L		
Trial 8	L	R				R	L		
Trial 9	R	L				R	L		
Trial 10	L	R				R	L		

Total learner responses to occlusion of the

Right eye (Trials 1, 3, 4, 6, and 9) _____ (If 4 or more responses are recorded, the right eye may be dominant.)

Left eye (Trials 2, 5, 7, 8, and 10) _____ (If 4 or more responses are recorded, the left eye may be dominant.)

Figure 11.3. Data sheet for recording the results of the cover test. Check marks in the "No response" column are not counted when summing the total number of learner responses. (Key: R = right eye, L = left eye.)

Table 11.6.   Steps for conducting the cover test

1. Using your nondominant hand, position a preferred object, your face, or a small bit of food (if necessary and appropriate) approximately 13 inches from the learner's face, at mid-line and at the level of the learner's nose tip.

2. Shake or tap the object to obtain the learner's visual localization on the object. Some learners may localize visually more readily if they hold the object jointly with you. This adaptation is appropriate if the learner will accept holding the object in the location in space described in Step 1.

3. Position an occluder just outside or peripheral to the learner's line of sight for the eye to be occluded in Trial 1. (If using your hand as an occluder, hold fingers together and palm out and orient vertically.)

4. Introduce the occluder into the line of sight of the eye to be occluded in Trial 1.

5. Observe continuously for any or all of the following responses:

   • The unoccluded eye rolls in any direction. A rolling movement may indicate that binocular vision is weak and that the occluded eye is dominant.

   • The learner moves his or her head around the occluder to continue viewing the preferred object.

   • The learner pushes the occluder out of his or her line of sight.

   • The learner closes one or both eyes.

   • The learner does not respond to the occluder's introduction into his or her line of sight. This may mean that the unoccluded eye is dominant.

6. Record the learner's response(s) in the space provided on the data sheet.

7. Repeat steps 1 though 6 for a total of ten trials, being sure to follow the progression of assessment trials that is designated on the data sheet. Note that the assessment trials specify that each eye is observed and occluded randomly.

From Utley, B.L. (1994). Providing support for sensory, postural, and movement needs. In L. Sternberg (Ed.), *Individuals with profound disabilities* (3rd ed., pp. 139–140). Austin, TX: PRO-ED; adapted by permission.

Table 11.7.   Steps for assessing convergence

1. Position a high-preference object, a peer's or an adult's face, or small pieces of food (if necessary and appropriate) approximately 18 inches from the learner's face at mid-line, and at the level of the tip of the learner's nose.

2. Shake or tap the object to obtain visual localization on the object with one or both eyes.

3. Move the object toward the learner's face at a pace that is rapid enough to sustain visual localization but not threatening.

4. Observe continuously for any or all of the following responses:

   • One or both eyes close.

   • One eye rolls nasally or temporally.

   • The learner turns his or her head laterally and watches the object approach with only one eye.

   • Responds in another way (to be described).

5. Record the learner's response(s) in the spaces provided on the data sheet.

6. Repeat Steps 1 through 5 a total of five times over several days.

Learner's Response				
Learner's name: _____ Date: _____				

	Closes eye(s)	Rolls one eye nasally or temporally	Turns head to watch object approach with one eye	Other
Trial 1	R L	R L Nasal Temporal	R L	
Trial 2	R L	R L Nasal Temporal	R L	
Trial 3	R L	R L Nasal Temporal	R L	
Trial 4	R L	R L Nasal Temporal	R L	
Trial 5	R L	R L Nasal Temporal	R L	

Figure 11.4. Data sheet for recording the results of the assessment of convergence. (Key: R = right eye, L = left eye.)

Summary of the Assessment Procedures for Binocularity versus Monocularity
The significance of all of the measures on binocularity versus monocularity is to assist team members with determining where in space a communication display or device should be placed for best visual regard. Data that reveal a learner's failure to converge with both eyes, combined with data from other procedures that also indicate monocularity, suggest that he or she might benefit from an AAC display that is narrowed to comprise the field of the preferred eye. To aid in the interpretation and synthesis of the four separate sets of results, an additional form has been created on which team members transcribe the separate assessment outcomes (see Figure 11.5). The team members may more easily see consistent results regarding the dominance of one eye if all four assessment procedures are summarized on a single data sheet. A medical professional can interpret the data from these observations, thereby either supporting the team members' impressions or providing an alternative explanation for the collected results. In this model of data-based decision making, monocularity versus binocularity is determined first. Thus, in subsequent assessments, the materials can be centered to the visual axis of one eye for those who are essentially monocular or at mid-line for those who are binocular.

The most significant implication of monocularity is a reduction of the visual field. A beginning communicator who is essentially monocular may respond in a more limited way to objects, people, and activities that are at near distance (within the length of the learner's arms and the width of his or her shoulders) due to a limited visual field. This may be particularly problematic

Learner's name: _____ Date: _____

Procedure 1: Assessment of pupillary consensual response

Instructions: Review the completed assessment of the pupillary consensual response data sheet and look for any pattern of responses with regard to pupillary constriction. If one eye constricts consistently and the other does not, circle the eye that constricts in the space provided under Procedure 1—Monocular in the table below. If both eyes constrict equally well, circle the term under "both eyes" in the space provided under Procedure 1—Binocular.

Procedure 2: Assessment of corneal light reflection

Instructions: Review the completed assessment of the corneal light reflection data sheet and look for any pattern that suggests that either one or both eyes deviate from a neutral position while viewing the lighted object or penlight. Circle the eye that *does not* deviate in the space provided under Procedure 2—Monocular in the table that follows. If neither eye deviates, circle the term "both eyes" in the space provided under Procedure 2—Binocular.

Procedure 3: The cover test

Instructions: Review the information at the bottom of the cover test data sheet and note whether the data suggests that either the left or right eye is dominant. In the space provided under Procedure 3—Monocular in the table that follows, circle the eye that is dominant. If no pattern of dominance emerges (i.e., learner consistently avoids introduction of the occluder in front of both eyes or neither eye), circle the term "both eyes" in the space provided under Procedure 3—Binocular.

Procedure 4: Assessment of convergence

Instructions: Review the completed assessment of convergence data sheet, paying particular attention to the data in the column "turns head to watch object approach with one eye." If the data recorded in this column indicate that one eye is used consistently to view the object as it approaches, circle that eye in the space provided in the table that follows under Procedure 4—Monocular. If the learner regards the object approaching with both eyes and fails to demonstrate an eye roll or a head turn, circle the term "both eyes" in the space provided under Procedure 4—Binocular.

Interpretation of the data

Instructions: Review columns 2, 4, 6, and 8 in the table that follows. If you have circled "both eyes" in all four columns, it is likely that the learner is binocular, and you may proceed to design the AAC system to be centered to the learner's midline. In the absence of data recorded in those columns, however, review columns 1, 3, 5, and 7 and note whether one eye is circled consistently. If so, it is likely that this eye is dominant, and the AAC system should be centered to that eye's visual field. Share these data with a medical professional for further clarification or refutation of these findings before a final decision is made.

1	2	3	4	5	6	7	8
Procedure 1 Monocular	Procedure 1 Binocular	Procedure 2 Monocular	Procedure 2 Binocular	Procedure 3 Monocular	Procedure 3 Binocular	Procedure 4 Monocular	Procedure 4 Binocular
L R	both eyes	L R	both eyes	L R	both eyes	L R	both eyes

Figure 11.5. Summary sheet for assisting team members in synthesizing the assessment procedure results to determine the presence or absence of binocularity. (Key: R = right eye, L = left eye.)

for learners who do not have head control and receive full head and neck support from a positioning device that limits the head to a mid-line orientation. Mid-line positioning may be important for the learner's comfort and have therapeutic value. Nonetheless, full external support of the head and neck may inadvertently prohibit the learner's ability to adjust his or her head and neck for full visual access to the typical work surface and area where close physical proximity and communication are likely to occur. If the team does not know that a learner's visual field is limited, then objects, people, and activities may continue to occur in a full 180-degree arc (i.e., the visual field of people with typical vision). A learner's failure to respond visually under these conditions may complicate interpretation of ongoing progress monitoring and decision making for AAC design.

Determining Presentation Distance

A second critical question for team members to answer is, "At what distance should a switch, object cue, or AAC system be positioned to promote the best visual regard?" A variation of the previously described convergence assessment may yield helpful data to answer this question. The procedures are implemented exactly as described in Table 11.7; however, the observed and recorded learner responses consist of where in space the learner's visual regard of the approaching object ceases (Campbell et al., 1989; Utley, 1994). Again, the assessment opportunities are distributed over several sessions and days to minimize fatigue or boredom with the assessment context. A preferred object, a favorite adult's or peer's face, or preferred food or drink (if appropriate) may be used as the visual stimulus. The learner is encouraged to actively regard the visual stimulus; then, the interventionist moves it toward the learner's face in a rapid but well-controlled, nonthreatening movement. The learner's visual response is observed carefully, and as soon as he or she ceases to regard the approaching stimulus, forward movement is stopped abruptly. Nonetheless, the adult does not move the object away from the learner until the precise distance at which the learner ceased fixation is recorded in inches on the data sheet (see Figure 11.6). That is, the interventionist records on the sheet the distance between the location of the object and the learner's face when visual regard was "broken." This assessment procedure is of great value to a team, as school professionals who suspect a visual impairment often place objects too close to a learner's face, hoping to increase the probability that the object will be the target of visual regard. It is important to remember that optimal viewing distance is no closer than 13 inches from the eyes. An object should only be presented closer than 13 inches when systematic, repeated data collection and analysis reveal that a closer viewing distance is optimal for that learner.

Learner's name: _____   Date: _____

	Distance in inches at which learner ceases to regard the approaching object
Trial 1	
Trial 2	
Trial 3	
Trial 4	
Trial 5	

Range of observed viewing distance: From _____ to _____ inches

Average observed viewing distance: _____ inches

Figure 11.6.   Data sheet for recording the results of the assessment of viewing distance.

Determining the Plane of Presentation and Arrangement of Stimuli on the Display   Assessment should be conducted to guide the team in answering two critical questions: 1) Which plane of presentation of the display surface (vertical, horizontal, or a point in between) contributes to a particular learner's fastest and most accurate visual responses? and 2) Which areas on a display surface are most physically accessible for the arrangement of a switch, an object cue, or a set of graphic or tangible stimuli? An essential factor in AAC design is the plane of presentation of the display surface relative to the learner's face and upper body. The presence of complex combinations of abnormal muscle tone, upper extremity function, head control, and reflex activity may make one plane of presentation superior to another regarding a particular learner's ability to visually gain access to a symbol display or a communication device. This assessment is designed to describe the highly dynamic visual processes that occur as a learner localizes visually to a switch, an object, or a symbol that is found in a variety of locations on a display surface that is presented in various planes. The assessment requires using a prototype communication display that is the approximate size and shape of the system that is being considered for the learner. The collected assessment data can guide decisions regarding the presentation of the device or display, as well as the arrangement of the tangible or graphic symbols to be used in the AAC system. At least two team members should conduct this assessment together. With the exception of AAC devices that are composed of transparent Plexiglas materials, positioning the prototype communication display in certain planes of presentation may partially block an observer's view of the learner's visual responses, thereby complicating data collection. A second team member can move flexibly to observe the learner's visual behavior while the first team member positions the prototype device or display; this may improve accuracy of data collection. Table 11.8 addresses the steps of this assessment proce-

---

Table 11.8. Steps for assessing visual localization within a display of stimuli presented in various planes relative to the learner's body

1. Select one or more high-preference stimuli that can be affixed to the prototype display surface. Examples include small toy people for young children, trading cards for somewhat older children, and a colorful CD insert or "jewel" box for adolescent learners.

2. If the object is not too heavy, attach it to the prototype communication display surface with two-sided adhesive tape. Heavier stimuli may need to be affixed to a piece of Velcro, with a small piece of the corresponding Velcro surface affixed in each quadrant of the display surface.

3. Determine prior to each assessment trial which of the three planes of presentation will be used for presentation of the stimulus. Record that information on the top of the data sheet in the space provided.

4. Determine prior to each assessment trial in which of the nine possible quadrants the tangible or graphic symbol will be located. Mark the trial number in the small square within the quadrant on the data sheet.

5. Alert the learner to the fact that you will be placing a large mirror or magazine (i.e., an occluder) between his or her face and the preferred object. If appropriate, you may tell the learner that his or her "job" will be to look for the object after the occluder is removed. It may also be important to tell the learner that he or she will have the opportunity to manipulate the object (with assistance, if needed) for a few minutes after he or she localizes on it visually.

6. Position the object in the predetermined location (i.e., affix on the display surface) and remove the occluder. Do not tap the object to gain the learner's attention, as that is atypical of the more static nature of graphic symbols that are arrayed on a communication display.

7. Observe continuously to determine how the learner behaves, sequentially, along two distinct dimensions: 1) how long (in seconds) the learner searches for the symbol and 2) if the learner successfully localizes the object visually, record whether he or she is able to sustain localization on the object visually for a minimum of two seconds. Each of these dimensions is recorded separately in the spaces provided on the data sheet. Record as well whether the learner exerted undue effort in localizing on the object.

8. Reward the learner's effort by providing a short break after each assessment trial during which the learner is free to manipulate the symbol (if appropriate) or receive access to the object or event that the symbol represents.

9. Proceed through the assessment a few trials at a time until you have observed and recorded the learner's behavior in all nine possible quadrants for each of the three planes of presentation (27 trials total).

dure and Figure 11.7 represents a data sheet to be completed for each assessment trial.

The team should pose the following questions as they review the data: 1) In which plane of presentation was the learner able to visually gain access to the greatest number of visual stimuli that were arranged on the display surface? and 2) In which plane of presentation was the learner's muscle tone and overall body position most normalized? It is hoped that the answers to these two questions are the same. If not, team members must experiment with various forms of physical guidance, handling techniques, and therapeutic positioning to ensure the learner's visual access to a system with minimal disruption to his or her overall physical well-being (Campbell, 2000; Sobsey & Wolf-Schein, 1996).

Learner's name: _____   Date: _____

Plane of presentation
Check the appropriate plane used during this trial.

___Vertical ___ Horizontal ___Intermediate (angle is approximately ___ degrees)

Location of visual stimulus according to the nine-part presentation field
Check the quadrant that indicates where the visual stimulus was presented during this trial:

Visual location response
Answer the following questions regarding the learner's responses to removal of the occluder:

* Did the student localize on the object?   YES   NO
* What was the approximate latency of the learner's response in seconds? ____
* Did the learner exert undue effort in
  localizing the object in this position?   YES   NO
* Did the learner sustain fixation on
  the object for a minimum of 2 seconds?   YES   NO

Figure 11.7.   Data sheet for recording the results of each trial during the assessment of visual localization in various planes of presentation. (From Utley, B.L. [1994]. Providing support for sensory, postural, and movement needs. In L. Sternberg [Ed.], *Individuals with profound disabilities* [3rd ed., pp. 135–136]. Austin, TX: PRO-ED; adapted by permission.]

Assessing Visually Directed Reach and Touch

This final assessment procedure requires that the team conduct systematic observation of a learner's physical responses to stimuli that are presented in a number of locations, including mid-line orientation and extending to the lateral right and left sides of mid-line. This assessment procedure is only intended for learners who may use an upper extremity movement to activate a switch, touch an object cue, or use direct selection to indicate a choice within a communication display. Although functional vision requires that a learner respond to objects of various sizes at different locations in space, it is also useful for the team to gather precise information regarding the learner's visual and physical accessibility within the width of the learner's shoulders and the length of his or her arms (i.e., the "work surface"). Assessment of visually directed reach and touch is structured to guide observation of a learner's visual and physical responses within the same nine-part grid that was used in the preceding assessment.

The grid, as used in this assessment, permits team members to determine the extent of the learner's visually directed reach and touch responses within the defined work surface. The grid consists of three presentation areas that extend across the front of the learner's body (defined by the width of the learner's shoulders) and three presentation areas that extend outward from the learner's body to the front (defined by the length of the learner's arms). The nine presentation areas in the grid consist of those at mid-line and at 6–9 inches to each lateral side of mid-line, as well as three locations that extend outward from the front of the learner's body. The presentation areas in front of the body are approximately 6 inches from the front edge of the work surface (i.e., the edge closest to the learner's torso) and approximately 12 and 18 inches in front of the learner's body. The presentation grid is shown on this assessment procedure's data sheet (see Figure 11.8). Table 11.9 lists the steps for conducting the assessment.

Team members may choose to repeat presentation of stimuli in certain quadrants of the grid on more than one trial, especially if the learner's response is difficult to observe or somewhat ambiguous. The learner may attempt to touch stimuli with either hand unless the team decides in advance to discourage this behavior through gentle restraint of the learner's hand and arm. A decision that one upper extremity should be used to the exclusion of the other, however, may suggest that the display should be centered in the arc that is accessible by the most readily used hand. This accommodation may reduce fatigue, improve motor accuracy, and mitigate abnormal reflex activity as well as undesirable changes in muscle tone. For more information, see Askvig (1990), which provides a detailed discussion of hand preference and its effect on visually directed reach.

Data that are obtained from this procedure permit the team to make a series of judgments regarding whether all nine quadrants of the presentation

Learner's name: _____   Date: _____

Location of visual stimulus according to the nine-part presentation field
Check the quadrant that indicates where the visual stimulus was presented during this trial:

Visual location response
Answer the following questions regarding the learner's physical responses to removal of the occluder:

• Did the student localize on the object visually?   YES   NO

• Did the learner reach and
  touch the object accurately?   YES   NO

• Which arm and/or hand was used
  to reach out and touch the object?   RIGHT   LEFT

  Was the object positioned on the same
  side of the body as the arm and/or hand
  that was used to reach and touch the object?   YES   NO

  Check here if the object was at mid-line for this trial _____

• Did the learner sustain visual attention
  during the entire reach-and-touch response?   YES   NO

• What was the approximate latency
  of the learner's physical response in seconds? _____

• Did the learner exert undue effort in
  reaching and touching the object in this position?   YES   NO

Figure 11.8. Data sheet for recording the results of each trial during assessment of the reach-and-touch response. (From Utley, B.L. [1994]. Providing support for sensory, postural, and movement needs. In L. Sternberg [Ed.], *Individuals with profound disabilities* [3rd ed., pp. 158–160]. Austin, TX: PRO-ED; adapted by permission.)

grid are equally accessible (physically and visually) for the beginning communicator. Some areas of the prototype may prove to be completely inaccessible, others may limit the accuracy of the learner's movements, and still others may occasion maladaptive movement patterns. Some researchers suggest that only symbols with high reinforcement value be placed in less desirable areas of the display surface (Orelove & Sobsey, 1996); however, an alternative viewpoint is that *no* symbols be placed in these areas. It may be undesirable

Table 11.9.   Steps for assessing visually directed reach and touch

1. Select one or more high-preference stimuli that can be affixed to the prototype display surface. Examples include small toy people for young children, trading cards for somewhat older children, and a colorful CD insert or "jewel" box for adolescent learners.

2. If the object is not too heavy, attach it to the prototype communication display surface with two-sided adhesive tape. Heavier stimuli may need to be affixed to a piece of Velcro, with a small piece of the corresponding Velcro surface affixed in each quadrant of the display surface.

3. Determine prior to each assessment trial in which of the nine possible quadrants the tangible or graphic symbol will be located. Mark the trial number within the quadrant on the data sheet.

4. Alert the learner to the fact that you will be placing a large mirror or magazine (i.e., an occluder) between his or her face and the preferred object. If appropriate, you may tell the learner that his or her "job" will be to look for the object after the occluder is removed. It may also be important to tell the learner that he or she will have the opportunity to manipulate the object (with assistance, if needed) for a few minutes after he or she localizes on it visually.

5. Position the object in the predetermined location (i.e., affix on the display surface) and remove the occluder. Do not tap the object to gain the learner's attention, as that is atypical of the more static nature of graphic symbols that are arrayed on a communication display.

6. Observe continuously to determine how the learner behaves, sequentially, along three distinct dimensions: 1) the learner's attempts to reach and touch the object in that location, 2) the learner's visual attention to guide his or her movement to the object during the reach and touch response, and 3) the accuracy of the reach-and-touch response. Each of these dimensions is recorded separately in the spaces provided on the data sheet.

7. Reward the learner's effort by providing a short break after each assessment trial during which he or she is free to manipulate the symbol (if appropriate) or receive access to the object or event that the symbol represents or the switch activates.

8. Proceed through the assessment a few trials at a time until you have observed and recorded the learner's behavior in all nine possible quadrants.

Note: Only conduct this assessment for learners who will use an upper extremity response to activate a switch, touch an object cue, or use direct selection.

to design a communication display that contains areas to which the learner has limited access, as the excess effort that is required to express a particular message may inadvertently (and inappropriately) determine the content of the learner's communication message. Such a design may also be inappropriate because a learner who is fatigued may be unable to gain access to the difficult areas and, thus, become discouraged from communicating his or her message. An alternative to this situation is to cluster multiple overlays of symbols within the learner's most accessible arc of movement. Different overlays can then be used for communication across various environmental contexts.

CONCLUSION

Teams of professionals must make many decisions to ensure the greatest probability of success when early communicators are introduced to graphic or tangible AAC systems. Some learners' physical and sensory disabilities interact to generate complex practice issues for the teams that are developing beginning AAC systems. Resolving these problems requires that team members engage in careful observation, high levels of role release (Utley & Rapport, 2000), and deference to an agreed-on set of data to best meet the complex needs that some learners bring to this essential skill area. Unfortunately, the research base is limited regarding AAC decision making for learners with combined sensory and physical disabilities. Therefore, the following questions are intended to guide future research in this challenging area:

- How can teams of professionals design supports for a learner's head and neck that provide comfort, therapeutic positioning, *and* optimal visual regard of an AAC device?
- What knowledge and which skills regarding vision assessment and intervention must be part of personnel preparation for school professionals who serve learners with multiple disabilities?
- What skills and processes facilitate communication between medical professionals and school-based teams regarding the results of formal physiological vision assessments (e.g., visual acuity, refractive errors) and the functional implications of those results?

In the future, answers to these and other research questions may assist school professionals during the complex process of designing AAC systems for beginning communicators with sensory and physical disabilities. In the short-term, however, it is hoped that this chapter's assessment procedures and data interpretation guidelines will serve school professionals as they respond to the unique assessment and design needs of individual beginning communicators.

REFERENCES

Askvig, B.A. (1990). Critical issues in assessing visual tracking and scanning, hand preference, and basic receptive language skills. In D. Baumgart, J. Johnson, & E. Helmstetter (Eds.), *Augmentative and alternative communication systems for persons with moderate and severe disabilities* (pp. 71–97). Baltimore: Paul H. Brookes Publishing Co.

Batshaw, M.L., & Shapiro, B.K. (1997). Mental retardation. In M.L. Batshaw (Ed.), *Children with disabilities* (4th ed., pp. 335–359). Baltimore: Paul H. Brookes Publishing Co.

Baumgart, D., Johnson, J., & Helmstetter, E. (Eds.). (1990). *Augmentative and alternative communication systems for persons with moderate and severe disabilities.* Baltimore: Paul H. Brookes Publishing Co.

Bayley, N. (1969). *Bayley Scales of Infant Development.* San Antonio, TX: The Psychological Corporation.

Campbell, P.H. (1987). Integrated programming for students with multiple handicaps. In L. Goetz, D. Guess, & K. Stremel-Campbell (Eds.), *Innovative program design for individuals with dual sensory impairments* (pp. 159–188). Baltimore: Paul H. Brookes Publishing Co.

Campbell, P.H. (2000). Promoting participation in natural environments by accommodating motor disabilities. In M.E. Snell & F. Brown (Eds.), *Instruction of students with severe disabilities* (5th ed., pp. 291–330). Upper Saddle River, NJ: Prentice Hall.

Campbell, P.H., Baumgarner, J., & Wilcox, M.J. (1989). *Guidelines for determining functional use of vision in school-based settings.* Talmadge, OH: Family Child Learning Center.

Cress, P. (1988). Visual assessment. In M. Bullis & G. Fielding (Eds.), *Communication development in young children with deaf-blindness: Literature review.* Monmouth: Oregon State System of Higher Education.

Dunn, W. (1996). The sensorimotor systems: A framework for assessment and intervention. In F.P. Orelove & D. Sobsey (Eds.), *Educating children with multiple disabilities: A transdisciplinary approach* (3rd ed., pp. 35–78). Baltimore: Paul H. Brookes Publishing Co.

Dunst, C.J. (1980). *A clinical and educational manual for use with the Uzgiris and Hunt Scales of Infant Psychological Development.* Baltimore: University Park Press.

Erhardt, R.P. (1986). *Erhardt Developmental Vision Assessment.* Fargo, ND: Author.

Giangreco, M.F., Edelman, S., & Dennis, R. (1991). Common professional practices that interfere with the integrated delivery of related services. *Remedial and Special Education, 12*(2), 16–24.

Guess, D., & Helmstetter, E. (1986). Skill cluster instruction and the individualized curriculum sequencing model. In R.H. Horner, L.H. Meyer, & H.D.B. Fredericks (Eds.), *Education of learners with severe handicaps: Exemplary service strategies* (pp. 221–248). Baltimore: Paul H. Brookes Publishing Co.

Johnson, J.M., Baumgart, D., Helmstetter, E., & Curry, C.A. (1996). *Augmenting basic communication in natural contexts.* Baltimore: Paul H. Brookes Publishing Co.

Musselwhite, C.R., & St. Louis, K.W. (1988). *Communication programming for persons with severe handicaps* (2nd ed.). New York: Little, Brown.

Orelove, F.P., & Sobsey, D. (1996). Communication skills. In F.P. Orelove & D. Sobsey (Eds.), *Educating children with multiple disabilities: A transdisciplinary approach* (3rd ed., pp. 253–299). Baltimore: Paul H. Brookes Publishing Co.

Pellegrino, L. (1997). Cerebral palsy. In M.L. Batshaw (Ed.), *Children with disabilities* (4th ed., pp. 499–528). Baltimore: Paul H. Brookes Publishing Co.

Rapport, M.K. (1995). Laws that shape therapy services in educational environments. *Physical and Occupational Therapy in Pediatrics, 15*(2), 5–32.

Rosen, S. (1998). Educating students who have visual impairments with neurological disabilities. In S.Z. Sacks & R.K. Silberman (Eds.), *Educating students who have visual impairments with other disabilities* (pp. 221–262). Baltimore: Paul H. Brookes Publishing Co.

Sacks, S.Z. (1998). Educating students who have visual impairment with other disabilities: An overview. In S.Z. Sacks & R.K. Silberman (Eds.), *Educating students who have visual impairments with other disabilities* (pp. 3–38). Baltimore: Paul H. Brookes Publishing Co.

Silberman, R.K., Sacks, S.Z., & Wolfe, J. (1998). Instructional strategies for educating students who have visual impairments with severe disabilities. In S.Z. Sacks & R.K. Silberman (Eds.), *Educating students who have visual impairments with other disabilities* (pp. 101–137). Baltimore: Paul H. Brookes Publishing Co.

Sobsey, D., & Wolf-Schein, E. (1996). Children with sensory impairments. In F.P. Orelove & D. Sobsey (Eds.), *Educating children with multiple disabilities: A transdisciplinary approach* (3rd ed., pp. 411–450). Baltimore: Paul H. Brookes Publishing Co.

Utley, B.L. (1993). Assessing the instructional environment to meet the needs of learners with multiple disabilities including students who are deaf-blind. *Deaf-Blind Perspectives, 1*(2), 5–8.

Utley, B.L. (1994). Providing support for sensory, postural, and movement needs. In L. Sternberg (Ed.), *Individuals with profound disabilities: Instructional and assistive strategies* (3rd ed., pp. 123–192). Austin, TX: PRO-ED.

Utley, B.L., & Nelson, G.L. (1992). Visual-motor efficiency of adults with multiple and visual disabilities: An assessment and intervention model. *Journal of Vocation Rehabilitation, 2*(1), 9–20.

Utley, B.L., & Rapport, M.K. (2000). Exploring role release in the multidisciplinary team. *Physical Disabilities: Education and Related Services, 28*(2), 89–118.

Utley, B.L., Roman, C., & Nelson, G.L. (1998). Functional vision. In S.Z. Sacks & R.K. Silberman (Eds.), *Educating students who have visual impairments with other disabilities* (pp. 371–412). Baltimore: Paul H. Brookes Publishing Co.

VORT Corporation. (1995). *HELP: Hawaii Early Learning Profile.* Palo Alto, CA: Author.

York, J., & Weimann, G. (1991). Accommodating severe physical disabilities. In J. Reichle, J. York, & J. Sigafoos (Eds.), *Implementing augmentative and alternative communication: Strategies for learners with severe disabilities* (pp. 239–255). Baltimore: Paul H. Brookes Publishing Co.

Appendix
Environmental Checklist

Name of learner: _____ Date: _____

I. Therapeutic positioning
1. Overall body positioning in sitting

_____ a. The learner is seated in a fully upright posture or the wheelchair/ seating equipment is at a slightly reclined seat-in-space angle; with hips, knees, and ankles at 90-degree angles. (Note: Some learners may require a different positioning angle at proximal joints of the body as recommended by an occupational or physical therapist.)

_____ b. The learner's head is in a neutral and full-upright position, with or without external supports provided through adaptive equipment or manual guidance.

_____ c. The tabletop or wheelchair tray supports the learner's arms so that his or her elbows are flexed between 90 and 120 degrees.

2. Overall body positioning in side lying

_____ a. The learner is supported therapeutically (i.e., lower shoulder is slightly forward of the spine; head is in alignment with the spine; hips, knees and ankles are flexed; soft, small pillows are placed between and below bony prominences as indicated).

_____ b. If the learner is monocular, he or she lies on the side that results in the better eye being on the upper lateral half of the body to facilitate visual regard of a communication partner and/or a communication device or display. (Note: An occupational therapist or a physical therapist should be consulted to determine whether side lying on a particular lateral half of the body is contraindicated.)

From Utley, B.L. (1993). Assessing the instructional environment to meet the needs of learners with multiple disabilities including students who are deaf-blind. *Deaf-Blind Perspectives, 1*(2), 6; adapted by permission.

3. Position of peers and adults
_____ a. Peers or adults position themselves for communication interaction at or near the learner's eye level.
_____ b. Peers or adults position themselves at mid-line or slightly to one lateral side of the learner to avoid eliciting abnormal reflex activity.

4. Plane of presentation for placement of the AAC device
_____ a. The AAC device is presented on a wheelchair tray, desk, or table (horizontal plane) if the learner's head erect behavior permits him or her to regard the device without loss of head control or poor visual regard of the device (e.g., eyes rolling upward into the bony orbits of the skull when the chin is flexed to the chest).

OR

_____ b. The AAC device is presented at eye level (vertical plane) if the learner's head erect behavior permits him or her to regard the device without loss of head control and if he or she is able to engage in antigravity movement of the hands to explore or activate the device.

OR

_____ c. The surface of the wheelchair tray is adjusted to an angle that is intermediate to full horizontal or vertical locations in space or a supplementary lightweight podium is placed on a table or desk to support presentation of the AAC device.

II. Lighting
1. Amount and type of lighting
_____ a. A combination of light sources (i.e., natural light plus incandescent light sources) is available to supplement typical fluorescent light sources.
_____ b. The entire communication display, or background surface for a switch or object cue, is illuminated evenly.
_____ c. Supplemental lighting is available (if indicated).

2. Position of light
_____ a. The learner and his or her communication partner are positioned so that all sources of natural light (e.g., windows) are to the side of both parties.
_____ b. The supplemental light source originates from over the learner's head so that the shade directs the light on the communication materials only.

OR

_____ c.   The supplemental light source originates from behind and over the shoulder opposite to the learner's dominant hand (i.e., over the left shoulder for those who use the right hand).

OR

_____ d.   If the learner is monocular, supplemental light source originates from behind and over the shoulder of the learner on the lateral side of the body with the functional eye.

12

Choosing Effective Selection Techniques for Beginning Communicators

Patricia Dowden and Albert M. Cook

Finding the most functional selection technique is sometimes considered the key to successfully using augmentative and alternative communication (AAC), particularly for individuals with severe sensory and/or motor impairments. AAC team members often believe that they can unlock an individual's ability to communicate with the world if only they can find the best access method. Yet, in reality, the selection technique is merely the first key to open the first door on the way to independent communication. There are too many possible access methods to try them out one by one as one might test keys on a key chain. Selection techniques encompass a nearly infinite set of variations that must be custom crafted for the individual. As with all other AAC decisions, the goal is not simply to provide access to a device but to allow an individual to participate in life's activities through communication (Beukelman & Mirenda, 1998).

This chapter focuses on selection techniques for beginning AAC users. It begins with definitions to illustrate some of the endless variations that are possible. A review of the available research on selection techniques shows what is known and what remains unknown about these methods and their impact on communication. From this perspective, this chapter addresses decision-making strategies that might assist AAC teams in this complex customization process for beginning communicators.

SELECTION TECHNIQUES AND INTERFACES: DEFINITIONS AND INVERVENTION PERSPECTIVES

There is some disagreement about how to describe the various selection methods, such as *direct selection* and *scanning*. The authors prefer to use the terms *direct selection* and *indirect selection*, focusing on the individual's degree of control

395

over the process. Briefly, *direct selection* means that the user specifically indicates the desired item in the selection set. *Indirect selection* includes single- and dual-switch scanning, directed scanning, and coded access. It involves intermediary steps by the device or the partner, usually to compensate for motor limitations of the user (Cook & Hussey, 1995). Individuals without disabilities engage in direct selection when typing on a computer keyboard, as they use their fingers to directly activate the letters of the alphabet or other characters. Individuals without disabilities have considerably less experience with indirect selection, except perhaps the "seek" button on a radio that scans each available station one by one. When a preferred station or song is reached, the scanning process is stopped by releasing the button or pressing it a second time.

Direct selection and *indirect selection* seem to be the most appropriate terms for four reasons. First, the contrast between the terms highlights the fact that direct selection has a one-to-one relationship between the motor act and the resultant selection, whereas indirect selection involves one or more intermediary steps (Cook & Hussey, 1995). Second, these terms emphasize the role of time in all indirect methods in which the additional steps introduce delays (Cook & Hussey, 1995). Third, these terms are easier to apply to new, emerging technologies. The popular dichotomy of direct selection versus scanning makes it difficult to discuss new interfaces, such as track pads, that are not direct selection and do not fit the scanning category particularly well. Finally, this terminology may encourage professionals to consider some of the less common indirect methods, such as coded access and multiswitch, directed scanning.

Direct Selection Techniques

As described previously, direct selection entails two fundamental features: 1) the motor act is direct, requiring no intermediary steps, and 2) the process of making a selection is not time dependent. The aforementioned keyboard example may seem like the prototypical example of direct selection, but there are some variations that should be noted. First, direct selection does not have to involve a large selection set; it includes even the activation of a single switch to achieve a single voice output message. Second, direct selection does not preclude encoding or the combinations of keys for meaning—for example, selecting the *control* and *s* keys together to save a computer file. These special cases do not change the motor aspects of the access method, in which there is a one-to-one relationship between the motor act and the selection. There are four primary types of direct selection (Beukelman & Mirenda, 1998; Lloyd, Fuller, & Arvidson, 1997): 1) pointing without physical contact (e.g., using eye gaze or a light pointer), 2) pointing with physical contact but without force (e.g., pointing on a book or board), 3) pointing with contact and force (e.g., depressing keys or switches), and 4) speech input (e.g., speech commands to a computer).

Intervention Perspectives on Direct Selection   Clinicians agree almost universally about the potential advantages and disadvantages of direct selection. They tend to focus on three characteristics: 1) speed, 2) ease of learning and use, and 3) motor requirements.

Clinicians agree that direct selection is the fastest method of selection as long as the individual's motor control is sufficient (Beukelman & Mirenda, 1998; Mustonen, Locke, Reichle, Solbrack, & Lindgren, 1991; Quist & Lloyd, 1997). The user simply reaches out or directs a light or pointer to the desired targets, so the speed of selection is limited only by the individual's motor abilities (Cook & Hussey, 1995).

Many clinicians have concluded that direct selection is also the easiest method to learn to use (Cook & Hussey, 1995; Gunderson, 1985; Ratcliff, 1994). This is due in part to the direct relationship between the motor act and the resultant selection (Cook & Hussey, 1995). It has been suggested that direct selection is the most natural method because it is used by infants and toddlers in their prelinguistic communication (Ratcliff, 1994).

Despite its potential advantages, direct selection has one disadvantage for some users: It places considerable demands on the user's motor abilities (Angelo, 1992; Cook & Hussey, 1995; Gunderson, 1985). Direct selection requires a greater *range of motion* (the extent of movement that is possible by a body part) so the user can reach all of the items in a selection set. It also requires a finer *resolution of movement* (the smallest separation possible between targets) to include as many items into that range as possible. When using the same body part, direct selection always requires more range and resolution than indirect selection, such as fingers on a keyboard (direct) compared with fingers on a switch (indirect). The motor requirement for a given direct selection method can be significantly reduced through control enhancements and other modifications to the technique, as shown in Table 12.1.

Indirect Selection Techniques

There are three categories of indirect selection: 1) scanning with single or dual switches, 2) directed scanning, and 3) coded access (Cook & Hussey, 1995). Each is discussed separately, with emphasis on the motor demands and precise timing requirements as well as on the potential speed of communication.

Scanning with Single or Dual Switches   Scanning with single or dual switches is the most common type of indirect selection (Cook & Hussey, 1995). In scanning, the selection set is presented sequentially, either by a communication device or by a communication partner (called *partner-assisted scanning*). The user must wait for the desired item before indicating a choice by either activating the switch or signaling to the partner (Mustonen et al., 1991). The selection set can be presented visually through graphic symbols, aurally

Table 12.1.   Control enhancers and technique modifications

Control enhancers: Devices or equipment to extend or enhance motor control for direct selection (or indirect selection, as indicated by *)

Postural support	At hands/arms	At head
Lap tray*	Finger splint/pointer	Mouth stick
Arm rests*	Universal cuff with typing stick	Head pointer
Hip belt*	Wrist strap pointer	Head light
Chest straps*	Mobile arm supports*	Head mouse
Lateral supports*	Hand brace*	Head rest*
Abductor/adductor*	Hand splint*	

Technique modifications: Changes to the selection technique to reduce the demands for direct selection (or indirect selection, as indicated by *)

Selection set design	Interface adjustments	Additional aids
Target size*	Acceptance time*	Keyguards
Spacing*	Delay until repeat*	Templates*
Array shape*	Repeat rate*	Shields*
Angle*	Cursor speed*	Hand rest*
Height*	Sensitivity*	
Order of items	Activation feedback*	

Sources: Cook & Hussey (1995) and Dowden (1999a).

through spoken words, or through both modalities in combination (Blackstone, 1989).

There are many types of scanning, differing in two primary ways: 1) the *scanning pattern* (i.e., how the cursor progresses through the selection set) and 2) the *selection control techniques* (i.e., how the user makes a selection). Some scanning patterns are *linear,* meaning that the cursor moves sequentially through each item in one or more rows. Scanning patterns can also be *circular.* Circular patterns present options sequentially either via a cursor that sweeps around the array similar to the second hand on a clock or lights that illuminate sequentially around the circle. There is some disagreement among clinicians as to which of these methods is easier for beginning communicators to learn and use. Some prefer linear scanning (Mustonen et al., 1991) while others believe circular scanning is easier (Beukelman & Mirenda, 1998). The third scanning pattern is *group-item* or *multidimensional scanning,* which is generally considered more difficult that the other two methods (Mustonen et al., 1991). In this technique, groups of items are presented and the user selects the group that contains the desired target. Items in that group are then presented individually until the user selects the target item itself (Lloyd et al., 1997). The most common group-item scanning technique is *row-column scanning,* in which the individual selects the row, then the specific item within that row.

There are also three different selection control techniques used in scanning, and each one places distinctly different demands on the user (Beukelman & Mirenda, 1998; Cook & Hussey, 1995). *Automatic scanning* is definitely the most common, although it is not necessarily the easiest to use. This method, also called *regular scanning* or *interrupted scanning*, requires the user to wait until the desired item is indicated by the cursor before activating the switch to select it. This approach requires the individual to identify the target item, wait while the cursor scans to it, and then activate the switch within a narrow window of time. This length of time is determined by the cursor speed or scanning rate–that is, the number of seconds that the cursor remains on each item as it moves through the array. *Inverse scanning* is very different from automatic scanning in many respects. When using inverse scanning, the individual activates a switch and maintains that activation until the cursor reaches the target item, then releases the switch to make a selection. This method requires one to identify the target item, activate the switch, maintain activation, and then release at just the right moment to select that item. Both types of single-switch scanning require little movement of the individual but also give the least control over the speed of selection because the user must wait until items are presented. Inverse scanning with a single switch is also sometimes called *directed scanning*, but this terminology causes some confusion in the field. The authors prefer to reserve the term *directed scanning* for a multiswitch scanning method that is described in the ensuing subsection. *Step scanning* is unlike other methods in that it requires the individual to activate the switch multiple times to move the cursor through each item in the selection set. For example, 15 activations moves the cursor to the 15th item in the display. The user makes a selection by activating a separate selection switch (in two-switch scanning) or by waiting a predetermined time for timed activation to occur. When contrasted with other single-switch methods, step scanning gives the user more control over the speed of the selection process, but it places comparatively greater demands on the individual's motor skills and causes greater fatigue.

Intervention perspectives on single- and dual-switch scanning have been very clear and consistent. These scanning methods require far less motor control than direct selection, but this comes at considerable cost (Angelo, 1992; Vanderheiden, 1988). First, scanning is generally slower than direct selection because the items in the selection set are presented sequentially to the user (Gunderson, 1985; Piché & Reichle, 1991). Second, scanning is considered more complex to learn (Ratcliff, 1994) because it involves complicated relationships between the cursor and the target and between the switch and the selection process (Light, 1993). Third, scanning may place greater cognitive demands on the user during selection, particularly in the areas of memory (Ratcliff, 1994) and attention to task (Cook & Hussey, 1995; Ratcliff, 1994).

Directed Scanning   Directed scanning, as distinct from inverse scanning, combines elements of direct selection and scanning (Cook & Hussey, 1995; Vanderheiden, 1988). The user must have access to multiple switches, such as an array of arrow keys or a joystick interface. He or she activates the interface to move the cursor in a particular direction toward the target. The cursor scans all of the items in that direction in a sequential manner until the user makes a selection by releasing the joystick and activating a separate selection switch or by waiting for timed acceptance. Similar to direct selection, this method requires the user to control the direction of movement to move the cursor toward the target (Vanderheiden, 1988). Unlike direct selection, however, there are additional steps and delays as the individual waits for the cursor to reach the target (Cook & Hussey, 1995). Individuals without disabilities are most familiar with directed scanning in the context of using a joystick to play computer games.

Little information exists about intervention perspectives on directed scanning because it is a comparatively rare technique. When contrasted with direct selection, directed scanning is generally considered slower, conceptually harder to learn, and cognitively more demanding to use. When compared with single- or dual-switch scanning, however, it is considerably faster for individuals who have sufficient motor control (Cook & Hussey, 1995).

Coded Access   The third type of indirect selection is termed *coded access* because the individual uses a sequence of movements as a code for each item in the selection set (Cook & Hussey, 1995). There is considerable confusion within the field about the difference between coded access, which is a selection technique, and *encoding*, which is a speed enhancement technique. The crucial difference is that coded access requires a *sequence of body movements* to make a selection (Cook & Hussey, 1995), whereas encoding uses a *sequence of selections* to make a message (Beukelman & Mirenda, 1998). It can be argued that when encoding becomes automatic, the individual may begin to combine access and encoding so that a sequence of body movements translates directly into a message. Yet, this is a short cut used by the most experienced individuals and does not change the fact that coded access and encoding are two distinct AAC strategies. It is significant that encoding can be used with all types of direct and indirect selection techniques, including coded access, to increase the speed of communication.

Individuals without disabilities have experience with coded access only if they use Morse code, in which each letter of the alphabet is represented by a different sequence of movements. In one-switch Morse code, the timing and duration of each switch activation selects the letter. For example *a* is selected with one short activation, immediately followed by one long activation. In two-switch Morse code, the direction of movement is also important, as the user activates first one then the other switch. Beukelman and Mirenda (1998) and Cook and Hussey (1995) described other coded access systems, from eight-switch codes via a joystick to eight-direction codes using the eyes. Many of these techniques rely on spelling, but the selection set can also be words or phrases that are assigned to a sequence of movements, such as "yes" and "no" being assigned to one or two eye blinks.

Clinicians have tended to avoid coded access for beginning communicators because of the confusion with encoding, which makes the technique appear too complex. Nonetheless, Goossens' and Crain (1987) taught coded access via the eyes even to very young children, and Culp and Ladtkow (1992) used it with "locked-in" adults following severe brain-stem strokes.

Interfaces

It would be impossible to mention all of the existing control interfaces. Even if that were possible at one point in time, the information would become outdated as soon as a new switch or computer interface appeared on the market. It is far more useful to give the reader a framework for evaluating control interfaces so that he or she can compare new ones with existing ones. Cook and Hussey (1995) described *control interfaces* in terms of the following features: spatial, sensory, and activation/deactivation characteristics. There are four spatial characteristics (Cook & Hussey 1995): 1) the overall size of the interface, 2) the number of targets available for activation, 3) the size of each target (direct selection) or the active part of a switch (indirect selection), and 4) the spacing between targets or switches. Clinicians often recognize the importance of the spatial characteristics but miss the role of sensory feedback even though it can increase the success of any interface (Barker & Cook, 1981). This feedback can be any audible sound upon activation, the visual position of the switch and any visible movement upon activation, and the somatosensory characteristics (tactile, kinesthetic, or proprioceptive information) upon activation (Cook & Hussey, 1995).

Activation and deactivation characteristics include the following:

- Effort, which is generally considered the force required to cause activation
- Displacement, which is the amount of travel in the interface from the rest position to the activated position
- Flexibility, or the number of ways in which the interface can be activated at a single location on the body
- Deactivation force, which is the amount of force necessary to end activation
- Durability, or the amount of use that a switch can withstand
- The method of activation, or the way in which the user activates the interface

The methods of activation can also be described by the type of action that activates the AAC device (Cook & Hussey, 1995). Mechanical switches are activated by pressure or force (e.g., keyboards, most switches). Electromagnetic interfaces are sensitive to light or radio waves (e.g., light pointers). Electrical sensors are activated by electrical signals from the body (e.g., electrodes, capacitive switches). Proximity switches are sensitive to the temperature increases near the body. Pneumatic switches are activated by changes in air pressure (e.g., sip-and-puff switches). Finally, sound switches (e.g., a whistle switch, speech-activated switch) are yet another method of activation.

RESEARCH ON SELECTION TECHNIQUES AND INTERFACES

Unfortunately, there is far too little empirical research about selection techniques, and replication of that research is nearly nonexistent (Beukelman & Mirenda, 1998; Mizuko & Esser, 1991; Ratcliff, 1994). This is due in part to the immense problems in participant selection, methodology, and replication that researchers face in such studies. The challenges of participant selection were described eloquently by Higginbotham (1995a, 1995b) and Bedrosian (1995). On one hand, it is relatively easy to conduct studies with individuals without disabilities who are readily available and show relative homogeneity as a population. However, Bedrosian (1995) raised serious concerns about the generalizability of such studies to individuals with disabilities, especially with so little empirical evidence. On the other hand, studies of people with disabilities are considerably more difficult to conduct logistically and are not necessarily more useful because of the extreme heterogeneity in individual characteristics and variability in performance.

In general, research into selection techniques has shown poor control of extraneous variables in the procedures, participant characteristics, participants' prior experience, and the definition and measurement of the dependent variable. The biggest flaw is defining and measuring the term *accuracy* in vastly different ways but then using it casually in discussions of intervention relevance as if it had a single, clear meaning. All of these methodological problems limit the value of many studies to the field. Even when the research is well conducted, questions regarding replicability often remain. The initial study must describe the participant criteria and the task in enough detail, and the replication study must adhere closely to those parameters. This is not easy in a "young" field, in which both the technology and the terminology change constantly.

Keeping these limitations in mind, the chapter authors have examined the available research on selection techniques. The following section reviews only studies that compare two or more selection methods by using participants and technology that have a bearing on beginning communicators. For this reason, the review does not cover research on certain interfaces (e.g., tongue-touch keypads) or participants (e.g., individuals with spinal cord injury). Research on speed enhancement techniques has likewise been excluded because this book focuses on beginning communicators.

Comparing Direct Techniques with Indirect Techniques

Several studies have compared direct techniques with indirect techniques. The first was Ratcliff's (1994) comparing direct selection via an optical head pointer with row-column scanning with a single switch. The researcher randomly assigned 100 typically developing elementary-school students to the two groups and taught them to participate in a symbol recall task. Participants were then tested in a direction-following task of increasing difficulty for finding geometric shapes in a 128-item array. Results across all grades suggested that the students who used row-column scanning made significantly more selection errors than students who used direct selection. The author concluded that row-column scanning was the more difficult access method but cautioned that replication of the results would be necessary.

Mizuko and Esser (1991) conducted a similar study with 12 typically developing children. Four-year-olds were taught to select two- or three-symbol sequences on a circular array, either by pointing or by using single-switch inverse scanning. Subsequent testing showed no significant differences in the number of correct sequences that were selected by the children who used either of the two selection techniques. The authors speculated that the results were different from those in Ratcliff's (1994) study due to subtle differences in participants' ages, the type of scanning used, the complexity of the task, and the size and type of array. These speculations only highlight the importance of exact replication. Yet, the findings from both studies cannot be generalized to individuals with disabilities because the impact of physical or other disabilities on the performance of this task remains unknown (Bedrosian, 1995).

Several authors subsequently conducted a joint study on selection techniques and the impact on short-term visual memory (Mizuko, Reichle, Ratcliff, & Esser, 1994). The participants were 22 children without disabilities, with a mean age of 55 months. The researchers randomly assigned the children to a direct selection or a row-column scanning group. Participants were shown pairs of line drawings and, after a demonstration, instructed to find the same symbols in the correct order on randomly arranged arrays of 10, 20, 30, and 40 items. For a response to be considered correct, both symbols had to be selected in the correct sequence via the assigned selection technique. Results showed no significant main effect for the selection techniques; however, one significant difference was identified. With a 40-item array, the mean level of accuracy was significantly greater with direct selection than with scanning, unlike results obtained in the original Mizuko and Esser (1991) study. The authors speculated that the larger array and using the row-column scanning method increased the processing demands on the user. Nevertheless, they cautioned strongly against generalizing these results to specific individuals with disabilities.

Horn and Jones (1996) conducted a study of selection techniques (an optical indicator and a single-switch circular scanner) with a 4-year-old boy with severe quadriplegic cerebral palsy. Using an alternating treatment design, the authors wanted to compare the child's accuracy, speed of response, and acquisition rate with each method on a symbol-matching task. Yet, the design only required the participant to use both selection methods in a task that involved one target item. Thus, the direct selection task only measured the child's ability to orient the light from the optical indicator onto a single target, whereas the indirect task measured his ability to wait and activate the switch within a narrow window of time. Consequently, this study did not predict the child's motor accuracy when symbol discrimination was required with either method.

Comparing Direct Selection Techniques

A larger body of research compares direct selection methods, but few of the studies involve AAC. Most studies have been in the domain of human performance and have used emerging computer access technologies (e.g., studies that compared the early mouse and keyboard). Such research is of limited applicability to the AAC field for several reasons: 1) the technologies have continued to evolve, making earlier studies incomparable to later research; 2) the studies have focused on extremely narrow tasks, which have often been more related to computer use than to communication (e.g., tracking a sine wave with a mouse); 3) many results have not been replicated; and 4) the few reported replication attempts have not been successful (Lin & Schmidt, 1993).

Two studies are relevant, however, because they compared alternate computer access methods that are commonly used for communication. Battenberg and Merbler (1989) compared the use of a touch screen with a standard keyboard with two groups of kindergartners. One group had developmental delays, the other did not. The participants were taught and tested in using the two access methods under counterbalanced conditions for letter-matching and spelling tasks. Measures of selection accuracy and speed of response suggested that the participants who used the touch screen were faster and made more correct selections than those who used the keyboard. Yet, the report did not specify the layout of the on-screen keyboard or the visual presentation of the computer stimuli; either of these factors could have favored the on-screen selection task for both measures, making the results difficult to interpret.

The second study was by Durfee and Billingsley (1999), who compared the touch screen and a computer mouse with an enlarged cursor for a 9-year-old boy with spastic quadriplegia, cognitive disabilities, and impaired visual acuity due to cerebral palsy. To examine accuracy, the authors used a within-subject replication design with four phases in which the child was taught to use access methods in a letter-matching task. Results indicated that this individual selected the correct letters more often by using the mouse than the touch screen, but he made correct selections faster with the touch screen than with the mouse. It is interesting to note that the child preferred the mouse although it was slower. The authors found the results to be useful in planning this child's computer access program, demonstrating that success cannot be measured by speed alone. The authors cautioned strongly against generalizing these results to any other individuals with disabilities unless replication has established the extent of generality.

Comparing Indirect Selection Techniques

It is not surprising that the research base regarding indirect selection techniques is also very limited. Nonetheless, a few studies have compared different scanning modes, scanning patterns, and switches and interfaces.

Comparing Across Scanning Modes   Angelo (1992) conducted a study of three indirect selection techniques, in part to replicate an earlier unpublished study by LeBlanc and Barker. That original study was not described in detail, but Angelo (1992) reported that individuals with athetoid cerebral palsy were less accurate with row-column scanning than with a user-driven two-switch system, a vertical scanning system, and a horizontal scanning system. The six participants in Angelo's study were diagnosed with cerebral palsy; three of the participants had spasticity and three had athetoid characteristics. The task was to use automatic-, inverse-, and step-scanning methods at both slow and fast scanning speeds to select a single target item from an array with otherwise empty boxes. After diagnostic intervention in which speeds were customized for all three scanning modes, the author measured accuracy on three separate trials using the modes in randomized order. In examining the results, Angelo found that the grouped data showed no significant differences among the scanning methods. Nonetheless, the author reported trends suggesting that the participants with spastic cerebral palsy were least accurate with automatic scanning and the participants with athetoid cerebral palsy were least accurate with step scanning. Yet, because of the considerable within- and between-subject performance variability (even within the diagnostic categories), it is difficult to draw clinically significant conclusions from this study. Angelo cautioned that the results have limited applicability to other individuals.

Comparing Scanning Patterns   Within a broader study, Venkatagiri (1999) used computer simulation to compare row-column scanning with linear scanning. The author used sentences that had been composed by college students for hypothetical communication situations. During the input process, dependent measures included characters per minute, words per minute, and, conversely, duration per character. Results showed that row-column scanning was significantly more efficient (in terms of duration per character) than linear scanning across all layouts, with a mean gain of 119% in efficiency (Venkatagiri, 1999).

Comparing Visual to Auditory Scanning   Only one study has compared the different presentation modalities in scanning: visual, auditory, or auditory-visual. Fried-Oken (1989) studied 90 typical adults as they produced sentences via visual, auditory, and auditory-visual scanning. Results suggested that selection accuracy and reaction times were highest for visual scanning and lowest for auditory scanning, with scores for auditory-visual presentation falling in between.

Comparing Interfaces   Swinth, Anson, and Deitz (1993) examined single hand switch use to activate pictures and music on a computer. The study participants were children between 6 and 17 months of age. This task was not actually indirect selection because each switch directly affected the software and no time dependency was involved, but the study has implications for selecting interfaces for indirect access. After no more than 5 minutes of intervention, the participants were tested in 10 consecutive opportunities. A correct response was defined as activation of the switch with or without cues from the examiner within 20 seconds after the pictures and music stopped playing on the computer. The authors concluded that some children as young as 6 months could perform this task accurately and most children were successful by 9 months of age. They found that children 15–17 months of age failed to learn this task, apparently due to boredom or disinterest. The authors cautioned against generalizing the results to children with disabilities due to the unpredictable effects that physical or other impairments may have in this task.

Glickman, Deitz, Anson, and Stewart (1996) conducted a partial replication and extension of this study by using two different switches with a similar task and dependent measures. The participants were 36 typically developing infants, 9–17 months of age. The researchers assigned them to a hand switch or a head switch group. After training the infants to use the switches, the authors compared the timing of switch activations across age groups and the types of switches. Results suggested that 1) all participants who used the hand switch responded more often within the 20-second time window than the participants who used the head switch, 2) the number of participants responding accurately increased with age for the hand switch but not for the head switch, and 3) fewer participants who used the hand switch lost interest or became distracted during the trials. Viewing this study as a partial replication of Swinth and colleagues (1993), the authors concluded that *some* infants as young as 6–9 months of age can use a single hand switch. Consequently, clinicians may be justified in attempting this task with young children. Nonetheless, the researchers cautioned that the results cannot be generalized to individuals with disabilities and that additional research is warranted.

Further research is needed on these topics, particularly studies that will help intervention decision making. Nevertheless, Higginbotham (1995b) cautioned researchers about the type of studies to pursue. First, participant selection must be based on the nature of the question as well as on the participant characteristics that will best answer that question. Researchers must specify very narrow inclusion criteria that have a direct, functional relationship to the research question. Second, the field needs considerably more studies with individuals who do not have disabilities to construct performance distributions, to be followed by comparative studies with individuals who have disabilities, to determine whether results can be generalized at all. It may be possible to design research that combines group and single-case design to address some of the most pressing research questions.

DECISION-MAKING STRATEGIES FOR ACCESS METHODS

There is tremendous pressure to translate research and intervention experience directly into decision making for the individual AAC user. Although each study may have limited applicability to individuals, research does provide general guidelines for selecting access techniques:

1. *There is a hierarchy of selection techniques.* One must first consider methods that can potentially give the individual the greatest control. Thus, direct selection should be considered before directed scanning, which should be considered before single- or dual-switch indirect selection.
2. *There is also a hierarchy of control sites.* Barker and Cook (1991) defined *control sites* as the potential locations on the body where an individual demonstrates purposeful movement. One should first consider sites with the greatest potential advantages and turn to other sites only as necessary— for example, fingers and hands before head before feet (Barker & Cook, 1981).
3. *Decisions must be based on actual trials with each individual.* Theoretical information from research studies or intervention trials with other individuals cannot be used to make decisions for a given AAC user.
4. *Initial trials with selection techniques should be optimized.* One must initially minimize cognitive and linguistic demands to determine whether the individual has the sensory and motor capabilities to use a given access method. Later, those factors should be added gradually to observe their impact on performance during symbol selection and communication

Given these guidelines, what are the first steps toward identifying a selection technique for an individual AAC user? Traditionally, interventionists begin by discussing seating and positioning, sensory abilities, and other factors that have a significant impact on the initial process. This seems particularly appropriate when focusing on beginning communicators. Practically speaking, however, the term *beginning* covers a wide range of individuals, from those who demonstrate no apparent communicative intent to those who use technology that provides multiple message capabilities. The term *beginning communicator* may blur whether the individual already has reliable access to AAC. In the following discussion, we present two groups of beginning AAC users—emerging communicators and context-dependent communicators—and the way in which their current expressive communication profoundly affects the evaluation and intervention process. Although these groups also apply to individuals with good motor control (Blackstone, 1999; Dowden, 1999a), the focus for this chapter is individuals with motor impairments.

Emerging communicators are individuals who currently have no reliable method of *symbolic* communication, no means of referring to the world around them through semantic reference (Dowden, 1999a). (Note that *symbolic communication* is used here in the sense of locutionary communicative acts [Reichle, 1991]. It is not synonymous with *graphic symbols* because it can also include the use of auditory scanning with no visual symbols.) Out of necessity, emerging communicators must rely on nonlinguistic methods such as gestures, body language, facial expressions, some vocalizations, and perhaps pointing to objects and people in the environment. There may be signals for "yes" and "no," such as a smile and frown, but they are reliable only in the sense of acceptance and rejection, not more abstract communication (i.e., confirming and denying the truth value of a statement). Thus, communication is confined to the "here and now" with familiar partners (Blischak, Loncke, & Waller, 1997), whether due to the individual's limitations (e.g., severe cognitive or linguistic delays) or poor AAC intervention (e.g., an adult with "locked-in syndrome" who is conscious but only able to control eye movements, which have not yet been identified as a communicative signal). For individuals with severe motor impairment, it may not be possible to determine the underlying cause of these limitations at this stage simply because cognitive and linguistic testing is not feasible until symbolic communication is established (Dowden, 1999a, 1999b).

Once symbolic communication has been established and determined to be reliable, AAC communication does not become instantly effective. In fact, the individual AAC user often begins as a *context-dependent communicator* (Blackstone, 1999; Dowden, 1999a). His or her communicative interactions tend to be severely constrained and effective only in specific physical, functional, and social contexts, as defined by Light (1997). On one hand, this may be due to the individual's intrinsic limitations (e.g., poor social skills, limited communication needs, an inability to attend to symbols). On the other hand, it may be due to inadequate AAC intervention that has provided a barely adequate access method, a limited or inappropriate vocabulary, or an output that is understood by few partners. This group may include individuals of all ages who use effective but severely limited systems of communication, such as children who use a symbol exchange technique, adults with aphasia who use simple communication boards, and adults with locked-in syndrome who use "yes" and "no" signals for daily communication.

These groupings do not relate in any way to an individual's age, diagnosis, receptive language, cognition, and, most important, his or her potential to succeed with AAC. Both emerging communicators and context-dependent communicators include individuals who are very young with congenital disabilities or older adults with acute impairments. Some individuals in each group may have untapped potential for using AAC.

Decision making about selection techniques differs significantly for these two groups of individuals in several fundamental ways. First, the goal of intervention and evaluation is different for each group. For an emerging communicator, the AAC team must identify a single, reliable method of communication—not necessarily the "best" or the fastest method. For a context-dependent communicator, the AAC team must give the user greater independence by improving his or her existing system. Second, the individual's participation in the process is different for each group. The individual with emerging skills has no means of communication beyond gestures and body language, whereas a context-dependent communicator can (and should) voice opinions about many aspects of the process when provided both the opportunity and the appropriate vocabulary. Finally, the definition of a successful outcome is different with each group. For an emerging communicator, one only needs to identify the first reliable method of symbolic communication. For a context-dependent communicator, there are many goals on the road toward independence, including expanding the vocabulary repertoire, improving the efficiency of communication, and increasing the effectiveness of communication with a wide range of partners (Dowden, 1999a, 1999b). For these reasons, the following detailed discussion of decision making with selection techniques addresses the two groups of communicators separately.

Identifying Access for Emerging Communicators

Emerging communicators have had little or no success with any methods of symbolic communication. Their strengths and weaknesses as well as their individual desires and needs remain largely hidden to team members. Some of their characteristics are most likely to be revealed within the context of a familiar and highly engaging activity. For this reason, AAC intervention for emerging communicators does not begin with equipment trials but with identifying activities or objects that engage the individual and then using those to screen sensory and motor abilities.

Identifying the Purpose for Interacting   Usually, it is most productive to begin by identifying powerful communicative functions (e.g., request objects or actions, protest objects or actions) or environmental controls (e.g., turn on music, turn off a fan) that will make this individual participate in assessment activities (Sigafoos & York, 1991). This particular topic is covered at length in Chapter 5, so it will not be discussed in depth in this chapter. Yet, two points need to be made regarding individuals with significant motor impairments. First, one must focus intervention activities on communicative functions that would add to, not reduce, the individual's current repertoire, so existing nonlinguistic communication must be honored at all times (Dowden, 1999a). Second, many children and youth with severe sensory and/or motor impairments may prefer to request an action rather than an object from partners because social closeness is more powerful than obtaining an object that they cannot manipulate (Hussey, Cook, Whinnery, Buckpitt, & Huntington, 1992).

Initial Sensory and/or Motor Screening   An individual's sensory and/or motor abilities can be observed in the context of familiar, pleasurable activities. For a child, this means one might begin with *play-based assessment* with activities that revolve around the child's favorite games (e.g., Peekaboo, dancing with music, playing with dolls or trucks, looking at books) (Casey, 1995). For older individuals, the intervention activities focus similarly on their special interests, from make-up to baseball cards to family photographs. During the course of these activities, the professional has an opportunity to examine sensory abilities, natural motor patterns, and the impact of seating and positioning, while keeping communication demands to a minimum.

Hearing and Vision   Children and adults with severe physical disabilities are at high risk for sensory deficits that can impede the development of AAC skills. Vision impairments are thought to occur in 75%–90% of all individuals with severe physical disabilities (Cress et al., 1981), and some degree of dual sensory impairments is very common in children with cerebral palsy (McCarthy, 1992; see also Chapter 11). These impairments are often undiagnosed in AAC users, particularly in emerging communicators who are difficult to test. Yet, even subtle impairments can interfere with the development of receptive language and AAC (Beukelman & Mirenda, 1998; Cook & Hussey, 1995; see also Chapter 14).

Seating and Positioning   Proper positioning is essential for an AAC user's long-term success, and this must be pursued as early as possible (Beukelman & Mirenda, 1998; Cook & Hussey, 1995; York & Weimann, 1991). Yet, this does not mean that AAC intervention depends on ideal seating and positioning. In fact, there are several reasons not to pursue optimum seating initially for an emerging communicator. The goal of intervention is to identify a single reliable method of symbolic communication. This means that, initially, the team does not have to provide access to communication for all positions throughout the day but that it should focus on select activities and the positions currently used for them. Second, the evaluator must fully engage the emerging communicator in the intervention activities. It would be an error to insist prematurely on positioning changes that might make the individual uncomfortable, either physically or psychologically. It is important to begin with the individual's most comfortable position for a given intervention activity and only make changes as necessary to keep the individual engaged or to obtain reliable communication. It can take many months or years for individuals with severe impairments to obtain optimum or even functional seating and positioning. The search for a reliable method of symbolic communication must not be delayed during that time.

Nonetheless, many circumstances do warrant seating and positioning changes for an emerging communicator. The team should consider making such changes under any of the following conditions:

- There is no current position that is comfortable for the individual. This requires immediate intervention by a physician and a physical therapist.
- The current position is not conducive to participation in a specific intervention activity. For example, a child might want to request bubbles but is unable to see them without better head support (York & Weimann, 1991).
- The individual is unsuccessful with all communication trials, and there is evidence that positioning is a contributing factor.

York and Weimann (1991) described two types of positioning that can facilitate communication. *Static positioning* involves aids or equipment that provide support to an individual (e.g., a laptray, footrests). Table 12.1 lists a number of such external supports along with other control enhancement techniques. Typically, the individual already has a number of these devices, even if they are not routinely used. The team should add them gradually for an individual's AAC intervention, depending on the individual's needs and comfort level. *Dynamic positioning* does not involve external aids or devices but physical assistance from a caregiver or a therapist throughout a specific trial or activity. For example, a therapist might provide head support or stabilize one arm during trials with direct selection. By constantly adjusting this support to meet the individual's needs, the interventionist can determine whether a static aid is appropriate for this purpose on a long-term basis.

Whether the team uses static or dynamic supports, it is essential to keep several principles in mind (Cook & Hussey, 1995; York & Weimann, 1991). A good positioning system should 1) enhance performance with AAC, 2) provide support without restricting necessary movement, 3) reduce abnormal reflexes or minimize the impact on volitional movement, 4) enhance the individual's ability to attend to the task, and 5) be compatible with long-term positioning goals for the individual. Adherence to these principles requires close collaboration among the entire team: the AAC user, occupational and physical therapists, the speech-language pathologist, the physician, and the family or caregivers.

Considering Direct Selection for the Emerging Communicator   As
discussed previously, both research and intervention experience suggest that
direct selection is preferable to indirect selection whenever possible because of
the degree of control that it affords the individual. Research has also suggested
that there are hierarchies within the control sites, with some parts of the body
theoretically providing access to more target items. This discussion begins
with an examination of this hierarchy before considering the interfaces and
possible trials with direct selection.

Identifying Control Sites   Table 12.2 shows various control sites on the
body that can be considered for direct selection along with their respective theoretical characteristics (Cook & Hussey, 1995). For each site, the table presents
the *potential range*, defined previously as the extent of possible movement, and
the *potential resolution,* which is the separation between targets. The maximum
size of the selection set is estimated and listed as the *maximum targets* for each
control site. For example, usually the fingers with hand and arm movement
can reach a greater number of direct selection targets than the head without a

Table 12.2.   Characteristics of control sites for direct selection (presented in order of potential number of targets in the selection set)

Control site	Example interface	Potential resolution	Potential range	Maximum targets
Fingers with hand or arm movement	Keyboard	High	Large	Numerous
Head with pointer	Keyboard	High	Large	Numerous
Eyes with head movement	Eye-gaze board	High	Moderate	Numerous
Eyes with no head movement	Infrared eye-position monitor	High	Small	Many
Fingers with hand movement	Mini keyboard at hand	High	Moderate	Many
Hand with arm movement	Large target, expanded keyboard	Moderate	Large	Many
Foot with leg movement	Expanded keyboard at foot	Moderate	Moderate	Many
Fingers with no hand or arm movement	Mini switches at hand	High	Small	Few
Arm with no fingers or hand movement	Arm slot switch	Low	Large	Few
Eyes with no head movement	Eye-gaze board	Moderate	Small	Few
Head with no pointer	Head switch (various locations)	Moderate	Small	Few

Source: Cook & Hussey (1995).

pointer. Of course, a given individual may not have sufficient control to perform at these maximum levels.

Interfaces   Table 12.3 shows some of the motor tasks that can be used to assess potential control sites and interfaces for communication. Using the individual's interests, tasks are designed with low linguistic or cognitive demands for eliciting these movements to show the following:

- Range of movement
- Resolution throughout the range
- Muscle tone and strength
- Relative endurance and the onset of fatigue upon repetitions
- Any evidence of reflexes and their impact on voluntary movement

Table 12.3.   Screening tasks for initial assessment of motor function

Movements with fingers, hands, and/or arms	Movements with the head	Movements involving the leg and/or foot	Movements with face and/or mouth
Play with toys of various sizes and shapes	Rotate head to the left or the right	Point with toe or touch a target with toe	Open and close jaw*
Grasp toys or objects of different sizes and shapes	Tilt head up or down	Kick toy or object*	Extend and retract tongue*
Point to and/or touch toys or objects	Flex or extend neck	Hold object between knees*	Vocalize on command*
Point to and/or touch targets on a visual display			Use straw to drink or blow air*
Touch therapist's finger in various positions			Blow against tissue*
Grasp and hand toys or objects			
Pour or drink from a cup or a glass			
Pick up and eat snack foods			
Use utensils or tools			
Draw or paint			
Write letters, words, or phrases			

Source: Cook & Hussey (1995).
These tasks can generally function for direct selection or indirect selection, although some tasks are for indirect selection only (indicated by *). When it is practical, tasks should be done in multiple planes, not just in the horizontal plane, and also in multiple locations in each plane.

- Any evidence of voluntary abnormal movement patterns
- The presence of overflow movements
- The individual's unilateral preference
- The use of compensatory strategies (Cook & Hussey, 1995).

This information should be compared with the previously discussed interface characteristics to identify the interface that would give the individual the greatest control for communication—with or without positioning changes, control enhancements, or modifications.

Nonetheless, decision making with emerging communicators must be guided by other principles as well. First, because the goal is to establish reliable symbolic communication, there is no reason to consider only control sites with the greatest potential number of targets. The team can establish initial communication via a physically easier strategy, even if it has fewer targets. Second, the drive for initial success means that there is a preference for strategies that are easy for both the user and the partner to learn. Third, the method that is selected initially does not have to be the fastest nor the most efficient technique possible. A slower or less efficient site may be used for initial training under some circumstances. Fourth, new techniques must not decrease current communication skills, so one should avoid sites that interfere with the individual's natural gestures or body language.

Communication Trials with Direct Selection   It is difficult to define and measure communicative success for an emerging communicator who is using a new access method. First, individuals with severe communication impairments, particularly those with sensory and/or motor disorders, may not demonstrate communicative intentionality in the conventional manner (Iacono, Carter, & Hook, 1998). For example, individuals with oculomotor or vision impairments may not demonstrate alternating eye gaze between a desired object and a partner. There are similar limitations in the use of the other behavioral criteria that were originally developed for individuals with cognitive impairments (Iacono et al., 1998). Second, an inappropriate selection technique may make communication unreliable and make it appear that the individual does not have communicative intent. For example, a child with poor pointing or an undiagnosed vision impairment may activate incorrect or unintended messages on a device even if he or she has the linguistic competence to communicate successfully. The third reason that success has been difficult to define and measure is that there has been too little effort in this direction by clinicians in the field (Dowden, 1999a). It is not uncommon for emerging communicators to use systems unreliably (e.g., children who do not look at symbols before reaching for them, children who use single-switch scanners and cannot time their switch activations). If the selection set is comprised solely of items that are both possible and positively reinforcing in a given context, then communication may appear more reliable and intentional than actually is the case.

One common technique for assessing intentionality and consistency of use in emerging communicators is to utilize structured elicitation techniques, sometimes called *communicative temptations* (Iacono et al., 1998). After optimizing all aspects of the selection technique, one can set up situations in which the individual is likely to be motivated to make a selection (e.g., request a desired activity). Foils should be included in the selection set to prevent the appearance of reliability when there is none. Foils can include any or all of the following: 1) blank items, 2) meaningless symbols, 3) items that are meaningless or irrelevant in this context (e.g., crayons at snack time), 4) items that are negative reinforcers for this individual (e.g., a toothbrush), or 5) items that are neutral to the individual (e.g., a piece of paper).

It should be noted, however, that changing preferences or unintentional reinforcement for some items can result in inappropriate conclusions from these tasks (Reichle, 1991). Clinicians should also use tasks that involve the exchange of verifiable information. These tasks invariably require skills in symbol discrimination that are not necessarily required for the previously mentioned communication temptations. One can use barrier tasks (Beukelman & Mirenda, 1998), in which the AAC user must convey information about an object or an action to a partner who cannot see the stimulus. This can range from playing "What's in the box?" with a young child to naming or describing pictures for an older individual. Reinforcement may make or break this task for many emerging communicators. One can also use team games (Dowden, 1999b), in which the AAC user makes choices or decisions with a speaking teammate and then must convey the choice to a third person, who is the communication partner. For example, the teammates might decide which snack to eat or which baseball card to request. Accuracy is measured only when the speaking teammate makes the choice and the AAC user conveys this choice to the partner. If the messages are conveyed correctly in multiple trials, then one can conclude that the communication technique is reliable and the individual has shown intentionality in this task.

When communication with direct selection fails for these types of tasks, it is tempting to consider changing to an indirect access method. Yet, this decision is not trivial for an emerging communicator because indirect methods place additional demands on memory, visual tracking, and other skills. Furthermore, many other factors may lead to an emerging communicator's lack of success with direct selection; thus, the first task is to eliminate any of these causes. Clinicians should consider all of the following possibilities:

- Sensory impairments: Could there be subtle sensory impairments that reduce symbol recognition?
- Excessive task complexity: Does performance improve if cognitive or linguistic demands are reduced?
- Distractions: Does performance improve when visual or auditory distractions are reduced or eliminated?

- Weak reinforcer: Is there greater success if the task is made more interesting for the individual?
- Insufficient training: Would additional instructional opportunities make direct selection successful?
- Conflicting training: Is the AAC user being taught contradictory skills for the same control site?

If the answer to any of these questions is "yes," then it is not yet appropriate to change to indirect selection for a given emerging communicator. Instead, these factors must be diligently improved with the existing direct selection technique. Yet, when these factors are well controlled and sensory and/or motor skills do not seem to support direct access, one must consider the possibility that indirect selection might be more successful.

Considering Indirect Selection for the Emerging Communicator The decision-making process with indirect selection is not a series of discrete steps but a process of homing in on the right combination of control site, interface(s), and indirect selection techniques. These three factors interact with each other for the individual user, so evaluation and intervention require consideration of all three simultaneously. Our discussion begins with a look at control sites and potential interfaces followed by a discussion about selection techniques.

Control Sites   There is a hierarchy of control sites for indirect selection just as there is for direct access. Table 12.4, which is based on Cook and Hussey (1995), shows the potential target size, strength, and number of targets for different control sites for indirect selection. For example, even limited movement of the fingers, arm, foot, or head can provide up to four switch sites. Other body parts are limited to two targets or fewer, even under optimal conditions. Of course it is not sufficient to identify *potential* control sites. The individual must be engaged in motor tasks, such as those listed in Table 12.3, to show his or her actual motor function at each anatomical site. As with direct selection, the interventionist needs to determine the range of movement, resolution, muscle tone and strength, endurance and fatigue, reflexes, abnormal movements patterns, overflow movements, unilateral preferences, and compensatory strategies. The expectations are more limited with indirect selection, however, because all of the methods require only a few reliable targets at any one control site.

Interfaces   The clinician can use information about the individual's actual motor control at different control sites to narrow the field of potential interfaces. Specifically, one must compare the individual's range, resolution, and strength to the previously discussed switch characteristics to rule out interfaces that are not appropriate for the individual. For example, a switch that has large displacement or requires considerable force would not be appropri-

Table 12.4. Characteristics of control sites for indirect selection (presented in order of potential number of targets in the selection set)

Control site	Example interface	Potential target size	Potential strength	Potential targets
Finger with no hand or arm movement	Switch or joystick at fingers	Small	Low	Up to four
Arm with no finger or hand movement	Switch or joystick	Large	Large	Up to four
Head with no pointer	Switch or joystick	Moderate	Moderate	Up to four
Foot with leg movement	Switch or joystick at foot	Moderate	High	Up to four
Hand with no finger or arm movement	Single or dual switches at hand	Moderate	Moderate	One or two
Mouth with respiration	Sip-and-puff switch	N/A	Low	One or two
Foot with no leg movement	Single or dual switches at foot	Small	High	One or two
Leg with no foot pointing	Single or dual switches at leg or knee	Moderate	High	One or two
Eye blink	Single switch at eye	Small	Negligible	One
Tongue	Tongue switch	Small	Low	One (for AAC)
Chin with no head movement	Single switch at chin	Small	Low	One

Source: Cook & Hussey (1995).

ate for activation by the tongue, which has small range and limited strength. Similarly, a switch with poor durability should not be considered at the knee or other location on the leg if the individual has great strength in those muscle groups.

Indirect Selection Techniques   Clearly, one cannot separate the control site and interfaces from the selection technique itself. A given individual may be able to use a single switch at the thumb for one scanning technique but not for another or may be better able to use his or her head than his or her hand for a given technique. Further complicating the matter, the individual may be able to use that switch and that selection technique only with control enhancers or other modifications. These factors are not separate parts of the process because each one works with the others to affect decision making. For these reasons, *each* combination of anatomical site and interface must be considered with *all* useful control enhancers and *every* indirect selection technique. This process may sound overwhelming, but it becomes simpler when one focuses on the subskills that are required for each selection technique.

Beukelman and Mirenda (1998) described a set of skills that are generally necessary for scanning techniques. These included 1) waiting for the right moment, 2) activating a switch, 3) maintaining switch closure, 4) releasing the switch at the right moment, and 5) reactivating the switch. Light (1993) and Ratcliff (1994) encouraged clinicians to select and to teach scanning techniques by observing the individual's abilities with these subskills. Dowden (1996) further described the specific subskills for the basic indirect access methods as follows:

- Automatic scanning: WAIT, ACTIVATE the switch (at the right moment), and RELEASE the switch.
- Inverse scanning: ACTIVATE the switch (at any time), MAINTAIN switch closure, and RELEASE the switch (at the right moment).
- Two-switch step scanning: ACTIVATE the correct switch, RELEASE it, ACTIVATE it again (repeatedly until the target is reached), and then ACTIVATE the other switch to accept the target.
- One-switch step scanning: This process is the same as that for two-switch step scanning except that WAITING for automatic acceptance replaces the use of the second switch.
- Directed scanning: ACTIVATE (correctly for the desired direction), MAINTAIN closure, and RELEASE (at the right moment).
- Coded access: ACTIVATE (or move in the correct direction), MAINTAIN position (until the right moment), RELEASE (or relax), ACTIVATE, MAINTAIN and RELEASE until the code is complete.

These subskills provide an important pattern for initial decision making with emerging communicators. Automatic scanning requires the user to time the *activation* of the switch precisely. Inverse and directed scanning require precision at the *release* of the switch. Step scanning and coded access require the ability to activate switches and/or to initiate movements in the right direction repeatedly with ease. Of course, all techniques also require additional cognitive and sensory skills, particularly the basic skill of waiting to use the switch until it is appropriate.

The first task for the interventionist is to determine which combination of control site and interface gives the individual the greatest control over activation or release. Initially, it is important to use activities that involve no symbol discrimination but require that the individual waits until it is appropriate to use the switch. The following discussion presents a hierarchy of intervention tasks to serve as trials for each of these methods: automatic scanning, inverse or directed scanning, and step scanning. (Each hierarchy lists manufacturers who provide equipment or software that can be of assistance. See the appendix at the end of the chapter for resource information.)

The tasks in the hierarchy for automatic scanning (see Table 12.5) are most successful for emerging communicators if interventionists and families

Table 12.5. Trials for automatic scanning

Level 1: Activities that require waiting

The individual must not activate the switch while the activity is ongoing but must WAIT (for an appropriate moment), ACTIVATE the switch, and RELEASE the switch. This trial can be done with the following devices:

- Switch activated devices with a switch latch and timer to keep device going, such as a tape recorder with music or a battery-operated toy or appliance (AbleNet, Crestwood Communication Aids, Enabling Devices/Toys for Special Children)
- Single message voice output communication aid (VOCA) with requests for actions (e.g., read the next page) or objects (e.g., give me another cracker) or any other repeatable task (AbleNet, Attainment Company, Don Johnston)
- Single-switch software that requires the user to activate the switch to hear music or to see moving graphics (Crick Software, RJ Cooper & Associates)

Level 2: Activities that require precise timing

The individual must WAIT, ACTIVATE the switch (at just the right moment), and RELEASE the switch. This trial can be done with the following devices:

- Single-message VOCAs with a message that must be spoken at just the right moment (e.g., completing a joke started by someone else, reading the repetitive line of a poem, singing the chorus of a song) (AbleNet, Attainment Company, Don Johnston)
- Scanning communication devices that are set up so that there is only one target symbol in an array of empty boxes; the function of the target item would be similar to any of the previous examples of single messages (ADAMLAB; DynaVox Systems, Communication Devices, Innocomp, Mayer-Johnson, Prentke Romich, Words+, Zygo Industries)
- Single-switch computer games that require the individual to activate the switch at just the right moment (e.g., to shoot down a fast-moving target, to stop a cursor at a particular spot on the screen) (Crick Software, Don Johnston, RJ Cooper, Soft-Touch Software)

Source: Dowden (1996).

follow a few simple guidelines. First, always give natural environmental cues to the AAC user, such as silence after someone sings part of a song. Using explicit commands such as "Hit the switch" will keep the individual dependent on that prompt and, thus, impede learning. Second, the individual must not repeatedly or continuously activate the switch in anticipation of the right moment. This would prevent him or her from learning to wait for the right moment in scanning, ultimately delaying success. Of course, using automatic scanning for actual communication requires an individual to engage in all of these sensory and motor acts *plus* DISCRIMINATE the target symbol and WATCH the cursor. For emerging communicators with motor impairments, it is unfair to expect communication before ensuring that the individual has reliable control over the interface itself.

Table 12.6 shows the hierarchy of tasks for inverse and directed scanning. Again it is best to engage the learner in these activities by using natural environmental prompts. Upon completion of Level 2 activities for inverse scanning, the individual has mastered the necessary motor skills and is now ready

Table 12.6.   Trials for inverse and directed scanning

Level 1: Activities that require maintaining switch closure:

The individual must not activate the switch repeatedly to reach the goal but must ACTIVATE the switch, MAINTAIN closure, and RELEASE the switch at any time. This trial can be done with the following devices:

- Power wheelchair in a safe, wide-open area; stopping on demand is not yet a crucial skill

- Single-switch toys without a switch or latch timer for which the switch closure must be maintained to keep the toy going (AbleNet, Crestwood Communication Aids, Enabling Devices/Toys for Special Children)

- Tape recorder or other electronic device without a switch latch and timer for which switch closure must be maintained (AbleNet, Crestwood Communication Aids, Enabling Devices/Toys for Special Children)

- Software that requires the user to press the switch and maintain closure to hear music or see graphics (Crick Software, Don Johnston, RJ Cooper, SoftTouch Software)

Level 2: Activities that require precise timing of the release:

The individual must have access to a single switch in an activity that requires him or her to ACTIVATE, MAINTAIN, and RELEASE the switch at just the right moment. This trial can be done with the following devices:

- Power wheelchair in an activity that only requires the individual to move forward (not in a particular direction) and then stop at just the right moment (e.g., go forward to get a snack from someone, go forward and stop just before an obstacle)

- Single-switch toys without a switch latch and timer that require the individual to stop them at the right moment (e.g., make the train bring a cookie to the user and have the user stop the train just in time) (AbleNet, Crestwood Communication Aids, Enabling Devices/Toys for Special Children)

- A communication device set up on inverse scanning so that there is only one target in an array of empty boxes; the target's function can be similar to those discussed for single-message devices (ADAMLAB, DynaVox Systems, Mayer-Johnson, Prentke Romich, Words+, TASH, Zygo Industries)

- Computer software that is set up with inverse scanning and designed to require no symbol recognition (e.g., a game that requires switch closure for the cursor to reach a desired target and then release at a precise moment) (SoftTouch Software, Intelli-Tools, Don Johnston)

Level 3 (for Directed scanning only): Activities that require correct direction and precise timing of the release

The individual must have access to an interface with two or more switches in an activity that requires him or her to ACTIVATE the switches in the correct direction, MAINTAIN the switches, and RELEASE them at the right moment. This trial can be done with the following devices:

- Power wheelchair in an environment in which obstacles or goals require movement in a specific direction and precise stopping (e.g., going through an obstacle course)

- Computer software that is set up with a joystick and targets but does not require symbol discrimination; the user must move the joystick until the cursor reaches a desired target, then release at a precise moment (SoftTouch Software)

- Communication device or software that is set up with a joystick or arrow keys and only one target that appears in different locations on the display (DynaVox Systems, Mayer-Johnson)

Source: Dowden (1996).

to learn to WATCH the cursor and to DISCRIMINATE symbols. For directed scanning, the users must be successful with Level 3 activities (see Table 12.6) before working on DISCRIMINATING symbols and WATCHING the cursor.

The hierarchy for step scanning appears in Table 12.7. To use step scanning, the individual would presumably practice ACTIVATION, RELEASE, ACTIVATION, RELEASE repeatedly until reaching the target item, then either ACTIVATE a second switch or WAIT for acceptance. In practice, it is difficult to set up an activity that teaches this pattern without encouraging the impulsivity and repeated switch activations that are seen with some emerging communicators. Step scanning should be considered for an emerging communicator only if 1) his or her motor skills strongly favor repeated activations over the precise timing of activiation or release and 2) the individual tends to be extremely passive. The intervention tasks are different for single- and dual-switch step scanning, as described in Table 12.7. In all tasks, however, it is imperative that the user is not reinforced for repeated activations after the goal

Table 12.7. Trials for step scanning

Single-switch step scanning: Activities that require repeated activations and waiting

The individual must ACTIVATE and RELEASE the switch many times until a goal is reached and then WAIT. This trial can be done with the following devices:

- Single switch voice output communication aid (VOCA) that plays prerecorded messages in a step-by-step manner; blank "messages" should initially be programmed in the first slots and one powerful target message in a later slot (e.g., "Dance with me"); the user ACTIVATES the switch repeatedly until the target message is produced, then WAITS for the partner to act (AbleNet, Adaptivation, Attainment Company)

- Simple environmental control systems that require two activations to make two appliances activate in sequence (AbleNet)

- Scanning communication device set for single-switch step scanning, with blanks in most squares except for one, which holds a single, powerful message (e.g., "Dance with me"); the user has to ACTIVATE the switch repeatedly until the cursor presents the target symbol, then WAIT for the output and for the partner to act (DynaVox Systems, Prentke Romich, Words+, Zygo Industries)

- Computer software that can be customized with a single target that is achieved only on a predetermined number of switch activations (e.g., a puzzle or dot-to-dot picture that is completed gradually with each switch closure); the user activates repeatedly but only until completion (SoftTouch Software, Don Johnston)

Two-switch step scanning: Activities that require repeated use of one switch, then a second switch

The individual must ACTIVATE and RELEASE one switch many times until a goal is reached and then ACTIVATE and RELEASE the second switch. This trial can be done with the following devices:

- Scanning communication device set for two-switch step scanning, with blanks in most squares except for one, which holds a single, powerful message (e.g., "Dance with me"); the user has to hit the switch repeatedly until the cursor presents the target symbol, then ACTIVATE and RELEASE the second switch (DynaVox Systems, Prentke Romich, Words+, Zygo Industries)

Source: Dowden (1996).

is accomplished. After learning initial activities that are designed to facilitate scanning, the communicator is ready to use these methods in more difficult tasks. He or she must learn to WATCH the cursor and DISCRIMINATE the symbols.

Communication Trials with Indirect Selection   Similar to direct selection, success with indirect selection is determined by the consistency and intentionality of true communication. One can use the previously described foils, barrier games, and team games to ensure that an individual is not making random selections. It is important to be sure that he or she understands the symbols, selects the target symbol accurately, and can use these skills in natural communication activities. If the individual fails to do so, the team must look at the same factors that were previously discussed for direct selection (sensory impairments, excessive task complexity, distractions, weak reinforcer, insufficient training, and conflicting training). However, it may also be necessary to revisit the switch site, the interface, the control enhancers and the particular selection technique in an effort to find one combination that will prove reliable for the individual.

Customizing Access for Context-Dependent Communicators

As discussed previously, a context-dependent communicator demonstrates intentional symbolic communication through at least one reliable means. This communication may be effective in only some activities or with a limited set of partners. There are many examples of beginning communicators who are context dependent, such as a child using multiple communication boards at school or an adult in an intensive care unit using an eye-gaze word board for basic physical needs. Intervention with these individuals must expand the physical, functional, linguistic, social, and cultural contexts (Light, 1997) in which communication is successful. For the purposes of this chapter, we focus only on situations in which changes to the selection technique can facilitate that development.

The methodology used to improve the selection technique for context-dependent communicators is quite different from that described previously for emerging communicators for three important reasons. First and foremost, the individual's current communication permits him or her to participate directly in all aspects of the assessment process in an age-appropriate way. The AAC team begins by understanding what the individual likes and dislikes about his or her current selection technique and then discusses each of the potential changes at an age-appropriate level. The team cannot proceed with any changes unless the user consents, so he or she must be given both the opportunity and the vocabulary to participate in this way. Second, the user's facility with communication means that the team does not have to emphasize powerful communicative functions during the entire assessment process. Instead, contrived tasks can be used to determine the user's sensory and motor abilities or to test possible access strategies. For example, it may be possible to assess hand control initially by having the individual point to colored dots or specific locations on an overlay. Finally, the overall intervention goal is much broader for a context-dependent communicator than for an emerging communicator. The ultimate purpose of intervention is independent communication that enhances participation in all contexts of daily life. For this reason, selection technique enhancements must be fully integrated into all contexts of the individual's life and prepare him or her for later independence.

Initial Sensory and Motor Screening   The fact that communication has been successful does not mean that the context-dependent communicator has no vision or hearing impairments that may interfere with AAC, but it does make testing considerably easier. The AAC team should encourage regular, routine vision and hearing screenings for these individuals as appropriate for their age and medical diagnosis (see Chapter 11). The team may have to work with hearing and vision specialists so that the assessment instruments can be modified to compensate for known motor impairments and/or limitations in vocabulary.

Just as for emerging communicators, there may be major concerns about positioning. These concerns must be addressed immediately by seating specialists and physicians, as small changes in positioning may enhance access to AAC. As with emerging communicators, current seating and postural supports are considered first, such as those shown in Table 12.1. The team must weigh the advantages and disadvantages of relying on supports for communication. One might find, for example, that a finger splint enhances accuracy for direct selection, but if the individual cannot or will not use the splint all day, it must be ruled out as a support option for communication. Similarly, a laptray cannot be used to support a switch if it interferes with an individual's ability to make independent transfers. Except perhaps for a very young individual, the AAC user is the final arbiter for these decisions; he or she must be given adequate time and vocabulary to fulfill this role.

Modifying Selection Techniques for Context-Dependent Communicators   Typically, a context-dependent communicator has at least one reliable method of communication, which meets some needs in some contexts. The team's first goal, then, is to identify small changes in any of these methods that might improve the efficiency or effectiveness of communication. For some individuals, the selection technique itself limits communication. For example, an adult may fatigue too quickly to use one AAC method all day. The team must examine the current control site and interface as well as potential enhancements and modifications. The options differ for direct and indirect selection methods.

In direct selection, small changes in the combination of control site and interface may increase the number of potential targets, the amount of effort necessary, or the speed or accuracy of access. For instance, a new keyboard with different interface characteristics might require a smaller range of movement or less force for activation, which could increase speed or decrease fatigue. Control enhancers—such as splints, pointers, and supports (see Table 12.1)—may have similar effects under some circumstances. The team must also consider modifications to the selection technique itself, such as changing the angle of the interface; redesigning the selection set; adjusting the interface; or adding keyguards, shields, and handrests (again, see Table 12.1).

The options for indirect selection differ somewhat as does the potential impact of any changes. On one hand, modifying the control site and the interface might result in more precise timing, permitting an increase in scanning speed and overall communication rate. On the other hand, a small change in the switch type or location might reduce fatigue or the effect of subtle positioning shifts over time, allowing the individual to use this method for longer periods of time. Similar effects may result with changes in the size of switches; the size and spacing of multiple switches; or adjustments to the interface in terms of sensitivity, feedback, or timing. As with direct selection, control enhancers and modifications (shown in Table 12.1) must be considered for the individual. For example, changing postural supports or adding splints or armrests may significantly improve timing for switch activation or release.

As mentioned previously, trials with a context-dependent communicator are often straightforward. Minor modifications, such as adding a keyguard, can usually be tested one by one during an evaluation, and the impact of each change can be discussed with the user. Whenever possible and when the user agrees to it, long-term trials should be conducted so that the individual can use the modification in natural communication. Gradually, the team should identify and resolve each obstacle to communication for this individual.

Changing Selection Techniques for Context-Dependent Communicator   Although minor changes are most common, there are circumstances in which radical change in the selection technique is necessary. A different method may be required only for certain positions, such as lying in bed, or for certain periods of time, such as late in the day when fatigue is an issue. A new method may become necessary because a degenerative disease has reduced motor control. In addition, it may be necessary to consider another technique simply because the original method was inappropriate, giving the individual less control than his or her motor abilities warrant. This happens occasionally with individuals who use single- or dual-switch scanning but have the ability to utilize directed scanning, coded access, or even direct selection with the addition of control enhancements or modifications.

In all of these situations, the team must reconsider the individual's entire selection method, from control sites to control enhancements. All possible techniques must be considered; any new access method must be compared to the individual's current communication strategy. The team must look at the individual's motor abilities to identify a control site that would give him or her more potential targets for communication. Potential interfaces must be considered next, as well as any enhancements and modifications that might give the individual greater control for communication (see Tables 12.2, 12.3, and 12.4). The team must also consider selection techniques, attempting to match each technique's motor subskills to the individual's specific motor abilities (see Tables 12.5, 12.6, and 12.7).

Trials with Different Selection Techniques   After completing the previously discussed steps, the team can then conduct trials to compare new and old techniques in terms of efficiency, which is a combination of speed and accuracy. Initially, this must be assessed during tasks that minimize the cognitive and linguistic demands of all selection techniques so that the focus is on sensory and motor demands only. For direct selection, the team can simply ask the AAC user to select different *locations* on the array, temporarily eliminating demands for symbol recognition or communicative interaction. For indirect selection, the team might use the previously discussed Level 2 and Level 3 activities for automatic scanning and inverse and directed scanning, as listed in Tables 12.5, 12.6, and 12.7. For example, to introduce multiswitch-directed scanning to a context-dependent communicator, one might use computer software that allows access by arrow keys for a task in which the individual must select particular targets on the screen. Cook and Hussey (1995) described many additional assessment approaches that can be used to compare the speed and accuracy of different techniques as well as the impact of training over time on both parameters.

Coded access is another option for context-dependent communicators who already have some method of communication, even if it is only reliable "yes" and "no" signals. The specific type of coding depends greatly on the results of the motor evaluation for control sites. For example, if the individual has considerable oculomotor control and good acuity, eye gaze is considered. The initial activities depend, in turn, on the type of coded access that is under consideration. Table 12.8 presents trials for two kinds of coded access: eye gaze and Morse code.

Eventually, of course, any new selection techniques must also be practiced and tested in natural communication exchanges, during which cognitive and linguistic demands are high. Blackstone (1989) recommended introducing such demands gradually to maximize success. The ultimate goal is to identify one (or more) selection technique(s) and communication system(s) that will maximize the individual's independence in communication. For a context-dependent communicator, it is essential to explore communication methods

Table 12.8. Trials for coded access

Eye gaze

The individual must first show success in using his or her eyes for direct selection before practicing with true eye codes. The following methods offer practice:

    Level 1: Introduce an eye-gaze communication board with symbols, words, or letters around the perimeter; reliability testing with direct selection is crucial to determine that the gaze is consistent and readable to partners

    Level 2: Introduce and practice the simplest eye codes requiring the fewest eye movements to the locations that are easiest for both the users and the partner; use reliability testing

    Level 3: Introduce and practice more complex codes utilizing multiple, complex eye movements; use reliability testing

Morse code

The individual must first show reliable control (including precise timing) in an inverse scanning task, which is similar to the automatic keying that is used in Morse code. Two opposing switch sites are preferred (e.g., both sides of the head, both hands), but one-switch Morse code is possible.

    Level 1: Introduce and practice inverse scanning at increasing speeds; reliability must be demonstrated with a scanning rate of 2 seconds or less

    Level 2: Introduce the simplest codes using one switch at a time (e.g., *e, i, o*), then practice use reliability testing

    Level 3: Introduce codes that require both switches (e.g., *a, b*), then practice; use reliability testing

    Level 4: Introduce codes that require multiple usage of both switches, (e.g., *c*), then practice; use reliability testing

that will meet Quist and Lloyd's (1997) principles for technology. Any new system must permit a full range of communicative functions with all potential partners, across all environments and positions, and without topic restrictions. At the same time, these systems must be affordable to implement and maintain as well as acceptable to the user and all communication partners.

CONCLUSION

Success with AAC has been described as being "magical" at times (Beukelman, 1991). When success occurs, AAC can look easy. Yet, AAC users and teams know that the true complexities are hidden from view. Decision making regarding access methods is a complex processes that, when successful, often appears transparent to the casual viewer. As has been shown in this chapter, however, an infinite number of variables must be considered, and the entire approach depends on the AAC user's current communication abilities. This chapter has presented some of the patterns in this complex task to assist teams in crafting a customized solution for each individual. As the AAC research base expands, more patterns will emerge to help AAC teams open this first door and move the individual toward independent communication.

REFERENCES

Angelo, J. (1992). Comparison of three computer scanning modes as an interface method for persons with cerebral palsy. *American Journal of Occupational Therapy, 46,* 217–222.

Barker, M.R., & Cook, A.M. (1981). A systematic approach to evaluating physical ability for control of assistive devices. *Proceedings from the Fourth Annual Conference of Rehabilitation Engineering* (pp. 287–289), Washington, DC.

Battenberg, J.K., & Merbler, J.B. (1989). Touch screen versus keyboard: A comparison of task performance of young children. *Journal of Special Education Technology, 10,* 24–28.

Bedrosian, J. (1995). Limitations in the use of nondisabled subjects in AAC research. *Augmentative and Alternative Communication, 11,* 6–10.

Beukelman, D.R. (1991). Magic and the cost of communicative competence. *Augmentative and Alternative Communication, 7,* 2–10.

Beukelman, D.R., & Mirenda, P. (1998). *Augmentative and alternative communication: Management of severe communication disorders in children and adults* (2nd ed.). Baltimore: Paul H. Brookes Publishing Co.

Blackstone, S. (1989). Visual scanning: What's it all about? and Visual scanning: Training approaches. *Augmentative Communication News, 2*(4), 1–5.

Blackstone, S. (1999). Different strokes for different folks. *Augmentative Communication News, 12,* 7–9.

Blischak, D.M., Loncke, F., & Waller, A. (1997). Intervention for persons with developmental disabilities. In L.L. Lloyd, D.R. Fuller, & H.H. Arvidson (Eds.), *Augmentative and alternative communication: A handbook of principles and practices* (pp. 299–339). Needham Heights, MA: Allyn & Bacon.

Casey, K. (1995). Play-based assessment for AAC. In G.M. VanTatenhove (Ed.), *Special Interest Division 12. Augmentative and Alternative Communication* (pp. 10–13). Rockville, MD: American Speech-Language-Hearing Association Publications.

Cook, A.M., & Hussey, S.M. (1995). *Assistive technologies: Principles and practice.* St. Louis, MO: Mosby.

Cress, P.J., Spellman, C.R., DeBriere, T.J., Sizemore, A.C., Northam, J.K., & Johnson, J.L. (1981). Vision screening for persons with severe handicaps. *Journal of The Association for Persons with Severe Handicaps, 6,* 41–49.

Culp, D., & Ladtkow, M. (1992). Locked-in syndrome and augmentative communication. In K. Yorkston (Ed.), *Augmentative communication in the medical setting* (pp. 59–138). San Antonio, TX: The Psychological Corp.

Dowden, P.A. (1996). Lesson 4: Assessing individuals with primary motor impairment In P.A. Dowden & K.M. Yorkston (1996), Speech and Hearing Sciences, C453: Augmentative and alternative communication: Implementation strategies [On line]. Available: http://www.extension.washington.edu/dl/courses/SPHSC453/.

Dowden, P.A. (1999a). Augmentative and alternative communication for children with motor speech disorders. In A.J. Caruso & E.A. Strand (Eds.), *Clinical management of motor speech disorders in children* (pp. 345–384). New York: Thieme Medical Publishers.

Dowden, P.A. (1999b). Lesson 6: Vocabulary selection. In P.A. Dowden & K.M. Yorkston (1999), Speech and Hearing Sciences C453: Augmentative and alternative communication: Implementation strategies [On line]. Available: http://www.extension.washington.edu/dl/courses/SPHSC453/.

Durfee, J.L., & Billingsley, F.F. (1999). Comparison of two computer input devices for uppercase letter matching. *American Journal of Occupational Therapy, 53*, 214–220.

Fried-Oken, M. (1989). Sentence recognition for auditory and visual scanning techniques in electronic augmentative communication devices. *Proceedings of the Rehabilitation Engineering Society of North America (RESNA) 12th Annual Conference* (pp. 67–68). Arlington, VA: RESNA.

Glickman, L., Deitz, J., Anson, D., & Stewart, K. (1996). The effect of switch control site on computer skills of infants and toddlers. *American Journal of Occupational Therapy, 50*, 545–553.

Goossens', C., & Crain, S. (1987). Overview of nonelectronic eye-gaze communication devices. *Augmentative and Alternative Communication, 3*, 77–89.

Gunderson, J.R. (1985). Interfacing the motor impaired for control and communication. In J.G. Webster, A.M. Cook, W.J. Tompkins, & G.C. Vanderheiden (Eds.), *Electronic devices for rehabilitation* (pp. 190–230). New York: John Wiley & Sons.

Higginbotham, D.J. (1995a). Use of nondisabled subjects in AAC research: Confessions of a research infidel. *Augmentative and Alternative Communication, 11*, 2–5.

Higginbotham, D.J. (1995b). Subject selection in AAC research: Decision points. *Augmentative and Alternative Communication, 11*, 11–13.

Horn, E.M., & Jones, H.A. (1996). Comparison of two selection techniques used in augmentative and alternative communication AAC. *Augmentative and Alternative Communication, 12*, 23–31.

Hussey, S.M, Cook A.M., Whinnery, S.E., Buckpitt, L., & Huntington, M. (1992). A conceptual model for developing augmentative communication skills in individuals with severe disabilities. *Proceedings from the RESNA International Conference* (pp. 287–289). Arlington, VA: RESNA.

Iacono, T., Carter, M., & Hook, J. (1998). Identification of intentional communication in students with severe and multiple disabilities. *Augmentative and Alternative Communication, 14*, 102–114.

Light, J. (1989). Towards a definition of communicative competence for individuals using augmentative and alternative communication systems. *Augmentative and Alternative Communication, 5*, 137–144.

Light, J. (1993). Teaching automatic linear scanning for computer access: A case study of a preschooler with severe physical and communication disabilities. *Journal of Special Education Technology, 2*, 125–134.

Light, J. (1997). "Let's go star fishing": Reflections on the contexts of language learning for children who use aided AAC. *Augmentative and Alternative Communication, 13*, 158–171.

Lin, C.H., & Schmidt, K.J. (1993). User preference and performance with three different input devices: Keyboard, mouse or touchscreen. *Educational Technology, 33*, 56–59.

Lloyd, L.L., Fuller, D.R., & Arvidson, H.H. (1997). *Augmentative and alternative communication: A handbook of principles and practices.* Needham Heights, MA: Allyn & Bacon.

McCarthy, G.T. (1992). *Physical disability in childhood.* London: Churchill Livingstone.

Mizuko, M., & Esser, J. (1991). The effect of direct selection and circular scanning on visual sequential recall. *Journal of Speech & Hearing Research, 34*, 43–48.

Mizuko, M., Reichle, J., Ratcliff, A., & Esser, J. (1994). Effects of selection techniques and array sizes on short-term visual memory. *Augmentative and Alternative Communication, 10*, 237–244.

Mustonen, T., Locke, P., Reichle, J., Solbrack, M., & Lindgren, A. (1991). An overview of augmentative and alternative communication systems. In J. Reichle, J. York, &

J. Sigafoos (Eds.), *Implementing augmentative and alternative communication: Strategies for learners with severe disabilities* (pp. 1–37). Baltimore: Paul H. Brookes Publishing Co.

Piché, L., & Reichle, J. (1991). Teaching scanning selection techniques. In J. Reichle, J. York, & J. Sigafoos (Eds.), *Implementing augmentative and alternative communication: Strategies for learners with severe disabilities* (pp. 257–274). Baltimore: Paul H. Brookes Publishing Co.

Quist, R.W., & Lloyd, L.L. (1997). Principles and uses of technology. In L.L. Lloyd, D.R. Fuller, & H.H. Arvidson (Eds.), *Augmentative and alternative communication: A handbook of principles and practices* (pp. 107–126). Needham Heights, MA: Allyn & Bacon.

Ratcliff, A. (1994). Comparison of relative demands implicated in direct selection and scanning: Considerations from normal children. *Augmentative and Alternative Communication, 10*, 67–74.

Reichle, J. (1991). Describing initial communicative intents. In J. Reichle, J. York, & J. Sigafoos (Eds.), *Implementing augmentative and alternative communication: Strategies for learners with severe disabilities* (pp. 71–88). Baltimore: Paul H. Brookes Publishing Co.

Sigafoos, J., & York, J. (1991). Using ecological inventories to promote functional communication. In J. Reichle, J. York, & J. Sigafoos (Eds.), *Implementing augmentative and alternative communication: Strategies for learners with severe disabilities* (pp. 61–70). Baltimore: Paul H. Brookes Publishing Co.

Swinth, Y., Anson, D., & Deitz, J. (1993). Single-switch computer access for infants and toddlers. *American Journal of Occupational Therapy, 47*, 1031–1038.

Vanderheiden, G.C. (1988). Overview of the basic selection techniques for augmentative communication: Past and future. In L.E. Bernstein (Ed.), *The vocally impaired: Clinical practice and research* (pp. 5–39). Philadelphia: Grune & Stratton.

Venkatagiri, H.S. (1999). Efficient keyboard layouts for sequential access in augmentative and alternative communication. *Augmentative and Alternative Communication, 15*, 126–134.

York, J., & Weimann, G. (1991). Accommodating severe physical disabilities. In J. Reichle, J. York, & J. Sigafoos (Eds.), *Implementing augmentative and alternative communication: Strategies for learners with severe disabilities* (pp. 239–255). Baltimore: Paul H. Brookes Publishing Co.

Appendix
Resources

Ablenet, Inc.
1081 10th Avenue, S.E.
Minneapolis, MN 55414
800-322-0956
www.ablenetinc.com

ADAMLAB
55 East Long Lake Road
PMB 337
Troy, MI 48098
248-594-6997
www.adamlab.com

Adaptivation, Inc.
2225 West 50th Street
Suite 100
Sioux Falls, SD 57105
800-723-2783
www.adaptivation.com

Assistive Technology, Inc.
7 Wells Avenue
Newton, MA 02459
800-793-9227
www.assistivetech.com

Attainment Company, Inc.
Post Office Box 930160
Verona, WI 53593
800-327-4269
www.attainmentcompany.com

Communication Aid Manufacturers
Association (CAMA)
Post Office Box 1039
Evanston, IL 60204
800-441-2262
www.aacproducts.org

Communication Devices, Inc.
4830 Industrial Way West
Coeur d'Alene, ID 83814
800-604-6559
www.comdevices.com

Crestwood Communication Aids,
Inc.
6625 North Sidney Place
Milwaukee, WI 53209
414-352-5678
www.communicationaids.com

Crick Software
35 Charter Gate
Quarry Park Close
Moulton Park
Northampton NN3 6QB
UNITED KINGDOM
44 (0)1604-67116991
www.cricksoft.com

Don Johnston, Inc.
26799 West Commerce Drive
Volo, IL 60073
800-999-4660
www.donjohnston.com

DynaVox Systems, Inc.
2100 Wharton Street
Suite 400
Pittsburgh, PA 15203
800-344-1778
www.dynavoxsys.com

Enabling Devices/Toys for Special
  Children
385 Warburton Avenue
Hastings-on-Hudson, NY 10706
800-832-8697
www.enablingdevices.com

Innocomp
26210 Emery Road
Suite 302
Warrensville Heights, OH 44128
800-382-8622
www.sayitall.com

IntelliTools, Inc.
1720 Corporate Circle
Petaluma, CA 94954
800-899-6687
www.intellitools.com

Mayer-Johnson, Inc.
Post Office Box 1579
Solana Beach, CA 94061
800-588-4548
www.mayer-johnson.com

Prentke Romich Company
1022 Heyl Road
Wooster, OH 44691
800-262-1984
www.prentrom.com

RJ Cooper & Associates
27601 Forbes Road
Suite 39
Laguana Niguel, CA 92677
800-752-6673
www.rjcooper.com

SoftTouch Software
4300 Stine Road
Suite 401
Bakersfield, CA 93313
877-763-8868
www.funsoftware.com/softtouch/in
dex.htm

Words+, Inc.
1220 West Avenue J
Lancaster, CA 93534
800-869-8521
www.words-plus.com

Zygo Industries, Inc.
Post Office Box 1008
Portland, OR 97207
800-234-6006
www.zygo-usa.com

13

AAC Strategies for Enhancing
the Usefulness of Natural Speech in
Children with Severe Intelligibility Challenges

Katherine C. Hustad, Toni B. Morehouse, and Michelle Gutmann

Communication, by its very nature, is multimodal (Kraat, 1987). Human beings communicate by simultaneously using a variety of both verbal and nonverbal means. During early language development, children rely extensively on nonverbal or prelinguistic forms of communication. As children develop language and speech production skills, using multiple modes of communication seems to become less crucial for successful communication. For children who have speech production challenges that result in reduced speech intelligibility, the use of a variety of communication strategies as part of a multimodal communication package is critical for successful communication. Augmentative and alternative communication (AAC) strategies and systems that serve to enhance the effectiveness of natural speech can become important components of a multimodal communication system for these children. In fact, we suggest throughout this chapter that natural speech and multimodal communication strategies that include AAC should not be mutually exclusive options but, rather, complementary strategies.

The purpose of this chapter is to describe communication interventions that incorporate AAC and natural speech for children who have reduced speech intelligibility in any or all communicative contexts. We advocate for an approach to intervention that includes both functionally oriented AAC strategies and more traditional developmentally oriented speech-language interventions. We demonstrate simultaneous use of these approaches through vignettes, which illustrate clinical decision making and prioritization of intervention objectives for three children.

CHILDREN WITH SEVERELY
REDUCED SPEECH INTELLIGIBILITY

The children to whom this chapter specifically refers are from diverse etiological groups. Nonetheless, these children share two important communication characteristics. First, all of them have relatively intact language and cognitive skills. That is, their language and cognition are not the primary areas of impairment underlying the communication disability. Second, intelligibility is compromised to such an extent that it is not sufficient for the child to meet his or her communication needs across all contexts. That is, reduced speech intelligibility is the primary communication disability that the child experiences, regardless of coexisting impairments. With varying degrees of success, these children attempt to use connected speech that consists of utterances that are two or more words in length. Implicit in the definition of this population is that these children have intentional, symbolic communication abilities but are unable to make themselves entirely understood via natural speech alone.

Reduced intelligibility is a heterogeneous construct that is defined subjectively in terms of the impact on functional communication. Two children with the same level of intelligibility may have very different functional capabilities. How reduced intelligibility affects a given child depends on a number of variables, such as chronological and/or developmental age, communication partners, context, language and cognitive skills, the use of gestures, the use of compensatory strategies, and previous experience with communication failure. There are no rules regarding what constitutes functionally compromised intelligibility; rather, each child must be considered individually.

Communication disability due to speech intelligibility challenges is always secondary to other underlying impairments, including phonological disorders, developmental apraxia of speech (DAS), cleft palate or other orofacial anomalies, cerebral palsy or other neuromotor disorders, Down syndrome, and mental retardation. Each of these impairments has unique characteristics, communication issues, and clusters of co-occurring impairments. As a result, intervention issues are unique to each etiological group. The intent of this chapter is to provide general principles for integrating natural speech with AAC strategies. Although issues that are specific to particular etiologies are beyond the scope of this chapter, clinicians should consider the characteristics of the underlying etiology and the individual child when designing interventions that target both AAC and natural speech.

Concomitant Communication Behaviors

The occurrence of challenging behavior in some children who have severe communication disorders secondary to mental retardation is well documented in the literature (Beukelman & Mirenda, 1998; Doss & Reichle, 1991; Parrish,

1997; see also Chapter 4). In fact, Reichle and Wacker (1993) devoted an entire book to assessment and intervention strategies for replacing challenging behavior with socially appropriate communicative behavior. Most of the literature on behavioral issues associated with severe communication disorders has focused on individuals whose primary disabilities are cognitive and/or emotionally based.

Little attention has been given to challenging behaviors that are associated with speech intelligibility challenges. Clinical observations and preliminary data suggest several patterns of behavior may be present in children with reduced speech intelligibility. Using parent and teacher surveys, Ball (1999) found that children with moderate to severe intelligibility challenges secondary to DAS consistently exhibited behavior differences relative to peers. Behaviors identified for these children included both social withdrawal and aggression. In addition, it has been observed that children with intelligibility challenges may also become excessively dependent on communication partners.

Our clinical observations suggest that children who exhibit social withdrawal or communication avoidance tend to do so with all but the most familiar communication partners (e.g., parents, siblings). When presented with new situations or even familiar situations that involve new speaking partners, children whose speech is severely unintelligible may choose not to participate in verbal exchanges or even nonverbal activities. Certainly, their experience with restating the same message to no avail reinforces the notion that verbal communication is a frustrating and unsatisfying process. Consequently, children with severely reduced speech intelligibility may appear withdrawn, shy, and unwilling to participate in activities that same-age peers seem to find interesting and intriguing.

Conversely, other children with severely reduced speech intelligibility may exhibit aggressive behavior patterns that are considered excessive in same-age peers. When these children experience communication challenges, rather than withdraw, they are inclined to extend their communicative attempts by expressing themselves in a less acceptable and often more physical manner. They may manifest their frustration with the communication process by hitting, kicking, biting, pushing, and engaging in other combative behaviors. Consequently, these children are forced to cope with the social stigma that is the result of inappropriate behavior.

Finally, children with intelligibility problems may show inordinate dependence on parents or siblings. In situations with unfamiliar listeners or with familiar listeners who do not understand a message, unintelligible children may come to depend on someone else to interpret for them or act as their spokesperson. This dependence can also extend to other areas, such as gross motor skills (e.g., wanting to be carried), fine motor skills (e.g., wanting assistance with eating), hygiene (e.g., not learning to use a tissue or a napkin), or adaptive skills (e.g., not being toilet trained until the later preschool years). Although some of these dependent behaviors may be unrelated to a communication disorder, we have observed functional dependence in these children even when the only overt disorder is severe unintelligibility.

It appears that these three patterns of behavior are not mutually exclusive but, rather, are context- and partner-specific for some children. Clearly, speech intelligibility challenges can have a serious effect on concomitant communication behaviors. Ideally, clinicians should provide means to support children with severe speech intelligibility challenges as functional communicators while they continue to work toward improving speech production. In essence, clinicians must strike a balance between encouraging ongoing work on speech goals while providing the scaffolding, by way of AAC strategies, for successful communicative interaction across communication environments.

Intervention Options

Historically, speech-language assessment and intervention for children with compromised speech intelligibility has taken a developmental approach with a focus on remediating underlying impairments, such as sound-specific errors and feature-specific processes, to improve speech production skills. Examples of resources for these types of interventions include Hodge and Wellman (1999) for childhood dysarthria; Yorkston, Beukelman, Strand, and Bell (1999) for DAS; Hodson and Paden (1991) for phonological processes; and Golding-Kushner (1995) for cleft palate and velopharyngeal incompetence. Yet, functional communication often remains markedly compromised when compensatory strategies, including AAC options that serve to enhance existing expressive skills, are not addressed as part of a comprehensive intervention package. For many children with speech intelligibility challenges, improvements in underlying impairments (i.e., articulatory, phonological, or motor skills development problems) are slow and may not result in short-term meaningful changes in functional communication. Conversely, using AAC to replace natural speech with intervention focused exclusively on AAC skill development may deprive the child of the chance to optimize speech production and speech intelligibility. Developmentally oriented speech-language interventions that focus on improving underlying speech-language impairments and compensatory communication approaches that focus on augmenting existing skills to improve functional communication need not be mutually exclusive. Both approaches can and should be integrated to best serve children with speech production deficits.

Natural speech is clearly the most efficient mode of communication for those who are able to use it effectively. As such, introducing AAC to children who have speech production capabilities, regardless of intelligibility issues, is often a "hard sell" for clinicians. Family members, educators, and others who are involved with these children often report concerns that introducing AAC options will have a deleterious effect on any progress that might be made in improving speech production and speech intelligibility. Although there is no definitive research examining the effects of AAC on speech development, the results of a meta-analysis of the AAC literature seem to suggest that implementing AAC systems did not have a negative effect on the development of speech (Millar, Light, & Schlosser, 1999). However, none of the studies that Millar and colleagues examined focused on speech outcomes when speech production and AAC strategies were targeted simultaneously. This is an area where future research is necessary.

Supporting children's ongoing communication needs provides a strong rationale for introducing AAC options, even when one avenue of therapeutic emphasis continues to be speech production. The types of AAC systems that are typically introduced follow a hierarchy of options. This hierarchy encompasses strategies that range from gestures that naturally accompany communication (e.g., pointing) to low-technology communication systems (e.g., communication displays) and on to high-technology AAC systems (e.g., voice output communication aids [VOCAs]).

Gestural Communication Strategies   Gestural communication systems and strategies require manual dexterity and are executed in relation to the body's axis. No external materials or aids are required to use gestures. There are, however, numerous gestural systems from which to choose (e.g., American Sign Language, Manually Coded English, Cued Speech, Amerind). In addition to formalized gestural systems, some gestures seem to be universally present across languages. Gestures such as waving for "good-bye" and head shakes/nods for "no"/"yes" fall into this category. These gestures are readily used and understood by speakers and listeners alike. When an adult speaker with severe dysarthria used gestures concurrently with speech, Garcia and Cannito (1996a, 1996b) found that the participant's speech intelligibility increased by approximately 23%, from 16% when no gestures were employed to 39% when iconic gestures were employed along with speech. In addition, Garcia and Cannito (1996b) found that when gestures alone were presented to listeners, sentence intelligibility was approximately 26%. That is, listeners were able to understand 26% of what the speaker said simply from hand gestures. Taken together, these results clearly indicate that gestures can contribute markedly to the utility of impaired speech. However, generalization of these results to children as yet remains unclear. The selection of gestures to include in a child's repertoire may be guided by the following principles:

- Follow the path of least resistance: Teach common gestures, and encourage the continued use of any socially acceptable gestures within the child's repertoire. Begin with gestures that will have a high payoff in terms of communicative gain across a number of communication environments.
- Capitalize on the child's manual dexterity: Choose gestures that the child can easily produce. Even if a child's manual dexterity is not perfect, ges-

tures should be "readable" enough that the meaning is clear. It is important for the child to produce gestures with enough motor accuracy so that they do not provide the listener with misleading information, which can then result in communication breakdown. In addition, for children with motor impairments, it is important to be certain that the communication benefit from gestures is worth the potential motor expenditure. These issues must be considered on a case-by-case basis with careful consideration of the child's motor skills profile.

- Use pointing as a means of deictic communication and as a clarification strategy: Teach the child to point to referents that are available within the environment to identify or clarify messages. Simply stated, take advantage of situational context with particular emphasis on the referent objects and people around which communication occurs.

- Select gestures to support the child in his or her most problematic communication situations: Teach gestures that alleviate or reduce the communication breakdowns that most frequently occur. Often, family members and others can identify the communication situations in which breakdowns occur regularly.

- Teach familiar and novel communication partners to understand gestural cues: By their very nature, many of the gestural cues used to supplement speech are relatively transparent and can be readily understood by familiar communication partners. When new gestures are incorporated into a child's repertoire, it is nonetheless important that they be introduced in a systematic manner to familiar communication partners. In this way, communication partners arc apprised of new additions to the child's repertoire and the flow of communication is not hampered. Beukelman and Mirenda (1998) suggested using gesture dictionaries in which a particular child's gestures are described and the meaning of each is defined.

Gestures often constitute the first tier in communication intervention for children with severe speech intelligibility challenges. Because gestures require only manual involvement for their execution, they are entirely portable and are always "on the child's person." Communication boards are another portable means of supplementing speech, although they are not always on the child's person.

Communication Boards   There are many different types of communication boards; this discussion focuses on two—topic boards and alphabet boards. These types of communication boards, or displays, are intended specifically for use as supplemental aids to communication that is principally conducted via speech.

Topic Boards   Topic boards are low-technology communication displays that consist of photographs, symbols, words/utterances, or all three, depending on the child's literacy skills. Items that are included on a topic board are usually environment or activity specific and are selected to represent common items, people, and events that occur within the target context. As such, children who use topic boards typically have a different board for each context in which speech is not sufficient to meet their communication needs. Individual topic boards can be either limited in size and scope of items or more detailed and specific, depending on the child's communication needs and the adequacy of natural speech in each context.

Topic boards can be used to indicate a referent or topic that pertains to a message. Hustad and Beukelman (2000) suggested that indicating a topic via written words or pictures serves as a preparatory set for the listener, thereby helping him or her anticipate and/or narrow expectations for the content of messages. In turn, providing this top-down knowledge to the listener serves to enhance the speaker's intelligibility. Research in this area has shown that topic cues increase the intelligibility of adult speakers' sentences by 4%–20% (Bruce, 1958; Carter, Yorkston, Strand, & Hammen, 1996; Dongilli, 1994; Garcia & Cannito, 1996a, 1996b; Monsen, 1983). Hustad and Morehouse (1998) examined how topic cues affected the intelligibility of speech in children with severe intelligibility challenges secondary to phonological disorders and/or DAS. This research showed that topic cues increased intelligibility by approximately 12% across four children.

In practice, implementing topic supplementation involves having the child point to a picture while speaking his or her message. The verbal message produced by the child would ultimately be more complex and elaborate than the topic picture. For instance, if a child were participating in a craft-making activity, to request scissors he or she would point to the picture of scissors on his or her topic board while saying, "Can I please have the scissors?" Should the child only point to the picture without using natural speech, he or she would be cued to "tell me with your speech, too." During initial implementation of this type of strategy, we have used highly structured activities, such as craft making, in which all of the referents are clearly known to all communication partners. This may seem counterproductive because the child could easily obtain the desired item by using gestural strategies rather than the more restrictive topic board. However, we have found this type of situation to be excellent for teaching the concurrent use of topic boards and speech. As children become increasingly successful in highly structured activities, the use of topic boards is introduced into activities that are more spontaneous. Speech production objectives can be easily implemented within topic supplementation activities through careful planning on behalf of the interventionist. That is, activities can be designed that incorporate target sounds and words so that as the child produces speech, he or she is working on speech production in a highly communicative and functional context.

Alphabet Boards   Alphabet boards are similar to topic boards in that they, too, are low-technology communication displays. As the name implies, however, alphabet boards contain orthographic representations of the letters of the alphabet, numbers, and, often, some conversational control phrases or picture symbols. The size and arrangement of alphabet boards is typically customized according to the child's motor skills. An example of an alphabet board is shown in Figure 13.1. The use of alphabet boards presupposes facility/familiarity with traditional orthography. Clearly, to use alphabet boards, the child minimally must have letter identification skills.

Alphabet boards can be used in several different ways. Perhaps their most obvious use is to spell out individual words and messages. Yet, this can be a very time- and motor-intensive strategy, requiring extensive literacy skills. We recommend this only as a last resort when other strategies have failed.

Alphabet boards can also be used to provide word initial orthophonetic context to listeners in conjunction with natural speech. This type of strategy is known as *alphabet supplementation*. To use alphabet supplementation, the speaker must point to the first letter of each word as he or she speaks it (Hustad & Beukelman, 2000). Consequently, the speaker is providing the listener with complementary information through two modalities simultaneously—the acoustic speech signal and orthographic information that supports decoding of the acoustic speech signal (Hustad, 1999). Alphabet supplementation can also involve the use of a partner-based technique called *shadowing* (Yorkston, Beukelman, & Hustad, 1999). Shadowing involves having the communication partner repeat the letter that the speaker indicates on the board as well as the spoken word. In this way, communication is followed on a word-by-word basis. Should an error in transmission occur, communication breakdown can be repaired at the level of the individual letter and/or word.

Alphabet supplementation also affects temporal properties of the speech signal, resulting in reduced rate of speech and increased word segmentation (Beukelman & Yorkston, 1977). Research suggests that the combined effects

I'll point to the first letter of each word I'm saying.

Please repeat each word after I say it.

A	B	C	D	E	F
G	H	I	J	K	L
M	N	O	P	Q	R
S	T	U	V	W	X
Y	Z	New word	Start over		

Figure 13.1. Sample alphabet board.

of reduced rate and orthophonetic cues can enhance speech intelligibility in adults by as much as 52% (Beukelman & Yorkston, 1977). Because the Beukelman and Yorkston study is the only one of its kind in the literature, additional research is necessary to replicate this effect with both adults and children.

Alphabet supplementation requires a number of prerequisite skills, such as the ability to identify word-initial letters, sound–letter correspondence, and the metalinguistic ability to segment words at their boundaries. There is no published research that examines the skills that are necessary to use alphabet supplementation successfully. Nevertheless, we have found that children as young as 6 years of age, who have intact cognitive and language skills, have been able to begin learning this strategy in structured contexts. Similar to implementing topic boards, we have found the use of structured activities for assessment and teaching to be highly productive. In addition, it is critical that clinician modeling of alphabet supplementation be provided during all initial teaching activities.

Empirical evidence suggests that alphabet supplementation results in greater intelligibility gains than topic supplementation (Hustad, 1999). Therefore, alphabet supplementation is a preferred strategy for children who have the necessary linguistic and literacy skills. Hustad and Beukelman (2001) examined adult speakers with cerebral palsy and demonstrated that using a combined cuing strategy that incorporates both alphabetic and topic cues is superior to either strategy in isolation. These results showed that intelligibility was approximately 15% higher for combined cues than for alphabet cues alone and approximately 23% higher for combined cues than for topic cues alone. From a developmental perspective, the use of topic cues seems to be the simplest speech supplementation strategy, followed by the use of alphabet cues, and, finally, combined cues. Therefore, we recommend that a combined cuing strategy be implemented only after a child has demonstrated successful use of both strategies in isolation.

Voice Output Communication Aids   In some situations, high-technology options such as VOCAs may be introduced to help compensate for speech intelligibility challenges. The range of available VOCAs is broad, such that some support text to speech and others support a limited number of prerecorded messages. For the purposes of this chapter, we discuss the use of VOCAs as speech supplementation strategies and as a means for clarifying messages when they are not understood by listeners. We emphasize situation-specific use of VOCAs as part of a hierarchical communication system.

For children who use speech as their primary means of communication, VOCAs confer some unique advantages over gestures and low-technology aids. With both gestures and communication boards, the communicative interaction must be face to face with the listener physically present and actively interpreting information as it is presented through the visual modality. A

VOCA, however, allows for the introduction of space between child and listener. For example, telecommunication and communication from a distance are possible with VOCAs, but they are difficult if the child uses gestures or communication boards. As speech supplementation strategies, VOCAs can be employed in a similar fashion as that described for topic or alphabetic supplementation. When VOCAs are employed, however, supplemental information is presented via the auditory modality or simultaneously through the auditory and visual modalities, depending on the type of device and the communication partner's position. Typically, supplemental cues are presented prior to the production of words and messages that are produced via natural speech.

In addition, VOCAs can be used to clarify messages for listeners when they are unable to understand what the child is saying via speech plus a supplementation strategy. In this way, the VOCA is used as a measure of last resort for the child to make him- or herself understood. There also may be some special situations in which it is necessary for the child to use his or her VOCA in lieu of natural speech. Examples of this type of situation include communication in extremely noisy situations, with individuals who are hearing impaired, or with novel communication partners. Situations in which the child uses his or her VOCA as a primary means of communication should be decided on a case-by-case basis, with careful consideration given to the severity of the child's speech intelligibility problems and to his or her success with speech supplementation strategies.

There are pros and cons to introducing a VOCA to a child who speaks but has intelligibility challenges. On the positive side, the child has an aid that is powerful and commands attention. On the negative side, the child has additional responsibility for part of his or her communication when using a VOCA. Successful implementation of a VOCA depends on appropriate programming and continued maintenance. Should the VOCA not work for some reason, it is important that the user have a low-technology back-up system handy (e.g., communication boards). Relying on technology can inadvertently leave a child with limited communication options if he or she does not have facility with a nontechnical system as well.

The information presented thus far describes several viable strategies that can be used to enhance the functionality of natural speech for children who have severe speech intelligibility issues. We advocate a hierarchical approach of moving from less to more in terms of strategy use. It is of the utmost importance to consider the individual child when implementing multimodal communication strategies to enhance the utility of natural speech. For children who have patient and capable communication partners and are capable of engaging in revisions that involve conversational repair, we recommend the following hierarchy for strategy use:

1. Say the message by using speech. If the listener does not understand, go to the next step.

2. Say the message by using speech while simultaneously producing gestures or pointing to environmental referents, if available. If the listener does not understand, go to the next step.

3. Say the message by using speech while simultaneously employing a supplementation strategy, either via communication board or a VOCA (use alphabet cues with topic cues if possible, or use alphabet cues alone or topic cues alone). If the listener does not understand, go to the next step.

4. Repeat the message by using a supplementation strategy. If the listener does not understand, go to the next step

5. Use a VOCA to produce the entire message or the components of message that the listener did not understand.

For beginning communicators who are not capable of conversational revision and repair or who have communication partners who are less patient and/or capable (e.g., other children), these guidelines should be modified. Although we advocate a less-to-more approach to communication augmentation, the needs of the individual child always take precedence. For instance, children with more pervasive intelligibility challenges may benefit from a more aggressive approach to communication augmentation in which VOCAs are introduced early in intervention and faded as speech production and intelligibility skills improve. For this type of communicator, the previous hierarchy may be most appropriately implemented in a backward fashion.

VIGNETTES

The three vignettes that follow illustrate the decision-making and intervention prioritization process for children with speech intelligibility challenges. These examples show the diverse skill profiles and issues that might be observed in children who would likely benefit from using speech supplementation strategies in conjunction with traditional speech production oriented interventions.

Assessment Measures

Four different assessment measures were selected to illustrate the ensuing decision-making processes. A number of other formal and informal instruments may be employed in comprehensive assessments of children. Yet, the following measures seem to be most illustrative with respect to the content of this chapter:

1. Khan-Lewis Phonological Analysis (KLPA; Khan & Lewis, 1986): This measure was used to determine the presence of typical and atypical phonological processes at the sound segment level according to age expectations.

2. Index of Augmented Speech Comprehensibility in Children (I-ASCC; Dowden, 1997): This measure was used to assess word intelligibility with and without topic cues. To accomplish this, tape recordings were made of each child as he or she produced 30 different words. Listeners were then asked to listen to the words and write down what they thought the child had said. To measure the effects of topic cues on word intelligibility, listeners were given a single topic word on their transcription forms that was associated with each target word that the child produced. They were asked to transcribe a series of 30 words that were produced by the child under this condition as well. For both measures, intelligibility was calculated as the number of words that were identified correctly from the total number of words.

3. Informal sentence intelligibility measure (Hustad & Morehouse, 1998): This measure was used to determine sentence intelligibility with and without topic cues and alphabetic cues. Similar to word intelligibility measures, recordings were made of each child repeating a collection of 20 short sentences, which were developed to be linguistically appropriate for children older than 3 years. Listeners were asked to transcribe each sentence with topic cues, alphabet cues, and no cues. For each cue condition, information regarding the first letter of each word (for the alphabet cue condition) and the topic of each sentence (for the topic cue condition) was provided on the transcription sheet that was given to the listeners. Intelligibility for each condition was calculated as the number of words that were identified correctly.

4. Informal Discourse Comprehensibility Measure (Hustad & Morehouse, 1998): This measure was used to assess discourse comprehension with and without topic cues. Again, recordings were made as each child repeated a 10-sentence narrative. Listeners were required to answer simple, factual comprehension questions regarding the narrative with and without topic cues, which were delivered as previously described.

Connor

Connor was a 5-year-old boy who had dysarthria secondary to cerebral palsy. He had mild cognitive and language impairments and moderate gross and fine motor impairments. Connor was a highly verbal and interactive child who frequently told stories and readily sought interaction with other children and adults. Although other children often had difficulty understanding Connor's speech, he was not easily deterred from communication attempts. When communication partners indicated that they did not understand him, Connor repeated his message or narrative, embellishing his verbal productions with gestures. Connor was a persistent communicator who continued his attempts until his partners understood his message. Yet, Connor often expended extensive amounts of time and energy in an attempt to convey his messages. Connor's speech intelligibility was moderately reduced overall, but when he became frustrated, intelligibility was further reduced because of increased spasticity and muscle tone in his speech musculature.

Formal and informal assessment measures at the sound segment level indicated that developmental articulation errors and phonological processes were not particularly prevalent for Connor. Because of the neuromotor etiology of Connor's disability, however, a number of dysarthric characteristics were present in his speech, such as mild consonant distortions, reduced respiratory support, and mild hypernasality. Overall, targeting developmental processes with Connor would not likely affect his speech intelligibility markedly in the short-term, as his underlying neurological impairments could not be alleviated. Yet, because Connor was a child, his gross and fine motor skills, including speech production, would continue to develop and change. Therefore, intervention should not entirely disregard sound segment and connected speech production skills.

Table 13.1 presents the results of the assessment measures for Connor. Measurement of speech intelligibility showed that Connor's word-level productions were 61% intelligible, sentence-level productions were 52% intelligible, and connected narratives were 43% understandable to unfamiliar listeners. When listeners were provided with topic cues, however, word intelligibility increased to 92% (a 31% gain), sentence intelligibility increased to 65% (a 13% gain), and narrative comprehensibility increased to 50% (a 7% gain). When alphabetic cues were provided to listeners, sentence intelligibility increased to 76% (an 11% gain from topic cues and a 24% gain from no cues).

These data suggested several important things. Connor's speech intelligibility decreased as length and complexity increased—words were most intelligible, followed by sentences, and, finally, connected discourse. We suspected that this finding may have been due to Connor's rapid rate of speech, his difficulty with word segmentation, and his motor-coordination problems. Connor benefited when topic cues were provided to his listeners; however, this benefit decreased as the length and complexity of his messages increased. Although the effectiveness of alphabetic cues was only measured at the sentence level, results suggested that Connor's speech intelligibility was optimal when alphabetic cues were provided to his listeners.

Table 13.1. Assessment measures for Connor

	Word intelligibility	Sentence intelligibility	Narrative comprehensibility
No cues	61%	52%	43%
Topic cues	92%	65%	50%
Alphabetic cues	—	76%	—

Overall, Connor's communication profile clearly indicated a need for AAC strategies to supplement speech, particularly for sentence and narrative length productions. In addition, speech intervention was necessary to focus on coordination and rate reduction. Because Connor did not yet have literacy skills that were sufficient for him to use alphabet supplementation accurately— cues were experimentally imposed for the previously presented measures—this strategy would not be addressed in intervention at this time. Yet, as Connor became increasingly literate, we would continue to assess the feasibility of having him use alphabet supplementation. Connor's intervention plan was prioritized as follows:

1. Introduce low-technology AAC topic boards. Teach the integration of natural speech and pointing to the referent or topic for addressing communication breakdowns.
2. Work on the segmentation of words in connected speech to improve listeners' ability to identify word boundaries.
3. Work on reducing the rate of speech to provide listeners with more processing time.
4. Introduce a VOCA as a backup and replacement for natural speech when listeners are unable to understand speech that is supplemented with pictures.
5. Teach the hierarchical use of communication strategies. Focus on enhancing an awareness of listeners' understanding.

Jenny

Jenny was a 6-year-old girl who had a primary diagnosis of DAS. Although Jenny's expressive language was moderately delayed, her cognitive and gross motor skills were within age-expected levels. Jenny had a history of chronic otitis media, allergies, hyperactivity, and challenging behavior that was associated with communication problems. Jenny's speech intelligibility was moderately compromised, and she experienced difficulty communicating effectively across all contexts. During communicative interactions when listeners did not understand her, Jenny often did not persist in her communicative attempts. In addition, she was somewhat socially isolated from peers because of their inability to understand her and because of her unconventional communication behavior. Jenny used behaviors to attain positive reinforcement as well as negative reinforcement. For example, she used physical aggression to gain attention and access to tangible items that were associated with specific activities. In addition, she became reluctant to attempt verbal communication to avoid communication failure with her peers. Jenny's behaviors tended to alienate her communication partners and further increased her social isolation.

Assessment at the sound segment level revealed that Jenny used a number of phonological processes. In fact, she incorrectly produced approximately 40% of target consonants. In addition to, and possibly because of, Jenny's sound production challenges, she also had difficulty with the syntactic and morphological aspects of spoken language. Her utterances contained multiple morphophonological errors that affected structures such as regular plurals (stridency deletion) and regular past tense (final consonant deletion). These errors seemed to further reduce her speech intelligibility.

Table 13.2 presents the results of the assessment measures for Jenny. Measurement of speech intelligibility showed that Jenny's word level productions were 38% intelligible, sentence-level productions were 60% intelligible, and connected narratives were 73% understandable to unfamiliar listeners. When listeners were provided with topic cues, word intelligibility increased to 82% (a 44% gain), sentence intelligibility increased to 75% (a 15% gain), and narrative comprehension remained at 73%. When alphabetic cues were provided to listeners, sentence intelligibility increased to 88% (a 13% gain from topic cues and a 28% gain from no cues).

These data showed that as the length and complexity of Jenny's production increased, her intelligibility and understandability increased. This pattern of results was quite different from the pattern observed with Connor, and it is what we would expect based on the intelligibility literature (Dongilli, 1994; Miller, Heise, & Lichten, 1951). For intelligibility tasks, Jenny showed a marked benefit when topic cues were provided to her listeners. For the narrative comprehension task, provision of cues did not differ from provision of no cues. Again, the effects of alphabet cues were measured only at the sentence level, but the results suggested that optimal intelligibility was obtained under this condition.

Jenny's communication profile clearly demonstrated that she benefited from the use of speech supplementation strategies, particularly at the word and sentence levels. In addition, her behavioral manifestations of communication frustration suggested an immediate need for intervention that focused on functional communication. Jenny's maximum intelligibility and comprehensibility levels were 88% (with alphabetic cues) and 73% (with topic cues), respectively; therefore, intervention with a VOCA did not seem to be warranted.

Table 13.2. Assessment measures for Jenny

	Word intelligibility	Sentence intelligibility	Narrative comprehensibility
No cues	38%	60%	73%
Topic cues	82%	75%	73%
Alphabetic cues	—	88%	—

Because Jenny showed age-appropriate literacy skills, the use of alphabet supplementation would be introduced in highly structured therapeutic contexts and, over time, generalized to broader conversational contexts. The use of alphabet supplementation could easily be combined with speech production objectives to target the remediation of sound segment errors. Jenny's intervention plan was prioritized as follows:

1. Introduce low-technology AAC topic boards. Teach the integration of natural speech and pointing to the referent or topic while speaking in words or isolated sentences.
2. Emphasize the provision of context through the verbal production of narratives or contiguous messages that maintain topical cohesion. This might be accomplished through partner dependent prompting (e.g., "Tell me more," "What else?").
3. Introduce alphabet supplementation strategies, and work on first letter identification of words in structured contexts.
4. Address phoneme- and process-specific speech production errors in word and connected speech.
5. Teach the hierarchical use of communication strategies as discussed previously. Focus on enhancing an awareness of listeners' understanding.

Eli

Eli was a 4-year-old boy who had typical cognitive skills, a mild language impairment, and severely impaired speech production skills. Eli's gross motor skills were within normal limits; however, he had difficulty with fine motor skills. He sought interaction with other children and adults, but his attempts to communicate were often unsuccessful because of his reduced speech intelligibility. In addition, Eli was easily frustrated by his unsuccessful communication attempts and often exhibited physically aggressive behavior toward peers and himself when others failed to understand him. Eli did not use gestures or environmental cues (e.g., pointing to referents in the environment, using universal gestures) to enhance his spoken communication.

Assessment measures at the sound segment level indicated that Eli frequently made developmental articulation errors and used phonological processes that followed an atypical pattern, with many nondevelopmental processes present. Oral-motor examination revealed motor planning difficulties that were characterized by oral groping behavior as well as coordination difficulty on repeated productions of single words and multisyllabic word productions. Eli had received speech-language intervention that specifically targeted phonological processes, articulation, and motor planning, but there was minimal progress and virtually no change in his functional communication skills.

Table 13.3. Assessment measures for Eli

	Word intelligibility	Sentence intelligibility	Narrative comprehensibility
No cues	3%	3%	3%
Topic cues	33%	11%	17%
Alphabetic cues	–	28%	–

Table 13.3 presents the results of the assessment measures for Eli. His speech intelligibility was measured to be 3% at the word-level and 3% at the sentence-level. His connected narratives were also only 3% understandable to unfamiliar listeners. When listeners were provided with topic cues, word-level intelligibility increased to 33% (an improvement of 30%), sentence-level intelligibility increased to 11% (an improvement of 8%), and narrative comprehension increased to 17% (an improvement of 14%). When alphabetic cues were provided to listeners, sentence intelligibility increased to 28% (a 25% gain from no cues and a 17% gain from topic cues).

Although the data indicated that speech supplementation strategies markedly enhanced Eli's intelligibility and understandability, his speech intelligibility and understandability continued to be severely impaired. Consequently, implementing these strategies might not provide meaningful functional improvement. Eli's communication profile suggested that a VOCA was necessary to enhance functional communication skills. Eli's intervention plan was prioritized as follows:

1. Introduce VOCAs immediately. Focus intervention on operational, social, linguistic, and strategic competencies (Light, 1989). Encourage the use of natural speech with VOCA for future integration of speech and AAC.
2. Encourage and increase the use of gestures and other paralinguistic cues, such as pointing to environmental referents to facilitate the exchange of meaning.
3. Work on speech production skills, including sound segments, coordination, and sequencing.
4. As speech production skills and, subsequently, speech intelligibility improve, reassess the usefulness of speech supplementation strategies.

CONCLUSION

In this chapter, we have described communication strategies and intervention options for children who have reduced speech intelligibility such that they are unable to meet their communication needs across all contexts. We have advocated for a communication approach in which natural speech, supplemented by AAC strategies, is regarded as the primary mode of communication for all but the most severe cases. In addition, we have recommended using a hierarchy of communication strategies that move from less to more dependency on AAC. Finally, we have emphasized that functionally oriented AAC interventions and developmentally oriented speech interventions should not be mutually exclusive options for children who have speech intelligibility challenges.

Only preliminary research exists on the efficacy of speech supplementation strategies for children with speech intelligibility challenges. Experimental as well as clinically based research is necessary to further the field's understanding of how these strategies influence speech intelligibility and the prerequisite skills that are necessary for the use of speech supplementation strategies. Other avenues of related investigation might include intervention paradigms to facilitate learning and the successful use of strategies, the partner's role in successful communication strategies, and the listener's perceptions of communicative competence and effectiveness when strategies are employed. Finally, the effects of supplementation strategies on the development of natural speech and speech intelligibility are important areas for future study.

REFERENCES

Ball, L.J. (1999). *Communication characteristics of children with DAS.* Unpublished doctoral dissertation, University of Nebraska–Lincoln.

Beukelman, D.R., & Mirenda, P. (1998). *Augmentative and alternative communication: Management of severe communication disorders in children and adults* (2nd ed.). Baltimore: Paul H. Brookes Publishing Co.

Beukelman, D.R., & Yorkston, K. (1977). A communication system for the severely dysarthric speaker with an intact language system. *Journal of Speech and Hearing Disorders, 42,* 265–270.

Bruce, D. (1958). The effect of listeners' anticipations on the intelligibility of heard speech. *Language and Speech, 1,* 79–97.

Carter, C.R., Yorkston, K.M., Strand, E.A., & Hammen, V.L. (1996). Effects of semantic and syntactic context on actual and estimated sentence intelligibility of dysarthric speakers. In D.A. Robin, K.M. Yorkston, & D.R. Beukelman (Eds.), *Disorders of motor speech: Assessment, treatment, and clinical characterization* (pp. 67–87). Baltimore: Paul H. Brookes Publishing Co.

Dongilli, P.A. (1994). Semantic context and speech intelligibility. In J.A. Till, K.M. Yorkston, & D.R. Beukelman (Eds.), *Motor speech disorders: Advances in assessment and treatment* (pp. 175–191). Baltimore: Paul H. Brookes Publishing Co.

Doss, L.S., & Reichle, J. (1991). Replacing excess behavior with an initial communicative repertoire. In J. Reichle, J. York, & J. Sigafoos (Eds.), *Implementing augmentative and alternative communication: Strategies for learners with severe disabilities* (pp. 215–237). Baltimore: Paul H. Brookes Publishing Co.

Dowden, P. (1997). Augmentative and alternative communication decision making for children with severely unintelligible speech. *Augmentative and Alternative Communication, 13,* 48–58.

Garcia, J., & Cannito, M. (1996a). Influence of verbal and nonverbal contexts on the sentence intelligibility of a speaker with dysarthria. *Journal of Speech and Hearing Research, 39,* 750–760.

Garcia, J.M., & Cannito, M.P. (1996b). Top-down influences on the intelligibility of a dysarthric speaker: Addition of natural gestures and situational context. In D.A. Robin, K.M. Yorkston, & D.R. Beukelman (Eds.), *Disorders of motor speech: Assessment, treatment, and clinical characterization* (pp. 89–103). Baltimore: Paul H. Brookes Publishing Co.

Golding-Kushner, K.J. (1995). Treatment of articulation and resonance disorders associated with cleft palate and VPI. In R.J. Shprintzen & J. Bardach (Eds.), *Cleft palate speech management: A multidisciplinary approach* (pp. 327–351). St. Louis, MO: Mosby.

Hodge, M.A., & Wellman, L. (1999). Management of children with dysarthria. In A.J. Caruso & E.A. Strand (Eds.), *Clinical management of motor speech disorders in children* (pp. 209–280). New York: Thieme Medical Publishers.

Hodson, B., & Paden, E. (1991). *Targeting intelligible speech: A phonological approach to remediation* (2nd ed.). Austin, TX: PRO-ED.

Hustad, K.C. (1999). *Effects of context on intelligibility and comprehensibility of severely dysarthric speech.* Unpublished doctoral dissertation, University of Nebraska–Lincoln.

Hustad, K.C., & Beukelman, D.R. (2000). Integrating AAC strategies with natural speech in adults. In D.R. Beukelman & J. Reichle (Series Eds.) & D.R. Beukelman, K.M. Yorkston, & J. Reichle (Vol. Eds.), *AAC series: Vol. 1. Augmentative and alternative communication for adults with acquired neurologic disorders* (pp. 83–106). Baltimore: Paul H. Brookes Publishing Co.

Hustad, K.C., & Beukelman, D.R. (2001). Effects of linguistic cues and stimulus cohesion on intelligibility of severely dysarthric speech. *Journal of Speech, Language, and Hearing Research, 44,* 497–510.

Hustad, K.C., & Morehouse, T.M. (1998, Nov.). *An integrated approach to improving communication effectiveness in unintelligible children.* Paper presented at the American Speech-Language-Hearing Association (ASHA) Annual Convention, San Antonio, TX.

Khan, L., & Lewis, N. (1986). *Khan-Lewis Phonological Analysis.* Circle Pines, MN: American Guidance Service.

Kraat, A. (1987). *Communication between aided and natural speakers: A state of the art report.* Madison, WI: Trace Center.

Light, J. (1989). Toward a definition of communicative competence for individuals using augmentative and alternative communication systems. *Augmentative and Alternative Communication, 5,* 137–144.

Millar, D., Light, J., & Schlosser, R. (1999, Nov.). *The impact of augmentative and alternative communication on natural speech development: A meta-analysis.* Poster presentation at the ASHA Annual Convention, San Francisco.

Miller, G.A., Heise, G.A., & Lichten, W. (1951). The intelligibility of speech as a function of the context of the test materials. *Journal of Experimental Psychology, 41,* 329–335.

Monsen, R.B. (1983). The oral speech intelligibility of hearing-impaired talkers. *Journal of Speech and Hearing Disorders, 43,* 286–296.

Parrish, J.M. (1997). Behavior management: Promoting adaptive behavior. In M.L. Batshaw (Ed.), *Children with disabilities* (4th ed., pp. 657–686). Baltimore: Paul H. Brookes Publishing Co.

Reichle, J., & Wacker, D.P. (Vol. Eds.). (1993). *Communication and language intervention series: Vol. 3. Communicative alternatives to challenging behavior: Integrating functional assessment and intervention strategies.* Baltimore: Paul H. Brookes Publishing Co.

Yorkston, K.M., Beukelman, D.R., Strand, E.A., & Bell, K.R. (1999). *Management of motor speech disorders in children and adults* (2nd ed.). Austin, TX: PRO-ED.

Yorkston, K.M., Beukelman, D.R., & Hustad, K.C. (1999). Optimizing communication effectiveness: Bringing it together. In K.M. Yorkston, D.R. Beukelman, E.A. Strand, & K.R. Bell (Eds.), *Management of motor speech disorders in children and adults* (2nd ed., pp. 483–537). Austin, TX: PRO-ED.

14

The Role of Language Comprehension in Establishing Early Augmented Conversations

Rose A. Sevcik and Mary Ann Romski

Language comprehension is the ability to understand what is said so that one can function as a listener in communicative exchanges. Conversely, language production is the ability to express information so that one can function as a speaker in conversational exchanges. For an individual to develop functional communication skills, he or she must be able to comprehend *and* produce language so that he or she can take on the reciprocal roles of both listener and speaker in conversational exchanges (Sevcik & Romski, 1997).

Augmentative and alternative communication (AAC) systems have typically provided an output mode so that an individual can produce communications and engage as a speaker in conversations with others to express his or her wants, needs, feelings, and ideas. Although this role is essential and permits the individual to have a visible communicative effect on his or her environment, it does not exist in isolation (Romski & Sevcik, 1993). There is the presumption that the individual can also take on the role of listener or receiver of messages in a conversation. To assume the role of message receiver, the individual must be able to understand the information that is being conveyed to him or her by a range of communicative partners. For beginning communicators, a primary focus on production may actually make learning to communicate via AAC systems extremely difficult. In these cases, the individual is asked to produce communications with the assumption that he or she has an adequate foundation of understanding on which to build these AAC productions.

In this chapter, we explore the role that language comprehension can play for beginning AAC communicators. The first section of this chapter provides

The preparation of this manuscript was funded by National Institutes of Health (NIH) Grant Nos. DC-03766 and DC-03799 and a Research Enhancement Grant from Georgia State University. The authors wish to thank Amy Hyatt for her assistance with library research and manuscript preparation.

a brief review of the literature on the early communication comprehension and production skills of young typically developing children and why these data are important as initial AAC use is considered. The second section characterizes who beginning communicators are and reviews the AAC literature with respect to speech comprehension abilities. Next, we discuss the role of comprehension in the AAC assessment process as well as its role in AAC interventions for beginning communicators. Finally, we provide some AAC research and practice directions for the future.

EARLY COMMUNICATION
DEVELOPMENT OF TYPICALLY DEVELOPING CHILDREN

Spoken language comprehension skills assume an extremely important role in the early communication development of typically developing children (Adamson, 1996). Young typically developing children first hear spoken language during rich social-communicative interactions that include recurring familiar situations or events (Bruner, 1983; Nelson, 1985). Prior to children's actually producing words, social and environmental contexts converge with the available linguistic information to produce understandings (Huttenlocher, 1974). Contextual, or situational, speech comprehension begins to emerge as early as 9 months of age (Benedict, 1979). This type of comprehension means that children learn to respond to words in highly contextualized routines that include situational supports (Platt & Coggins, 1990). For example, a child touches the ball after her mother says "Go get the ball" and simultaneously points to the ball. By the time typical children are 12–15 months of age, they understand, on average, about 50 words without contextual supports (Benedict, 1979; Miller, Chapman, Branston, & Reichle, 1980; Snyder, Bates, & Bretherton, 1981). These words progress developmentally from person and object names to actions and from present to absent person and object names. Fenson, Dale, Reznick, Bates, and colleagues (1994) described the most common compositions of the first 50 receptive words as including people, games and routines, familiar objects, animals, body parts, and actions.

As children move through their second year of life, the character of their word learning changes. By 24 months of age, they rely more on social cues than on perceptual cues (Hollich, Hirsh-Pasek, & Golinkoff, 2000). They also quickly expand their understanding from single words to relational commands, such as "Give daddy a kiss," and can carry them out (Goldin-Meadow, Seligman, & Gelman, 1976; Hirsh-Pasek & Golinkoff, 1996; Roberts, 1983). Golinkoff, Hirsh-Pasek, Cauley, and Gordon (1987) reported that typically developing children as young as 17 months of age, who were characterized as one-word communicators and who were not producing word order, actually comprehended word order (e.g., "Big Bird tickle Ernie," "Ernie tickle Big

Bird") when a video-based preferential looking paradigm was employed to assess their skills. During this procedure, a child was seated on his or her mother's lap, midway between two television monitors. A central speaker played a linguistic stimulus that matched the video scenario on only one of the two television screens. The child's task was to visually choose the video screen that matched the linguistic stimulus that he or she heard by looking at the screen. Thus, before the typically developing child is 24 months of age, he or she understands the meanings of single words and the role that word order plays in understanding some phrases and sentences.

The relatively modest literature on early word comprehension has focused on describing the emergence of word comprehension in development (e.g., Benedict, 1979; Huttenlocher, 1974) and experimentally examining the contextual influences on its development (e.g., Halle & de Boysson-Bardies, 1994; Oviatt, 1980; Resnick & Goldfield, 1992). The findings from both of these methodologies provide strong evidence that early word comprehension precedes early word production. Snyder and colleagues (1981), for example, reported on the vocabulary development of 32 children who were 13 months old. They had comprehension vocabularies of 11–97 words (mean = 45 words) compared with production vocabularies of 0–45 words (mean = 11 words). It is interesting to note that Fenson, Dale, Reznick, Bates, and colleagues (1994) reported overlap between the words young children comprehended and produced, though comprehension was shown to have a developmental advantage in the majority of the children. Young typically developing children quickly move on to word production, and their ability to comprehend words, and even sentences, becomes simply a "given" to the adults in the children's environments. Because word production skills emerge so quickly in typically developing children, they may mask and overshadow the continuing role that speech comprehension plays in the early language development process. After a young typically developing child starts talking, it is difficult, if not impossible, to independently examine speech comprehension skills without considering the impact of word production skills on the findings. Based on her study of 18 children (ages 12–24 months), however, Nelson (1973) proposed that those typically developing children who, very early in the language development process, have few productive spoken words may rely on an internal processing of the language that they hear to advance their underlying linguistic competence. She reported a positive relationship between speech comprehension skills at 15 months of age and all later indices of language maturity. Nonetheless, the words that a child comprehends may not be the exact words that the child wants or needs to use in his or her own productions.

What, then, does comprehension provide the young child who is learning language? Comprehension skills draw the young language learner's attention to word forms and their referents in the environment. New methodologies suggest that, from the outset, the young child relies on comprehension to build a foundation for later productive word use (Hollich et al., 2000). Word input from the caregiver to the child also permits the caregiver to create new learning opportunities by capitalizing on well-established routines and the child's understanding of them (Oviatt, 1985).

AAC BEGINNING COMMUNICATORS

Who are beginning communicators? From our perspective, beginning communicators are heterogeneous in composition and bring a broad range of communicative skills to the task of learning to communicate symbolically. Their profiles vary depending on the blend of their biological status, the environment in which they operate, and their experiences. Individual profiles, in turn, will interact differentially with AAC instructional strategies to influence intervention outcomes. It is also likely that individuals with congenital disabilities that have been present since birth will be beginning communicators, because they may have encountered difficulty with spoken communication from the onset of development. It is possible, however, that some children and adults with acquired disabilities, such as traumatic brain injury, could have profiles that also are consistent with the beginning stages of communication development. Chronological age (CA) may also vary for beginning communicators. The range can span from infants and toddlers with little experience to adults who have had a number of years of sometimes unsuccessful communication experiences and/or interventions. Among the factors that contribute to an individual's beginning communicative profile are cognitive development and related disabilities, communicative experience, vocal production skills, and speech comprehension skills.

Cognitive Skills and Related Disabilities

The cognitive skills that a beginning communicator brings to the intervention task can vary from no evidence of cognitive disabilities to that of severe cognitive disabilities. The likelihood, however, is high that a beginning communicator will evidence some degree of cognitive disability. At one time, individuals with severe cognitive disabilities were frequently excluded from AAC instruction because their assessed cognitive and sensorimotor development were not commensurate with cognitive and sensorimotor skills that had been linked to early language development (Chapman & Miller, 1980; Mirenda & Locke, 1989; Romski & Sevcik, 1988a). Although one may argue that some basic cognitive skills are essential for language to develop, the precise relationship between the domains of cognition and language have not been specified clearly (see Rice, 1983, and Rice & Kemper, 1984, for reviews). Thus, investigators have argued against excluding children from AAC instruction based on cognitive performance and/or prerequisite sensorimotor skills (Kangas & Lloyd, 1988; Reichle & Karlan, 1988; Romski & Sevcik, 1988a). Given the overall impact that language exerts on cognitive development, a lack of productive language skills may put an individual at a distinct developmental disadvantage (Rice & Kemper, 1984). Developing language skills through AAC may be of critical importance if the individual is to make functional cognitive gains as well.

A range of related disabilities may accompany severe levels of cognitive disability. These may include though need not be restricted to autism, cerebral palsy, seizure disorders, sensory impairments, or challenging behaviors. Each of these disabilities may have additional influences on the individual's communicative profile (Guess & Horner, 1978; Snell, 1987). An individual with severe physical disabilities, for example, may encounter significant difficulty in gaining access to an AAC output mode. Thus, it may also be a formidable task to gain an accurate estimate of the individual's cognitive abilities.

Communicative Experience

As noted in Chapter 1, experience is often overlooked as an influence when characterizing the factors that may affect communication profiles. Because beginning communicators often do not demonstrate productive language skills, it is frequently presumed that they are functioning below a 12- to 18-month-old developmental level, although they sometimes may be well beyond that age. This assumption often provides an inaccurate, or at least incomplete, description of their competencies. In many respects, such individuals function well beyond the sensorimotor stage of development, as they have frequently developed and/or utilized a range of alternative ways, including some idiosyncratic means, with which to communicate in familiar environs (Romski, Sevcik, Reumann, & Pate, 1989). These natural communicative repertoires may have been employed for prolonged periods of time and have included multiple conversational experiences, communicative partners, and environments and often do not resemble those of 12- to 18-month-old typically developing children. Rather, the repertoires are used in more variable contexts and perhaps less flexibly than those of young typically developing children. The effect of life experience beyond that of the early developmental period must be overlaid and considered as well.

Vocal Production Skills

As noted in Chapter 1, beginning communicators also bring a wide range of vocal production skills to the task. One of the most striking observations of the Romski and colleagues (1989) study was the extent to which the children vocalized naturally, though unintelligibly, prior to the introduction of an AAC device. Although vocal skills are not necessary for learning to communicate via an AAC system, the ability to vocally imitate may play a role in the child's subsequent gains with speech in the context of the AAC system (e.g., Romski, Sevcik, Robinson, & Wilkinson, 1990; Yoder & Layton, 1988).

Speech Comprehension Skills

As part of their language profile, beginning communicators may evidence speech comprehension skills that range from no or minimal comprehension to comprehension skills that are equivalent to their chronological age (Nelson, 1992). As stated in Chapter 1, individuals who do comprehend some speech may have knowledge about the relationship between words and their referents in the environment (Romski & Sevcik, 1993). Consequently, their auditory processing skills may be quite distinct from those of individuals who do not have such a foundation on which to build AAC skills. Individuals who do not understand spoken words confront a very different task. They must establish conditional relationships between the visual symbols to be learned and their real-world referents while relying, almost exclusively, on the visual modality (Romski & Sevcik, 1996). Consequently, AAC systems can serve as both the input and output modes.

These four factors—cognitive skills and related disabilities, communicative experience, vocal production skills, and speech comprehension skills— vary across individuals who may be considered beginning communicators. Each factor is intrinsic to the individual as a function of his or her biological makeup and experiences and can combine in different ways with the selected AAC instructional approach to influence how the individual profits from AAC experience.

Speech and Language Comprehension and
Beginning AAC Conversations: What Do We Know?

Why is speech comprehension an important underpinning for AAC system development and use? Speech comprehension provides an essential foundation on which individuals can build productive language competence. The ability to comprehend spoken words permits the young typically developing child to bootstrap his or her way into the world of productive spoken language. The same opportunities should be true for an individual who uses an AAC communication mode. The comprehension of words and, ultimately, sentences can be developing even when an individual is not speaking and can be a link between the auditory and visual symbol modalities when speech is not a viable productive mode. Speech comprehension plays a silent yet critical role in the language development process (Romski & Sevcik, 1993; Sevcik & Romski, 1997). When beginning communicators do not have a speech comprehension repertoire with which to build, their productive language learning may be slow and constrained even when an AAC mode for productive communication is made available to them (Romski & Sevcik, 1993; Sevcik & Romski, 1997). In addition, they may not be able to understand another's spoken or augmented communications. If an individual does not comprehend spoken words, intervention that focuses on teaching the individual to comprehend the meanings of visual-graphic symbols or manual signs can provide the individual with an alternative foundation on which to build productive AAC use.

In this section, we provide a review of the AAC literature, highlighting studies that contribute to our understanding of the role of speech comprehension in beginning AAC use. Three types of studies have informed the field about AAC and the role of comprehension. The first type addresses the relationship between language comprehension abilities and symbolic representational skills. The second type of studies considers what we know about the language comprehension skills of beginning communicators. Finally, a third type of studies focuses on the role of language comprehension and AAC instructional outcomes.

Symbols and Representation   Very little symbol research has been conducted in which beginning AAC communicators have served as participants. Of the studies that have been reported, the focus of investigation has been on describing the participants' symbolic representational abilities. Sevcik and Romski (1986) examined the representational matching skills of 8 individuals with severe mental retardation (mean CA = 14 years, 6 months; range = from 9 years, 2 months, to 22 years, 6 months). They found that the four individuals who lacked functional language skills (operationally defined as a minimum vocabulary of 10 spoken words, manual signs, or visual-graphic symbols used spontaneously in comprehension and production) encountered more difficulty with identity (e.g., photograph to photograph) as well as nonidentity (e.g., photograph to line drawing) matching for photographs and line drawings than comparable participants with functional language skills (see Chapter 9 for a discussion of matching). Mirenda and Locke (1989) studied the symbolic representational abilities of 40 nonspeaking children and adolescents (ages 3 years, 11 months, to 20 years, 10 months) with a range of cognitive disabilities (e.g., autism, cerebral palsy, moderate or severe mental retardation) by using a verbal receptive language protocol ("Show me [spoken word]" from a choice of two symbols) *or* a visual matching assessment task (object or photograph to symbol). For the majority of the participants (75%), the verbal receptive language protocol was used to assess representational skill. For participants who encountered difficulty in using the receptive language protocol, the nonverbal nonidentity matching task was utilized. Mirenda and Locke reported that a hierarchy of symbol representation was found from objects to Blissymbols and written words for all of the participants. The use of these two distinct protocols (verbal versus visual matching) highlights the heterogeneity of beginning communicators' linguistic comprehension skills. The absence of expressive language skills does not necessarily imply the presence of adequate comprehension skills. The importance of language comprehension skills to performance on the verbal and visual matching protocols was corroborated by Franklin, Mirenda, and Phillips (1996). They examined the performance of 20 participants with severe intellectual disabilities and functional or nonfunctional language comprehension skills on five tasks that assessed object and photograph matching by using verbal or visual matching protocols. With results paralleling those of Sevcik and Romski (1986) and Mirenda and Locke (1989), Franklin and colleagues found that participants who comprehended the verbal labels for the symbols performed significantly better on all tasks than the participants who did not demonstrate such comprehension skills. Furthermore, they reported distinctly better performance patterns on the visual matching protocol than on the verbal protocol, suggesting again that participants with this type of profile do not always bring comprehension skills to the augmented language learning task.

Language Comprehension Skills   Typically, little is known about the speech comprehension skills that beginning AAC users bring to the task. In a study of an 8-year-old girl with a severe expressive communication impairment, Roth and Cassatt-James (1989) reported that the child's severe expressive communication limitations actually masked concurrent significant language comprehension difficulties. Attention had been focused exclusively on the girl's production difficulties and it was assumed that her comprehension skills were adequate. In fact, although her comprehension skills were better than her production skills, they were not adequate for her chronological age.

Sevcik, Romski, and Adamson (1998) characterized the language comprehension skills of 16 toddlers (mean CA = 29.7 months, range = 22 to 44 months) who had significant developmental disabilities and were not speaking, by using three measures: 1) the MacArthur Communicative Development Inventories (CDI; Fenson, Dale, Reznick, Thal, et al., 1994), a receptive and expressive parent report vocabulary inventory; 2) the Peabody Picture Vocabulary Test–Revised (PPVT-R; Dunn & Dunn, 1981), a standardized test of single word vocabulary comprehension; and 3) the Emerging Language Stage items of The Clinical Assessment of Language Comprehension (Miller & Paul, 1995), an informal assessment of speech comprehension development. At the time of the study, none of the children had begun to talk or had demonstrated behaviors that suggested they were on the verge of talking (e.g., vocal behavior, appropriate oral-motor reflexes). All children demonstrated at least primitive intentional communication skills (e.g., physically manipulating a person to obtain a desired item). Gestural abilities ranged from none to a point with the index finger.

On the CDI, parents reported that all 16 children responded to their names, "No-no," and "There's Mommy (or Daddy)." They also reported that the children comprehended 5–28 phrases (mean = 16.3 phrases) and 16–289 words (mean = 134.2 words). The children's performance on the PPVT-R, however, did not reflect the parental report. In general, the children were at the very beginning of the age range at which a standard score could be obtained on the PPVT-R; nevertheless, only 2 of the 16 children obtained a basal score. One of these two children received a moderately low standard score for his chronological age, whereas the other child's standard score was considered low average for his chronological age.

Although all of the children had similar productive language profiles, there was a wide range of overall performance (range = from 8% to 100% correct, mean correct = 46%) on the Emerging Language Stage items on The Clinical Assessment of Language Comprehension. This stage consists of six items, which are described in Table 14.1. Children performed best on a joint reference activity. All children responded correctly on at least one trial for this item, and nine of the children answered correctly in 100% of the trials. This performance level was followed by performance on the comprehension of familiar routines, on which 8 of the 16 children performed with 100% accuracy. Comprehension of object and person names, action words, words for absent persons and objects, and early two-word relations clustered together in terms of mean percent correct performance. Only one child received an 100% correct score on these items, whereas the majority of the children encountered some difficulty with these items. Even within the Emerging Language Stage, performance on The Clinical Assessment of Language Comprehension items evidenced an increased difficulty for these children, suggesting that they were following the developmental hierarchy hypothesized by Miller and Paul (1995).

These three comprehension assessment tools each tapped distinct dimensions of the children's comprehension, from phrase and single word vocabulary comprehension in context to a standardized task that employed a 2 × 2 array of four of black-and-white line drawings in informal yet structured interactions that permitted the observation of comprehension skills. In addition, they each employed a different method of measurement, from parental

Table 14.1. Items from the Emerging Language Stage of The Clinical Assessment of Language Comprehension

Comprehending familiar routines
Establishing joint reference
Comprehending object and person names
Comprehending action words
Comprehending words for absent people and objects
Comprehending early two-word relations (e.g., kiss doggie)

Source: Miller & Paul (1995).

report to behavioral compliance to pointing. The range of comprehension profiles exhibited by these 16 young children, who all presented with extremely limited productive spoken language skills, ranged from minimal to fairly advanced. The less formal comprehension measures (i.e., CDI and The Clinical Assessment of Language Comprehension) provided a means by which to characterize a range of the children's emerging speech comprehension skills. These distinct profiles give important information about where to begin the augmented language intervention process to achieve the most efficient and effective communication gains.

In another descriptive study, Sutton and Gallagher (1995) explored the utility of two tasks (a discourse task and a nonsense-enactment task) for assessing the past-tense comprehension of a girl with severe physical disabilities who was 4 years, 8 months old. They compared this child's performance on these two experimental tasks with the performance of chronologically age-matched peers. Similar performance among the peers was reported on the nonsense-enactment task. Differences in performance on the discourse task were attributed to discourse use differences among the mothers and limitations in the response options and opportunities that were available on the child's AAC device. Sutton and Gallagher suggested that these two tasks can be employed to provide additional tools for assessing the knowledge of grammatical rules in children who encounter difficulty with standardized measures. In sum, all of these studies indicate that a range of tools is available to assess comprehension. These tools should be incorporated into the AAC assessment process.

Language Comprehension Skills and Instructional Outcomes   Augmented language intervention studies are another area that can provide information about the role of receptive language in AAC instructional outcomes. Romski and Sevcik (1996) studied the communication abilities of school-age youth with moderate or severe mental retardation over a 2-year period. They introduced the System for Augmenting Language (SAL) to 13 school-age youth with moderate or severe mental retardation (mean CA = 12 years, 3 months; mean nonverbal mental age = 3 years, 6 months). Each participant had moderate or severe cognitive disabilities and severe spoken language impairments, resided at home, and attended a special education program at his or her local public school. All participants demonstrated intentional communication abilities (e.g., gestures, vocalizations), no more than 10 intelligible word approximations at the onset of the study and an unsuccessful history of learning to communicate via other means (i.e., speech, manual signs, communication boards). As described in Chapter 1, the SAL included five integrated components: 1) speech-output communication device; 2) an individually chosen arbitrary visual-graphic symbol vocabulary; 3) naturalistic communicative experiences during which the youth were encouraged, but not required, to communicate; 4) partners (teachers, parents, and siblings) who were taught how to use the device and how to provide both a symbol model and input via speech + symbols to the youth; and 5) a resource and feedback mechanism from investigators to monitor progress across the study. The youth had opportunities to employ a range of communicative functions from greeting, requesting, and attention directing to answering and questioning during the day at home and school.

It was found that the 13 youth integrated their use of the SAL with their extant vocalizations and gestures, resulting in a rich multimodal form of communication that they used to both successfully and effectively communicate with adults (Romski, Sevcik, Robinson, & Bakeman, 1994) and peers (Romski, Sevcik, & Wilkinson, 1994). These youth developed a vocabulary that integrated referential and social-regulative symbols (Adamson, Romski, Deffebach, & Sevcik, 1992). Some of the youth also then combined their symbols to form more sophisticated symbol meanings as well as intelligible spoken words and rudimentary reading skills (Romski & Sevcik, 1996; Wilkinson, Romski, & Sevcik, 1994).

By the end of the study's first year, however, considerable variability was evident in the quantity of different symbols that each participant employed in comprehension and production. More than half of the 13 participants' symbol vocabulary was comprehended and produced. Yet, individually, the participants fell into one of two nonoverlapping categories that was based on the proportion of symbol vocabulary that they did *not* understand or produce. Nine of the 13 participants comprehended and produced the majority of their referential symbol vocabularies. These participants were described as having an advanced achievement pattern, composed of the rather swift acquisition of symbols and followed by the emergence of symbol combinations and other symbolic skills (e.g., printed word recognition). The participants used basic symbol skills as a firm foundation to progress from and develop skills in other related domains (e.g., reading, spoken words). The remaining four participants were more likely to comprehend a symbol than to produce it. Their performance also included a much larger proportion of symbol vocabulary that they neither comprehended nor produced. They evidenced a second distinct pattern that was described as a *beginning achievement pattern*. This pattern consisted of the slow acquisition of a small set (< 35) of single visual-graphic symbols in comprehension and production and was labeled *beginning* because it suggested that the participants were in the process of developing a set of basic skills from which they could build additional communication skills. Although they had not, as yet, generalized their skills to spoken words and printed English recognition, two of these participants were showing signs of skill development in these two areas.

In addition, Sevcik, Romski, Watkins, and Deffebach (1995) reported that parents and teachers spontaneously increased the amount of augmented communication input (speech + symbol) that they employed when communicating with the beginning achievers than with the advanced achievers. Comprehension skills can serve as the foundation not only for productive symbol learning but also as a vehicle for language instruction. Similarly, Peterson, Bondy, Vincent, and Finnegan, (1995) reported that two school-age boys with autism and no speech made better communicative gains with a communicative input intervention that included speech + pictures and gestures than with one that was speech input alone.

Romski and Sevcik (1996) suggested that the extant spoken language comprehension skills that the advanced achievers brought to the language learning task allowed them to rapidly acquire and use symbols for communication. Their performance was in sharp contrast to the beginning achievers, who did not evidence testable speech comprehension skill at the onset of the study. If only symbol production performance had been measured, then the conclusion would be that these individuals had learned no symbol vocabulary meanings. Additional support for this achievement distinction was provided by Romski, Sevcik, and Pate (1988), who studied older adolescents and young adults with severe cognitive disabilities. The participants were explicitly taught visual-graphic symbol production skills without speech output. The researchers reported distinct symbol acquisition and generalization patterns that were linked to the participants' extant speech comprehension skills.

With the SAL approach, a participant was not directly taught relationships between symbols and their referents. Instead, the participant had to extend existing abilities to acquire new relationships that involve the learning of the rule that "symbols refer." If the relationship between a spoken word and its referent was established during a participant's previous life experience and the SAL was subsequently provided, existing comprehension and cognitive skills may have served as a foundation on which the participant could build a relationship between the visual symbols that he or she was acquiring and already established understandings of spoken words. Given the small number of symbols that were learned and the lack of generalization to other domains, the beginning achievers may have been using a different, less sophisticated, learning strategy than the advanced achievers.

Although the overall knowledge base is, at best, modest, these studies consistently demonstrated that comprehension skills vary across individuals who are beginning AAC intervention. In addition, these different comprehension abilities may influence how beginning communicators respond to AAC intervention.

AAC Assessment and Comprehension   By definition, AAC is an intervention approach (Glennen, 2000). Typically, AAC assessment has focused primarily on determining which device to recommend for an individual (Beukelman & Mirenda, 1998). Another goal of AAC assessment is gaining knowledge about the individual's communication skills, which is used to outline goals for the course of AAC intervention so that the individual can develop functional communication skills. The AAC assessment process, however, has typically not focused on an examination of the individual's comprehension skills, although a number of authors have suggested that it should be an important and included component (Gerber & Kraat, 1992; Light, 1997; Nelson, 1992; Sevcik & Romski, 1997).

With respect to AAC systems, there are at least three routes to understanding another's message: 1) through the comprehension of speech, 2) through an understanding of the meanings of AAC symbols (manual signs, visual-graphic symbols) themselves, or 3) through a combination of speech and symbols. Two areas of comprehension must be included in the assessment process: 1) the comprehension of speech and/or symbols (either manual signs or visual-graphic symbols) words, semantic relations, word order, grammatical morphemes, and/or sentence structure and 2) the individual's ability to take on the role of the listener in AAC communicative interactions. When comprehension is assessed for beginning communicators, the focus is often on single word comprehension. Traditionally, more advanced comprehension skills have not been assessed because the formats of the available standardized measures have made the tasks too difficult. Yet, alternative experimental tools to standardized tests are being developed to assess the comprehension skills of very young typically developing children (see Hirsh-Pasek & Golinkoff, 1996, for a detailed description of one such procedure) and should be considered for beginning communicators as well.

Tools for AAC Assessment of Comprehension

There are at least two types of tools that are available for the assessment of comprehension. These include standardized assessment tools and informal assessment tools (Romski, 2000). Standardized tests are norm-referenced and the most formal, decontextualized way of assessing language skills (e.g., Peabody Picture Vocabulary Test–Third Edition [PPVT-III]; Dunn & Dunn, 1997). These tests have clear administration and scoring criteria, validity, reliability, standardization, measures of central tendency and variability, a standard error of measurement, and norm-referenced scores (both standard comparisons and equivalent scores). Adaptations can be made to standardized tests when assessing someone who cannot otherwise respond conventionally. Wasson, Arvidson, and Lloyd (1997) listed five examples of adaptations, including 1) altering the test instructions and feedback, 2) allowing an alternative response type (e.g., eye gaze rather than pointing), 3) altering the test stimuli, 4) altering the position of the test stimuli, and 5) altering the amount of test time. The drawback to utilizing these adaptations, however, is that they invalidate the test's results and do not permit standard comparisons with the standardization group. Such adaptations do provide some indication of the individual's comprehension skills. At the beginning of the 21st century, there are no standardized AAC language tests.

Developmental scales are interview or observational instruments that sample behaviors from a specific period of development (e.g., CDI, Sequenced Inventory of Communication Development [Hedrick, Prather, & Tobin, 1984]). They are used to help establish how children's language development compares with that of children their own chronological age. Such developmental scales usually cover the developmental period from birth to, at most, 48 months of age. The CDI has been shown to provide a stable report of lexical comprehension in very young children with developmental disabilities (Yoder, Warren, & Biggar, 1997). The Nonspeech Test for Receptive/Expressive Language (Blake-Huer, 1983) is a developmental scale that has been used when testing children with AAC needs. It was designed to provide a systematic means for observing, recording, and summarizing the variety of ways through which an individual may communicate, whether speech or other modes are utilized for communication. It provides comprehension and production language age equivalencies from birth to 48 months of age for typically developing preschool children, public school children with multiple disabilities, and individuals with multiple disabilities who are in institutions.

Criterion-referenced procedures are another type of measure that are devised to examine a particular form of communicative behavior (e.g., comprehension, production), not with reference to other children's achievement but only to determine whether the child can attain a certain level of performance. The Clinical Assessment of Language Comprehension, for example, permits a systematic observation of comprehension within familiar routines and activities. It does not rely on the identification of photographs or pictures nor on an accurate pointing response—both of which can, at times, hinder performance.

Finally, formal and informal behavioral observations are employed to gain information about the individual's language skills. Formal observational checklists, such as the Interaction Checklist for Augmentative Communication (INCH; Bolton & Dashiell, 1991), provide a systematic way to examine communication interaction skills with an AAC system. The INCH provides a consistent way to assess communication interaction on the part of the AAC communicator. It does not, however, directly measure the individual's skill as a listener or a message receiver in the conversational exchange. Informal observations include descriptions of the individual's natural environments (home, school, community, work) and the range of familiar and unfamiliar communicative partners with whom he or she communicates. Experimental measures, developed to answer research questions, may provide a framework that aids in gathering information about the individual's comprehension skills in natural environments (Romski & Sevcik, 1988b).

When planning an AAC assessment, it is important to determine the goal (e.g., planning intervention, recommending an AAC device) to determine the types of measures that should be employed. It is critical that a systematic examination of comprehension skills be incorporated into AAC assessment protocols for beginning communicators and all other AAC communicators (Romski, 2000).

AAC Interventions

Once it is known which comprehension skills the individual brings to the AAC task, the interventionist can utilize that information to develop intervention strategies that match the individual's extant language skills. For individuals who are first learning to use AAC, the field has not yet addressed how to inculcate both comprehension and production in AAC intervention efforts. In practice, beginning AAC intervention has focused on physical access to a device and the production of messages (Beukelman & Mirenda, 1998). The sequence of introduction and the relationship between comprehension and production in beginning AAC intervention has not been specified. Similar to the process observed in typically developing children's first words (Huttenlocher, 1974), a shift in focus to comprehension may permit the child to observe and actively engage in the communicative process prior to actually taking on the role of speaker. Again, similar to very young typically developing children, beginning communicators should be exposed to augmented language before they are asked to produce it. There is very little information about the speech comprehension abilities that individuals with challenging behaviors, who have an immediate need to communicate a message in a conventionally appropriate way, bring to the AAC intervention task and the role that understanding what is said plays in remediating such challenging behaviors.

The role of spoken language input, sometimes referred to as *motherese,* has received considerable attention in the literatures on language acquisition in typically developing children (Gallaway & Richards, 1994; Snow, 1984) and the language development in and intervention for speaking children with developmental language disorders (e.g., Fey, 1986). Although the specific role of spoken language input in the language development of typically developing children is still under debate, it is a natural part of the communicative exchange. The term *total communication* refers to a teaching approach that incorporates both signs and spoken language as input (Kretschmer & Kretschmer, 1978). The input to which children and adults who use AAC systems are typically exposed has been termed *aided language stimulation* (Goossens' & Crain, 1986) or *augmented communicative input* (Romski & Sevcik, 1988b). Goossens' and Crain (1986) defined *aided language stimulation* as being, in many ways, analogous to the total communication and simultaneous communication approaches that appear in the manual sign training literature. When providing aided language stimulation, the facilitator (e.g., parent, clinician) points to picture symbols on the child's communication display in conjunction with ongoing language stimulation. Goossens' (1989) noted that the type of display format and the child's selection techniques are irrelevant to the facilitator's use of the technique. Romski and Sevcik (1988b) defined *AAC input* as the incoming communication/language from the individual's communicative partner, which includes speech and is supplemented by AAC symbols, the speech output that is produced by the AAC device when the symbol is activated, and the environmental context. Augmented communication input requires that the communicative partner use AAC symbols and the speech-output device to give the beginning communicator language input. It models how an AAC device is used, as well as for what contexts and purposes during communicative exchanges. It also can reinforce the effectiveness of using the AAC device by illustrating its utility and power. In addition, it demonstrates that the AAC device is an acceptable vehicle for communication interactions. It provides real-world experiences that illustrate the meaning of AAC symbols and the varied functions that they serve. Finally, its use by partners makes an implicit statement to the AAC user that the AAC system is an accepted and encouraged form of communication.

As part of their longitudinal study of youth with moderate or severe cognitive disabilities who learned language through augmented means, Romski and Sevcik (1996) instructed the participants' adult partners to model AAC use by supplementing spoken communicative input with symbols from the communication system. Sevcik and colleagues (1995) then examined the quantity and quality of the symbol input that the partners employed. They reported that only a small percentage (mean = 10%) of the partners' overall spoken communicative utterances that were directed to the youth contained symbol input. The sophistication of the youths' speech comprehension skills, however, differentially affected the amount of AAC symbol input that they received. Partners were more likely to use AAC symbol input with the beginning achievers who had poor speech comprehension skills than with the advanced achievers who demonstrated comprehension skills at or greater than 24 months of age.

Romski and colleagues (1999) completed a pilot study to examine the effects of an augmented input intervention that focused on teaching the parent to use the strategy. The participant in the study was a 34-month-old boy with a diagnosis of partial trisomy 13, cerebral palsy, significant developmental delay, and speech comprehension skills at about 15 months. He had some undifferentiated vocalizations and a laugh that he did not use communicatively. He did not comprehend the meanings for any of the symbols to be taught (e.g., MORE, ALL DONE, BOOK, SNACK). The intervention increased his symbol and speech comprehension skills for the target vocabulary from 0 to 10 words across a 12-week period. After 6 weeks, there was also a steady increase in his spontaneous use of symbols to communicate messages. There was no comparable change in spoken language production skills, however, over the course of the 12-week intervention. The boy's mother spontaneously reported that she appreciated the intervention because it did not place demands on her to make the child use the device. This input strategy permitted the parent to be successful regardless of the child's response. That is, the child did not have to perform a specific action in order for the parent to think that he or she had implemented the intervention strategy (Romski, Sevcik, & Forrest, 2001). This pilot study suggests that augmented input may yield not only increased comprehension but also the productive communicative use of symbols. Clearly, additional studies of augmented input are needed to evaluate the effects of providing AAC input to beginning communicators.

FUTURE RESEARCH AND PRACTICE DIRECTIONS

Although interventions typically focus on the productive use of AAC systems, speech or symbol comprehension is an essential component of AAC acquisition and/or use. An adequate empirical accounting of comprehension's relative role in early and later AAC system acquisition is required particularly if a focus on comprehension is to be incorporated into practice (for both assessment and intervention). Three areas for future research direction are suggested: 1) the relationship between speech comprehension skills and visual-graphic symbol representation, 2) assessment and measurement of comprehension, and 3) the development and evaluation of augmented input interventions.

First, studies are beginning to link comprehension skills with an individual's achievement using a range of visual-graphic symbols. They do not, however, address the interaction of extant participant language skills (e.g., speech comprehension skills) with learning and using pictographic or arbitrary symbols for beginning AAC users. Direct comparisons of arbitrary symbols and "guessable," less arbitrary, more pictographic symbols have not been made. To learn arbitrary symbol meanings, the relationship between the symbol and its referent must be internalized as there is no overt relationship between symbol and referent (Sevcik, Romski, & Wilkinson, 1991). Nonarbitrary, pictographic symbols can be learned by associating the guessable symbol with its referent. If an individual has not yet established an understanding of the symbol–referent relationship in comprehension, then the individual may not benefit from the help that guessable symbols may provide. It is important, then, to examine the relationship between symbol acquisition and the symbol set that is employed, taking into account the speech comprehension skills that the participants bring to the learning task. In concert with quantifying the child's speech comprehension skills, this type of comparison may provide data that will disentangle the intrinsic and extrinsic components of symbol learning, which address a central issue in initial symbol acquisition (Sevcik et al., 1991).

Second, because speech comprehension can serve as a foundation for AAC acquisition and use, detailed examinations are needed of the continuation of speech comprehension abilities of children and adults who may use AAC output modes. In addition, the development of tools by which to measure comprehension of beginning communicators must be examined and refined. Cauley, Golinkoff, Hirsh-Pasek, and Gordon (1989), for example, applied the video-based preferential-looking procedure to children with motor impairments. Their initial findings suggested that this systematic procedure had potential as an assessment tool for evaluating the comprehension skills of beginning AAC users with accompanying physical disabilities. Because many individuals who use AAC systems encounter difficulty in demonstrating their comprehension via traditional standardized assessment methods, new and innovative measures must continue to be developed and appraised.

Third, evaluating augmented input or aided language stimulation as an AAC intervention strategy is sorely needed. Aided language stimulation, for instance, has been used in clinical practice since the mid-1980s without experimental examination of its efficacy. Research must specify the precise roles that input can play in developing comprehension and production of language with AAC systems by AAC users who have varying abilities at the onset of intervention. Intervention studies are needed that specify the exact effects of augmented input on AAC learning and use. Perhaps most essential are investigations that focus on the role that augmented input can play in beginning AAC use. Very little is known, for example, about the effects of augmented language input for infants and toddlers who are at extremely high risk for severe oral language impairments or for individuals who use challenging behaviors to communicate.

With respect to clinical implications, there are at least two important considerations for clinicians. First, beginning AAC users present a broad range of language comprehension skills. Thus, AAC language assessment must include measurement of language comprehension skills through a range of tools to obtain an accurate and complete profile of spoken language understanding. Second, if an individual has limited speech comprehension, augmented language intervention may first need to incorporate a comprehension and input focus before demands are placed on the individual to produce symbols. In addition, research is needed to examine whether individuals with challenging behaviors may benefit from this intervention approach.

CONCLUSION

Language comprehension has been a forgotten partner in the acquisition of conversations for beginning AAC users. Similar to the process observed in the development of spoken language by young typically developing children,

AAC intervention approaches require a carefully balanced blend of the comprehension and production experiences, which are based on the language skills that the individual brings to the task. As a field, we have directed only modest amounts of attention toward understanding the roles that comprehension (of both speech and AAC symbols) can play in the AAC assessment and intervention process. In the future, researchers and practitioners alike must consider how language comprehension influences beginning AAC users to advance the communication skills and abilities of these individuals.

REFERENCES

Adamson, L.B. (1996). *Communication development during infancy.* Boulder, CO: Westview Press.

Adamson, L.B., Romski, M.A., Deffebach, K.P., & Sevcik, R.A. (1992). Symbol vocabulary and the focus of conversations: Augmenting language development for youth with mental retardation. *Journal of Speech and Hearing Research, 35,* 1333–1344.

Benedict, H. (1979). Early lexical development: Comprehension and production. *Journal of Child Language, 6,* 183–200.

Beukelman, D.R., & Mirenda, P. (1998). *Augmentative and alternative communication: Management of severe communication disorders in children and adults* (2nd ed.). Baltimore: Paul H. Brookes Publishing Co.

Blake-Huer, M. (1983). *The Nonspeech Test for Receptive/Expressive Language.* Volo, IL: Don Johnston.

Bolton, S.O., & Dashiell, S.E. (1991). *Interaction Checklist for Augmentative Communication (INCH).* Bisbee, AZ: Imaginart Press.

Bruner, J. (1983). *Child's talk: Learning to use language.* New York: Norton.

Cauley, K., Golinkoff, R., Hirsh-Pasek, K., & Gordon, L. (1989). Revealing hidden competencies: A new method for studying language comprehension in children with motoric impairment. *American Journal on Mental Retardation, 94,* 53–63.

Chapman, R., & Miller, J. (1980). Analyzing language and communication in the child. In R.L. Schiefelbusch (Ed.), *Nonspeech language and communication: Analysis and intervention* (pp. 159–196). Baltimore: University Park Press.

Dunn, L.M., & Dunn, L.M. (1981). *Peabody Picture Vocabulary Test–Revised (PPVT-R).* Circle Pines, MN: American Guidance Service.

Dunn, L.M., & Dunn, L.M. (1997). *Peabody Picture Vocabulary Test–Third Edition (PPVT-III).* Circle Pines, MN: American Guidance Service.

Fenson, L., Dale, P., Reznick, J.S., Bates, E., Thal, D., & Pethick, S. (1994). Variability in early communicative development. *Monographs of the Society for Research in Child Development, 59*(Serial No. 242).

Fenson, L., Dale, P., Reznick, J.S., Thal, D., Bates, E., Hartung, J., Pethick, S., & Reilly, J. (1994). *MacArthur Communicative Development Inventories (CDI): User's guide and technical manual.* San Diego: Singular Publishing Group.

Fey, M. (1986). *Language intervention with young children.* San Diego: College-Hill Press.

Franklin, K., Mirenda, P., & Phillips, G. (1996). Comparison of five symbol assessment protocols with nondisabled preschoolers and learners with severe intellectual disabilities. *Augmentative and Alternative Communication, 12,* 63–77.

Gallaway, C., & Richards, B.J. (1994). *Input and interaction in language acquisition.* New York: Cambridge University Press.

Gerber, S., & Kraat, A. (1992). Use of a developmental model of language acquisition: Applications to children using AAC systems. *Augmentative and Alternative Communication, 8,* 19–32.

Glennen, S. (2000, January). *AAC assessment myths and realities.* Paper presented at the American Speech-Language-Hearing Association (ASHA) Special Interest Division (SID) 12 Leadership Conference on Augmentative and Alternative Communication, Sea Island, GA.

Goldin-Meadow, S., Seligman, M.E.P., & Gelman, R. (1976). Language in the two year old. *Cognition, 4,* 189–202.

Golinkoff, R.M., Hirsh-Pasek, K., Cauley, K.M., & Gordon, L. (1987). The eyes have it: Lexical and syntactic comprehension in a new paradigm. *Journal of Child Language, 14,* 23–46.

Goossens', C. (1989). Aided communication intervention before assessment: A case study of a child with cerebral palsy. *Augmentative and Alternative Communication, 5,* 14–26.

Goossens', C., & Crain, S. (1986). *Augmentative communication intervention resource.* Volo, IL: Don Johnston.

Guess, D., & Horner, R. (1978). The severely and profoundly handicapped. In E.L. Meyen (Ed.), *Exceptional children and youth: An introduction* (pp. 218–268). Denver, CO: Love Publishing.

Halle P.A., & de Boysson-Bardies, B. (1994). Emergence of an early receptive lexicon: Infants' recognition of words. *Infant Behavior and Development, 17,* 119–129.

Hedrick, D., Prather, E., & Tobin, A. (1984). *Sequenced Inventory of Communication Development.* Los Angeles: Western Psychological Services.

Hirsh-Pasek, K., & Golinkoff, R.M. (1996). *The origins of grammar: Evidence from early language comprehension.* Cambridge, MA: The MIT Press.

Hollich, G., Hirsh-Pasek, K., & Golinkoff, R. (2000). Breaking the language barrier: An emergentist coalition model of word learning. *Monographs of the Society for Research in Child Development, 65*(3, Serial No. 262).

Huttenlocher, J. (1974). The origins of language comprehension. In R.L. Solso (Ed.), *Theories of cognitive psychology* (pp. 331–368). Mahwah, NJ: Lawrence Erlbaum Associates.

Kangas, K., & Lloyd, L. (1988). Early cognitive skills prerequisites to augmentative and alternative communication use: What are we waiting for? *Augmentative and Alternative Communication, 4,* 211–221.

Kretschmer, R., & Kretschmer, L. (1978). *Perspectives in audiology series: Language development and intervention with the hearing impaired.* Baltimore: University Park Press.

Light, J. (1997). "Let's go star fishing": Reflections on the contexts of language learning for children who use aided AAC. *Augmentative and Alternative Communication, 13,* 158–170.

Miller, J.F., Chapman, R.S., Branston, M., & Reichle, J. (1980). Language comprehension in sensorimotor stages V and VI. *Journal of Speech and Hearing Research, 23,* 284–311.

Miller, J.F., & Paul, R. (1995). *The Clinical Assessment of Language Comprehension.* Baltimore: Paul H. Brookes Publishing Co.

Mirenda, P., & Locke, M. (1989). A comparison of symbol transparency in nonspeaking persons with intellectual disabilities. *Journal of Speech and Hearing Disorders, 54,* 131–140.

Nelson, K. (1973). Structure and strategy in learning to talk. *Monographs of the Society for Research in Child Development, 38*(Serial No. 149).

Nelson, K. (1985). *Making sense: The acquisition of shared meaning.* San Diego: Academic Press.

Nelson, N. (1992). Performance is the prize: Language competence and performance among AAC users. *Augmentative and Alternative Communication, 8,* 3–18.

Oviatt, S.L. (1980). The emerging ability to comprehend language: An experimental approach. *Child Development, 51,* 97–106.

Oviatt, S.L. (1985). Tracing developmental change in language comprehension ability before twelve months of age. *Papers and Reports on Child Language Development, 24,* 87–94.

Peterson, S., Bondy, A., Vincent, Y., & Finnegan, C. (1995). Effects of altering communicative input for students with autism and no speech: Two case studies. *Augmentative and Alternative Communication, 11,* 93–100.

Platt, H., & Coggins, T. (1990). Comprehension of social-action games in prelinguistic children: Levels of participation and effect of adult structure. *Journal of Speech and Hearing Disorders, 55,* 315–326.

Reichle, J., & Karlan, G.A (1988). Selecting augmentative communication interventions: A critique of candidacy criteria and a proposed alternative. In R.L. Schiefelbusch & L.L. Lloyd (Eds.), *Language perspectives: Acquisition, retardation, and intervention* (2nd ed., pp. 321–339). Austin, TX: PRO-ED.

Resnick, J.S., & Goldfield, B.A. (1992). Rapid change in lexical development in comprehension and production. *Developmental Psychology, 28,* 406–413.

Rice, M. (1983). Contemporary accounts of the cognition/language relationship: Implication for speech-language clinicians. *Journal of Speech and Hearing Disorders, 48,* 347– 359.

Rice, M., & Kemper, S. (1984). *Child language and cognition.* Austin, TX: PRO-ED.

Roberts, S. (1983). Comprehension and production of word order in stage I. *Child Development, 54,* 443–449.

Romski, M.A. (2000, January). *Language assessment and AAC.* Paper presented at the ASHA SID 12 Leadership Conference on Augmentative and Alternative Communication, Sea Island, GA.

Romski, M.A., & Sevcik, R.A. (1988a). Augmentative and alternative communication systems: Considerations for individuals with severe intellectual disabilities. *Augmentative and Alternative Communication, 4,* 83–93.

Romski, M.A., & Sevcik, R.A. (1988b). Augmentative communication system acquisition and use: A model for teaching and assessing progress. *NSSLHA Journal, 16,* 61–74.

Romski, M.A., & Sevcik, R.A. (1993). Language comprehension: Considerations for augmentative and alternative communication. *Augmentative and Alternative Communication, 9,* 281–285.

Romski, M.A., & Sevcik, R.A. (1996). *Breaking the speech barrier: Language development through augmented means.* Baltimore: Paul H. Brookes Publishing Co.

Romski, M.A., Sevcik, R.A., Adamson, L.B., Browning, J., Williams, S., & Colbert, N. (1999, November). *Augmented communication input intervention for toddlers: A pilot study.* Poster presented at the ASHA Annual Convention, San Francisco.

Romski, M.A., Sevcik, R.A., & Forrest, S. (2001). Assistive technology and augmentative and alternative communication in inclusive early childhood programs. In M.J. Guralnick (Ed.), *Early childhood inclusion: Focus on change* (pp. 465–479). Baltimore: Paul H. Brookes Publishing Co.

Romski, M.A., Sevcik, R.A., & Pate, J.L. (1988). The establishment of symbolic communication in persons with severe retardation. *Journal of Speech and Hearing Disorders, 53,* 94–107.

Romski, M.A., Sevcik, R.A., Reumann, R., & Pate, J.L. (1989). Youngsters with moderate or severe retardation and severe spoken language impairments I: Extant communicative patterns. *Journal of Speech and Hearing Disorders, 54,* 366–373.

Romski, M.A., Sevcik, R.A., Robinson, B.F., & Bakeman, R. (1994). Effects of augmented language use by children with mental retardation on their communicative success and effectiveness. *Journal of Speech and Hearing Research, 37,* 617–628.

Romski, M.A., Sevcik, R.A., Robinson, B.F., & Wilkinson, K.M. (1990, November). *Intelligibility and form changes in the vocalizations of augmented language learners.* Paper presented at the ASHA Annual Convention, Seattle.

Romski, M.A., Sevcik, R.A, & Wilkinson, K. (1994). Peer-directed communications of augmented language learner. *American Journal on Mental Retardation, 98,* 527–538.

Roth, F., & Cassatt-James, E. (1989). The language assessment process: Clinical implications for individuals with severe speech impairments. *Augmentative and Alternative Communication, 5,* 165–172.

Sevcik, R.A., & Romski, M.A. (1986). Representational matching skills of persons with severe retardation. *Augmentative and Alternative Communication, 2,* 160–164.

Sevcik, R.A., & Romski, M.A. (1997). Comprehension and language acquisition: Evidence from youth with severe cognitive disabilities. In L.B. Adamson & M.A. Romski (Eds.), *Communication and language acquisition: Discoveries from atypical development* (pp. 187–202). Baltimore: Paul H. Brookes Publishing Co.

Sevcik, R.A., Romski, M.A., & Adamson, L.B. (1998, April). *Communication profiles of toddlers with severe spoken communication impairments.* Poster presented at the biennial International Conference on Infant Studies, Atlanta, GA.

Sevcik, R.A., Romski, M.A., Watkins, R., & Deffebach, K. (1995). Adult partner–augmented communication input to youth with mental retardation using the system for augmenting language (SAL). *Journal of Speech and Hearing Research, 38,* 902–912.

Sevcik, R.A., Romski, M.A., & Wilkinson, K. (1991). Roles of graphic symbols in the language acquisition process for persons with severe cognitive disabilities. *Augmentative and Alternative Communication, 7,* 161–170.

Snell, M. (1987). *Systematic instruction of persons with severe handicaps.* Columbus, OH: Charles E. Merrill.

Snell, M. (1993). *Instruction of students with severe disabilities.* Columbus, OH: Merrill/Macmillan.

Snow, C. (1984). Parent–child interaction and the development of communicative ability. In R.L. Schiefelbusch & J. Pickar (Eds.), *The acquisition of communicative competence* (pp. 69–107). Baltimore: University Park Press.

Snyder, L., Bates, E., & Bretherton, I. (1981). Content and context in early lexical development. *Journal of Child Language, 8,* 565–582.

Sutton, A., & Gallagher, T. (1995). Comprehension assessment of a child using an AAC system: A comparison of two techniques. *American Journal of Speech-Language Pathology, 4,* 60–68.

Wasson W.A., Arvidson, H.H. , & Lloyd, L.L. (1997). AAC assessment process. In L.L Lloyd, D.R Fuller, & H.H. Arvidson (Eds.), *Augmentative and alternative communication: A handbook of principles and practices* (pp. 169–198). Needham Heights, MA: Allyn & Bacon.

Wilkinson, K., Romski, M.A, & Sevcik, R.A. (1994). Emergence of visual-graphic symbol combinations by youth with moderate or severe mental retardation. *Journal of Speech and Hearing Research, 37,* 883–895.

Yoder, P., & Layton, T. (1988). Speech following sign language training in autistic children with minimal verbal language. *Journal of Autism and Developmental Disorders, 18,* 217–229.

Yoder, P., Warren, S., & Biggar, H. (1997). Stability of maternal reports of lexical comprehension in very young children with developmental disabilities. *American Journal of Speech-Language Pathology, 6,* 59–64.

Index

Page references ending in *t* denote tables; those ending in *f* denote figures.

Two more outstanding resources devoted to AAC...

Building Communicative Competence with Individuals Who Use Augmentative and Alternative Communication

By Janice C. Light, Ph.D., & Cathy Binger, M.S., CCC-SLP

Quick and easy to use, this hands-on instructional guide offers goal-setting, teaching, and coaching methods for the communication partners of people who depend on augmentative and alternative communication (AAC) systems. You'll find carefully designed and tested strategies you can use to help AAC users build 3 specific skills conducive to communicative competence: use of an introduction strategy, nonobligatory turn taking, and asking partner-focused questions. This program improves the communicative skills of children, adolescents, and adults—at any stage of communicative development.

Price: $37.95 • 1998 • 336 pages • 7 x 10 • spiral-bound • ISBN 1-55766-324-6

Speaking Up and Spelling It Out

Personal Essays on Augmentative and Alternative Communication
Edited by Melanie Fried-Oken, Ph.D., CCC-SLP, & Hank A. Bersani, Jr., Ph.D.

Twenty-seven diverse individuals who use AAC, from teens to senior citizens, give first-person accounts of how living with AAC has affected them. Through their personal essays and interviews, you'll hear their perspectives on the issues that matter most to them, including education, employment, technology, and family. The contributors reveal what using AAC is all about and what works for them as they face the daily challenges of communication.

Price: $24.95 • 2000 • 288 pages • 6 x 9 • paperback • ISBN 1-55766-447-1

Please send me ____ copies of **Building Communicative Competence** / Stock #3246 / Price $37.95
____ copies of **Speaking Up and Spelling it Out** / Stock #4471 / Price $24.95

Name: _____

Street address *(orders cannot be shipped to P.O. boxes)*: _____ ❑ Residential ❑ Commercial

City/State/ZIP: _____

Daytime phone: _____   E-mail address: _____
❑ *Yes! I want to receive special web site offers!*
My e-mail address will not be shared with any other party.

____ Check enclosed (payable to Brookes Publishing Co.)   ____ Purchase Order attached (please bill my institution)

____ Please charge my ____ American Express ____ MasterCard ____ Visa

Card No.: _____   Exp. date: _____/_____/_____

Signature *(required on all credit card orders)*: _____

Within Continental U.S. Shipping Rates for UPS Ground delivery*	
If your **product total** (before tax) is:	
$0.00 to $49.99 add $5.00	
$50.00 to $399.99 add 10% of product total	
$400.00 and over add 8% of product total	
*For rush orders call 1-800-638-3775 For international orders call 410-337-9580	

Product Total	$_____
Maryland Orders add 5% sales tax *(to product total only)*	+ $_____
Shipping Rate (see chart at left)	+ $_____
Grand Total U.S.	$_____

Photocopy this form and mail it to **Brookes Publishing Co.,** P.O. Box 10624, Baltimore, MD 21285-0624;
FAX **410-337-8539;** call toll-free (8 A.M. – 5 P.M. ET) **1-800-638-3775** or 410-337-9580 (outside the U.S.)
or order online at **www.brookespublishing.com**

Browse our entire catalog at www.brookespublishing.com

Prices subject to change without notice and may be higher outside the U.S. You may return books within 30 days for a full credit of the product price.
Refunds will be issued for prepaid orders. Items must be returned in resalable condition.

Your source code is: BA 5

DATE DUE

GAYLORD			PRINTED IN U.S.A.